Nursing KNOWLEDGE & PRACTICE

Environmental safety

Stress & anxiety

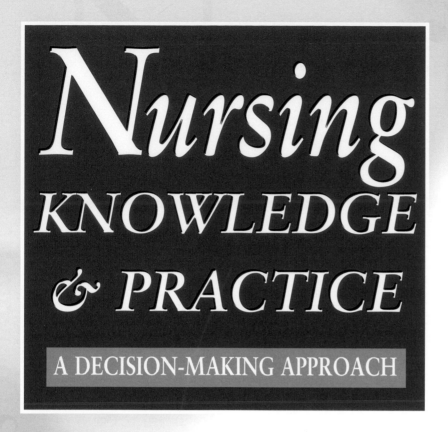

Nursing KNOWLEDGE & PRACTICE

A DECISION-MAKING APPROACH

EDITED BY

Maggie Mallik MPhil, BSc(Hons), DipN(Lond), Cert Ed, RGN
Lecturer in Adult Nursing (Acute/Critical),
University of Nottingham, Nottingham (UK)

Carol Hall BSc(Hons), DipN(Lond), Dip Ed, Dip(Res), RSCN, RGN
Teacher/Researcher (Child Health),
University of Nottingham, Nottingham (UK)

David Howard, MEd, Cert Ed, DipN(Lond), RMN, RGN
Nurse Teacher (Mental Health),
University of Nottingham, Lincoln (UK)

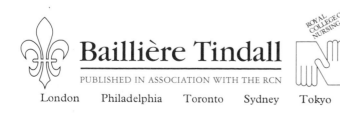

Baillière Tindall

PUBLISHED IN ASSOCIATION WITH THE RCN

ROYAL COLLEGE OF NURSING

London   Philadelphia   Toronto   Sydney   Tokyo

Baillière Tindall   24–28 Oval Road
London NW1 7DX

The Curtis Center
Independence Square West
Philadelphia, PA 19106-3399, USA

Harcourt Brace & Company
55 Horner Avenue
Toronto, Ontario, M8Z 4X6, Canada

Harcourt Brace & Company, Australia
30–52 Smidmore Street
Marrickville
NSW 2204, Australia

Harcourt Brace & Company, Japan
Ichibancho Central Building
22-1 Ichibancho
Chiyoda-ku, Tokyo 102, Japan

A catalogue record for this book is available from the British Library

ISBN 0-7020-1991-7

Typeset by Wyvern 21 Ltd, Bristol
Printed and bound in Great Britain by The Bath Press, Bath

The publishers have made every effort to trace the copyright holders of borrowed
material. If they have inadvertently overlooked any, they will be pleased to make
the necessary arrangements at the first opportunity.

Contents

Section One: Safe Practice

1.1 Environmental Safety   C. Weaver and C. Hall

1.2 Handling and Moving   L. Aston and J. Wakefield

Section Two: Immediate to Supportive Practice

2.1 Resuscitation   *R. Cable and H. Swain*

2.2 Homeostasis   *H. Dobbins and G. Adams*

2.3 Pain   *K. Jackson*

2.4 Skin Integrity   *K. Lewis and L. Roberts*

Section Three: Supportive Practice

Section Four: Supportive to Restorative Practice

4.4 Sleep and Rest   *M. Reet*

4.5 Rehabilitation   *J. Barker*

Contributors

Gary Adams BSc(Hons), Dip Ad Ed, RGN
Nurse Teacher (Adult)
University of Nottingham
School of Nursing
Queen's Medical Centre
Nottingham NG7 2UH

Liz Aston BSc, SRN, RCNT, RNT
Nurse Teacher (Adult)
University of Nottingham
School of Nursing
Queen's Medical Centre
Nottingham NG7 2UH

Janet Barker BSc(Hons), Dip Ad Ed, SRN, RMN
Nurse Teacher (Mental Health)
University of Nottingham
School of Nursing
Lincoln County Hospital
Lincoln LN2 5QY

Roderick Cable BSc, Dip Ad Ed, RN
Associate County Training Officer
St John Ambulance, Nottinghamshire
Nurse Teacher (Adult)
University of Nottingham
School of Nursing
Queen's Medical Centre
Nottingham NG7 2UH

Helen Dobbins Cert Ed, RGN
Nurse Teacher (Adult)
University of Nottingham
School of Nursing
Queen's Medical Centre
Nottingham NG7 2UH

Steve Eastburn BSc(Hons), Dip Ed, RGN, NDN
Nurse Teacher (Adult)
University of Nottingham
School of Nursing
Lincoln County Hospital
Lincoln LN2 5QY

Moonee Gungaphul MSc, BSc(Hons), Cert Ed,
RGN, OND, RMN
Nurse Teacher (Mental Health)
University of Nottingham
School of Nursing
Lincoln County Hospital
Lincoln LN2 5QY

Carol Hall BSc(Hons), Dip N(London), Dip Ed,
Dip(Res), RSCN, RGN
Teacher/Researcher (Child Health)
University of Nottingham
School of Nursing
Queen's Medical Centre
Nottingham NG7 2UH

David Howard MEd, Cert Ed, Dip N(London),
RMN, RGN
Nurse Teacher (Mental Health)
University of Nottingham
School of Nursing
Lincoln County Hospital
Lincoln LN2 5QY

Terence Hoyle BSc, RNT, RGN
Nurse Teacher (Adult)
University of Nottingham
School of Nursing
Pilgrim Hospital
Boston
Lincolnshire PE21 9QS

Karen Jackson MSc, NDN(Cert), Dip Ad Ed,
RSCN, RGN
Nurse Teacher (Child Health)
University of Nottingham
School of Nursing
Derbyshire Royal Infirmary
Derby DE1 2QY

Alison Kelley BSc(Hons), Dip N(London), Dip Ed, RGN
Nurse Teacher (Programme Leader Promotion of Continence, and Adult)
University of Nottingham
School of Nursing
Queen's Medical Centre
Nottingham NG7 2UH

Kerry Lewis MSc, BA, PGCE, RGN
Nurse Teacher (Adult)
University of Nottingham
School of Nursing
Pilgrim Hospital
Boston, Lincolnshire PE21 9QS

Maggie Mallik MPhil, BSc(Hons), Dip N(London), Cert Ed, RGN
Lecturer in Adult Nursing (Acute/Critical)
University of Nottingham
School of Nursing
Queen's Medical Centre
Nottingham NG7 2UH

Dave Nichol BA, Dip Ad Ed, RGN, ONC, RNT
Nurse Teacher (Adult)
University of Nottingham
School of Nursing
Queen's Medical Centre
Nottingham NG7 2UH

Rachel Peto BSc(Hons), RGN
Nurse Teacher (Adult)
University of Nottingham
School of Nursing
Queen's Medical Centre
Nottingham NG7 2UH

Mary Reet MSc, Dip N(London), Cert Ed, RSCN, RGN
Nurse Teacher (Child Health)
University of Nottingham
School of Nursing
Pilgrim Hospital
Boston
Lincolnshire PE21 9QS

Lorraine Roberts BSc(Hons), RGN
Nurse Teacher (Adult)
University of Nottingham
School of Nursing
Pilgrim Hospital
Boston
Lincolnshire PE21 9QS

Sheryll Shepherd RGN
Continence Advisor
Nottingham Healthcare NHS Trust
Nottingham

Helen Swain MSc, BSc,(Hons), Dip Ed, RSCN, RGN
Nurse Teacher (Child Health)
University of Nottingham
School of Nursing
Queen's Medical Centre
Nottingham NG7 2UH

Mike Taylor BA(Hons), Dip N(London), CertEd, RMN, RGN
Recently: Nurse Teacher (Mental Health)
University of Nottingham
School of Nursing
Now: Mental Health Counsellor
Lincolnshire and Louth District NHS Trust

Jill Wakefield BSc, Dip N(London), Cert Ed, RGN,
Nurse Teacher (Adult)
University of Nottingham
School of Nursing
Queen's Medical Centre
Nottingham NG7 2UH

Chris Weaver RGN
Staff Nurse and RCN Lead Steward
Nottingham City Hospital
Nottingham NG5 1PB

Linda Wilson MA(Medical Ethics), Cert Ed(FE), RGN, OND
Nurse Teacher (Adult)
University of Nottingham
School of Nursing
Grantham Centre
Grantham Hospital
Grantham NG31 8DE

Editors' Introduction

The original idea for writing this book arose from our experiences in facilitating and teaching *Nursing Theory and Practice* within a new curriculum for the Diploma in Higher Education in Nursing (P2000). We noted a shift towards subject based teaching and that even with a coherent curriculum model, students were often struggling to link up the various topics within the subjects covered to the core elements of nursing practice. Modularization of subject content further fragmented this knowledge. Books already available have concentrated on the classic subject subdivisions of the nursing curricula which are covered in the early generic phase of the courses (Common Foundation Programme). These subjects include the biological and social sciences as well as health, ethico-legal, communication and professional nursing studies. The pattern was to present subject knowledge leaving the students to make the necessary connections between this knowledge and their practice in nursing. Books which developed the core knowledge base of nursing practice within these curricula models were not available.

Regardless of the level of theory taught in the classroom, the ongoing challenge for the student is how to select and use the appropriate knowledge in order to make decisions in practice. The level of cognitive skills needed to apply generic principles to specific practice issues can often be underestimated. When knowledge is supplied through subject discipline work, the application of that knowledge is potentially difficult. Practice issues are generally much more complex and multifactorial so that often the student is left confused as to why a particular choice of action was made which according to the 'textbook' should not occur. Making the knowledge specific to students' particular branches of nursing, when it is taught in a generic manner, is also complex. Teaching through classroom work and the use of textbooks will always be limited in the context of practice knowledge.

If nursing students are to be encouraged to think critically about situations they encounter there is a need to integrate knowledge from theory to the observed practice. It has been argued that cognition is the process of linking observed behaviours and subjective impressions to a substantiated and well-delineated knowledge base. Such linkage will allow students to debate existing theory, observe variety in its practice application and possibly propose new solutions to the nursing care problems they meet. This development of critical thinking skills will allow students to interpret and integrate data from several perspectives so that they can arrive at their own 'truth' about practice situations.

This book integrates the knowledge base from the many subject areas within a nursing curriculum through the focus on areas of patient/client needs/problems which are generally considered within the primary domain of nursing knowledge and nurses' decision making across all fields of nursing practice.

As stated above, knowledge derived from the practice experience is an important element of learning to be a nurse. In fact, the preoccupation of the new student when in the practice setting is firmly focused on learning how to *do* nursing and also on being able to cope with the interpersonal experiences involved. Evaluating what has been learnt while in practice is now being encouraged through recording and reflecting on experience. The general approach of this book and the student exercises within the text aims to encourage and foster these reflective processes.

With the above issues in mind, our intention was to provide a book which:

- enabled students to understand how knowledge from subjects taught within a nursing curriculum is focused towards the theory and practice of nursing;
- illustrated for students how knowledge from classroom subjects and knowledge from practice experience can be integrated in order to make decisions in nursing practice;
- provided an appropriate level of foundation knowledge of client/patient problems/needs which is applicable across all fields of nursing;
- stimulated the student to critically appraise current research based evidence for and from practice;
- encouraged the student to reflect on learning from both classroom material and practice experience and to integrate this knowledge into their decision making processes.

▶ STRUCTURE OF THE BOOK

Knowledge in any textbook has to be presented in a reductionist form for the sake of clarity. In the organization of this book, it is hoped that by bringing the separate subject knowledge bases together to deal with core nursing issues, the reader is helped to identify the application of the knowledge needed for decision making in practice. The topic areas covered in the book focus on aspects of care that are primarily a nursing responsibility. Exercises are set which will have a critical incident/case study approach. However, it should be recognized that patients/clients have multiple problems in varying contexts and cope with these in very individual ways.

The individual chapters are organized and presented in four sections. Section headings reflect the main focus of nursing activity for these particular needs/problems.

Section 1, *Safe Practice*, includes chapters which present knowledge needed to promote health and practice safely in order to protect self, the client and society. Topics addressed are Environmental Safety (1.1); Handling and Moving (1.2) materials and clients/patients; protecting self and clients from infection, (Infection Control, 1.3); and finally the storage and administration of medicines (Medicines, 1.4). Nurses are important decision makers and policy makers in these areas and have roles in education as well as in prevention and maintenance of safe practice.

Section 2, *Immediate to Supportive Practice*, focuses more on patient/client needs/problems which require immediate decisions to be made quickly and correctly in order to deal with the acute situation. Supportive care involves ongoing assessment and problem solving to restore health. Topics in this section include Resuscitation (2.1); Homeostasis (2.2); Pain (2.3); Skin Integrity (2.4); and Aggression (2.5).

Section 3, *Supportive Practice*, deals with those topic areas which generally form the primary daily concern of nurses in multiple contexts and with many different client groups. Although there are multidisciplinary team decisions and other specialists involved, nurses are often the key decision makers in Hygiene (3.1), Nutrition (3.2), Continence (3.3) Mobility (3.4) and Death and Dying (3.5).

Section 4, *Supportive to Restorative Practice*, has a particular emphasis on those areas of practice which deal with restoring the patient/client to health. Although supportive care continues to be necessary, the focus is on the knowledge needed to help the client/patient develop their own rehabilitative processes. Chapters in this section cover Stress and Anxiety (4.1), Confusion (4.2), Sexuality (4.3), Sleep and Rest (4.4) and Rehabilitation (4.5).

All chapters have the same format which subdivides the material presented into four main parts. The subdivisions in each chapter subsume areas of theory within nursing curricula and also knowledge derived from the practice of nursing. These include:

- Subject Knowledge, which incorporates two subdivisions:
  - Biological knowledge focuses on the related applied biology for the chapter topic;
  - Psychosocial knowledge covers both psychological and social dimensions as well as appropriate cultural issues.
- Practice Knowledge presents material relevant to the assessment and management of patient/client care.
- Professional Knowledge focuses on ethico-legal, political and policy issues related to the chapter topic. This section also reviews nursing roles and specific educational needs related to client care.
- Reflective Knowledge reviews knowledge gained through experience in the practicum and consolidates learning through case study exercises.

Integrated within each chapter are the student exercises and information boxes. These include:

- reflective exercises;
- decision making exercises;
- research based evidence;
- case studies from each of the nursing fields (Reflective Knowledge)

How to use this book

The Editors' Introduction has described how this book is organized into sections and chapters and how each chapter is structured into four sections as follows:

- ▶ **Subject Knowledge** *which incorporates two subdivisions*
  Biological knowledge
  Psychosocial knowledge
- ▶ **Practice Knowledge**
- ▶ **Professional Knowledge**
- ▶ **Reflective Knowledge**.

In addition, each chapter is designed to contain a number of features which will guide you around the topic as well as encourage you to reflect on your learning and your experiences in practice.

▶ EACH CHAPTER BEGINS WITH:

KEY ISSUES. This list provides a succinct menu of topics covered within the chapter for quick and easy reference.

The INTRODUCTION and OVERVIEW provide a guide to the chapter indicating how and why this topic is an important component in nursing practice.

▶ WITHIN THE CHAPTER:

Each chapter contains a number of different types of information and activities which are highlighted within the text. They are designed to help you reflect on your own knowledge, consider the basis of nursing decisions, and demonstrate the research base for practice.

▶ *Reflective Exercises*

Reflection is a very important process to develop in order to aid your learning. You can learn from your practice experience and also from your reactions to the knowledge presented in texts and the classroom. The main focus of the reflective exercises in this text is on yourself and your reactions and how these interact with the particular situation observed or reflected upon. Many of the exercises will focus on dilemmas where there is no right or wrong answer but one which is negotiated to suit the specific situation. You may find these exercises particularly useful as a basis for discussion and debate in a group.

▶ *Decision-making Exercises*

Decision-making exercises are generally related to material presented in the chapter. However, they may ask you to complete further work which will take you outside the scope of the text. Based on the philosophy of problem based learning where you are given a short scenario/critical incident from practice (broadly defined) you are requested to review information already obtained from whatever source, collect further information and then make decisions as to what actions you would take, supporting this with the rationale for your actions.

▶ Guidance may be given, and helpful references, but some exercises will be open-ended as textbooks and articles go out of date quickly. It is important to do a literature search for up-to-date and local material which may be relevant to the topic being explored.

▶ There is an assumption that you are able to use the appropriate library facilities and find the relevant material. These are skills you should develop and maintain throughout your professional career.

▶ Discussion with your peers, teachers and practitioners will help you to focus your learning within the exercises.

▶ Research Based Evidence

Brief summaries of a research study or several studies are presented in order to provide support for evidence based practice. Although not explicitly stated in the book, you are encouraged to obtain a copy of the full report, read and critically appraise the study. You should also, where possible, link these studies with your practice experiences. Research evidence, where at all possible, is from studies completed in the late 1980s and the 1990s. However, you must remember that these research briefings can quickly become out of date, so they should act as the starting point for further investigation.

▶ Case Studies

In the Reflective Knowledge section of each chapter you will find four or more case studies. These are designed to show how core nursing knowledge is relevant across all four branches of nursing. Each case study provides an opportunity for you to consider nursing decisions and to appreciate how knowledge from different sources is integrated in nursing practice. They may also act as a stimulus for you to explore in more depth issues related to your chosen branch of nursing. You may also wish to read them before reading the chapter.

▶ AT THE END OF EACH CHAPTER:

FURTHER READING provides guidance on sources of relevant information if you wish to pursue particular interests further. Each suggested item has a brief commentary explaining why it has been recommended. These resources are in addition to the extensive list of REFERENCES.

Authors' Acknowledgements

Given the unique structure and layout of this book, we are very grateful to all our individual authors for their hard work and patience with our editorial comments through the many re-writes. All of their individual expertise was needed to fulfil the broad remit of each chapter. As the writing was completed in their own personal time, we would like to take this opportunity to thank their families for their support during the long process of getting each of the chapters successfully completed.

Thanks also to all those teaching colleagues who in the course of conversations in 'coffee breaks' provided information and advice over specific issues. A special thanks to both Anne Bacon and Helen Laverty, teachers in Learning Disabilities Nursing, who provided information and guidance on their specific branch related case studies.

A special thanks goes to Jacqueline Curthoys of Baillière Tindall who listened to the original ideas for the book, took them on board and steered us through from the initial proposal writing to the final production. Jacqueline has been positive and enthusiastic throughout the lengthy writing and editing period and the regular contact over 'lunches' has inspired us and kept us on track. Our thanks to Robert Langham (formerly of Baillière Tindall) our Development Editor who resolutely ensured we met our deadlines. Carol Parr, Senior Production Editor, has been very positive and supportive in the final stages of getting the book into production. Our thanks to the whole team at Baillière Tindall.

▶ PERSONAL ACKNOWLEDGEMENTS

The planning, writing and editing of this book has been done in our out of work time. This would not have been possible without the constant support and inspiration of our loving families. Many thanks go from

Maggie: to my husband Alak and daughter Cathy, to my mother, Mabel O'Hara who supported my decision to become a nurse at a time when she needed me most, and to my first mentor, my grand-aunt, Bridget Meehan, ex-ward sister, St Andrews Hospital, Bow, London.

Carol: To my husband Rich and our children James and Rachel for all their patience, and to Pauline Wells (ex Sister, Leicester Royal Infirmary) without whom I probably would have never discovered the many challenges of a career in nursing children.

David: to my wife Penny and to our boys Simon and Peter.

SECTION ONE

Safe practice

1.1 Environmental Safety

C. Weaver and C. Hall

KEY ISSUES

■ SUBJECT KNOWLEDGE
▶ exploration of the concept of internal and external environments
▶ the relationship between man and his environment
▶ basic human requirements for life
▶ hazards to human safety
▶ psychological and social concepts of risk
▶ barriers to maintaining safety
▶ environmental and occupational safety

■ PRACTICE KNOWLEDGE
▶ risk assessment in nursing
▶ control of substances hazardous to health
▶ managing strategies for ensuring client safety

▶ implementing strategies for a safe environment
▶ reporting accidents

■ PROFESSIONAL KNOWLEDGE
▶ the development of British legislation in health and safety
▶ European guidelines for safety
▶ the employer's responsibility for safety at work
▶ the nurse's responsibility for safety at work
▶ education needs in ensuring safety
▶ upholding the law in the work environment

■ REFLECTIVE KNOWLEDGE
▶ case studies applying principles of health and safety in branches of nursing

▶ INTRODUCTION

A safe environment is something many of us take for granted. Florence Nightingale (1860) highlighted the importance of ensuring that patients were safe when she stated in her instructions to nurses, *Notes on Nursing*, that nursing should 'Do the patient no harm'. She also offered advice on the design of hospital wards in an attempt to ensure an optimum environment for hospital patients (Nightingale, 1863).

However, to view the promotion of a safe environment as simply something nurses can do for their patients is simplistic. This perspective, alone, fails to recognize the sociological components of maintaining a safe environment, that is, the need for clients (and nurses) to be aware of potential threats to health within their personal environments and to behave in a safe manner. Nursing has a responsibility to understand and promote both the concept of maintaining client safety in care environments and the notion of safe client behaviour through health promotion.

Although patients have always featured as a prime concern with regards to health and safety, the safety of the nurse at work has not always received as much attention. The last 100 years has seen many legislative attempts at improving the health of the worker in society. Many people, including health service workers, were not given legal protection while at work until the last decade. For many, the establishment of the *Health and Safety at Work Act* (1974) was the first real opportunity for ensuring safe working premises and practices. The National Health Service became subject to the new law, but avoided the need for implementation because of Crown Immunity. After a number of well publicized incidents of poor standards, this immunity was finally lifted by the NHS (Amendment) Bill in 1986.

Today, the provision and maintenance of an optimum environment for both clients and health care staff is a major concern. Laws, regulations, local procedures and policies at European, national and local levels offer guidance for safe practice. Under these acts, nurses have a responsibility to ensure that the work place is a safe place for themselves and their clients. Some nurses, in particular, occupational health nurses and those who represent unions with regard to health and safety have additional responsibility to ensure that the workplace of the workforce is a safe place for all employees.

This chapter explores issues in the provision of a safe environment for clients and carers. Safety in the care environment includes the introduction of risk management, exploring the roles of both the nurse and client. Health and safety at work is a key feature of the day-to-day management of a workload and the relationship between professional practice and the law is illustrated. The scope of this first chapter presents a broad overview as other chapters in this book contain sections that focus on specific areas of safety such as handling and moving (see Chapter 1.2), infection control (see Chapter 1.3) and medicines (see Chapter 1.4). Food safety will be addressed under nutrition (see Chapter 3.2) and stress arising from multiple external environmental sources will be explored in stress and anxiety (see Chapter 4.1). The functions and maintenance of the body in dealing with environmental threats are addressed in homeostasis (see Chapter 2.2).

▶ OVERVIEW

▶ *Subject Knowledge*

The concept of 'environment' and the meanings of internal and external environment are explored. Threats to safety that are either part of the natural world or manmade are outlined.

In the psychosocial knowledge section, our interaction with the world around us is considered and there is discussion about the basic human needs for maintaining safety and wellbeing. Behavioural issues are addressed, with a particular reference to factors that may compromise safety. These factors include theories of risk behaviour and individual and societal noncompliance in maintaining a healthy environment.

▶ *Practice Knowledge*

Ways to facilitate an optimum environment for clients are explored with reference to specific regulations identified within the *Health and Safety at Work Act* (1974). Emphasis is placed on risk assessment and the management of threats to safety to both clients and carers within health settings.

▶ *Professional Knowledge*

The development of law in relation to health and safety is outlined and the responsibilities of both employers and employees are reviewed. Consideration is given to ways in which health and safety law may be upheld in practice.

▶ *Reflective Knowledge*

Throughout the chapter you will be encouraged to apply information reflectively through exercises and by considering examples. In this final section case studies from the four branches of nursing help you reflect further and apply the knowledge you have gained.

On pp. 30–32 there are four case studies, each one relating to one of the branch programmes. You may find it helpful to read one of them before you start the chapter and use it as a focus for your reflections while reading.

SUBJECT KNOWLEDGE
Biological

▸ A SAFE ENVIRONMENT

It is important to clarify what is meant by the 'internal' and 'external' environments, for it is within these domains that threats to well-being and safety take place. Although both have potential dangers for human life and wellbeing, they are discretely different, both in the likely risks to safety and in the way in which threats may be managed (Roper, 1976).

For the purposes of this chapter, the internal environment can be described as the functions and workings of the human body. The body's ability to maintain a homeostatic (stable) internal environment is essential to wellbeing (see Chapter 2.2). The essential consideration of the internal environment in relation to health and safety is concerned with its interaction with the external environment and the effects which may result. The external environment is the world surrounding the human body. In order to function, the human body has essential requirements, which must be met externally. Conversely the actions of individuals can influence the safety and ambience of the external environment for all who live in it. Both environments are highly dependent upon one another for their own maintenance.

Reflect on your own body.

- *List all the requirements you can think of that the outside world must provide in order to enable your body to function.*
- *What would happen if these requirements were not sufficiently met?*
- *Now think about other ways that the external environment in which you live may impact on your body. Try to identify both positive and negative impacts.*
- *Finally, think about how your body may impact upon the external environment. What kind of things can you do to help or damage our world?*

▸ BASIC NEEDS OF HUMAN LIFE

The basic requirements of living are well known and you probably identified them in the exercise above. Physiological needs include:

- ▸ air;
- ▸ water;
- ▸ food;
- ▸ shelter.

Without these basic needs, higher order psychological needs such as belonging and esteem cannot be easily achieved (Maslow, 1970). Over thousands of years of development, however, an increasingly complicated way for meeting basic needs has developed. This has resulted in modifying the external environment to suit our needs.

Table 1.1.1 illustrates how individuals interact within the external environmental system. It demonstrates how components essential for life support are taken from the external environment and how the two environments interact through activities of living. Waste and residues are contributed to the external environment as a byproduct of human existence.

Throughout life activities, individual's may find threats to safety both to and from the external environment. These are also summarized in the categories outlined in Table 1.1.1. Compare this with your findings from the above reflective exercise.

Life Support	Activities	Residues and waste
Air	Home	Solids
Water	Work	Liquids
Food	Recreation	Gases
Shelter	Transportation	

Environmental Hazards			
Type	Example	Type	Example
Biological	Animal	Psychological	Stress
	Insect		Boredom
	Microbiological		Anxiety
			Discomfort
Chemical	Poisons and toxins		Depression
	Allergens		
	Irritants	Sociological	Overcrowding
			Isolation
Physical	Vibration		Anomie
	Radiation		
	Forces and abrasion		
	Humidity		

Table 1.1.1 The environmental system. (Adapted from Purdom and Walton, 1971.)

▶ POTENTIAL HAZARDS IN MEETING BASIC REQUIREMENTS FOR LIVING

▶ *Air*

The air that we breathe usually contains 21% oxygen and 78% nitrogen with the other 1% being made up of trace gases such as carbon dioxide, xenon and neon. If the oxygen concentration was to drop below 16%, anoxia would develop resulting in effects on the brain and other body functions. If the oxygen level decreased further to 6%, life could not be sustained, and immediate loss of consciousness results from exposure to a zero oxygen atmosphere.

Air can also act as a vehicle for microorganisms, allergens, waste gases and dust, all of which enter the body via the lungs (Harrington and Gill, 1992). These pollutants may cause damage or illness if present in sufficient quantity or if an individual develops an allergic response to them. Air quality is particularly compromised in large urban areas when the temperature rises and there is little wind movement. Threats to health have been acknowledged in the increasing rates of respiratory disease, especially in young children (Keely *et al.*, 1991). There is evidence to suggest that children exposed to lead in exhaust fumes arising from the increased use of the car in our society have exhibited symptoms (such as decreased intelligence) consistent with the expected neurological sequelae identified in those with high levels of lead exposure via other sources such as contaminated drinking water (Hendrikson, 1994; Krowchuk, 1995).

▶ *Water*

Life for individuals without water can be measured in days, but it is not only individuals who suffer if water is in short supply. A civilization cannot develop or prosper without sufficient water to grow crops, develop industries or establish communities for people to live in. Water for human consumption must be clean and free from toxins and microorganisms.

In developing countries and in areas affected by war or disaster the greatest risk to the population may be contamination of the drinking water, resulting in life-threatening infections such as cholera and amoebic dysentry. In developed countries, most residents have access to water purification systems that have been in place for many decades (Ineichen, 1993). We have now become preoccupied with water contaminants arising from the original source of the water and from the old (sometimes lead) pipework through which water is delivered to each household. Water companies are under pressure from their regulating body to produce cleaner water at a time when water demand is growing with increasing ownership of dishwashers, and washing machines. This has led to the introduction of water metering and a proposed 'smart card' for the pre-payment of water in the UK. In these initiatives, water is paid for by volume rather than by the traditional method, which used a standard rate. Measures such as these, however, are controversial, since those most in need of clean water for health and wellbeing could be those least able to afford it under this scheme (Cohen, 1996).

Preoccupation with contamination of supplies among the wealthier population has spawned a large water bottling industry. This development in the provision of water for drinking, however, is not without problems, as it is not suitable for everyone. Small babies cannot physically manage the increased mineral content found in many bottled waters due to renal immaturity. Care is required in educating parents about the provision of water for consumption by infants and young children.

In nursing, there are occasions when water must be sterile. This is especially important when water is being used for the preparation of feeds for those who are immunosuppressed as a result of illness. Infants require sterile feeds because they have not developed resistance to infective organisms. Sterile water is also essential where water is used to irrigate wounds or in the preparation of medication via infusion, to protect patients from absorbing harmful contaminants.

▶ *Food*

DECISION MAKING
What information about 'sterile' feed preparation would you need to offer Julie, a new mother, who wishes to bottle feed her baby?
• *How would she ensure that the feeding implements are sterile?*
• *How would she ensure that the water she is using is safe for her baby?*
• *Where would you obtain information to give to Julie?*

For dietary provision to be considered safe, it must be free from contaminants such as harmful bacteria (e.g. *Salmonella*, *Escherichia coli*) or disease (e.g. bovine spongiform encephalopathy), (Kimberlin, 1993) which may be passed to humans. Additionally, food should be in adequate supply, and this is not always the case in the developing world or in some instances in developed countries such as the UK.

Within nursing, providing adequate nutrition for clients is important to promote healing and recovery. Health promotion is also important to prevent malnutrition and obesity.

Although the main impact of nutrition on health is discussed in greater detail in Chapter 3.2, it is important to recognize that modern systems for developing food sources need to be monitored closely. Contamination of food at any stage in the external 'food chain' processing will be a potential threat to the wellbeing of the internal environment.

▶ *Shelter*

Shelter is essential for survival. It provides protection from both excessive heat and cold, from the weather, and from other environmental hazards. However, shelter should be safe for the resident and should not itself be contributory to disease. These two aspects are surprisingly difficult to achieve within the home and institutional setting.

Care institutions are often work settings and there is an increasing interest in how the design of individual workplace buildings can have an effect on the health of the individual workers within the building (Raw and Goldman, 1996). Sick building syndrome (SBS) has been linked to a group of symptoms developed by people in certain buildings, notably office blocks. Symptoms of SBS include physical and behavioural problems such as irritation of the eyes, nose, throat and skin, headaches, lethargy and lack of concentration. Features of the buildings that appear to cause problems are associated with the air-conditioning systems, office layouts, windows and light, furnishings and decorations (Raw and Goldman, 1996).

▶ ENVIRONMENTAL HAZARDS

As we have seen above, an individual's basic needs can be threatened by insufficiency or excess or poor management leading to the occurrence of identified hazards to health such as food poisoning or respiratory illness.

Potential hazards in our environment may be naturally occurring or result from manmade conditions, including the production of wastes and residues. Production of waste is unavoidable within communal societies and with modern technology and the production of consumer goods. Safe waste removal and disposal strategies are of vital importance to the survival of a community. Within nursing the type of waste is different from that produced domestically or industrially because of its clinical nature. Sharps and dressings need to be treated separately from paper and glass, because of the risks to health associated with cross-infection. Policies for the safe disposal of clinical waste and environmental policies ensure the safe disposal of clinical and non-clinical waste in care settings.

Apart from waste products, other hazards can seriously compromise the safety of the internal and external environments. They may be categorized into the following five groups:

- ▶ biological;
- ▶ chemical;
- ▶ physical;
- ▶ psychological;
- ▶ sociological.

▶ *Biological Hazards*

Biological hazards are concerned primarily with the entry of disease-producing infectious agents into the body, thus causing a risk to the stability of the internal environment. Such organisms include bacteria, viruses and fungi as well as parasites, which may additionally carry harmful pathogens.

▶ *Chemical Hazards*

Chemical hazards are not new: the gaining of knowledge into knowing which plants are safe to eat and which liquids are safe to drink must have been fraught and littered with many accidents. Even though our predecessors may not have known the finer physiological details of any particular poison, they would have learnt to avoid it. Chemical agents may be synthetic or derived from natural substances and can affect the internal or the external environment beneficially or detrimentally. The most important consideration related to chemical hazard is regarding knowledge about the substance and the judicious application of this knowledge in using chemical substances safely and effectively. It is important to consider the impact of improper use or exposure to substances by clients. Nurses have a large role to play in caring for the public who may have become poisoned by chemicals. However, there is also a nursing role in the management and education of the public in maintaining a safe home environment for themselves and their families.

▶ Physical Hazards

Physical hazards are all around us and may cause disease, disability or fatality, and are manifest in many different ways. Certain dusts can be dangerous to the internal environment if they are inhaled and then absorbed, while other powders can be used therapeutically in the form of inhalers. Temperature in the external environment can also be a physical hazard. Extreme external temperatures can lead to a loss of the internal homeostatic balance (see Chapter 2.2). Contact with an extreme hot or cold source can cause extensive physical damage (burning) and potentially, death.

Electromagnetic radiation, which includes x-rays, ultraviolet, infrared, and microwaves, can cause skin burns, an elevation in temperature and fatality with prolonged exposure. Understanding of the dangers related to uncontrolled exposure to these radiations is vital for nurses since controlled ionizing radiation such as x-rays and gamma rays can be used beneficially to produce radiographic pictures and in the treatment of neoplastic disease (cancer).

Human inventions such as equipment and machinery can cause accidents as well as offering the intended benefit. Modern machinery, including all nursing equipment, is being continually made safer as it is evaluated through use. Equipment that is used inappropriately or without regard to the manufacturer's instructions may provide a hazard to safety; even if it is functioning correctly technically. In the community, everyday machinery such as motor vehicles, drills, or gardening equipment can be dangerous if not used appropriately.

▶ Accidents

The above hazards, are associated with a risk of accident, or an undesirable interaction between the internal and external environment. The risk may be higher if an individual is unable to physically meet the demands of the world in which he or she is living, for example an elderly frail individual may be more likely to fall, or a small child may tumble while trying to reach an object from a high shelf. Additionally, accidents may occur if the individuals are unable to appreciate the effect of their behaviour either as a result of their stage of cognitive development or because of their disease process. Such examples would include a baby who becomes burned as a result of pulling a cup of hot tea from a nearby table onto himself because he is too young to understand the hazard associated such contact with extremes of heat and an individual with senile dementia who wanders out into a busy road and is knocked down by a car because he is confused about his environment. Nurses have a responsibility to define and assess risks for their clients and this is addressed further in the Practice Knowledge section of this chapter.

Accidents are a major concern for health carers since it is estimated that more than 2.5 million people attended accident and emergency departments for accidents occurring in the home in the survey year 1992, and a further 2.88 million attended for accidents occurring outside the home. There is particular concern by those responsible for the care of children since although accounting for only 19% of the total UK population, children under 14 years of age account for 41% of reported accidents (The Dettol Report, 1994).

Some accidents can be prevented if carers are aware of the hazards and able to offer health and safety education. Clients and their families need to clearly understand the outcomes of risky behaviour and the implications that may arise. This may require imaginative education for the most vulnerable groups to communicate this information in a way that can be easily understood and accepted.

DECISION MAKING

This scenario illustrates an unsafe interaction between a child and his immediate external environment that resulted in a serious risk to his internal environment.

Paulo Vincenti is a four-year-old boy, who when playing in his grandmother's house found what he thought looked like red sweets. After eating several Paulo was found by his mother, who to her horror found that he had consumed iron tablets. She rushed him to hospital where treatment commenced to retrieve the sugar-coated tablets before Paulo became ill.

1. *What lessons may be learned about the safety of individuals within different external environments and Paulo's vulnerability with regard to any chemical agent?*
2. *Using the information above, how could you offer health education to Paulo and his family in order to try and prevent a similar incident happening again ?*

Simon Whitaker is 17 years old and has been admitted to casualty following a collapse after inhaling butane gas with some friends. His family are in attendance and say that it is not the first time that Simon has abused solvents, and say that in spite of advice about the dangers of such practices he continues because he enjoys the feeling that it gives him. Compare this incident with that of Paulo. This time Simon knowingly abused a substance designed for use in his external environment for the effect he found it had on his internal environment.

1. *What are the issues related to the knowledge and judicious use of substances on this occasion?*
2. *Decide what should be different about the way in which health promotion advice may be offered to Simon and his family compared to that offered for Paulo?*

▶ *Psychological and Sociological Hazards*

Psychological and sociological hazards are closely linked to human interactions with the environment. The next section explores the influence of psychosocial factors in the promotion of a safe and healthy environment.

Psychosocial   There are many ways in which individuals strive to understand risks in their daily lives and factors influencing how they may act in the light of such perceptions (Bloor, 1995). Fallowfield (1990) suggests that quality of life and therefore ultimately perceived health and wellbeing is directly related to the quality of the environment in which life exists. The environment must not only satisfy physiological needs, but also psychological and sociological needs. Fallowfield (1990) further identified four areas where the perception of life quality is paramount as follows:

- ▶ psychological – related to the perception of mental wellbeing;
- ▶ social – related to involvement in social activities;
- ▶ occupational – related to functional ability to achieve work (paid or voluntary);
- ▶ physical – related to pain, comfort, sleep, physical ability.

These areas are useful for exploring factors associated with determining life quality. However, it should be remembered that the way you view something may be very different from the way another person may perceive it. Culture, social class, gender, age, level of education, and emotional state should be acknowledged. Toxic effects from drugs and general level of health are also important.

DECISION MAKING

Mrs James, a widow who lives alone has been admitted with a severe chest infection that has made her acutely short of breath. On arrival to the ward you are involved with her immediate nursing needs and are very busy assisting the medical team in her care. However, Mrs James remains agitated and anxious. Further discussion leads you to identify that she has left home without feeding her cat,. She is also depressed about her admission, commenting that none of her friends will visit her as they do not have transport to make the journey.

1. *Which of the areas identified by Fallowfield (1990) in Mrs James environment are causing concern to (a) the medical team and (b) Mrs James?*
2. *What effect does this difference in priorities have in relation to Mrs James' health and wellbeing?*
3. *As Mrs James' nurse, decide what intervention you can make to help resolve the situation to the satisfaction of all concerned.*

For Mrs James, whose case is considered in the decision-making exercise, it can be seen that her personal perception of danger was related more to her inability to function in the area associated with occupational ability than with the concept of personal risk associated with the physical illness, which was causing the medical and nursing staff concern. Although she had a knowledge of her physical health as a danger, her perception of risk associated with the illness appeared to be a lower priority.

Finally, there may be differences in the perception of priorities between clients and their carers. A knowledge of these differences may be critical in facilitating the provision of appropriate care.

▶ PSYCHOLOGICAL STRESS

Using Chapter 4.1 as a guide, identify how your external environment can be made less safe as the result of stress. You may include poor concentration leading to a lack of attention to safe practice for example.

How may knowing that a client is anxious influence your assessment of their care?

Stress can alter an individual's perceived environment, which can ultimately become hazardous.

The main issues associated with psychological stress and its effects on the internal environment are addressed elsewhere (see Chapter 4.1). However, it is important to consider how the effects of stress on an individual can impact on their immediate external environment.

▶ RISK PERCEPTION

Risk perception is different from the knowledge of a danger as it does not necessarily cause people to worry. Risk perception may result from the personal orientations that guide an individual to make commitments consistent with one specific political culture and inconsistent with others. At the same time cultures may select those individuals who support their way of life. Individuals may choose what to fear in supporting their preferred way of life (Royal Society Study Group, 1992). For example, a religious sect propounding a particular set of beliefs may attract new members who are sympathetic to the views of that sect. Gabe (1995) identifies that in this sense risk cannot be objectively 'measured', but must be viewed as a social construct. This draws from the original anthropological work by Douglas (1966), which addressed questions about why different cultures select different risks for particular attention using beliefs to rationalize behaviour. Given that such interpretations of risk perception are valid, then points of cultural difference are extremely important in nursing. If a client has different social expectations and selects different risks from the nurse's social expectation then a true assessment could be difficult and treatment could fail to meet the expectations of both parties. There may even be open conflict between the client and carer. For instance, Jehovah's Witnesses can present a challenge because they may refuse to receive blood transfusions. Where clients are severely ill and unable to give informed consent to treatment or where children require urgent blood transfusion, nurses may then face moral dilemmas in respecting the cultural beliefs of such individuals while acting in their best interest to maintain their safety.

Finally, individuals may react differently in different environments. A perception of risk and knowledge of danger are important in the care setting because clients may rely on the carer to protect them (Simpson, 1991). Those who are particularly vulnerable include:

 ▶ children and people with a learning disability, who may not perceive risks to their wellbeing as they are unable to understand them;
 ▶ people with a mental health problem whose perception of danger may be reduced as the result of their illness or because of the treatment they are receiving;
 ▶ people who are critically ill and unable to determine dangers.

Within the hospital setting most clients are away from their known environment and are therefore unable to perceive risks in what amounts to an 'alien' environment. It is the responsibility of the carer to ensure that individuals are aware of hazards wherever possible and are protected by either their own action or action on their behalf by the carer. The nurse's role is to ensure the safety of the environment by assessing the potential risks and facilitating action for change.

▶ PSYCHOSOCIAL HAZARDS IN THE WORK ENVIRONMENT

Up to this point there has been an emphasis on the individual's responsibility within their personal environment and some discusssion in relation to the behaviour of people when interacting within the health care environment. It is important to recognize that the organization has some influence in creating a safe and healthy environment. According to Cox and Griffiths (1996, p. 128) a 'safe' environment might be relatively easy to define, but perceptions of a 'healthy' work environment are usually narrowly focused on physical threats to health. These authors argue that healthy work can be defined as 'work that does not threaten but which helps maintain and enhance physical, psychological and social well-being'.

A 'hazard' has been defined as an event or situation that has the potential to cause harm (Cox and Griffiths, 1996). Besides the physical hazards referred to in the previous section, the International Labour Organization (1986) has defined psychosocial hazards arising from interactions between job content, work organizational, management and environmental conditions, and the employee's competencies and needs. Those interactions that can be defined as hazardous influence the health of employees through their 'perceptions' and 'experiences' of these conditions (International Labour Organization, 1986; Cox et al., 1995). Exposure to psychosocial hazards in particular is often chronic and cumulative except when a particular acute traumatic incident occurs. Table 1.1.2 outlines the common psychosocial hazards associated with the work environment and the conditions that define the potential level of hazard for the individual employee.

It is important to remember the synergistic nature of the physical and psychosocial hazard in the work environment. Significant interactions can occur between the different types of hazard and their consequent effects on the health of the individual (Levi, 1984). Stress in the workplace from whatever cause may inadvertently lead to risk-taking behaviour by the individual worker.

Category	Conditions
Content of work	
Job content	Lack of variety or short work cycles, fragmented or meaningless work, underuse of skills, high uncertainty
Workload and work pace	Work overload or underload, lack of control over pacing, high levels of time pressure
Work schedule	Shift working, inflexible work schedules, unpredictable hours, long or unsocial hours
Interpersonal relationships at work	Social or physical isolation, poor relationships with superiors, interpersonal conflict, lack of social support
Control	Low participation in decision making, lack of control over work
Context of work	
Organizational culture and function	Poor communication, low levels of support for problem solving and personal development, lack of definition of organizational objectives
Role in organization	Role ambiguity and role conflict, responsibility for people
Career development	Career stagnation and uncertainty, underpromotion or overpromotion, poor pay, job insecurity, low social value of work
Home work interface	Conflicting demands of work and home, low support at home, dual career problems

Table 1.1.2 Psychosocial hazards in the work environment. (Reproduced by kind permission of John Wiley and Sons Ltd from Cox and Griffiths, 1996.)

▶ MANAGEMENT OF HAZARDS AND DANGERS

When it comes to dealing with safety issues, particularly in the workplace environment, there have been three common approaches to the problem (Landy, 1989) as follows.

- ▶ The 'engineering' approach assumes that by modifying the environment or the equipment used that safety can be enhanced and accident rates reduced. Modifying the environment should include both physical and psychosocial factors.
- ▶ The 'person psychology' approach in which the psychologist attempts to identify particular individual characteristics that might lead a person to be more accident prone or to take risks. Within this particular approach the focus is on training programmes that will highlight individual behaviour and will attempt to influence change in unsafe behaviour.
- ▶ The 'industrial–social' approach makes the assumption that unsafe behaviour is linked to group motivation. Individual motivation is linked with conditions in the environment which might support unsafe behaviour, for example it might be that taking risks is considered the 'macho' thing to do or that safe behaviour takes a lot more energy than careless behaviour. The focus in this approach is to try and change group behaviour so that people prefer safe practices (Landy, 1989)

Each of the above three approaches can be applied to reduce risks and promote health in other environments besides the workplace. It is interesting to note that although health promotion approaches (Naidoo and

Wills, 1994) recognize the multiple factors that influence the health status of an individual they often focus on changing individual behaviour.

For individuals in society, the desire to manage hazards relies on many factors. It is possible to relate to Bandura's concept of self-efficacy (Bandura, 1977) which suggests that to make behavioural changes (and thus promote personal safety), the individual needs to have an awareness or risk perception of the danger or threat, to have the competence and incentive to change in order to avert the hazard and a feeling that change would be beneficial with few adverse consequences. According to Naidoo and Wills (1994) Bandura's model (Bandura, 1977) has been incorporated into Becker's Health Belief Model (Becker, 1974), which focuses on demonstrating the functions of personal beliefs in decision making regarding health.

When exploring 'how' individuals may change their behaviour to avert hazards to their external or internal environment nurses must also be aware about 'why' individuals behave the way they do and also that individuals may not carry out their stated intentions (Ajzen and Fishbein, 1980). The nurse's role in health education and promotion of safety is reliant upon the client's willingness to listen, understand and comply with the information he or she is being offered. Information must be presented by the carer in a way that is appropriate for the client's needs and sensitive to the client's likely reaction if it is to be successful.

The main factors influencing an individual's response to health advice include:

- readiness;
- motivation;
- maturity;
- level of education (Akinsola, 1983).

Readiness

Human beings will only respond positively when they are physically, socially and psychologically ready to respond. For instance, the mother of an acutely ill two-year-old child may not be ready to learn what caused her child's illness until the physical condition of the child improves, or an elderly client may be reluctant to mobilize independently in hospital because the floor is too slippery or is unsure of the ward layout.

Motivation

To gain a better client outcome client involvement and active participation are essential. Client motivation requires an explanation about the importance of treatment and the use of equipment. Teaching clients with newly diagnosed diabetes mellitus to test their own blood sugar and to give their own insulin will mean that they can regain their self-esteem by being independent. Gaining a client's involvement in his or her treatment requires insight into the illness. This can be difficult if the nature of the illness affects perception, as in some mental illnesses where the client has no insight or when there is apathy due to low self-esteem.

Maturity

Because of differences in the maturity of individuals, carers need to be able to choose their words carefully so as not to either patronize clients or relatives or use words or concepts that are inappropriate. Careful consideration also has to be given to clients with learning disabilities or adolescents who appear physically more mature than the chronological age. Although they may appear adult, their perceptions and experiences and understandings may be limited. Initiatives, such as *A Campaign with Street Cred* (Lowery, 1996) have successfully targetted teenagers with asthma, aiming information and support directly at the adolescent age group in order to resolve risk-taking problems associated with poor compliance.

If clients are not used to medical terminology, using complex ideas or words can leave them frustrated and isolated. It is wise to avoid the use of medical jargon with clients.

Theories of risk taking are of interest to psychologists and health educators alike because they can help to explain major barriers to the effective provision of health care advice. Campaigns to encourage individuals to stop smoking or to reduce the number of people drinking and driving cars are two examples where individuals may be aware of the risk to safety in their own (and others) environment, but still persist in risk-taking behaviour.

How would you deal with information about which you have little or no understanding? Find a book at random from a section of your university library containing books addressing a different discipline (e.g. engineering or advanced mathematics). Read a few pages of text and try to make sense of it. How do you feel about the subject? Try to explain the content you have read to someone else. Did he or she understand you? What strategies might you employ to learn more about the subject?

DECISION MAKING

Staff Nurse Baker had just completed five shifts on day duty and was just about to finish her final shift before taking two days off work. When leaving the ward she is approached by the ward manager who asks her to fill in for a colleague who is 'off sick' that night. Staff Nurse Baker agrees as she welcomes the idea of earning some extra money for her holidays. Her manager also emphasizes that she can find no-one else to complete the shift. During the night shift, one of Nurse Baker's patient's slips to the floor when attempting to sit on the commode, which had been by her bedside. She is unhurt and Nurse Baker attempts to move her from the floor back to the commode. The client is 66 kg and feeling weak due to her illness.

- *Identify the potential risk factors to Nurse Baker's health through her decision to complete the night shift.*
- *Decide on what factors may motivate Nurse Baker in how she copes with her client's fall.*
- *Decide on what staff training or health promotion strategy is needed in this situation for all of the workforce involved in the incident.*

PRACTICE KNOWLEDGE

This section explores the ways in which a safe external environment may be facilitated. Assessment of clients and the care environment are included as well as managing strategies for ensuring and evaluating safety.

▶ RISK ASSESSMENT

Risk assessment in nursing falls within two main remits. First, there is a need to assess individual clients in relation to their own safety and the safety of others. This is an essential part of nursing care and is important in all branches of nursing. The need for cognitive understanding of risk and physical compatibility within the environment has already been illustrated in relation to accidents in the community, and these features are equally applicable in the care setting. In caring for children these two considerations are particularly important. For clients with learning disabilities, an assessment of individual ability and understanding is essential in order to ensure a safe environment for care. It cannot be assumed that an individual will behave in a way consistent with someone of a similar chronological age. Nurses in mental health have to assess and plan care for their clients ensuring the safety of the client, other clients within the care setting and personal safety. Nurses are also becoming involved in ensuring that patients who are released into the community do not pose a hazard to themselves or anyone else (Noak, 1997). Finally, in caring for adults, there is a need for all of the above, because adult individuals develop to different stages of maturity both physically and psychologically and the effects of disease can impair individual ability to maintain a safe environment. Adults have uniquely different motivations for their behaviours, which may not necessarily be predictable or rational. In relation to personal safety, there are risks of violence to nurses by clients (Bibby, 1995)

The second remit for nurses in risk assessment is more general in nature and relates to the care environment. The outcome of risk assessment must be the identification and implementation of risk management strategies to ensure that particular risks are eliminated or adequately controlled. However, there is evidence that accidents do happen and that many result from the failure of control systems, such as policy failure, deficent working practices and inadequate communication, as well as poorly defined responsibilities and staff working beyond their competence (UKCC, 1994; National Health Service Management Executive, 1994). Within the care setting evidence of nosocomial (hospital-acquired) disease suggests that nurses are not always completely successful in protecting their clients from environmental hazard.

Nurses need to know what the risks are and develop appropriate control systems. Risk assessment is not a 'once and for all' activity; it must be revised as changes occur such as new equipment, revised systems of work and different approaches to patient care. In the employment setting it is the employer's role to carry out risk assessment; however, in relation to individual client care, this role is firmly within the nursing domain.

▌ *Defining a Risk*

Before carrying out the risk assessment, a distinction must be made between 'hazard' and 'risk'. You will have already seen that a hazard can be defined as something with the potential to cause harm (Griffiths, 1996) and the concept of hazard has been widely discussed. A risk can be defined as the likelihood that the harm from a particular hazard is realized, (Control of Substances Hazardous to Health (Amendment) Regulations, 1990). The relationship between risk and hazard can be illustrated by the use of glutaraldehyde, which is a hazard in nursing. The risk of industrial asthma resulting from inhalation of glutaraldehyde is high if it is used in areas without adequate ventilation and personal protective clothing (i.e. inappropriately). However, with effective ventilation and a defined safe system of work, the risks associated with glutaraldehyde can be reduced, although it still remains a hazard.

There are a number of approaches to general risk assessment, but the underlying principles and steps involved are similar. An example of an approach proposed by the Royal College of Nursing (Brewer, 1994) is shown in Figure 1.1.1. Another related more generally to health care can be found in the National Health Service Management Executive's manual *Risk Management in the NHS* (1994).

RESEARCH BASED EVIDENCE

Wall et al. (1996) investigated outbreaks of intestinal infectious disease in England and Wales between 1992 and 1994. Of the 1590 reported cases 15% were accounted for by infections aquired in hospitals. Closer examination of outbreaks caused by Salmonella in hospital indicated that in 12 of the 22 outbreaks the mode of transmission was person to person and resulted from poor ward and personal hygiene. This study highlights the need for good ward and personal hygiene to ensure that spread of infection to staff and patients is minimized.

DECISION MAKING

Some risks and hazards associated with common problems in nursing are lifting and handling clients, back injury in nursing, violence to nurses by clients, pathogens, nosocomial disease and injury from assault

1. *Decide which of these are hazards and which are risks.*
2. *Using the hazards you have* identified, follow the principles of risk assessment illustrated above.
3. *Use your examples to decide whether the hazards identified have acceptable or unnacceptable risks.*

(You may like to record your assessment and a proforma for assessment recording is shown in Figure 1.1.1).

For each work activity and workplace identify all the hazards and record.
This should reflect what currently happens, not what should happen. Remember that different hazards may face different groups of staff or the hazard may vary according to the time of day.

Hazard identified	Location					Date of this assessment						Date of last assessment					Risk
	Persons at risk					Worst case outcome						Likelihood/probability					acceptable
	E	P	V	C	S	F	MI	Min Inj	No Inj	Plant	Cum effect	L/F	Prob	Poss	Rem	IP	Y/N

Persons at risk
E   = employee
P   = patient
V   = visitor
C   = contractor
S   = students

Worst case outcome
F   = fatal
MI   = major injury
Min Inj   = minor injury
No Inj   = no injury
Plant   = damage to plant/equipment
Cum effect = cumulative effect, i.e. where damage builds up over time

Likelihood/probability
L/F   = likely/frequent
Prob   = probable
Poss   = possible
Rem   = remote
IP   = improbable

The final judgement of whether the risk is deemed to be acceptable is obtained by reviewing the answers you have gained. If the worst case outcome is 'fatal' and this is a 'likely' occurrence then risk is clearly not acceptable. If on the other hand the worst case outcome is 'minor injury' and the occurrence is 'remote' then the risk may be deemed to be acceptable.

Figure 1.1.1. An approach to risk assessment proposed by the Royal College of Nursing (Brewer, 1994). (Reproduced by kind permission of S. Brewer.)

Assessment tools for psychosocial hazards at work, particularly with a focus on the organization's ability to investigate interventions, have been devised by Cox and Cox (1993).

▶ PLANNING AND IMPLEMENTING A STRATEGY FOR RISK MANAGEMENT

Planning care relates to the promotion of a safe environment for clients. There are two levels to planning. First, planning care in relation to the safety of the individual client. Secondly, planning daily work in relation to controlling of risks or hazards in the environment.

▶ *Issues in Planning Related to Clients*

The need for a hospital admission may bring about physical hazards for clients associated with the strangeness of the environment and an unknown ward layout. They may demonstrate anxiety and an unnatural response as a result of their situation. The nurse should identify and address these problems when making the assessment of a client's needs and in negotiating a safe and acceptable plan of care. Talking with the client about how to best address his or her needs is an important starting point, since compliance with a safe plan for care is critical. An example could relate to a hospital 'no smoking' policy. If a client usually enjoys

DECISION MAKING

In your next practice setting, look at a client's plan of nursing care. Take a particular note of any assessment that includes areas where safety may require nursing care planning.

- *What measures would you plan for this client?*
- *How do your ideas compare with those of the nurses?*
- *Have both psychological and physical safety issues been addressed?*
- *Has the plan been updated to incorporate any changes in the client's situation?*

cigarettes at home and will not entertain giving up smoking in hospital, it is not helpful to include in the nursing care plan that smoking is prohibited. For the client, this may lead to anger and frustration and potential noncompliance, either overtly or covertly. In a setting where there are inflammable substances (such as oxygen) this can create a serious risk both for the client and all others in the vicinity. It is safer to negotiate a plan with the client which agrees where cigarettes can be smoked safely, also ensuring that the client is able to gain access to this area. Information can also be given about the hazards of smoking in no-smoking areas, and there may be an opportunity for health education, leading to a reduction in smoking.

▶ Risk and Hazard Control in the Care Setting

Once hazards in the care setting have been identified where the risk is not acceptable, the next stage is to systematically plan control. For risk control the options listed in Table 1.1.3 are ranked in priority with one being the most effective and ten being the least effective.

Rank	Priority (1, most effective; 10, least effective)
1	Elimination of hazard entirely
2	Substitution by something less hazardous and risky
3	Enclosure
4	Guarding or segregation of people
5	Safe systems of work that reduce risk to an acceptable level
6	Written procedures known to be effective
7	Adequate supervision
8	Identification of training needs
9	Information or instruction (signs)
10	Personal protective equipment

Table 1.1.3 Options for controlling risk (Brewer, 1994). (Reproduced with kind permission of S. Brewer.)

DECISION MAKING

Managers opened an acute mental illness admission ward on the fourth floor of a general hospital to replace the admission facility of the local psychiatric hospital, which was due to close. The ward was previously used as an acute surgical ward and there were numerous cubicles, several exits, and the windows opened without restriction and were not glazed with safety glass. Shortly after the ward opened, the managers were surprised by the occurrence of a number of suicides.

- *How might a risk assessment have identified potential hazards in this situation?*
- *Using methods of hazard control, how could you address the hazards of poor observation from cubicles, exits and windows.*

Note that the amount of management or supervisory effort needed to maintain the controls shown in Table 1.1.3 is in inverse rank order with ten needing the most effort.

▶ Safe Equipment and Safe Systems of Work

In order to ensure an optimum working environment for nursing, it is important that all equipment in use is well maintained and all practices are safe and without risks to health as outlined by section 2(2)(a) of the *Health and Safety at Work Act* (1974). This is a general requirement, defined by the *Health and Safety at Work Act* as including machinery, equipment and appliances used at work, as well as the establishment of safe systems or practices while working.

In caring for clients, nurses use a wide variety of equipment. The following criteria apply to the way in which all equipment is used:

- ▶ equipment must meet all the current health and safety standards;
- ▶ equipment must be regularly inspected and serviced;
- ▶ the system of work must be safe;
- ▶ repair and maintenance operations must have a safe system of work identified;
- ▶ personal protective equipment should be provided if required.

DECISION MAKING

In your next placement, choose one piece of equipment that is regularly used.
Find out as much information as you can about it from workshop manuals, service records, and records of faults and repairs.
1. *Decide whether the equipment meets the criteria in Figure 1.1.1 as established by the Health and Safety at Work Act*
2. *If the evidence is not available then how would you proceed?*

Further information can be found from the Safety Action Bulletins produced by the Department of Health.

▌ *Managing Safety in the Care Environment*

Ensuring client safety while receiving care is ultimately an employer's responsibility in all settings, but nurses have a direct role in ensuring the implementation of safe care for their clients. Since clients are all individuals they all bring different situations to the care setting. Fear or anxiety may mean a client is not willing to comply with planned procedures of care regardless of how content they may have appeared with the negotiated plan. For example, a patient with a stroke may not like the hoist used to transfer him or her from the bed to the chair. There will always be dilemmas about how clients should receive intervention that is appropriate and safe. Discussing interventions with the client can air anxieties, and in this case finding a different lifting system that the client would feel happier with could be safer for all concerned. Other examples include critically ill patients who may have numerous treatments and monitoring equipment around them and the nurse should endeavour to make the area as safe as possible. If there is a lot of electrical equipment, extension sockets should not be used as the number of electrical items could overload the socket and result in a fire. Oxygen cylinders and wall points must have 'No smoking' signs in view to make everyone aware of the danger. There should be cot sides available for children, confused clients, and patients with poor muscle control.

In general, the nurse identifying a risk must ensure that action is taken. Further investigation may reveal that the problem has already been recognized and a solution is being sought; a policy decision may be required or the solution may have cost implications and the money is being found. The nurse has a responsibility to establish the current position and if necessary to facilitate change for improvement. Change must be implemented with the cooperation of all staff to ensure maximum benefit. If working with managers and staff to resolve a risk to the environment is ineffective, then advice may be required from outside agencies with a remit for the facilitation of health and safety at work. A safe policy for practice should exist and be readily available for most of the procedures that a nurse will perform.

▌ *Repair and Maintenance of Equipment*

A safe system of work needs to be identified for repair and maintenance operations themselves and this can have implications for nurses. For instance, the safe decontamination of equipment before maintenance must be specified. This may be especially important in areas where equipment has been used with clients carrying infectious organisms. At a simple level, working with children for instance, this may mean that there should be a procedure for cleaning toys safely after they have been used by a child who has an infection such as diarrhea and vomiting before checking their safety for offering to another child. It may also mean the appropriate cleaning of equipment or even rooms after use by clients. While the appropriate disposal of contaminated linen and sharps are further areas where a nurse's decision making involves procedures which are required to maintain the employers reponsibility for the safety of other employees.

It is important to remember that the employer's duty to provide a safe system of work applies to all nurses, including community nurses as well as those based in hospitals. The fact that the nurse will be working in a patient's home does not diminish the employer's duty.

▶ *Managing Safe Handling and Storage of Substance*

Within nursing practice, handling of potentially hazardous substances may be a regular occurrence. Issues related to the safe handling of substances are addressed in section 53 of the *Health and Safety at Work Act* and are developed further by the *Control of Substances Hazardous to Health (COSHH) Regulations*, 1988.

▶ *Control of Substances Hazardous to Health (COSHH) Regulations*, 1988

This was the most significant piece of health and safety legislation after the *Health and Safety at Work Act* (1974). It applies to all work where people (including nurses) are exposed or liable to be exposed to substances hazardous to health. The regulations give both a general description of the types of substances that are hazardous to health and a specific list of materials currently regarded as hazardous. There are 19 regulations, which include key duties such as assessment and training and a related *Approved Code of Practice* is given for each regulation.

Any 'substance' should be regarded as hazardous to health in the form in which it occurs in the work activity, whether or not its mode of causing injury to health is known and whether or not the active constituent has been identified. A substance hazardous to health is not just a single chemical compound but also includes mixtures, for example of compounds, microorganisms, or allergens. The *Approved Code of Practice* further defines what is hazardous. Among the key points are that:

- ▶ different forms of the same substance may present different hazards, for instance when a solid is ground into dust;
- ▶ impurities may create hazards;
- ▶ fibres of a certain size or shape can be hazardous.

▶ Summary of Duties of Employer Under the *Control of Substances Hazardous to Health (COSHH) Regulations*

The employer must:

- ▶ assess the risks;
- ▶ assess the steps needed to meet the regulation;
- ▶ prevent or at least control exposure;
- ▶ ensure controls are used to monitor exposure;
- ▶ provide health surveillance;
- ▶ examine and test control;
- ▶ inform, instruct and train employees and non-employees (Brewer, 1994).

The storage of substances on the ward should follow the principles of 'good housekeeping' to improve safety. This may mean storing glass bottles on the back of a low shelf to avoid breakages, or keeping the stock of substances to a minimum to avoid stock expiring and the dangers of major spillages. There should be procedures and policies in relation to the handling of substances, and these should be readily available.

DECISION MAKING

A five-gallon container of glutaraldehyde is knocked over accidentally and its contents spill over the clinic room floor. A nurse tries to mop it up, but is overcome by a coughing fit and is off sick for three months. *Using the above summary of the Control of Substances Hazardous to Health (COSHH) Regulations (1988) what questions could be asked in attempting to establish liability?*

▶ EVALUATING SAFETY

Nursing care must be regularly evaluated to ensure that it is effective, and this should include the provision of a safe environment. If safety is breached then a further evaluation will be necessary. Additional requirements would include the completion of an accident report form, which is a legal requirement under the *Reporting of Injuries, Diseases and Dangerous Occurrences Regulations (RIDDOR)* (1985). The breach in safety and the effect on the client would be noted, the circumstances in which the incident occurred, the outcome and any action that ensued to amend the situation.

Employers need information about accidents so that an investigation can take place and action can be taken to prevent a recurrence. The information can be used by the Health and Safety Executive (HSE) for national monitoring of occupational incidents. For nurses, accurate reporting will protect individual rights and benefits in the event of loss of income or personal injury. Occupational injuries should be reported to the occupational health department and injured workers may require an assessment of fitness before returning to the work environment.

Accident forms provide essential information and may be referred to in the event of any litigation (Rogers and Salvage, 1988). If a nurse suffers a back injury while moving a client then bland statements such as 'hurt her back while moving a patient' should be avoided because it offers no indication of specific issues of concern. Evaluative information is required, and examples of questions that may be asked include the following:

- ▶ What lifting procedure was involved?
- ▶ Who decided the system for lifting the patient? ·
- ▶ What was the weight, height and name of the patient?
- ▶ What part of the body was injured?
- ▶ Were mechanical aids used? If not, why not?
- ▶ Was anyone else involved? If yes, record names and addresses.
- ▶ Was there a written care plan on the lifting procedure to be used?

After completing an accident report, you must ensure that you have your own copy of the statement or incident form. Your personal record of the events that have taken place must be kept safely for future referral. This is particularly important if legal action is pursued by any party. Within the health services, employers are required to keep an accident book under *Social Security Regulations* (1979). In spite of the benefits of accident reporting, there is evidence to suggest that in hospital settings it is not performed well and underreporting is a serious problem (Sutton *et al.*, 1994).

▶ *Evaluating Changes to Working Practices*

Once an acceptable solution to a risk has been identified then some way of ensuring that all staff involved are making the necessary changes to their practice should be established. It is also necessary to evaluate the effectiveness of the new intervention. This might require a short questionnaire or informal chats with or observation of people, or even a small evaluative research project. Examples include the evaluation of a no-fault reporting system for drug errors achieved by Bourns (1996) and, in relation to patients, an evaluation of patient compliance related to self administration of medicines (Sutherland *et al.*, 1995). There are also updates in regulations and law to keep in line with European Community

RESEARCH BASED EVIDENCE

A study by Sutton et al. (1994) aimed to discover the incidence of unreported accidents. It was carried out in ten wards in a large acute hospital, 575 clients were included in the study, and 75 accidents were identified. Of these accidents only 65% were reported. In some instances multiple incidents were left unreported, and patient reponses suggested that in the majority of cases staff knew about the accidents that were not reported.

directives and the Health and Safety Commission reports. To ensure that a health and safety issue is being properly resolved can be complex. The nurse has a duty to inform the employer of any health and safety risk and to ensure that the risk thereafter is no longer present. Conversely with recent legislation, the manager now has an obligation to involve the employee in the management of health and safety issues.

PROFESSIONAL KNOWLEDGE

This section illustrates the development of current health and safety legislation and considers its overall impact upon decision making in nursing practice. Particular emphasis is placed upon the effect of the law on the role and responsibilities of the nurse. To appreciate the context in which today's law has emerged, it is important to review UK law before the signing of the Maastricht Treaty (1992) and the acceptance of European legislation. Before proceeding however, you will need to recall the UKCC *Code of Professional Conduct* (UKCC, 1994) with reference to health and safety issues, which is summarized in Table 1.1.4). These particular requirements are reflected in current health and safety legislation.

Part of *Code of Professional Conduct*	Requirement
Part 1	Act always in such a way as to promote and safeguard the wellbeing and interests of patients and clients
Part 2	Ensure that no action or omission on your part, or within your sphere of responsibility, is detrimental to the interests, condition or safety of patients and clients
Part 11	Report to an appropriate person or authority, having regard to the physical, psychological and social effects on patients and clients, any circumstances in the environment of care which could jeopardize standards of practice
Part 13	Report to an appropriate person or authority any circumstances where it appears that the health and safety of colleagues is at risk, as such circumstances may compromise standards of practice and care

Table 1.1.4 Health and safety issues from the UKCC's *Code of Professional Conduct* (1994)

▶ HISTORY OF HEALTH AND SAFETY IN THE UK

In 1970, a Committee of Inquiry on Health and Safety at Work was set up under the chairmanship of Lord Robens. The job of the Committee was to examine existing health and safety legislation and make any recommendations for change. This finished in 1972 (the Robens Report), and the inquiry's findings became the basis of the *Health and Safety at Work Act* (1974), which came into force on 1st April 1975, and which currently underpins health and safety legislation in Britain. The act comes in four parts, which highlight different aspects and address the major principles and objectives of health and safety (Table 1.1.5). The Act insisted that any implementation of the law by the employers would be done so with consultation of the employees, i.e. nurses, although there are general duties that the employer and others must carry out.

How do you see the points in Table 1.1.5 applying to your particular field of nursing?

Write down your thoughts on each of the points.

To secure the health, safety and welfare of people at work

To protect people other than those at work against risks arising out of activities of others

To control the storage and use of explosive, highly flammable or dangerous substances

To control the release into the atmosphere of noxious or offensive substances from premises

Table 1.1.5 The four parts of the *Health and Safety at Work Act* (1974)

The *Health and Safety at Work Act* (1974) applies throughout England, Scotland and Wales with the exception of certain building regulations, which do not apply in Scotland. It does not cover Northern Ireland (minor exceptions) or the Isle of Man and Channel Islands, each of which have their own laws. In section 2(1) it establishes the duty of employers and of employees, which is a fundamental principle of health and safety at work as 'It shall be the duty of every employer to ensure, so far as is reasonably practicable, the health, safety and welfare at work of all his employees'.

The general duties often come with the expressions 'so far as is reasonably practicable', or 'so far as practicable'. These expressions do play an important role in the law's implementation. 'Reasonably practicable' is a narrower expression than 'physically possible' and it implies that risks must be measured against the time or money required to avert them. This idea is very important as this calculation must be made before an accident or dangerous occurrence. Think of it this way – if a safety measure is practicable (i.e. physically possible) it could financially cripple a Trust because of the cost involved. So therefore 'reasonably' allows the employer to find a safe compromise. Conversely if the employer insists that a cheaper machine is used in a manufacturing process but it comes without safeguards then it is not practicable to use it for all the reasonableness the employer asks for. So assessment is made on two levels – is it 'practicable', and is it 'reasonable'?

▶ *The Change in Health and Safety Legislation Since 1992*

The European Community in 1992 agreed that several legislations had to be adopted by member States. These legislations have been interpreted by member states into additional regulations. In the UK these are known quaintly as the 'six pack', because there are six new regulations in force and these are identified in Table 1.1.6.

All the regulations have implications for safe working practices in nursing and should be included within policies for employment practices. They should be considered as useful supplementary reading for this chapter.

DECISION MAKING

You are the defendant in a court case involving the *Health and Safety at Work Act* (Department of Health, 1974) after you received a back injury from slipping on a wet floor. Although the floor dryer was broken and had been sent for repair, the cleaners did possess warning cones to advise employees about wet floors. There were none in evidence on the day that you slipped. The onus of proving that an employer has not fulfilled the statutory obligation by being 'reasonably practicable' is placed on the defendant (i.e. you). The court would then have to decide what is or was reasonable or practicable in your case.

Decide how you could convince a court that the employer had broken the law.

The Management of Health and Safety at Work Regulations, 1992

Manual Handling Regulations (Health and Safety Executive, 1992)

Workplace (Health, Safety and Welfare) Regulations, 1992

Health and Safety (Display Screen Equipment) Regulations, 1992

Provision and Use of Work Equipment Regulations, 1992

Personal Protective Equipment (PPE) at Work Regulations, 1992

Table 1.1.6 The 'six pack' regulations for health and safety – UK interpretations of the European Community directives

▶ EXTENDING THE REGULATIONS

The construction of *Health and Safety at Work Act* (1974) allows the Act to be extended by the development of regulations more specific to areas of needs within its scope. These regulations directly affect nursing and are outlined below. Where there is no duty for the nurse, but the regulation is generally pertinent to nursing it is listed for further reference, as are regulations that have been reviewed extensively elsewhere in the chapter.

▶ Health and Safety (First Aid) Regulations, 1981

The employer has a duty to provide, or ensure that there is provided, personnel, equipment and facilities appropriate in the circumstances for enabling first aid to be rendered to his employees (including nurses) if they are injured at work or become ill at work.

A suitable person is someone who holds a current first aid certificate (approved by HSE). The *Code of Professional Practice* also states that practising nurses whose names are entered on Parts 1, 2 or 7 of the UKCC Register (1992) can be regarded as first aiders. The regulations also describe the need for and contents of a first aid room and first aid kits.

▶ Health and Safety Information for Employees Regulations, 1989

Employers have a duty to either display posters or give leaflets containing up-to-date information on health, safety and welfare legislation, including the address of the local HSE office.

▶ Electricity at Work Regulations, 1989

These are designed to help prevent injury or even death from an electric shock. The regulations state who may or may not carry out any work on electrical installations and equipment. Invariably this would be the Estates Department, but in the community nurses have to be careful about using their equipment with the patient's electrical supply or with using the patient's own equipment.

▶ The Management of Health and Safety at Work Regulations, 1992

Nurses must make full and proper use of any arrangements established by the employer for health and safety at work, and must report to the employer details of any work situation that might represent a serious and imminent danger.

▶ Manual Handling Operations Regulations, 1992

These regulations require a fundamental change in attitude to the handling of clients. The many implications for nurses are addressed in Chapter 1.2.

▶ Health and Safety (Display Screen Equipment) Regulations, 1992

These regulations will have greater impact on nursing as more areas and hospitals use computers. The aim is to prevent health problems by encouraging good ergonomic design of equipment, furniture, the working environment and the job. They not only apply to office-type equipment such as visual display units (VDUs), but also to some display screen technology specific to the health care field. Certain items are, however, excluded, such as portable systems not in prolonged use and any equipment having a small data or measurement display required for direct use of the equipment, for example cardiac monitors, oscilloscopes and instruments with small displays showing a series of digits.

▶ *Personal Protective Equipment (PPE) at Work Regulations, 1992*

The main aim of all the new regulations is to eliminate hazards and remove the need for PPE. The duties relate to the assessment, selection, provision, maintenance and use of PPE to ensure that equipment and clothing worn by people at work protects them against risk to their health and safety. Nurses must make full and proper use of PPE provided and take all reasonable steps to ensure that it is returned to the storage provided for it after use. They should report any loss or obvious defect in PPE to their employer.

▶ *Other regulations*

These include the *Provision and Use of Work Equipment Regulations, 1992 Control of Substances Hazardous to Health (COSHH) Regulations, 1988,* and *Workplace (Health, Safety and Welfare) Regulations,* 1992.

▶ HEALTH AND SAFETY – EDUCATION REQUIREMENTS FOR NURSING

Within the educational preparation for becoming a nurse, broad issues related to ensuring safe and competent practice are addressed. These include an understanding of maintaining a safe internal and external environment for nurses, their clients, and their peers. Principles relating to law and ethical considerations are also considered. In practice placements the student should work within the parameters of their education addressed to date and not attempt practices with which they are not familar. Policies are often established between health trusts and schools of nursing and midwifery to clarify policy position in relation to ensuring safe practice for students. If there is uncertainty about whether students can participate in an aspect of practice not identified within their practice guidelines, then the issue should be addressed to the school of nursing and midwifery concerned and the matter clarified. Students are urged not to participate in procedures for which they have not been educated. Clear procedural guidance must also be evident.

Once qualified, employers are legally obliged to provide nurses with appropriate education and training for procedures and equipment in their work setting as defined in section 2(2)(c) of the *Health and Safety at*

DECISION MAKING

You may like to discuss some or all of this exercise with practice colleagues or your tutor.

You are at work when the fire alarm sounds. The fire doors shut automatically.
1. *What would your action be?*
2. *Staff and visitors continue to go through the doors and do not respond to the alarm. How would you deal with this situation?*

You are advised by the fire officer that the ward should be evacuated. While making arrangements for evacuation a patient has a cardiac arrest.
3. *What would be the priority? The patient who has arrested or the other patients?*
4. *What action would you need to take in both cases?*
5. *What questions may you need to ask (a) at the time? (b) afterwards?*

Work Act (1974). This may include provision of information about drugs and chemicals in use and instruction and training in safe ways of handling these substances (e.g. antiseptics) and in the use of equipment (e.g. hoists). Where nurses are expected to participate in activities that expand on their initial education and training, for instance in taking blood samples, then extra training and assessment must be provided. The UKCC supports this view in it's document on *Guidelines for Professional Practice* (1996). Mandatory updates in relation to safety aspects such as fire evacuation procedures or emergency life support are also included.

▶ RESPONSIBILITIES OF THE EMPLOYER

In addition to providing education and training, it is the responsibility of your employer to make sure that the area in which you work is a safe place to be and that adequate facilities are provided as outlined by sections 2(2)d and 2(2)e of the *Health and Safety at Work Act* (1974). Community nurses are exempt from this section as the patient's home is not 'under the employer's control'. However, if the working environment is at all hazardous to the nurse the employer must decide what action to take to ensure the nurse's safety. Withdrawing the nursing service must be seen as a last option.

▶ *Points to Consider When Assessing the Safety of Work Environs*

The points to consider are as follows:

- ▶ Is general cleanliness and housekeeping adequate?
- ▶ Are fire exits clearly identified and kept free from obstruction?
- ▶ Are fire extinguishers provided and maintained and do staff know how to use them correctly?
- ▶ Is the fire alarm system working and checked regularly and are fire drills held?
- ▶ Are buildings safe?
- ▶ Are other sources of danger (e.g. radiators, stairways) guarded where necessary?
- ▶ Are there hazards associated with doors, such as visibility or a heavy to open door?
- ▶ Are there any problems in connection with heating, lighting, ventilation?
- ▶ What are the arrangements for first aid?
- ▶ Are there policies for managing the employee who is human immuno-deficiency virus (HIV) positive?
- ▶ Are hepatitis B vaccinations available?
- ▶ Is there access to a counselling service?
- ▶ Is there a smoking policy?
- ▶ Are there adequate rest facilities?
- ▶ Do night staff have access to a hot meal when on duty?

▶ *Visitor Safety*

A subsection of the *Health and Safety at Work Act* (1974) adds responsibilities to the employer to protect other people who are not employees, for example patients, visitors and non-health service employees working on the premises. Section 3(3) places a duty on employers to give information to persons who are not their employees about aspects of the way in which they conduct their undertaking that might affect health and safety. For example, an agency nurse or employees of a contractor will need to know the safety rules for the area in which they are to work.

Finally, although your employer has duties relating to the control of premises, they may not be responsible if you are seconded to another care setting such as general practitioner's premises or a clinic not owned or contracted by your employer. You would in this case be protected by section 4 of the *Health and Safety at Work Act*. Here duties are established with respect to health and safety for those who are in control of non-domestic premises where people work who are not their own employees or where these people use equipment and substances provided for their use while working.

▶ THE NURSE'S RESPONSIBILITY IN HEALTH AND SAFETY

▶ *The Duties of Employees*

The *Health and Safety at Work Act* (1974) defines the duties for employees, which include members of management. Sections 7 and 8 lay out the duties. The employer has many duties to ensure nurses' health and safety while at work, but this would have no impact on the workforce if they had no legal duty. So sections 7 and 8 are there to ensure that 'you' as a part of the workforce have a duty under this act. Horseplay and practical jokes often breach section 7 because of the possible tragic consequences.

If protective or manual handling equipment is provided the nurse must cooperate and wear or use the equipment. Failure to do so would legitimately lead to disciplinary action; however, this aspect may be ignored by workers if the organizational commitment is not perceived to be strong.

> A nursing auxiliary in a care of the elderly ward thought that her good humoured jokes cheered everyone's day. One day she thought it would be fun to remove the supports from the chairs in the staff room leaving just the cushions. It would be fun to see the nursing staff slipping through the chairs as they sat down for their morning break.
>
> Unfortunately one nurse sat down heavily, fell through the chair to the floor, sustained a back injury and was no longer able to work. Compensation for loss of earnings was sought through the courts.
>
> *What are the issues in this case? Who would be liable? Could prosecution and compensation be pursued?*

▶ UPHOLDING THE LAW

▶ *HSE Inspectors*

The purpose of a visit to an institution by an HSE inspector is to ensure the observance, maintenance and improvement of health and safety standards, and to make sure that they comply with the law. During a visit the inspector will have discussions with management and safety representatives, and perhaps other employees.

The inspector may rely on informal methods to improve health and safety or eliminate hazards. They may give advice verbally, send follow-up letters. or provide more information. If a risk is serious, the law is being blatantly ignored or the organization's methods for dealing with health and safety are inadequate, the inspector will use formal procedures, which comprise improvement notices, prohibition notices or prosecution.

RESEARCH BASED EVIDENCE

Gershon et al. (1995) surveyed 1716 American care workers about their compliance with universal safety precautions. They found that compliance varied according to activity, but was overall strongly correlated to several key factors, including perceived organizational commitment to safety and perceived conflict of interest between the workers need to protect themselves and the need to provide care for their patients. Risk-taking personality, perception of risk, and knowledge and training were also noted to be influential factors.

Within the health care profession a variety of additional strategies are established to ensure that the law as described above is adhered to and to provide a monitoring and referral system in relation to health and safety. Nurses should be aware of the function and composition of strategy and monitoring groups that enforce the law since they offer a resource for support and advice.

▶ *Health and Safety Committees*

These provide a forum for employees (including nurses) to work with management in improving health and safety standards. This is done through recognized trade union and other professional organizations' safety representatives.

▶ *Health and Safety Policies*

Employers are required by section 2(3) of the *Health and Safety at Work Act* (1974) to prepare and update or revise a written statement of general policy covering the health and safety of employees and the arrangements for carrying out that policy. Written statements of policy should be made available to all employees and should be updated. The Health and Safety Commission regards this as an important requirement, as it underpins the Act's whole approach – that health and safety is not a marginal technical issue, but an integral part of management, organization and how people do their work. This does not negate the importance of detailed regulations, for example for the handling of pathogens, but detailed regulations are unlikely to work properly if the organization as a whole does not actively promote health and safety at work.

It is the employer's duty to update and revise safety policies in the light of safety committees' recommendations, changes in responsible personnel, and any new guidance or legislation from the relevant authorities, such as the HSC and HSE.

▶ *The Composition and Procedures relating to a Health and Safety Committee*

Membership and structure should be settled through negotiation, though management must have representatives who have adequate knowledge and experience of the policy and plans of the organization (e.g. medical, nursing, finance, administration); at least one of the management representatives must have adequate authority to give proper consideration to views and recommendations to help give the committee effective power.

Representation for employees is a matter for the unions to determine. Generally, the unions representing the largest groups should have one or more safety representatives on the committee. Relevant specialists such as safety officer, occupational health nurse or fire officer, should be ex officio members of the committee; other specialists can be co-opted for certain meetings. The formal definition of the committee's function is 'keeping under review the measures taken to ensure the health and safety at work of employees and such functions as may be prescribed' in accordance with section 2(9) of the *Health and Safety at Work Act* (1974).

Safety committees should establish broad objectives such as promoting cooperation between employer and employees (including nurses) in investigating, developing and carrying out health and safety measures. Within these objectives, committees then define specific functions such as studying accident and disease statistics and trends to identify problem areas, devising appropriate measures and reporting these to management, or examining safety audits. They may consider reports and other factual information provided by HSE inspectors or safety representatives and assist in the development of safety rules and safe systems of work. They help monitor the effectiveness of the safety content of employee training or assess the adequacy of health and safety publicity in the workplace, providing a good link with the local HSE. Other functions may include overseeing a programme of planned preventive maintenance or approving the purchase of equipment and products.

Finally, from the nurse's point of view, possibly the most significant part of the *Health and Safety at Work Act* is the ability of unions to appoint safety representatives with wide ranging legal rights. If you are a union member you can approach your union representative to discuss an issue of concern. The safety representative has access to relevant information regarding safety issues and may be able to exert union pressure to ensure that safety is addressed if a line management approach proves ineffective.

If you suffer financial loss as a result of an industrial accident a range of benefits may be available. It can be complicated, so you should seek advice as soon as possible. Each case must be considered on its own merits. If you have any concerns any of the following would be happy to help:

▶ the department of human resources;
▶ your local union representative;
▶ the employment service – disability services branch.

REFLECTIVE KNOWLEDGE

It is evident that all nurses have a major responsibility for ensuring the safety of clients and of peers. This responsibility is underpinned professionally within the Code of Professional Conduct (UKCC, 1992), and legislated within all the regulations. Additionally, nurses have a legal duty of care to their patients and this includes ensuring the provision of safe practice. To fulfil such a responsibility it is essential to understand concepts associated with physical, psychological and social perceptions of safety and possible motivations in determining risk and behaving in a safe manner. Nurses also need to have an appreciation of the particular health and safety needs of the client group for which they are predominantly responsible. In each branch of nursing there are particular roles for the nurse related to assisting their clients. These may be related to understanding the limited cognitive development in child and learning disability nursing or understanding the impact of mental or physical disorder in nursing adults and those with mental illness.

Some nurses have a greater responsibility for ensuring the safety of individuals in the workplace (for example occupational health nurses or those undertaking a union or employment role with a remit for health and safety representation or those in managerial positions.

Application of the concepts introduced within this chapter will enable you to begin to understand the complexities of ensuring safety in many individual circumstances and allow nursing decisions to be made through reflection over the concepts underpinning such differences.

Finally the seriousness of health and safety in the workplace cannot be underestimated, the provisions made within the *Health and Safety at Work Act* (1974) and the extending regulations are there to protect you, your colleagues and your clients in your day to day activities. If these are breached through neglect or ignorance then an optimum environment is compromised. It is the responsibility of every individual at work to insist on the highest standards of safe practice and to report situations of compromise to the appropriate health and safety regulator. This may be your manager or union or employment safety representative, or, if necessary, the HSE. Without the integrity of individuals in practice, the provision and promotion of health and safety would be an impossible feat.

▶ CASE STUDY: MENTAL HEALTH

Jeremiah Jacobs is 62 years old. He has lived in a large rural hospital for the mentally ill for the last 30 years and is diagnosed as having moderate learning disabilities and schizophrenia. Jeremiah remains in a long-term care facility because as yet no appropriate community facility has been found. In the hospital where he lives many patients have been moved into community homes and wards have been closed. The hospital is now a small facility where all clients are well known by the resident staff. Jeremiah enjoys sitting on the main ward corridor trying to trip passers-by up. As everyone knows him, they know to keep out of tripping distance. One day a visitor comes into the hospital and is tripped up by Jeremiah. The visitor sustains a number of bruises and sues the hospital.

■ Do you think the visitor will be successful in her claim?

■ Who was responsible for ensuring the vistor's safety?

■ Which section of the *Health and Safety at Work Act* (1974) may be referred to in this case?

■ Decide how you could have prevented this situation from arising.

▶ CASE STUDY: ADULT

Mrs Smith is a 95-year-old woman who has arrived at the accident and emergency department after a fall at her home. She had been found by neighbours after crying out for some hours. On arrival in hospital Mrs Smith is cold and in pain and appears confused. She is to have a radiograph of her femur as a fracture is suspected. A nurse takes Mrs Smith to the radiography department and then goes on a coffee break. Mrs Smith attempts to get off the trolley while left alone in the radiography department and falls again.

■ Using the information gained from this chapter write down the questions that you think should be asked, in the event of an inquiry into the incident. For example, did the nurse inform the radiographer that the patient was there? If no, why not? If yes, why was there no-one with her?

■ Were the trolley sides up or down? What system of work is there for transferring patients from the accident and emergency department to the radiography department? Is there one? Was it followed?

▶ CASE STUDY: CHILD

As a school nurse you are attempting to reduce the number of home accidents among school children. This means that you plan to attend the children's school and talk to a group of 5–7-year-olds about the types of accidents that may occur in the home.

■ What factors may influence the way in which you help to ensure that the children can participate actively in their own risk assessment and hazard management?

■ Decide on a plan of action that could help get the safety message across to this group.

■ Who is ultimately responsible for ensuring your safety while you are visiting the school to talk to the children. Which section of the *Health and Safety at Work Act* (1974) would apply in this instance?

▶ CASE STUDY: LEARNING DISABILITIES

Benny Wong is a 25-year-old Chinese man with moderate learning difficulties. He is unable to care independently for himself and tends to be noisy and aggressive at times. Benny's parents are elderly and although they have been caring for him at home they have recently been finding him an increasing challenge. Benny has now been accepted into a community home, which provides full time care for a few clients with learning disabilities. For Benny the move is a great change since he is used to living with his Chinese-speaking parents in a quiet house in a small village where he is well known to the community. His new home is in a suburban estate close to a main road.

■ **Using the principles of risk assessment, identify the hazards that may be a problem for Benny in his new home.**

■ **Try to decide what the main safety risks are for Benny.**

■ **Now decide what strategies may be appropriate for tackling the risks that you have identified.**

■ **Finally, identify what barriers may need to be overcome in making Benny safe in his new home.**

▶ ANNOTATED FURTHER READING

AKASS, R. (1994) *Essential Health and Safety for Managers: Guide to Good Practice in the EC.* Cambridge. Gower Publishing Ltd.
A book covering, for employees and especially for employers, the ways to comply with the demands needed.
HEALTH AND SAFETY COMMISSION (1992) *Monitoring Strategies for Toxic Substances. Guidance Note EH42.* London. Her Majesty's Stationery Office.
This guidance covers essential thoughts behind all safe practice by using assessment as a tool.
ROGERS, R., SALVAGE, J. (1989) *Nurses at Risk: A Guide to Health and Safety at Work.* Guildford. Heinemann Nursing.
A book specifically for nurses, giving the principles of health and safety.
GARRICK, B.J. GEKLER, W.C. (1991) *The Analysis, Communication, and Perception of Risk.* New York. Plenum.
This deals extensively with the problems associated with people's understanding of health and safety.

▶ ACKNOWLEDGEMENT

Special thanks must go to Richard Przystupa and Sheelagh Brewer.

▶ REFERENCES

AJZEN, I., FISHBEIN, M. (1980) *Understanding Attitudes and Predicting Social Behaviour.* Englewood Cliffs. Prentice Hall.

AKINSOLA, H.Y. (1983) *Behavioural Science for Nurses.* Singapore: Churchill Livingstone.

BANDURA, A. (1977) *Social Learning Theory.* Englewood Cliffs. Prentice Hall.

BECKER, M.H. (1974) (ed.) *The Health Belief Model and Personal Health Behaviour.* Slack Thorofare. New Jersey.

BIBBY, P (1995) *Personal Safety for Health Workers.* Vermont. Arena.

BLOOR, M. (1995) *The Sociology of HIV Transmission.* London. Sage.

BREWER S. (1994) *Royal College of Nursing Safety Representatives' Manual.* Southampton. The Royal College of Nursing of the United Kingdom.

BOURNS (1996) Errors but no trials. *Nursing Times* **92(42)**: 50–51.

COHEN, P (1996) Water companies threaten to return to Victorian Times. *Health Visitor* **69(7)**: 259.

Consumer Protection Act (1987) London. Her Majesty's Stationery Office.

Control of Substances Hazardous to Health (COSHH) Regulations (1988) London. Her Majesty's Stationery Office.

Control of Substances Hazardous to Health (COSHH) (Amendment) Regulations (1990) SI 2026 and (1991) SI 2431. London. Her Majesty's Stationery Office.

COX, T., COX, S. (1993) Psychosocial and organizational hazards: control and monitoring in the workplace. *European Occupational Health Series no.5.* Copenhagen. World Health Organization Regional Office for Europe.

COX, T., GRIFFITHS, A., COX, S. (1995) *Work-related Stress in Nursing. Managing the Risk.* Geneva. International Labour Organization.

COX, T., GRIFFITHS, A. (1996) Assessment of psychosocial hazards at work. In. Schabracq, M.J., Winnubst, J.A.M., Cooper, C.L. (eds) *Handbook of Work and Health Psychology.* John Wiley and Sons 127–143.

THE DETTOL REPORT. *Child Accidents in the UK* (1994) Dettol Care Network in association with the Child Accident Prevention Trust.

DOUGLAS, M. (1966) *Purity and Danger; An Analysis of Concepts of Pollution and Taboo.* London. Routledge and Kegan Paul.

Electricity at Work Regulations (1989) SI 635. London. Her Majesty's Stationery Office.

FALLOWFIELD, L. (1990) *The Quality of Life: The Missing Measurement in Health Care.* London. London University Press.

GABE, J. (1995) *Medicine, Health and Risk: Sociological Approaches.* Norwich. Blackwell.

GERSHON R.R.M, VLAHOV, D., FELKNOR, S.A., VESLEY, D., JOHNSON, P.C., DELCLOS, G.L., MURPHY, L.R. (1995) Compliance with universal precautions among health care workers at 3 regional hospitals. *American Journal of Infection Control* **23**(4): 225–236.

HARRINGTON, J.M., GILL, F.S. (1992) *Occupational Health* (3rd edition). Oxford. Blackwell Scientific Publications.

Health and Safety at Work etc. Act (1974) London. Her Majesty's Stationery Office.

HEALTH AND SAFETY EXECUTIVE (1992) *Manual Handling Operations Regulations, SI 2793 and Guidance on Regulations, L23.* London. Her Majesty's Stationery Office.

HEALTH AND SAFETY (Display Screen Equipment) Regulations SI 2792. (1992) London. Her Majesty's Stationery Office.

Health and Safety (First Aid) Regulations SI 917. (1981) London. Her Majesty's Stationery Office.

Health and Safety Information for Employees Regulations SI 682. (1989) London. Her Majesty's Stationery Office.

HENDRIKSON, E (1994) Lead exposure in migrant children in Northern Colorado. *Journal of American Academy of Physicians Assistants* **7**(10): 707–710.

HYNDMAN, S.J. (1990) Housing dampness and health among British Bengalis in East London. *Social Science Medicine* 30: 131–141.

INEICHEN, B (1993) *Homes and Health – How Housing and Health Interact.* London. E & FN Spon.

INTERNATIONAL LABOUR ORGANIZATION (1986) *Psychosocial Factors at Work: Recognition and Control. Occupational Safety and Health Series no.56.* Geneva. International Labour Organization.

KEELEY, D.J., NEILL, P., GALLIVAN, S. (1991) Comparison of the prevalence of reversible airways obstruction in rural and urban Zimbabwean children. *Thorax* **46**: 549–553

KIMBERLIN, R.H. (1993) *Bovine Spongiform Encephalopathy.* Rome. Food and Agriculture Organization of the United Nations.

KROWCHUK, H.V. (1995) Neurobehavioural effects of childhood lead exposure. *Annual Review of Nursing Research* **138**: 87–114

LANDY, F. (1989) *Psychology of Work Behaviour* (4th edition). California. Brooks Cole Pub. Co.

LEVI, L (1984) Stress in Industry: Causes, Effects and Prevention. Occupational Safety and Health Series no. 51. International Labour Organization, Geneva.

LOWERY, M (1996) A campaign with street cred to target teenagers with asthma. *Nursing Times* **92**(42): 34–37.

LOWRY, S (1991) Housing and Health. *British Medical Journal* **299**: 1261–1262

Maastricht Treaty (1992) London. Her Majesty's Stationery Office.

Management of Health and Safety at Work Regulations SI 2051. (1992) London. Her Majesty's Stationery Office.

MASLOW, A.H. (1970) *Motivation and Personality* (2nd edition). New York Harper Row.

NAIDOO, J. and WILLS, J. (1994) *Health Promotion: Foundations for Practice.* London, Baillière Tindall.

NATIONAL HEALTH SERVICE MANAGEMENT EXECUTIVE (1994) Risk Management in the National Health Service (NHS). London. National Health Service Management Executive.

NHS (Amendment) Bill (1986) London. Her Majesty's Stationery Office.

NIGHTINGALE, F. (1860) *Notes on Nursing – What It Is and What It Is Not.* London. Harrison.

NIGHTINGALE, F. (1863) *Notes on Hospitals* (3rd edition). London. Longman Roberts and Green.

NOAK, J (1997) Assessment of the risks posed by people with mental illness. *Nursing Times* **93**(1): 1–8

Personal Protective Equipment (PPE) at Work Regulations SI 2966. (1992) London. Her Majesty's Stationery Office.

PLATT, S.D., MARTIN, C.J., HUNT, S.M. and LEWIS (1989) Damp housing,

mould growth and symptomatic health state. *British Medical Journal* **298**: 1673–1678

Provision and Use of Work Equipment Regulations SI 2932. (1992) London. Her Majesty's Stationery Office.

PURDOM, P. (1971) Walton *Environmental Health.* London. Academic Press.

RAW, G., GOLDMAN, L. (1996) Sick building syndrome: a suitable case for treatment. *Occupational Health* **48**(11): 388–392.

Reporting of Injuries, Diseases and Dangerous Occurrences Regulations SI 2023. (1985 amended 1995) London. Her Majesty's Stationery Office.

ROGERS R. & SALVAGE J. (1988) *Nurses at Risk: A Guide to Health and Safety at Work.* Guildford. Heinemann Nursing.

ROPER N. (1976) *Mans Anatomy, Physiology, Health and Environment.* 5th Ed. Edinburgh. Churchill Livingstone,.

ROYAL SOCIETY STUDY GROUP (1992) *Risk Analysis Perception and Management.* London. Royal Society.

Safety and Health at Work. The Report of the Robens Committee. (1972) London. Her Majesty's Stationery Office.

Safety Representatives and Safety Committee Regulations SI 500. (1972) London. Her Majesty's Stationery Office.

Single European Act (1987) London. Her Majesty's Stationery Office.

SIMPSON, G.C. (1991) *Risk Perception and Hazard Awareness as Factors in Safe and Efficient Working. Report for the Commission of the European Community.* Eastwood. British Coal Corporation.

Social Security Regulations (1979) London. Her Majesty's Stationery Office.

SUTHERLAND K, MORGAN J, SEMPLE S. (1995) Self administration of Drugs: An introduction. *Nursing Times* **91**(23): 29

SUTTON, J., STANDEN, P. and WALLACE, A. (1994) Unreported accidents to patients in hospital. *Nursing Times* **90**(39): 46–49

UKCC (1994) *Code of Professional Conduct.* London. UKCC.

UKCC (1996) *Guidelines for Professional Practice.* London. UKCC.

WALL, P.G., RYAN, M.T., WARD, L.R., ROWE, B. (1996) Outbreaks of Salmonellosis in British Hospitals. *Journal of Hospital Infection* **33**(3): 181–190.

WILLIAMS, H.C., STRACHAN, D.P., HAY, R.J. (1994) Childhood eczema; disease of the advantaged? *British Medical Journal* **308**: 1132–1135.

Workplace (Health, Safety and Welfare) Regulations SI 3004. (1992) London. Her Majesty's Stationery Office.

1.2 Handling and Moving

L. Aston and J. Wakefield

KEY ISSUES

■ SUBJECT KNOWLEDGE

▪ the relevance of spinal anatomy and physiology in relation to back care
▪ the concept of ergonomics and its relevance for nursing
▪ factors that may contribute to back injury
▪ the epidemiological background to back injury in nursing
▪ why individuals may participate in risk behaviours when handling clients

■ PRACTICE KNOWLEDGE

▪ the four main areas for assessment in moving and handling
▪ assessing handling situations
▪ plans for moving a client effectively
▪ equipment available to aid the moving and handling of clients
▪ factors affecting the effectiveness of a handling situation

■ PROFESSIONAL KNOWLEDGE

▪ the legislation guiding safe practice in moving and handling
▪ guidance in nursing related to the performance of safe moving and handling
▪ moral and ethical dilemmas that may occur in moving clients
▪ strategies for personal back care

■ REFLECTIVE KNOWLEDGE

▪ personal capacity for moving and handling clients
▪ factors affecting the response to moving and handling situations
▪ the principles of moving and handling to professional practice across all branches of nursing

▌ INTRODUCTION

Handling situations are experienced in all aspects of life, from childhood to old age. The National Back Pain Association have identified that much adult back pain can be traced to the posture and practices of childhood (National Back Pain Association, 1990). Within this context, load handling is recognized as a problem in both nursing and industry (Stubbs and Osborne, 1979). In nursing, however, it is important to stress that the occurrence of back injury resulting from patient handling is not a new phenomena. Although there have been attempts for many years to gain legislation to protect employees (including a European Community directive leading to the development of manual handling regulations, 1990), until recently the occurrence of back pain and injury was, according to Hardicre (1992), 'part and parcel of being a nurse'.

Today, the emphasis of managing load movement is not on lifting, and some areas are now emphasizing the advent of 'no lifting policies' being implemented (Moore, 1993a). The assessment of any task that may require manual handling is also a vital consideration (Corlett, 1992) and such assessment includes the need to take an ergonomic approach. In spite of these changes, however, there are still back injuries occurring and many of these are as a result of poor handling practices involving the continued use of 'banned' lifts (National Back Pain Association, 1992). Those injured are not always staff who have not received recent updating, as there is a wealth of evidence suggesting that back injury is a particular problem among student nurses (Griffiths, 1988; Hearn, 1988;

Gladman, 1993). Studies carried out among student nurses found that although they were aware of unsafe practices from input by nurse teachers, they had performed unsafe lifts in practice (Kane and Parahoo, 1994).

The principles of safe handling include the need to use a systematic approach to all handling situations. General principles of load handling include:

▶ knowledge of the patient;
▶ deciding on the most appropriate method;
▶ agreeing commands;
▶ identifying a leader for the task;
▶ explaining to the patient what is to happen;
▶ competence in using any handling aids;
▶ preparing the environment;
▶ keeping your spine in normal alignment;
▶ being relaxed with the lead foot pointing in the direction of movement;
▶ always lifting or sliding towards yourself.

It is the aim of this chapter to enable you to learn about safe principles of moving clients using an ergonomic approach and to understand why in spite of education poor practice can still be a problem. It is anticipated that personal recognition of the antecedents of poor practice, combined with a clear understanding of safe principles will enable you to become an effective (and uninjured!) practitioner.

It is important to realise that attending handling sessions in a classroom situation or reading and learning about safe practice is not enough to equip someone to handle effectively in practice. This chapter aims to help you develop skills in practice through assessment of handling situations, adequate planning and continuing evaluation.

The development of handling techniques is a process that should continue throughout your career. It should also be appreciated both inside and outside the work setting in order to be truly effective in reducing injury. Because of this, it is intended to address issues related to handling in a holistic way. This means that all areas of knowledge will be applied to encourage decision making and the questions encourage reflection and application in your personal circumstances.

▶ OVERVIEW

▶ *Subject Knowledge*

You will learn about the practical aspects of back structure. The anatomy and physiology of the spine and posture is addressed and the implications of this knowledge are applied in relation to developing an ergonomically-friendly work environment. The epidemiology of back pain and injury is highlighted, and psychosocial considerations are discussed.

▶ *Practice Knowledge*

Application of a systematic approach to the principles of handling is examined in developing a strategy for optimum handling practice in nursing.

▶ *Professional Knowledge*

Current legislation and professional issues are presented for discussion both in relation to ensuring safe practice and in seeking recompense for injured parties should an incident occur. Support agencies are included at this point for further reference. Finally, some of the dilemmas faced by nurses in providing individualized care related to moving and handling are presented for discussion.

▶ *Reflective Knowledge*

The case studies within this section will enable you to develop your ability to make decisions in handling situations while encouraging reflection on practice experiences. Depending on the situation, there may be straightforward solutions to the problems encountered. However, other situations may lend themselves to a variety of options, the choice of which may depend on the individuals concerned, the environment and the client.

On pp. 54–60 there are four case studies, each one relating to one of the branch programmes. You may find it helpful to read one of them before you start the chapter and use it as a focus for your reflections while reading.

SUBJECT KNOWLEDGE: *Biological*

The purpose of this section is to examine spinal anatomy and physiology and relate these to the prevention of problems caused by poor posture and poor load handling techniques. A consideration of the provision of an ergonomically-friendly environment for moving and handling clients is also explored. 'Ergonomics aims to design appliances, technical systems and tasks in such a way as to improve human safety, health, comfort and performance' and '...as a consequence of its applied nature the ergonomic approach results in the adaptation of the workplace or environment to fit people, rather than the other way around' (Dul and Weerdmeester, 1993).

▶ THE SPINAL CORD

The spinal column is composed of 33 vertebrae. It acts as a protective cover for the spinal cord and provides attachments for ligaments, muscles and ribs (Figure 1.2.1).

The spinal cord has five sections (Figure 1.2.2). Note that the vertebrae shape and size change according to their type and function. For instance, the cervical vertebrae are smaller and their shape is designed to facilitate movement of the head and neck, whereas the lumbar vertebrae have larger bodies in order to sustain more weight.

From Figure 1.2.3 you can see that each vertebra is composed of a main body of bone and this is the anterior aspect of the vertebra. Bony projections are situated posteriorly. These provide the attachment for muscles and ligaments.

The human spine, of which the spinal column and cord are component parts, has a unique design: it is constructed to withstand tremendous pressure and to facilitate a variety of movements (Figure 1.2.4). It can be seen that the spine is quite flexible. For good posture, the spine needs to be maintained in normal alignment, and forward bending, extension, side bending and rotation of the spine avoided. Persistent poor posture, not sitting correctly, standing incorrectly, slumping, twisting the back, and pulling, pushing and handling loads incorrectly will eventually damage the spine.

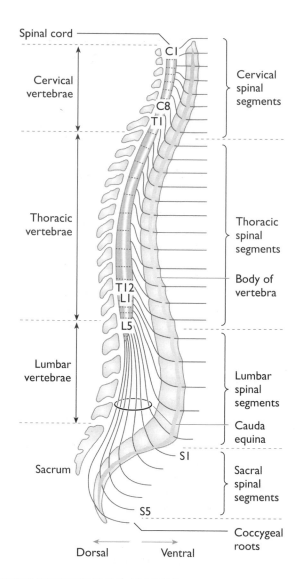

Figure 1.2.1: The spinal cord. (Redrawn from Hinchliffe and Montague, 1988.)

Spinal cord

Cervical vertebrae

Thoracic vertebrae

Lumbar vertebrae

Sacrum

C1

C8
T1

T12
L1
L5

S1

S5

Cervical spinal segments

Thoracic spinal segments

Body of vertebra

Lumbar spinal segments

Cauda equina

Sacral spinal segments

Coccygeal roots

Dorsal   Ventral

▶ INTERVERTEBRAL DISCS

Between each vertebra is a disc consisting of an outer fibrous elastic ring and a soft jellylike nucleus. The function of the disc is to act as a 'shock absorber', and provided it is not subjected to undue persistent pressure, it will serve this function well. Figure 1.2.5 indicates how the disc modifies its position to take account of this pressure. If the pressure on the disc is too great, it will herniate and acute pain may be felt if the nerves that emerge from the spinal cord become trapped by the herniation.

▶ BACK INJURY

Injury to the back results from activities that involve:

▶ stooping;
▶ twisting;
▶ uneven loads;
▶ forward bending;
▶ prolonged, fixed postures.

Figure 1.2.2: The five sections of the spinal cord.

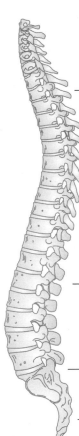

Cervical region
This consists of seven vertebrae, which are small and designed for maximum movement of the head and neck.

Thoracic region
This region consists of 12 vertebrae, which are slightly larger with a smaller range of movement. These vertebrae also provide attachment for the ribs.

Lumbar region
This region consists of five vertebrae. These are the largest vertebrae to allow maximum weight bearing. They also provide a wide range of movement.

Sacral region
This consists of five fused vertebrae and provides support for the spine.

Coccyx
This consists of four fused vertebrae and forms the base of the spine.

DECISION MAKING

Take 30 minutes for this exercise.
1. *Think of daily life events and tasks and compile a list of activities during which you might put your back at risk. You may be surprised at how extensive this list will be.*
2. *Look at your list and decide which of the above actions (i.e. those identified in the bullet list) may be involved.*
3. *Many health trusts are now advocating a 'non-lifting policy' at work. However, it is important that good handling practices are pursued both in and out of work to protect your back from injury. Look at your list again and decide what alternative actions may be possible to protect your back.*

In fact any activity that increases pressure on the intervertebral discs, particularly if the pressure is one-sided, will increase wear and tear on the discs and may ultimately contribute to disc herniation.

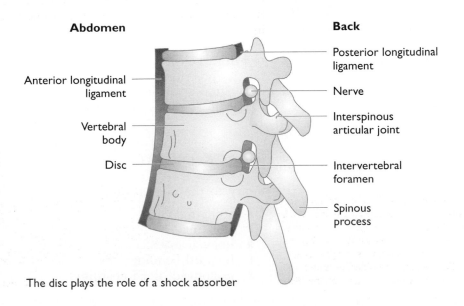

Figure 1.2.3: Anterior aspect of the vertebral unit.

The disc plays the role of a shock absorber

▶ CUMULATIVE STRAIN

Walsh (1988) explores the concept of human kinetics in more detail in the article *Good Movement Habits*, in which the importance of correct body movement is highlighted. This is also important in relation to the concept of cumulative strain, which in nursing is becoming recognized as a contributing factor to ultimate injury (Moore, 1993b). Poor practice may not result in one identifiable injury but rather to ongoing gradual wear and tear, which may cause pain and disability.

Psychosocial

▶ THE EPIDEMIOLOGY OF BACK INJURY

Although it is important to understand what may contribute to back injury, it is also essential to have some notion of the extent of the problem both in the population generally and in nursing. Information to aid your understanding and perspective of this problem includes the following:

- ▶ in nursing every year '80 000 nurses injure their backs and an estimated 3600 hurt themselves so seriously they are invalided out of the profession' (Snell, 1995);
- ▶ the health service union Confederation of Health Service Employees (COHSE) conducted a survey among their members and found that up to one in four nurses experience back pain either at work or at the end of the working day (Confederation of Health Service Employees, 1992);
- ▶ almost 70% of the 4500 health service accidents reported to the Health and Safety Executive between 1988 and 1990 involved nurses handling patients (Johnson, 1992);
- ▶ it is estimated that the average cost of a claim for back injury compensation is £60 000 (Barker *et al.*, 1994);
- ▶ damages of £184 603 have been awarded for a back injury sustained by a nurse while involved in handling a patient (Sadler, 1991).

The nursing profession is deeply concerned about the above situation. What cannot be calculated from these figures is the personal misery, loss of independence and chronic illness that may additionally result. A 'knock-on' effect, which is also difficult to quantify, is the cost of treatment and welfare benefit needed to support people who become injured.

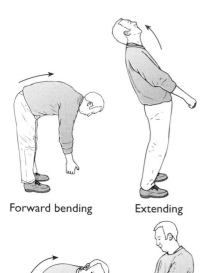

Forward bending   Extending

Side bending   Rotating

Figure 1.2.4: Movements of the spine.

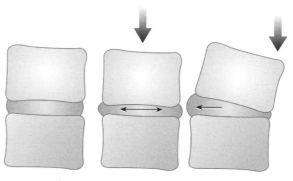

Without pressure   Under pressure

Figure 1.2.5: Under pressure, the disc is compressed and shapes itself to the angle and impact of pressure. When the pressure is released the disc returns to its original shape. Permanent one-sided pressure will cause wear and tear of the disc.

Take a few minutes to imagine that your back is injured and you are in constant pain and can no longer work.

What would you do?

Could you afford your current lifestyle?

How would you cope with the pain?

Who would you depend upon for help?

How would you feel?

▶ BEHAVIOURAL ISSUES

When all of the above is taken into consideration it seems inconceivable that much of this suffering arises out of poor practice; however, nurses' attitudes are identified as being slow to change. Much evidence of routine and ritual prevails in the area of manual handling in spite of documented research to inform nursing practice (McGuire and Dewar, 1995). Pearce (1992) comments that nursing needs a change in culture in relation to moving and handling practices. In relation to student learners, Johnston (1987) has observed that when student nurses are assessing, it is evident that they do not apply theory to practice. There is a reluctance to change existing practices in ward areas in spite of knowing about the principles of safe handling. Students on hospital wards appear to become socialized into ward practices – student nurses on wards do what trained nurses do.

DECISION MAKING

Consider the following for a few minutes. You are working for three weeks in a nursing home. The staff there have really made you feel welcome, involving you in many social activities with the clients, and as a common foundation programme student you are at last getting the 'hands on' nursing experience you have been waiting for. Two of the care assistants (who normally work together) are assigned to different duties for one shift and one of them asks you to participate in a banned lift that she proposes to use on a client.

1. Ask your practice teachers about 'banned' lifts. Identify which these are so that you know not to use them.

2. Jot down strategies you might use in order to respond assertively and protect your back.

3. Knowing that 'banned' lifts endanger both carers and clients, what action could you take in preventing similar future incidents?

It is here that you require assertiveness skills as you may need to acknowledge your limitations in this area and to decline to participate in unsafe practices with respect to handling situations. A good definition of self-assertion has been drawn up by Gerrard et al. (1980) 'this involves standing up for our own legitimate rights without violating the rights of others'.

Obviously, being assertive means making your point while keeping control of the situation. You will need to explain why you cannot participate in this particular task and you might even turn the situation to your advantage (with the advice of a qualified member of staff) to indicate an alternative safer approach. You will, however, have to decline to participate in this task. A further discussion related to the aspect of accountability is included in the Professional Knowledge section of this chapter.

▶ PREVENTING BACK INJURY

Obviously, everyone needs to take care of their backs and the logical point at which to start would be to encourage good posture from early childhood (National Back Pain Association, 1990). The notion 'prevention is better than cure' is well acknowledged. Organizations such as the Health Education Authority with its *Look After Yourself* project (1994) aim to educate people into preventive measures.

Certain predisposing factors help identify those who are at greatest risk of developing low back pain. People at greatest risk are likely to have one or more of the following characteristics (Kraus, 1972):

▶ excess weight;
▶ extreme lordosis;
▶ absence of regular exercise;
▶ weak abdominal muscles;
▶ tight hamstrings or hip flexors;
▶ weak or tight back muscles;
▶ general muscular tension.

▶ CARING FOR YOURSELF

You need to know how to care for yourself and your own back both at work as a nurse and in your lifestyle generally. Keeping yourself fit using gentle exercise programmes can help. Regular walking and swimming are to be recommended. Keeping to your desirable weight can prevent back problems, and problems can also be avoided by sensible footwear. Further reading on exercising to strengthen your back and keeping fit generally can be found in Braggins (1994).

In your practice placements you should always wear flat lace-up shoes. This type of footwear will give you maximum support for your feet. The type of footwear worn by someone who sustains a back injury would be investigated to see whether it has been a predisposing factor to the injury and the wrong type of footwear could nullify or reduce a claim for compensation.

> Take a few minutes to consider whether any of the above factors apply to you. Given the above information, which of your clients may be at particular risk of injuring their backs? Design a list of health promotion tips for use with clients you perceive 'at risk' on return to their own homes.

PRACTICE KNOWLEDGE

This part of the chapter will turn to the decision-making approach that handling situations now require of professional nurses. This section intends to address general aspects of assessment while specific assessment issues are addressed within the case studies.

▶ ASSESSMENT

Alexander (1989) observes that 'In our society we are overconcerned with getting things done and that not enough emphasis is placed on the way in which we do things'. This is true of many nurses in relation to handling situations. It is often argued that there is not time to assess patients as the work needs to be done. However, thorough assessment of a situation is the key to successful handling and requires knowledge, time and a framework for a systematic approach. The National Back Pain Association (1991) state that the task, load, environment and the individual need to be assessed, and these are now considered in more detail.

▶ *Assessing the Task*

For each individual client there may be several tasks to take into account, and manual lifting should be avoided if at all possible. Separate assessments will be necessary for each task. For example transferring a patient from a bed to the commode, from a chair to the bathroom, or from a wheelchair into a car will probably require the use of different strategies. Depending on the manoeuvre, different numbers of handlers may be required as well as a variety of techniques and postures. It is important to take into account the weight of the load and this is as important in lifting as it is in pushing, pulling, transferring or sliding. There is a tendency to acknowledge the risk of back injury, but other injuries due to repetitive strain or excess strain such as those utilized in sliding can be as injurious and debilitating to the nurse. It has been documented that prolonged postures and repetitive movements are tiring and in the long term can lead to muscle and joint injuries (Dul and Weerdmeester, 1993). Other important factors are positions used for handling, unsatisfactory or prolonged static postures, the height at which the manoeuvre is carried out (Royal College of Nursing, 1996a), or repetition rates over a period of time (National Back Pain Association, 1992, p. 16). All these factors can increase the cumulative stress on the body that may subsequently lead to injury.

▌ *Assessing the Load or Client*

The weight of the load is an important consideration and lifting should be avoided if at all possible. Identification of any factor that makes the load difficult to handle should be taken into account, for example, the psychological state of the client. Clients who are unpredictable in their responses to their situation will increase the risks in handling situations to both carers and themselves (Royal College of Nursing, 1993). In addition, the use of certain pieces of equipment may be socially unacceptable to the patient, and this is where good communication skills as well as the rights of the nurse to protect themselves from injury can be extremely important. This can be even more crucial in a community setting where the health carer is a guest in the client's home and not able to implement changes that one may automatically be able to make in a ward setting (Hemple, 1993).

▌ *Assessing the Environment*

As discussed already, the optimum working environment is one that is ergonomically sound. However, since caring for clients takes place in many different settings (including the client's own home) it may not always be possible to control the setting in this way. Additionally, it is important to note that since all individuals are different an ergonomically-friendly environment for one individual may be dangerous for another. All environments for moving and handling must therefore be assessed before a manoeuvre takes place.

Obstructions or hazards within the working area need to be assessed as well as specific environmental problems. Environmental problems can be interpreted as the wider physical environment (e.g. the room or bed area). Alternatively, they may pertain to the client's immediate environment. This may include a wide variety of such factors, from the presence of a urinary catheter to the client's painful joints that are aggravated by movement. All these aspects may require specific planning and careful assessment is perhaps especially pertinent in areas where clients have a learning disability, are young children or are unconscious and so are unable to contribute their views to the assessment.

▌ *Assessing the Equipment*

In utilizing any equipment for a manual handling situation, the first question that must be asked is whether the equipment is appropriate for the task you wish to undertake. This may include assessing such things as whether the equipment has the capacity to cope with the weight of the client you wish to move or whether the equipment is suitable to use in that particular environment. If appropriate equipment is not available it may be pertinent to obtain this equipment either from another area or through local protocols that are in place.

Specific equipment checks need to be employed in order to ensure client safety. Checking that the equipment is in working order and that there are no apparent defects in the equipment are essential. Specific equipment checks will vary according to the type of equipment employed, for example, cracks in a plastic transfer belt, brakes that are not efficient on a hoist or clasps that are worn on a transfer belt will mean that this equipment is unsafe and should not be used.

If appropriate, the last occasion on which the equipment was serviced (i.e. a hoist) should be noted and should not be used if the date does not comply with local protocols.

For all equipment, social cleanliness needs to be observed to prevent the risk of cross-infection between patients; if soiled, the equipment will require cleaning in accordance with local policy.

▶ *Assessing the Individual Handler*

In assessing any handling situation the capabilities of the individuals undertaking the handling is vital. What may be an appropriate handling plan for an experienced nurse may be beyond the capabilities and competence of the junior student. In addition, the individual may have limitations due to factors other than their nursing experience. Carers may feel discomfort adopting recommended positions or postures for particular techniques and in some instances may need referral to occupational health for assessment for such discomfort. Also many female nurses are of childbearing age and if they are or think they may be pregnant, they need advice for manual handling. Such advice is offered by the Royal College of Nursing (1995) in their guide *Hazards for Pregnant Nurses – An A–Z Guide*). In addition, the drive to recruit more mature staff into nursing may mean that some have existing back problems, which may be compounded by the practices they are undertaking. This has implications for student recruitment (Gladman, 1993).

Assessment factors to take into account may seem daunting at first, but the planning and safety of any manoeuvre depends upon accurate assessment. Handling assessment skills can be likened to learning to drive a car. Initially, this requires careful thought and learner drivers may be slow because of all the things that need to be taken into account and their actions may be uncoordinated. However, as with practice, driving theory and skills become second nature, so it is to some extent with client handling. If an assessment is initially completed thoroughly, then on subsequent occasions discomfort for the client and risk of injury to the nurse can be reduced. However, it must be acknowledged that assessment tools are simply an aid to nurses. Knowledge and professional judgement are also needed to select the appropriate manoeuvre. Once it is established that the risk is low, medium or high, then planning the handling task will follow more easily. However, no handling situation is without risk. The risk of injury can only be minimized. Two examples of assessment tools are the Pilling lifting/handling risk calculator (Pilling and Frank, 1994) and the patient handling assessment.

▶ The Pilling lifting/handling risk calculator (Pilling and Frank, 1994)

In assessing mobility, body weight, psychological state, environment, staff, carer and other risk factors, an appropriate numerical score is allocated to the patient and these are added together (Figure 1.2.6). If the score is over ten, specific actions need to be planned for the patient. The reverse side of the calculator gives carers guidance on actions and aids that may need to be used. Using the score and the guidance offered, carers can begin to formulate a handling plan specific to the client's needs. This form was originally developed for use in the community setting, but can be adapted to any area.

MOBILITY		BODY WEIGHT		PSYCHOLOGICAL	
Fully mobile	0	Below 8 stone	0	Well motivated	0
Minimal assistance required	1	Above 8 stone	5	Confused/dementia	5
Walks with aids/carer	2	Oedema/rigid	5	Irrational behaviour	5
Unstable gait/uncoordinated	5	Patient height greater than staff/		Apprehensive/anxious	5
Can stand but unable to walk	5	carer's height	5		
Unable to assist 'dead weight'	10				

ENVIRONMENT		STAFF/CARER		OTHER RISK FACTORS	
Spacious, well designed	0	Handlers trained in correct		Spinal injuries	5
Low bed, low chair	5	techniques	0	Motor/sensory deficit	5
Restricted space/obstacles	5	Non-trained staff/carer	5	Orthopaedic conditions	5
Constraints on posture/over-reaching	5	Staff pregnant/health problems	5	Heavy sedation	5
Cold, hot, humid conditions	5			Prone to falls	5
Poor lighting	5			Pain	5

Copyright   CONSIDER – NO HANDLING SITUATION IS EVER TRULY RISK FREE
S. Pilling 1993   Score of 10+ needs specific action planning

PREVENTIVE ACTION FOR PATIENT SAFETY
Discuss with patient/carer aspects of home safety.
Explanation/teaching in safe transfers.
Referral to physiotherapist, occupational therapist, GP
for: treatment, rehabilitation, mobility aids.
Review medication (e.g. sedation, pain control).

Social Aspects Heating, clothing, footwear, changing
environment, diet, benefits, outside help.
Consider: Waterlow score

AIDS/ADAPTATIONS FOR PATIENT'S USE
Stair rails/lifts
Grab handles
Toilet frames, raised toilet seats.
Walking aids, frames, trolleys etc.
Monkey poles, rope ladders
High seat chairs
Bath aids
Special beds, baths, showers
Wheelchairs

PREVENTIVE ACTION FOR STAFF/CARER SAFETY
Avoid physical lifting if you can
Assess size of load, staff capabilities, equipment available,
number of staff required. Consider constraints (e.g.
environment, clothing, untrained staff).
Gain patient cooperation.
Use approved lifting techniques. Equipment in use.
Trained staff/carer.
PLAN – EXPLAIN – PERFORM – REVIEW.
Leave written advice for emergency use.

LIFTING AIDS STAFF/CARER
Lifting straps
Joney belts
Turn table
Easy slide (for patients in bed)
Use of towels, blanket, lifting net.
Hoists mobile/ceiling track
Special rise/fall beds etc.

PLAN TO INCLUDE:

Weight of patient
Patient's ability to help
Number of staff required
Lifting technique in use
Equipment
Advise patient/carer

The Pilling Lifting/Handling Risk Calculator: Several scores may be ringed from each section, then work out the total.

Figure 1.2.6: The Pilling lifting/handling risk calculator. (Redrawn from Pilling, S and Frank, J, 1994.)

▷ Patient handling assessment

This form (Figure 1.2.7) does not use a numerical scoring and is therefore a less objective system than one using a numerical score. However, numerical scoring systems can sometimes be inflexible and are not recommended as it is not justifiable to simply ignore any risks under a certain score (Royal College of Nursing, 1996c). By not using a numerical score, the nurse needs to take into account the whole picture of the patient and has to use professional knowledge of patient handling to make a considered judgement about the level of risk. As such the more experienced the nurse the more accurate the assessment of risk is likely to be. If when using this form you are in doubt as to the level of risk it is advisable to identify the higher risk and take this into account when planning care.

Figure 1.2.7: Patient handling assessment.

PATIENT HANDLING ASSESSMENT

NAME: _____

HOSPITAL NO: _____

WEIGHT	Actual [ ]		Estimate [ ]	

MOBILITY	Able to mobilize unaided. If no, walking aid if used: _____ If yes, proceed no further.		YES | NO

WEAKNESS	If yes, specify type: _____ _____	YES | NO
PARALYSIS	If yes, specify type: _____ _____	YES | NO
UNSTEADY	If yes, give details _____ _____	YES | NO
TOTALLY IMMOBILE	If yes, give details _____ _____	YES | NO

MENTAL STATE	CONFUSED	YES | NO
	LEVEL OF COOPERATION: Partially cooperative	YES | NO
	Unpredictable at times	YES | NO
	Totally uncooperative	YES | NO

GENERAL CONDITION   _____
                     _____

HANDLING PROBLEM	YES | NO

DO YOU CONSIDER THE HANDLING RISK TO BE

(Please tick appropriate box).   LOW [   ]   MEDIUM [   ]   HIGH [   ]

Signature of Nurse _____   Date _____

If problem identified, proceed to Planning.

DECISION MAKING

Take a few minutes for the following.
1. *Identify a client in your practice.*
2. *Using the Pilling risk calculator, assess this client's risk.*
3. *Now use the patient handling assessment to make a repeat assessment.*
4. *How do these assessments compare?*
5. *Discuss your findings with a qualified carer working with the client.*

▶ PLANNING

Once an assessment has been undertaken the information is used to form the basis of planning (Figure 1.2.8). A major factor to consider here is the resources available in human terms and in relation to the equipment available. Equipment may include:

- ▶ hoists;
- ▶ sliding equipment;
- ▶ transfer equipment;
- ▶ turning equipment.

Figure 1.2.8: Planning.

PLANNING

Using the assessment information, consider the most appropriate handling method for each task you undertake with the patient.

a)   ASSISTANCE REQUIRED   1 nurse   ☐

                              2 nurses   ☐

                              Other (specify)   ☐ _____

b)   AIDS   Hoist (specify type) ☐ _____

                              Sliding equipment ☐ _____

                              Transfer belt/aid ☐ _____

                              Other (specify)   ☐ _____

c)   TYPE OF TURNING   30° tilt   ☐ _____

                              Other (specify)   ☐ _____

d)   TRANSFER   Stroke patient   ☐ _____

                              Other (specify)   ☐ _____

IMPLEMENTATION (Any additional instructions for carrying out the procedure): _____

_____

_____

_____

SIGNATURE OF COMPLETING NURSE: _____   DATE: _____

EVALUATION

Successful procedure _____   Unsuccessful procedure _____

_____   _____

_____   _____

_____   _____

SIGNATURE OF COMPLETING NURSE: _____   DATE: _____

IF UNSUCCESSFUL OR PROBLEMS ENCOUNTERED, RE-ASSESS.

RESEARCH BASED EVIDENCE

McGuire et al. (1996) highlight that if mechanical aids are to be useful manual handling tools it is important that they do not cause additional manual handling problems.

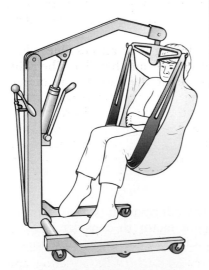

Figure 1.2.9: Hoisting using a sling to take the full weight of the patient. (Redrawn from the National Back Pain Association, 1992, with permission.)

Many types of equipment are available, some of which is sophisticated and expensive while other equipment is simple and relatively inexpensive. Some examples of handling aids are given below.

▶ Hoist

A hoist (Figure 1.2.9) takes the full weight of a patient, but hoists have specified weight limits and it is still important for the nurse to adopt a safe posture when putting a sling onto a patient and while using the hoist.

▶ Sliding Equipment

When using sliding equipment (Figure 1.2.10) it is important to think carefully about the safety of the patient and the handlers. Although the

Figure 1.2.10: Using an Easy-slide. (Redrawn from the National Back Pain Association, 1992, with permission.)

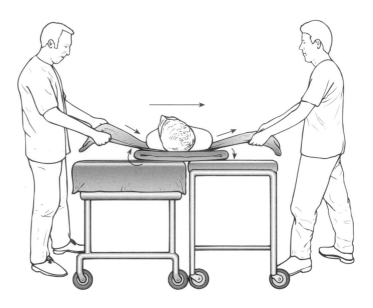

nurse is not handling the full weight of the patient, effort is required to complete the manoeuvre and therefore this task should be planned carefully and carried out in manageable stages.

▶ Transfer Equipment

There are many types of transfer equipment. Although transfer aids may assist the transfer, individual capacity, the weight and cooperation of the patient will affect whether the choice of a transfer aid is appropriate.

It is sometimes argued that equipment should not be used as the patient does not like to be handled using a mechanical aid. However, it must be remembered that although patient preferences are important, the safety of the handlers needs to be considered.

In planning, a key principle is to avoid lifting if at all possible while making a move as easy as possible for both client and handler. The solution needs to be chosen using knowledge about the patient and professional judgement. Any assistants need to agree to the manoeuvre and it must be ascertained that the handlers have the capacity and expertise to undertake the procedure. Handling aids such as hoists or sliding equipment can reduce the risk of injury to the handlers, but can injure both handler and patient if the individuals concerned are not familiar with its function and safe operation.

▶ Coordinating a Moving Strategy

A decision needs to be made about how many people are required to undertake the chosen procedure. If more than one handler is required, a leader must be appointed to avoid confusion during the handling and so reduce the risk of injury. Any commands to be used during the procedure need to be agreed in advance. This ensures the handling is coordinated and weight will be evenly distributed between handlers, thereby reducing the risk of injury.

▶ *Preparing the Environment*

The environment and equipment also need to be prepared. Note that the environment includes the route and the area in which the patient is to be handled or moved. This will help to facilitate good posture and will ensure removal of any potential hazards within the environment. Checks will also need to be made to ensure that the equipment is in good working order and is safe to use.

The checklist when planning is as follows:

- ▶ assessment information is available;
- ▶ resources are reviewed;
- ▶ avoid lifting if at all possible;
- ▶ choose the appropriate method for all concerned;
- ▶ ensure all staff involved are familiar with the equipment and procedure;
- ▶ choose a leader if appropriate;
- ▶ decide on commands to be used;
- ▶ communicate with the patient;
- ▶ check the environment and the equipment.

▶ RECORDING THE TASK

Once the procedure has been decided upon it is the nurse's responsibility to document each handling task to create a handling plan. The importance of record keeping cannot be overemphasized as records are an essential and integral part of care (UKCC, 1993). Records should provide accurate, current, comprehensive and concise information about a patient, including a record of any problems that arise and the action taken in response to them (UKCC, 1993). The Health Service Commissioner's annual report (National Health Service Training Directorate, 1994) has stated that poor record keeping continues to crop up in cases he investigates. Therefore comprehensive records are a necessary requirement in relation to manual handling.

A handling plan for the client must include the task being addressed, the type of equipment to be used, the number of staff required and the level of expertise necessary to make the procedure as safe as possible. Inexperienced handlers must take care not to act beyond their level of competence when participating in the planning of client care. If any problems arise these must be recorded in the plan together with the actions taken to resolve problems.

▶ IMPLEMENTATION

Every handling situation carries a potential risk to the handler and care must be taken to reduce the risk. Assessment and forward planning will help to reduce the risk as will sound knowledge regarding handling loads or patients. Two additional points that need to be taken into consideration when implementing handling plans are optimum height for handling and handling in confined spaces.

▶ *Optimum Height for Handling*

The optimum height for handling is between the knee and shoulder (National Back Pain Association, 1991, p. 12). This is to minimize the

---

DECISION MAKING

As previously discussed all moving and handling manoeuvres should be assessed and planned with care to ensure safety for both the handler and the load. This should apply in whatever setting handling takes place.

1. *Before you next go shopping take a few minutes to devise a plan for handling your shopping safely between the store and your home.*
2. *Consider each handling task that you may have to make and note down an action plan.*
3. *What does this tell you about your everyday activities in moving and handling?*
4. *Now devise a handling plan for a client in your care.*

risk of poor posture that may lead to stress on the spine. If variable-height beds are available, they should be adjusted for the height of the handler so that when moving, the handler's pelvis is level. This avoids one-sided pressure on the vertebral column. If two handlers are working together the bed should be adjusted so that the pelvis of the shorter individual is level when moving. Fixed-height beds or specialist beds and cots can present a hazard due to the adoption of unsafe postures when handling patients. If assessment and planning have been adequate hazards should be avoided through the choice of an appropriate handling method for the situation.

Hoists should be used when moving an adult or large child from the floor. If such equipment is not available a sliding sheet may be an alternative provided there are sufficient handlers to minimize the risk of back injury due to lifting heavy loads. A good method for handling babies who may wriggle and therefore present a hazard can be found in the guide *The Handling of Patients* (National Back Pain Association, 1992, p. 114)

▶ *Handling in Confined Spaces*

As it is impossible to optimize all environments completely, it may be best to identify areas that are not suitable for handling dependent patients. This will help to avoid unsafe postures and reduce the risk of injury to carers. If a patient falls in a confined space, it may be necessary to slide the patient into a more accessible area so that a safe procedure can then be planned.

▶ *Dilemmas in Handling Practice*

When implementing handling plans situations can arise that pose additional problems for carers. Such problems may be of a physical nature or an ethical dilemma. This is addressed more thoroughly in the Professional Knowledge section of this chapter.

▶ EVALUATION

Evaluation is an integral part of the systematic approach to handling situations and is necessary to identify the level of success of the handling plan that has been implemented. If problems are identified they need to be documented and acted upon. Evaluation can provide the basis for reassessing, re-planning or altering the methods used. Evaluation can also assist nursing staff in building up a body of knowledge that can be of great value in future situations.

PROFESSIONAL KNOWLEDGE

Recently there have been legal changes within care settings with respect to the handling of patients. Before January 1993 in the United Kingdom, the *Health and Safety at Work Act* (1974) was in place to prevent industrial accidents. This Act had some weaknesses, thereby rendering it somewhat inadequate, with a major area of weakness related to assessment of risk (Love, 1995).

In 1992, the British government adopted the European Community Directive 90/269/EEC (Commission of the European Communities, 1990). This requires greater attention to be given to all aspects of any handling situation and stated that assessment should be used to avoid risk of injury.

In your next practice placement find the manual handling policy used by the area.

1. *How does it compare with the guidelines outlined by the European Community Directive 90/269/EEC (Commission of the European Communities, 1990)?*

2. *How does it compare with practice in the setting?*

DECISION MAKING

Take 30 minutes to think of ways in which you can participate safely in handling operations, taking into account the above-mentioned requirements. It may be useful to reflect upon any situations in which you may have already been involved.

Managers of care settings are now required to establish and implement safe policies and procedures with respect to handling. They must ensure that regular training and updating are given and reinforced to all employees. Careful records should be kept of this training. Attention must be paid to the environment in which handling takes place and an ergonomic approach is recommended.

Nurses in supervisory positions (i.e. qualified nurses) are responsible for carrying out a comprehensive risk assessment of each handling situation and must ensure that the handling task is completed safely. Information related to technique, equipment and load involved must be communicated to other parties and also documented in nursing records. Consideration must be given to the capacity of the individual handlers in every situation as this will affect any technique selected.

▶ GUIDELINES FOR SAFE PRACTICE

The first Royal College of Nursing *Code of Practice for Handling of Patients* (Royal College of Nursing, 1993) advocated a 50 kg (8 stone) weight limit for a patient being lifted by two nurses under ideal conditions. The second edition (1996a) advocates eliminating hazardous manual handling in all but exceptional or life-threatening situations. Obviously, clients may still need to be handled manually. However, this should only be done if it does not involve lifting all or most of the client's weight. As far as possible aids should be used to assist client handlers. Supporting or transferring a client can still pose a hazard to carers and care should be taken when selecting the appropriate method. The client should always be encouraged to assist in the manoeuvre as much as they are able. This will not only reduce the risk of injury for the carer, but will also promote client independence and therefore increase self-esteem.

▶ LOCAL POLICY

Those organizations that have introduced safer handling policies since the legislation in 1992 have recognized the improvements in handling practice and also minimized the risk of large compensation claims for back-injured employees (Royal College of Nursing, 1996b).

▶ THE CODE OF PROFESSIONAL CONDUCT

The UKCC *Code of Professional Conduct* (1992) guides both qualified and student nurses in deciding whether to participate in a handling situation if there is any uncertainty regarding professional accountability. You are personally accountable for your practice and you must not involve yourself in anything that you know to be dangerous (such as a banned lift). The first clause of the code of conduct states that we should always act in such a manner as to promote and safeguard the interests and well-being of patients and clients. As such, we need to be knowledgeable and up to date in all aspects of our current practice. By being up-to-date with regard to manual handling we will be better equipped to choose appropriate handling methods that will ensure that we fulfil clause one (UKCC, 1992).

▶ MANAGING UNTOWARD INCIDENTS IN HANDLING AND MOVING

In spite of the careful provision of both legislation and professional and local guidelines and policies, incidents leading to compensation claims for back injuries are still occurring. It is estimated that the National Health Service loses approximately 50 million pounds each year as a result of inability to work due to back injuries (Williams, 1996). Case studies show that the fight for compensation is a slow process with detrimental effects on many aspects of an individual's life (Cowell, 1996).

The following list indicates the areas that are likely to be investigated should a claim for compensation be pursued through the law courts:

- ▶ staff training, updating and attendance;
- ▶ hazards, loads;
- ▶ footwear and clothing at the time of the incident;
- ▶ written policies for handling;
- ▶ written plans for handling particular loads;
- ▶ equipment provided or used to assist in load handling;
- ▶ incident reporting;
- ▶ follow-up treatment at the time of the injury;
- ▶ any history of previous injury;
- ▶ current work practices, staffing, workload.

▶ DOCUMENTATION

The previous section on nursing practice highlighted the need for careful documentation of handling plans and evaluation of practices. Documentation communicates to all effective techniques or those that have been tried and found to be unsuccessful. There can be serious implications on any claim for compensation if an employee has ignored their employer's handling plan.

Additionally there is a requirement for adverse incidents to be clearly documented and such documentation can provide essential information in the event of an incident investigation.

The Health and Safety at Work Act (1974) has defined responsibilities for both employer and employee in this respect, as outlined in Chapter 1.1 of this book. However, it would appear that health care staff need to improve record keeping considerably. The National Health Service Training Directorate (1994) indicate that more than one-third of the complaints upheld in 1992/1993 regarding patient care involved lack of or incorrect information (i.e. poor record keeping). Often the problem is not writing down the wrong thing, but not writing anything.

▶ MONITORING ACCIDENTS

A final aspect related to safety in moving and handling is the monitoring of accidents and incidents. This falls within the remit of the occupational health department: they monitor accidents and incidents that occur; they also monitor follow-up care and the outcomes of care and treatment. This information can then be of use should an injured party seek compensation.

As a nurse you are at risk of injury and an occurrence such as back

---

DECISION MAKING

Take 30 minutes to consider the following situation.

While in a short placement with an occupational health nurse you learn that an employee of the company has sustained a shoulder injury while handling loads in the stores. He has been unable to work for three months and is submitting a claim for compensation against the company.

1. *List the factors you think will need to be investigated by the occupational health nurse in connection with the claim.*
2. *Look at your list. Why have you included each item?*

pain unrelieved by a night's rest should be documented on an appropriate incident form and reported to your local occupational health service. Follow-up advice should be obtained to protect yourself from further injury.

Monitoring also enables occupational health to identify areas where practices should be investigated. Where staff are reporting high levels of injury and absenteeism through back injury specific support may be beneficial, and in some hospitals ergonomists have been appointed to provide advice. In some situations it may be appropriate for the Health and Safety Executive to investigate working practices.

▶ PROFESSIONAL DILEMMAS IN THE PROVISION OF SAFE HANDLING

Within any handling situation that involves the movement of clients it is paramount that wherever possible their wishes are respected: however, one must recognize that at times this may have unacceptable consequences for carers (e.g. a possible injury to carers as a result of not using a hoist). This is one example of a moral and ethical dilemma with which carers may be faced when planning to move clients. There are no easy answers and careful negotiation is required to achieve an acceptable outcome for all concerned.

DECISION MAKING

Mrs Townshend is an obese 65-year-old diabetic lady who has just undergone an above-knee amputation of her right leg. It is proposed that she sits out of bed in a chair for a while and the nurses propose to use a hoist to help transfer her from bed to chair. However, Mrs Townshend refuses to get out of bed saying she is worried that she will fall out of the hoist and end up on the floor.

Try to answer the following questions.
1. *Does the use of handling aids such as a hoist infringe on a client's rights?*
2. *If a client states that he or she does not wish to be moved using a hoist, do carers have any right to insist that the aid is used?*
3. *What might you do in the above circumstances?*

This chapter has introduced you to the varied aspects of knowledge required to make effective nursing decisions in moving and handling situations. The importance of accurate assessment has been emphasized as it is the basis for effective planning and implementation of skills. Safe practice requires you to be a knowledgeable professional and to develop the appropriate skills for your particular client population. These require continual development and updating throughout your career. Moving and handling practice is no exception. A safe practitioner must keep up to date with the latest legislation, guidelines and practices in order to move clients most effectively and safely. It is also essential to participate in the ongoing evaluation and development of equipment used in moving and handling clients in their own particular setting.

By the end of this chapter you should be able to:

▶ appreciate spinal physiology;
▶ describe the effects of cumulative back strain;
▶ discuss how a back injury can affect a person's lifestyle;
▶ discuss the importance of record keeping in relation to manual handling;
▶ explain the consequences of inadequate documentation with respect to handling situations;
▶ discuss the importance of manual handling legislation;
▶ use an assessment tool for handling situations;
▶ produce a handling plan;
▶ identify how evaluation can contribute to safer handling of patients.

You have already reflected on your personal needs in relation to caring for yourself and ensuring optimum personal performance in the light of the knowledge offered in this chapter and reflective practice requires practitioners to review their nursing actions and interventions critically. This can be carried out either while practising, or subject to practice (Schon, cited in Bailey, 1995). From reflection, nurses can identify future strategies that may be utilized and, in relation to manual handling, appropriate support agencies may be of help in formulating strategies for the future.

Should you experience an injury in relation to manual handling, the following organizations can provide advice and support.

▶ The National Back Pain Association is a charity specifically concerned with the back pain sufferer and their family. Its address is National Back Pain Association, 16 Elmtree Road, Teddington, Middlesex TW11 8ST. Telephone: 0181 9775474.
▶ The Work Injured Nurses' Group (WING) is affiliated to the Royal College of Nursing and can also offer advice and support. The address is c/o Royal College of Nursing, 20 Cavendish Square, London W1M 0AB.
▶ A final useful organization for general information about back care (multi-disciplinary) is National Back Exchange, 82 Muswell Hill Road, Highgate, London N10 3JR. Telephone 0181 4445386.

Reflection on practice can be achieved by a comprehensive consideration of the four main branches of nursing. Case studies and reflective exercises are provided for you to consider these issues. Because of the practical nature of this chapter, a 'worked' discussion is included for each case study. It is envisaged that this will allow you to compare your thoughts with those of the authors and generate ideas for your own practice.

REFLECTIVE KNOWLEDGE

▶ CASE STUDIES

The following case study scenarios will be used in the next section so that you can explore the importance of assessing the task, load, environment and individual handler's capabilities. All names used are pseudonyms.

▶ CASE STUDY: LEARNING DISABILITIES

Martin Richards is a 15-year-old boy with learning disabilities. He weighs 8 stone (50.8 kg), lives at home with his parents, and attends a day centre during school periods. His mobility needs are met by transporting him in a wheelchair both at home and in the day centre, but he does need transferring from wheelchair to the toilet and vice versa on a regular basis. At the day centre he receives regular physiotherapy to prevent joint contractures. He is subject to bouts of anger, which make him uncooperative at times. Both Martin's home and the day centre have been adapted to allow access for equipment.

1. In relation to Martin:
   (a) Identify factors to take into consideration regarding the 'load' to be handled.
   (b) List all the tasks that require assessment.
   (c) Jot down any pertinent environmental factors that may affect Martin's handling situation.
   (d) Consider equipment that may be useful and why you would choose to use it.
   (e) Are there any additional factors relating to individual handlers that need to be taken into account?

2. Using the scenario make notes on the handling plan you might make for Martin.

3. In the middle of a bout of anger, Martin indicates that he needs to use the toilet. He is shouting at carers and making punching gestures at anyone who approaches him. How would you deal with this situation?

4. Compare your ideas with the thoughts of our authors outlined below.

▶ *Suggested Management for Martin Richards*

1. Assessment:
   (a) Load: Martin is unpredictable at times, although in ideal conditions his weight is acceptable for handling.
   (b) Tasks: Manouevring the wheelchair; pivotal transfer will be necessary from wheelchair to the toilet and vice versa.
   (c) Environment: Suitable access for wheelchairs and transfers.
   (d) Equipment: A transfer belt could assist the pivotal transfer. No equipment is necessary for manoeuvring the wheelchair but good posture needs to be taken into acount here.
   (e) Factors affecting individual handlers: Staff need to be aware of signs that precede Martin's bouts of anger that lead to his difficult behaviour. It has already been established that the environment is suitable for clients in wheelchairs and those who require transfer. The main focus for Martin is his unpredictability. Therefore, it is vital that staff have identified and documented both verbal and nonverbal cues that

precede his bouts of anger. These warning signs must be made known to all carers so that they can avoid situations that carry a high risk of resulting in injury.

2. Handling plan:

■ Transfer: Martin does not usually have to be lifted. In using a pivotal transfer the nurse uses the principles of leverage and the patient takes some weight through their legs and feet. The choice here may be for one or two nurses to transfer Martin, possibly using a transfer belt or board. It must be remembered that the individual's capabilities in relation to handling are important here. It is also often recommended by employers that two people should be present for any handling situation and it is vital that you check the local policy about this. It is usually useful to have a second person strategically placed to assist in the transfer should the need arise. Using a transfer belt or board will also assist the individual who has reduced or absent muscle tone. The joints of such patients can be damaged if the nurse's grasp is at the joints. In addition, if the patient suddenly becomes a 'dead weight' through not taking some weight through their lower limbs the nurse may be put at risk. A transfer aid enables the assistant to help take some weight from the main transfer person.

■ Unpredictable behaviour: Martin's bouts of anger leading to uncooperative behaviour are a key factor. Careful observation may mean that subtle signs of developing anger can alert the nurse to potentially hazardous situations when manual handling should be avoided until the situation has been defused or resolved. If problems are encountered during the transfer it may be appropriate to use controlled fall techniques (National Back Pain Association, 1991) to lower Martin to the floor until he can be handled safely. As long as Martin is not a danger to himself or others the nurse should let him vent his anger and only attempt to handle him once the situation is over and he is cooperative again.

■ Communication: Nursing staff must not rely on recognizing the signs of Martin's anger intuitively: they must be recorded. This is particularly important for students who may be in placements for short periods of time and so do not know the patients as intimately as the permanent staff. Close supervision of a student by experienced staff can form the basis of a positive learning experience for the student in this sort of situation.

3. Dealing with Martin's anger and his need to use the toilet: An occurrence like this will pose a dilemma for the carers. To maintain Martin's dignity and promote normality it is important to help him meet his physical needs. However, the carer has to balance meeting his immediate needs with the possibility that Martin or his carers may sustain injuries as handling under these circumstances would be less than ideal.

▶ CASE STUDY: CHILD

Emma Newton is a two and a half-year-old girl who is being treated at regular intervals in hospital for leukaemia. The treatment leaves her feeling very weak, but in spite of this she is a determined little girl who dislikes staying in her cot and becomes distressed if she cannot continue to play with her toys on the floor. She weighs 2 stone (12.7 kg). Her drugs are given intermittently through a line inserted into a major vein in the upper thorax and care needs to be taken not to dislodge this.

Her mother stays with her while she is an inpatient and she is visited regularly by her twin brothers who are five years old. The environment is a happy cheerful setting and provides many toys and equipment for the children to play with. Friends are encouraged to visit and the ward is often full of children.

1. **In relation to Emma:**
   (a) **Identify factors to take into consideration regarding the 'load' to be handled**
   (b) **List all the tasks that will require assessment.**
   (c) **Jot down any pertinent environmental factors that may affect Emma's handling situation.**
   (d) **Consider any equipment that may be used and why you would choose to use it.**
   (e) **Are there additional factors relating to the individual handlers that need to be taken into account?**

2. **Using the scenario make notes on how the handling plan you might make for Emma.**

3. **Emma's mother comments to you that she is concerned that Andrew, one of Emma's twin brothers spends a lot of time trying to pick Emma up and cuddle her. Although she says she can understand that he wants to make her better, she is concerned about him dropping her and also about the long-term effects on his back from carrying her around. Given that spinal damage often begins in childhood (National Back Pain Association, 1990), devise a programme to help educate Emma's brothers about the importance of caring for their backs.**

4. **Compare your ideas with the thoughts of our authors outlined below.**

▶ *Suggested Management for Emma Newton*

1. **Assessment:**
   (a) **Load: Emma's weight should be acceptable for one nurse to manage under ideal conditions, but assistance may be required because of attachments.**
   (b) **Tasks: Moving from cot to floor and chair, moving from floor to cot, assisting with toileting and hygiene needs.**
   (c) **Environment: May be cluttered with toys. Other children present may be a hazard. Cot is fixed height and has side bars to negotiate.**
   (d) **Equipment: Equipment may not be necessary, but wrapping Emma in a blanket may make her more secure.**
   (e) **Factors affecting individual handlers: Fitness for task and assistance required. Although Emma's weight may make it easy for one nurse to manage her, other factors such as taking care not to displace the intravenous line mean that additional help may be required. If Emma's mother is involved in Emma's care, it is important to consider the educational needs of the mother in relation to handling. The nurse should also consider her own posture when lifting the child from the cot. Does this mean reaching forward, forward bending or rotation of the spine, or can the cot sides be lowered to allow a good posture? In addition, when lifting from the floor, the handler's knees are fully bent, which reduces the handler's lifting capacity. These factors, together with possible clutter and hazards of other children present, create a high-risk manoeuvre that requires careful thought and planning by the nurse. However, as Emma is cared for regularly in this setting it may be pertinent for the nurse to consult previous assessments and plans that have been formulated for Emma. They could provide invaluable information about how Emma has been handled successfully in the past. Alternatively, the evaluations may provide information about which manoeuvres have been unsuccessful.**

2. **Handling plan:**

■ **Movement in bed:** Moving Emma within her cot poses little risk due to her weight, but could be hazardous if the height of the cot is unsuitable as the nurse may find it difficult to adopt a safe posture. It may help to lower the cot side and put one knee on the cot to get close to Emma and to help keep the spine in normal alignment. Forward bending must be avoided.

■ **Movement from cot to floor:** This could be quite hazardous. The nurse needs to ensure that there are no obstacles in the way and may need assistance to protect the venous line. Moving from an upright position to the floor needs to be carried out with care to maintain normal spinal posture. Holding Emma close to the trunk will help reduce spinal loading on the nurse.

3. **An educational strategy for Emma's brother:** This could include making up a game or rhyme to help the children think about bending their knees and keeping the spine in alignment when reaching for items on the floor. Also, obtaining leaflets and posters that are appropriate for children would be helpful for the ward Emma is on. This type of information would also help Emma's mother handle her daughter safely.

▶ CASE STUDY: ADULT

Robert Sinclair is a 70-year-old man who has always had a problem with his weight. He weighs 20 stone (127 kg) and over the years this excess weight has caused degeneration in his joints. The net result is that he is unable to stand and take his own weight. This is the main reason why he is living in a nursing home. Mr Sinclair is an articulate gentleman who pays a great deal of attention to his personal hygiene and likes to bath on a daily basis. He likes to sit in the conservatory as he has enjoyed gardening in the past. The nursing home is modern and the nurse managers have taken account for the need for access for specialized equipment in the design of the building.

1. **In relation to Robert:**
   (a) Identify factors to take into consideration regarding the 'load' to be handled.
   (b) List all the tasks that will require assessment.
   (c) Jot down any pertinent environmental factors that may affect Robert's handling situation.
   (d) Consider equipment that may be of use and state why you would choose to use it.
   (e) Are there additional factors relating to individual handlers that need to be taken into account?

2. Using the scenario make notes on the handling plan you might make for Robert.

3. While you are working on placement in the nursing home you hear that a care assistant has transferred Robert from his bed to a chair using the hoist and sling that is normally used for his transfer. After the manoeuvre Robert complains bitterly that he was extremely uncomfortable and that the sling has scraped the skin on the back of his thighs. It becomes apparent that the care assistant has only been shown once how to use the hoist by another care assistant.

(a) What should the qualified nurse in charge of the shift need to do about this situation?

(b) What measures could have been implemented to prevent this type of occurrence?

4. Compare your ideas with the thoughts of our authors outlined below.

▶ *Suggested Management for Robert Sinclair*

1. Assessment:
    (a) Load: Robert's weight is far too heavy for even two nurses to handle without using aids.
    (b) Tasks: Moving Robert from bed to a chair, chair to the toilet and transfer to other areas in the home, moving Robert up the bed and turning him on his side.
    (c) Environment: The home is well adapted for the residents, but may become cluttered with the residents' personal belongings. Carpets may mean that hoists and wheelchairs will be difficult to manoeuvre.
    (d) Equipment: A hoist with sling suitable for Robert's weight would be used to move him from bed to chair, chair to toilet, and transfer within the home. A sliding sheet could be used for turning Robert and sliding him up the bed.
    (e) Factors affecting individual handlers: Staff will need education in the use of hoists and other equipment. In using equipment there may be a risk of repetitive strain injury. Because Robert is able to cooperate he will be able to participate in the assessment process. This will be helpful as the pain in his joints may vary in intensity. The ability to communicate this will enable the variations in handling techniques to be employed, i.e. the type of sling to use with the hoist for maximum patient comfort. Adequate pain relief also needs to be provided to ensure patient comfort.

2. Handling plan:

■ The options to choose in most handling situations are to avoid lifting. To promote Robert's quality of life it is necessary to make him as mobile as possible without lifting and putting the nursing staff at high risk of injury.

■ Moving in bed: Sliding may be an option for movement up the bed or the use of the 30° tilt (Preston, 1988) for turning. However, Robert is rather heavy and it is unlikely that two nurses could manage these manoeuvres without risk. If enough staff are available these may be viable options.

■ Movement from bed to chair or toilet: A hoist would be the most appropriate piece of equipment and would also be the safest way to move Robert up and down the bed. There are many hoists available and it is important to choose within any area the one that is most versatile and useful for the type of patients nursed. Other considerations are the weight limit of the hoist and the selection of slings available for use with the hoist. Noise levels produced, the way the hoist is operated, and how easy it is to manoeuvre in the environment are other important factors. In relation to the nursing staff, the postures adopted when operating the hoist and the type of operating controls can result in repetitive strain injury to the wrists, shoulders and spine. Also strain when pushing or pulling the hoist (e.g. on carpeted areas) may put the nurse at risk of injury. Some hoists may require additional force to move them. It is vital that nurses have adequate training and supervision for operating any equipment used. This prevents discomfort for the patient and reduces the risk of injury to both nurses and patients.

■ Environment: Clearing the environment of patients' personal belongings as well as other equipment is vital to reduce potential hazards. Timing of procedures may help with this and can contribute to the safety of all involved. In addition, preparing things such as the chair the patient is to sit in will save time and minimize distress for the person being moved. It can be most undignifed to be left supported in a hoist while nurses look for a suitable chair for the patient to sit in.

3. Managing Robert's 'transfer' problem:
   (a) The nurse in charge of the shift on this occasion would have a duty to ensure that any treatment and care necessary for the skin abrasion was carried out and documented. An untoward incident form would require completion, detailing all aspects of the incident, including the outcome of interviews with the care assistant and any other witnesses to the incident. Robert's relatives would need to be informed and also the manager of the nursing home.
   (b) The provision of training for staff should be considered to prevent such an incident. Training is required under the *Health and Safety at Work Act (1974)*.

▶ CASE STUDY: MENTAL HEALTH

Doreen Jones is a 66-year-old lady with advanced dementia. She has extremely limited communication skills and is really only able to communicate pain by screaming at the nurses. Doreen weighs 11 stone (69.9 kg) and is unable to perform activities of living unaided as her body is permanently rigid with arms and legs flexed and in a fixed position. She frequently slips down the bed, but is unable to sit out in a chair because when she does she arches her back and is at risk of falling out of the chair and injuring herself. The care setting is purpose built, but to make it as homely as possible, much of the area is taken up by bedside tables, chairs and personal belongings for the residents.

1. In relation to Doreen:
   (a) Identify factors to take into consideration regarding the 'load' to be handled.
   (b) List all the tasks that require assessment.
   (c) Jot down any pertinent environmental factors that may affect Doreen's handling situation.
   (d) Consider equipment that may be of use and state why you would choose to use it.
   (e) Are there additional factors relating to individual handlers that need to be taken into account?

2. Using the scenario make notes on the handling plan you might make for Doreen.

3. Compare your ideas with the thoughts of our authors outlined below.

▶ *Suggested Management for Doreen Jones*

1. Assessment:
   (a) Load: Doreen is 11 stone (69.9 kg) and will require an appropriate handling plan or the use of handling aids.
   (b) Tasks: Moving Doreen up and down the bed, turning from side to side.

(c) **Environment:** The environment is cluttered and will therefore pose a hazard to staff that needs to be eliminated.

(d) **Equipment:** A sliding sheet to move Doreen up the bed or a sheet for the 30° tilt (Preston, 1988).

(e) **Factors affecting individual handlers:** Staff need to be aware of maximizing communication with Doreen. Awareness of the signs of pain that Doreen demonstrates and analgesia available for her are important factors to take into consideration. For Doreen, continuous slipping which will result in repetitive tasks will increase the risk of injury considerably, particularly as communication is difficult. These factors, together with a cluttered environment, pose a potential hazard. Therefore, the assessment in this type of situation will need to be detailed to allow effective planning.

2. **Handling plan:**

■ **Movement in bed:** Doreen is a high-risk handling situation. This is compounded by communication difficulties, her flexed, rigid posture, and the level of pain she suffers. The most sensible option for Doreen would be to use a sliding sheet to move her up and down the bed and the 30° tilt to turn her to prevent pressure sore formation. Utilizing these manoeuvres will reduce the pain she suffers and will help to prevent joint injuries due to poor grasp of the patient by nursing staff. Use of the same techniques by nursing staff may help to reduce some of Doreen's fear about what is happening to her. Another important factor is the use of prophylactic pain relief rather than waiting for Doreen to scream out in pain before analgesia is administered. Slipping down the bed frequently not only means that Doreen will have to be handled frequently, but can also contribute to the development of pressure sores. To help prevent slipping down the bed it is important to check that the lumbar curve of the spine is well supported. This can be done by inserting your hand between the pillows and lumbar curve. If there is a gap between the pillows and the spine, the pillows need to be rearranged to fit comfortably into the lumbar curve. If this is not done, the lack of support will give Doreen backache and make her fidget to get comfortable, and as a result she will slip further down the bed. In addition, a soft pillow support underneath her flexed legs will fulfil a similar function to the lumbar curve support. Alternatively, using a hoist with an appropriate sling may be another option. Due to difficulties in communicating with Doreen the sight of a large piece of mechanical machinery may increase her fear. Over time though, the efficient use of the equipment with minimal discomfort to Doreen may help alleviate this. However, it is vital that nursing staff know how to use the equipment correctly as one disastrous attempt with such equipment will lead to further patient fear, distrust and lack of cooperation.

▶ ANNOTATED FURTHER READING

BRAGGINS, S. (1994) *The Back: Functions, Malfunctions and Care.* London. Mosby–Year Book Europe Ltd.
   The first section of this book contains excellent information about the anatomy and physiology of the spine, including the injury process and how injuries heal. The second section looks specifically at back care in a variety of situations. It includes exercises for specific problems, but also advises complete and appropriate assessment of an individual before embarking on exercise programmes. The final section examines treatments that are available together with advice on how to access credible practitioners.
DUL, J., WEERDMEESTER, B. (1993) *Ergonomics for Beginners (A Quick Reference Guide).* London. Taylor and Francis Ltd.
   This book is a useful introduction to ergonomics. It contains a very comprehensive chapter on posture and movement that includes useful diagrams that

are referred to within the text. Chapter 2 in particular contains information that will add to the information you have already acquired about posture and movement from the chapter in this book. The book also covers ergonomics from a variety of aspects such as seating, work height, postures when performing a variety of work tasks and making the workplace suitable for lifting activities.

NATIONAL BACK PAIN ASSOCIATION. (1991) *Lifting and Handling – An Ergonomic Approach*. London. National Back Pain Association.

This is a key text that covers aspects of back pain at work, body mechanics, ergonomics, risk assessment, training and special lifting procedures. The risk assessment checklist is particularly useful. The diagrams are clear and the text provides useful principles for handling a variety of loads.

NATIONAL BACK PAIN ASSOCIATION (1997) *The Handling of Patients* (4th edition). Middlesex. National Back Pain Association in collaboration with the Royal College of Nursing.

This is an extremely useful publication that gives a comprehensive outline of all aspects of manual handling from legal and professional responsibilities to special patient needs. It is an important text in that it covers manual handling in acute hospitals and community settings. It can be used as a quick reference guide or as a basic text to expand knowledge about manual handling. The diagrams are clear and are particularly useful in explaining the text.

▶ REFERENCES

ALEXANDER, J. (1989) The Alexander technique. *Nursing Times* **85(42)**: 55–57.

BAILEY, J. (1995) Reflective practice: implementing theory. *Nursing Standard* **9(46)**: 29–31.

BARKER, A., CASSAR, S., GABBETT, J. (1994) *Handling People: Equipment, Advice and Information*. London. Disabled Living Foundation.

BRAGGINS, S. (1994) *The Back; Functions, Malfunctions and Care*. Chapter 18. London. Mosby Year Book, Europe Ltd.

COMMISSION OF THE EUROPEAN COMMUNITIES (1990) Council Directive on the minimum health and safety requirements for the manual handling of loads where there is a risk of Back Injury to Workers. Fourth Directive 90/269/EEC. *Official Journal of the European Communities* **156**: 9–13.

CONFEDERATION OF HEALTH SERVICE EMPLOYEES (1992) *Backbreaking Work*. Banstead. Confederation of Health Service Employees.

CORLETT, N. (1992) Ergonomics and back pain. *Nursing Standard* **6(32)**: 51.

COWELL, R. (1996) Case study. *Nursing Standard* **10(28)**: 27.

DEPARTMENT OF HEALTH (1974) *Health and Safety At Work*. p. 2, p. 7. London. Her Majesty's Stationery Office.

DUL, J., WEERDMEESTER, B. (1993) *Ergonomics for Beginners* (9th edition). p. 1, p.2, p.7. London. Taylor and Francis Ltd.

GERRARD, B.A., BONIFACE, W.J., LOVE,

B.H. (1980) *Interpersonal Skills for Health Professionals*. Virginia, U.S.A. Reston Publishing Company.

GLADMAN, G. (1993) Backpain in student nurses – the mature factor. *Occupational Health* **45(2)**: 47–51.

GRIFFITHS, B.L. (1988) Have you ever had a pain in your back? *Professional Nurse* January: 125–129.

HARDICRE, J. (1992) Put your back out of danger. *Nursing Standard* **7(5)**: 54.

HEALTH EDUCATION AUTHORITY (1994) *Look After Yourself Tutors' Manual*. London. Health Education Authority.

HEARN, V. (1988) Safe lifting and moving for nurse and patient. *Nursing* **3(30)**: 9–12.

HEMPLE, S. (1993) Home truths. *Nursing Times* **89(15)**: 40–41.

HINCHLIFFE, S., MONTAGUE, S. (1988) *Physiology for Nursing Practice*. London. Baillière Tindall.

JOHNSON, P. (1992) Handle with care. *Nursing Times* **88(42)**: 28–30.

JOHNSTON, M. (1987) Handle with care. *Senior Nurse* **6(5)**: 20–22.

KANE, M.E., PARAHOO, K. (1994) Knowledge and use of lifting techniques among a group of undergraduate student nurses. *Journal of Clinical Nursing* **3(1)**: 35–42.

KNIBBE, H. (1992) Overcoming resistance. *Nursing Times* **88(52)**: 46–47.

KRAUS, H. (1972) Evaluation of muscular and cardiovascular fitness. *Preventive Medicine* **1**:178.

LOVE, C. (1995) Managing manual handling in clinical situations. *Nursing Times* **91(2)**: 38–39.

McGUIRE, T., DEWAR, B.J. (1995) An

assessment of moving and handling practices amongst Scottish nurses. *Nursing Standard* **9(40)**: 35–39.

McGUIRE, T., MOODY, J., HANSON, M. (1996) An evaluation of mechanical aids used within the NHS. *Nursing Standard* **11(6)**: 33–38.

MOORE, W. (1993a) Reporting back. *Nursing Times* **89(22)**: 26–28.

MOORE, W. (1993b) The last straw. *Nursing Times* **89(22)**: 29–30.

NATIONAL BACK PAIN ASSOCIATION (1990) *Better Backs for Children – A Guide For Teachers and Parents*. London. National Back Pain Association with British Petroleum.

NATIONAL BACK PAIN ASSOCIATION (1991) *Lifting and Handling – An Ergonomic Approach*. London. National Back Pain Association.

NATIONAL BACK PAIN ASSOCIATION (1992) *The Handling of Patients* (3rd edition). National Back Pain Association in collaboration with the Royal College of Nursing.

NATIONAL HEALTH SERVICE TRAINING DIRECTORATE (1994) *Formal Investigation and Legal Issues. Just for the Record*. pp. 8–9. Leeds. National Health Service Executive.

PEARCE, R. (1992) Linking backcare and safe handling. *Nursing Standard* **6(32)**: 54

PHEASANT, S., STUBBS, D. (1991) *Lifting and Handling: An Ergonomic Approach*. London. National Back Pain Association.

PILLING, S., FRANK, J. (1994) Evaluation back-up. *Nursing Standard* **8(35)**: 22–23.

PRESTON, K.W. (1988) Positioning for comfort and pressure relief: the thirty degree alternative. *Care, Science and Practice* **6(4)**: 116–119.

ROYAL COLLEGE OF NURSING (1993) *Code of Practice for the Handling of Patients.* London. Royal College of Nursing.

ROYAL COLLEGE OF NURSING (1995) *Hazards for Pregnant Nurses – An A–Z Guide.* London. Royal College of Nursing.

ROYAL COLLEGE OF NURSING (1996a) *Code of Practice for the Handling of Patients.* p. 3. London. Royal College of Nursing.

ROYAL COLLEGE OF NURSING (1996b) *Introducing a Safer Patient Handling Policy.* London. Royal College of Nursing.

ROYAL COLLEGE OF NURSING (1996c) *Manual Handling Assessment in Hospitals and the Community.* London. Royal College of Nursing.

SADLER, C. (1991) Back up. *Nursing Times* **87(11)**: 16–17.

SNELL, J. (1995) Raising awareness. *Nursing Times* **91(31)**: 20–21.

STUBBS, D.A, OSBORNE, C.M. (1979) How to save your back. *Nursing (Oxford)* June: 116–124.

UKCC (1992) *Code of Professional Conduct* (3rd edition). London. UKCC.

UKCC (1993) *Standards for Records and Record Keeping.* London. UKCC.

WALSH, R. (1988) Good movement habits. *Nursing Times* **84(37)**: 59–61.

WILLIAMS, K. (1996) Handle with care. *Nursing Standard* **10(28)**: 26–27.

1.3 Infection Control

R. Peto

KEY ISSUES

■ SUBJECT KNOWLEDGE
▷ the six main groups of microorganisms
▷ the routes of spread of infection
▷ physical and physiological aspects related to infection control
▷ the influence of behaviour, attitude and culture on the prevention and control of infection
▷ the epidemiology related to identification and control of infection
▷ a problem solving approach to the practice of infection control
▷ health promotion

■ PRACTICE KNOWLEDGE
▷ the assessment, planning, implementation and evaluation of nursing care in relation to infection control
▷ five specific nursing practices related to the

prevention and control of infection: handwashing, disposal of clinical material, wearing of protective clothing, aseptic technique and personal hygiene

■ PROFESSIONAL KNOWLEDGE
▷ personal, professional, ethical and political issues
▷ the role of the infection control team in hospital and the environmental health team in the community

■ REFLECTIVE KNOWLEDGE
▷ decision making exercises and reflective exercises related to the section
▷ four case studies related to the four branches of nursing with decision making exercises to apply subject matter

▶ INTRODUCTION

Infection control, the prevention of spread of disease caused by infection, is fundamental to all nursing care. It is one of the most challenging aspects of care as it demands both an understanding of the causes and self-discipline to apply the theoretical knowledge to a variety of practice settings (Gould, 1987).

Outbreaks of infection have occurred for centuries, often generating great fear in people, and have been attributed to a variety of causes as diverse as witchcraft and bad air (Parker, 1990). It is only just over one hundred years ago that the relationship between disease and microorganisms was discovered by Pasteur. However, despite great technological advances such as antibiotics and vaccines, infection remains a major threat in developed countries.

Central to the concept of infection control is the frequently quoted statement 'Hospitals should do the sick no harm' (Nightingale, 1854). Today 140 years on, hospital staff are still traditionally recognized and respected as the authority on infection control and on the problems of cross-infection affecting hospital patients. Research indicates that one patient in every ten will develop an infection while in hospital (Meers et al., 1981). Conversely, the control of communicable diseases has traditionally been the prerogative of community staff (Worsley et al., 1994) and environmental health teams. However, increasing attention is being paid to the control of infection in the community. This is particularly because inpatient hospital stays are shorter, increasing numbers of ill people are being cared for in the community, often in their own homes, and invasive procedures such as minor operations are increasingly performed in health centres and GP surgeries (Worsley *et al.*, 1994).

Infection control is part of every nurse's clinical practice and so nurses of all branches (adult, children's, mental health and learning disabilities) have a role to play with their specific patient or client groups. Whether nursing in an institution (hospital or nursing home) or in the community (individual homes, health centres or shared housing) it is necessary to recognize the sources and modes of spread of infectious microorganisms and know how to apply practices to control infection.

▶ OVERVIEW

This chapter aims to provide you, the student, in whatever branch of nursing you have chosen to study, with an understanding of what infection and infection control means for individual patients and clients (sick or well) and their carers (health professional or informal family and friends), whether this care is in a home or community setting or in a hospital or institution.

▶ *Subject Knowledge*

The biological aspects of infection are introduced and the five main groups of microorganisms – bacteria, viruses, fungi, protozoa and worms – are considered. The routes and modes of spread and sources of physiological and physical control are discussed.

The complex psychosocial issues related to the control of infection are also considered, with particular reference to the influence of personal and group behaviour, attitude and culture. This section also considers epidemiology and its importance in the identification and control of infection, with particular reference to health promotion.

▶ *Practice Knowledge*

A range of nursing practices are explored using a problem solving approach of assessment, planning, implementation and evaluation. Five specific practices to prevent and control infection are considered with the aim of enabling you to apply them in practice in whatever branch of nursing you are studying and in a range of practice placements.

▶ *Professional Knowledge*

Both personal and professional issues are highlighted with specific sections on ethical and political issues. The roles of the infection control team in the hospital and the environmental health team in the community are considered.

▶ *Reflective Knowledge*

The care of individuals who may have an infection or who are particularly susceptible to an infection has important decision-making implications for the nurse providing that care. Throughout this chapter there are reflective questions and decision-making exercises related to the section they are included in. They are provided to allow you to reflect upon practices you have observed or been involved with while in a clinical placement or to use when you have been exposed to such an experience.

On pp. 96–97 there are four case studies, each one relating to one of the branch programmes. You may find it helpful to read one of them before you start the chapter and use it as a focus for your reflections while reading.

▶ CLASSIFICATION OF INFECTIVE AGENTS

An infection is caused by the invasion of a person's immunological defences by the deposition of infective agents called microorganisms within the body tissues. They are responsible for approximately half of all known human diseases (Gould, 1987). Bacteria, viruses, fungi, protozoa and worms are the five main groups of organisms capable of causing disease (Table 1.3.1).

The main cause or source of hospital-acquired (nosocomial) infections are bacteria, while viruses are the most common cause of infectious conditions in the community (Gould, 1987). However, not all microorganisms cause infection or disease. Many live quite harmlessly in soil,

Organism	Infections and diseases
Bacteria	
Staphylococcus aureus	Wound infections, pneumonia, osteomyelitis, food poisoning
Staphylococcus epidermidis	Wound infection
Streptococci (group A)	Streptococcal throat, impetigo, rheumatic fever, scarlet fever
Streptococci (group B)	UTI, wound infection
Neisseria gonorrhoeae	Gonorrhoea, pelvic inflammatory disease, conjunctivitis, infective arthritis
Mycobacterium tuberculosis	Tuberculosis
Pseudomonas aeruginosa	Wound infections, chest infections
Klebsiella	UTI, wound infections, respiratory infections
Escherichia coli	Wound infections, UTI, pelvic inflammatory disease
Proteus	UTI, wound infections
Campylobacter	Diarrhoea
Acinetobacter	UTI, wound infections, respiratory infections
Salmonella	Food poisoning
Clostridium welchii	Gas gangrene, food poisoning
Viruses	
Hepatitis A	Infectious hepatitis
Hepatitis B	Serum hepatitis
Herpes (type 1)	Cold sores, sexually transmitted disease
Herpes (type 2)	Genital lesions
Human immunodeficiency virus (HIV)	Acquired immunodeficiency syndrome (AIDS)
Fungi	
Candida albicans	Vaginal thrush, UTI
Tinea	Athlete's foot
Protozoa	
Trichomonas vaginalis	Sexually transmitted disease in women
Plasmodium falciparum	Malaria
Entamoeba	Amoebic dysentery
Worms	
Roundworms: threadworms, *Ascaris*	
Flatworms: flukes, tapeworms	

Table 1.3.1 Common organisms and infections and diseases they cause. (UTI, urinary tract infection.)

water and the air, and some are vital in the production of antibiotics (bacteria) and in cake, alcohol and cheese making (yeasts).

Microorganisms capable of causing disease are called pathogens, but the presence of a pathogen does not necessarily mean that an infection will ensue. Everyday the body excretes millions of microorganisms through the intestinal system and there is a large population of resident bacteria on the skin. Pathogens that can live harmlessly in a specific body site such as the gut or on the skin are called commensals. They only become pathogenic and cause an infection when transferred to an abnormal body site. For example, the bacteria *Escherichia coli* lives harmlessly in the gut and aids digestion, but if transferred to an abnormal body site such as a wound or the urinary tract it becomes pathogenic and causes infection and disease.

For disease to ensue pathogens need to be able to multiply and to do this a chain or series of events has to take place (Figure 1.3.1). Infection control principles are based on disrupting this chain.

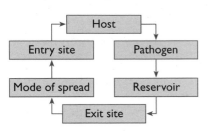

Figure 1.3.1: Chain of infection.

▶ SOURCES OF INFECTION

▶ *Bacteria*

Bacteria are unicellular organisms that evolved millions of years ago. They are visible under the high magnification of an ordinary light microscope using an appropriate stain. Surrounding the bacterial cell is a membrane made up of proteins and phospholipids and surrounding the membrane is a hard cell wall, which gives the organism its shape. Bacteria are most commonly classified according to their shape (Figure 1.3.2). They are also classified according to their laboratory reaction when treated with a dye called Gram's stain. The response is determined by a chemical present in the bacteria's cell wall. Bacteria are termed gram positive

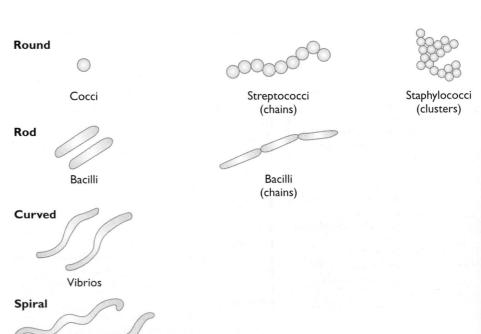

Figure 1.3.2: Bacterial classification according to shape.

if they stain blue/purple, and gram negative if they fail to take up the stain and remain the red colour of the counterstain.

▶ Viruses

Viruses are minute particles and rather than having a cellular structure like bacteria they consist of genetic material and protein. They are therefore not usually defined as living organisms (Gould, 1987). Instead of growing and dividing like cells, they infect cells. For example the human immunodeficiency virus (HIV) infects T cells of the human immune system, while viruses that cause the common cold attach themselves to the epithelial cell membrane of the mucous membrane and invade the cell, releasing new virus particles and destroying the host cell. The structure of a virus only becomes apparent when looked at with a high-powered electron microscope. Unlike bacterial cells, viruses have a poor survival rate outside of living cells.

▶ Fungi

Fungi have a more complicated structure than bacteria and contain a nucleus. They are either branch shaped (e.g. mushrooms) or form buds (e.g. yeasts). Only a few species of fungi cause disease (see Table 1.3.1). *Candida*, the yeast that is responsible for causing thrush, destroys the normal bacteria of the area it infects, namely the mouth, large bowel and vagina. The most common, *Candida albicans* causes vaginal thrush. *Tinea* is a fungus that produces a superficial infection. It is responsible for athlete's foot and causes a painful and irritant rash in the folds of skin, most commonly between the toes. Deeper fungal infections are more common in hot climates.

▶ Protozoa

Protozoa are microscopic single-celled animals (see Table 1.3.1). One of the most common is *Trichomonas vaginalis*, which is a sexually transmitted infection and causes a foul-smelling, green-yellow vaginal discharge. Malaria, caused by the protozoan *Plasmodium falciparum*, remains an endemic disease in many parts of the African, Indian and Asian continents. Neither *Trichomonas* or malaria poses any risk of cross-infection in hospitals. A third protozoan, *Entamoeba histolytica* is responsible for amoebic dysentery and is present in the stools of infected patients. This does carry cross-infection risks as it can be passed from one patient to another if staff do not wash their hands after handling equipment such as bedpans and bedclothes contaminated with the infected stools.

▶ Worms

Worms are multicellular animals and numerous species cause infections in humans. They broadly fall into two main groups – roundworms and flatworms (see Table 1.3.1). They mostly live in the large bowel of the human host having invaded the digestive system as a result of eating infected and uncooked foods. Worm infections can be avoided by hygenic food preparation and adequate sanitation.

Reflecting upon a placement you have experienced, consider the patients and clients you knew had an infection and try to decide what type of microorganism was responsible. For example, you may have been involved in the care of a patient with a wound infection, which is commonly caused by the bacteria *Staphylococcus aureus*.

Site	Anatomical or physiological barrier	Mechanism of action
Skin	Layers of skin Sebaceous glands	Mechanical and waterproof barrier Secrete sebum, which has bactericidal properties and fatty acid, which kills bacteria
Eyes	Tears	Contain lysozyme, which digests and destroys bacteria
	Eyelashes	The blinking reflex protects the cornea from injury
Mouth	Mucosa Saliva	Mechanical barrier White blood cells destroy bacteria
Stomach	Gastric secretions	High acidity destroys bacteria
Duodenum	Bile	Alkaline pH inhibits bacterial growth
Small intestine	Lymphatic tissue Rapid peristalsis	Destroys bacteria Prevents bacteria from remaining in the intestine
Nostrils	Hairs Turbinal bones	Trap inhaled particles and microorganisms Trap inhaled particles and microorganisms
Pharynx and nasopharynx	Tonsils	Lymphoid tissue traps inspired particles
Respiratory tree (except alveoli)	Cilia	Beat mucus and particles away from lungs
	Mucus Lung tissue	Traps particles during inhalation Isolates focus of infection
Vagina	Secretions	Acid pH inhibits bacterial growth
Urethra	Male length	Prevents migration of bacteria to bladder
Urine	Flushing action	Washes away microorganisms

Table 1.3.5 The body's passive defence mechanisms.

▶ RISK OF INFECTION

The decision as to whether an item requires cleaning, disinfection, or sterilization depends upon whether it carries a low, medium or high risk of causing infection to the patient or client.

▶ *Low Risk*

Cleaning, the removal of 'soil', may be sufficient to control the microorganism population and so prevent the transfer of infection. There are two methods of cleaning – dry and wet (Table 1.3.6). After cleaning, any article should have fewer microorganisms on it. The dry method, however, may simply redistribute the microorganisms into the air, while the wet method may distribute and increase the microorganisms through the use of contaminated articles such as mop heads and cloths or contaminated water.

▶ *Medium Risk*

Disinfection, the destruction of vegetative microorganisms to a level unlikely to cause infection is usually acceptable (Ayliffe *et al.*, 1982,

p. 89). It does not necessarily kill bacterial spores. However, the pathogens remaining following disinfection may pose an infection risk to particularly susceptible patients, for example patients with an impaired immunity, such as patients on cytotoxic therapy. The two main methods of disinfection are heat and chemicals (see Table 1.3.6). Heat is the preferred method for disinfecting articles (e.g. surgical instruments) as it is more penetrative and easier to control than chemicals. However, disinfection by chemicals may be required if heat is unsuitable (e.g. for skin disinfection or for items that are heat sensitive such as fibreoptic endoscopes). The choice is therefore a complex matter and requires a working knowledge of the disinfectants available and what requires disinfecting (see Table 1.3.6).

▶ *High Risk*

Sterilization, 'the complete destruction or removal of all microorganisms' (Ayliffe *et al.*, 1982, p. 83) involves the use of either heat (dry or moist), gas, chemicals or irradiation (see Table 1.3.6). Items requiring sterilization are described as being a high risk to patients. Such items are used during invasive procedures (e.g. intravenous cannulas, surgical instruments, urinary catheters). As with disinfection the choice of method used depends upon the item being sterilized (see Table 1.3.6).

▶ OTHER METHODS OF INFECTION CONTROL

Other methods of control that are very important in the prevention of cross-infection between patient and health care worker include personal hygiene, waste disposal and correct food handling (cooking and serving). These will be discussed in detail in the Nursing Knowledge section

▶ INDIVIDUAL SUSCEPTIBILITY TO INFECTION

Individual susceptibility to infection can be caused when a person's immunity is impaired, either active or passive. Particular groups of patients are at particular risk (see Table 1.3.7). Although patients in hospital are generally at a greater risk of getting infections, partly due to the increased risk of cross infection from other patients, individuals being cared for in the community, for example in their own home, still remain at risk from many of the identical risk factors as the individual in hospital. For example, wound infections, urinary tract infection whilst catheterized.

Pyschosocial   It is important to recognize not only the causal relationship and influence of physical sources and controls of infection and disease, but also the complex psychosocial issues that can be involved.

System	Type and mechanism of action	Examples and comments
Cleaning	Dry: mechanical action to loosen and remove large particles, but may increase airborne bacterial count up to tenfold. Does not remove stains.	Sweeping redisperses bacteria in dust and larger particles.
		Dry mops may be specifically treated to attract and retain dust particles. Vacuum cleaning should not increase airborne counts of bacteria. Expelled air from the machine should not blow dust from uncleaned surfaces back into the air. Dry dusting increases the air count of dust and bacteria and recontaminates cleaned surfaces
	Wet: water containing detergents or solvents is used to dissolve adherent dirt and dust. Dispersal of micro-organisms into the air is less likely than with dry cleaning, but the cleaning fluids may grow bacteria due to contamination.	Damp dusting is less likely to disperse bacteria into air, but need to rinse after cleaning with detergents to prevent build up of detergent film. All surfaces need to be dry before use to prevent contamination from bacterial growth.
Disinfection	Heat	80°C for one minute or 65°C for 10 minutes kills vegetative organisms. Steam heat is most effective (e.g. autoclave). Damage relates to time and temperature. Disinfection at a lower temperature for a longer time is possible for heat-sensitive equipment.
	Chemical	Phenolics are widely used for disinfecting inanimate objects, but are not active against bacterial spores or some viruses. They are toxic and unsuitable for living tissue until thoroughly rinsed. They should not be used for food preparation or storage surfaces. Hypochlorites (bleach) (e.g. Milton, Sanichlor) are mainly used for environmental disinfection. They are active against many microorganisms including viruses and may corrode metals and bleach fabrics. Chlorhexidine is used clinically, but should not be used to disinfect inanimate objects. It is active against gram-positive cocci (*Staphylococcus aureus*), and less active against bacilli and spores. It has little virucidal activity and is inactivated by soap. Alcohol (70% ethyl or 60% isopropyl) is rapidly active against vegetative bacteria, but is a poor sporicidal. It acts rapidly and is a useful surface disinfectant for physically clean surfaces (e.g. trolley tops, injection sites, hands). It evaporates rapidly to leave a dry clean surface. Glutaraldehyde is used to disinfect heat-sensitive inanimate objects. It is very toxic and all equipment requires thorough rinsing. It is more commonly used as a method of sterilizing.

System	Type and mechanism of action	Examples and comments
Sterilization	Heat	Autoclaves sterilize using moist heat (steam at increased pressure, 134°C, for three minutes). They are suitable for most metal instruments, plastics, glass and fabrics. Sterilizing ovens use dry heat (160°C, for 45 minutes, 190°C for 60 minutes). Heat distortion can occur, and materials may become brittle or scorched.
	Gas	Ethylene oxide is very toxic and requires careful control of temperature, humidity, gas concentration and pressure. It is used to sterilize manufactured goods.
	Chemicals: used when heat or other methods are not possible, but reliable sterilization is difficult as grease, proteins (blood, tissue) or air will prevent fluids coming into contact with all surfaces and prolonged immersion times are required to kill bacterial spores	Glutaraldehyde is most commonly used, but is very toxic and is unpleasant to handle.
	Irradiation	Gamma rays are used industrially (e.g. for disposable plastics after packaging), but repeated irradiation causes plastics to become brittle and is expensive and uneconomical to use in hospital.

Table 1.3.6 Physical systems of infection control.

Group	Examples
Extremes of age	Very young and elderly
Critically ill	Patients in ITU, multiple injuries
Chronically sick	Patients with heart and respiratory disease
Surgical patients	Abdominal surgery, trauma
Patients with underlying diseases	Patients with diabetes mellitus or malignancy
Immunosuppressed patients	Patients on glucocorticosteroids or chemotherapy and transplant patients

Table 1.3.7 Patients at greatest risk of infection.

▶ BEHAVIOUR

Behaviour is influenced by personal beliefs and attitudes and is now recognized as one of the many determinants of disease (O'Boyle Williams, 1995). In the past disease and infections were normally perceived as being outside an individual's own control. For example, 100 years ago dirty water was associated with infections and diseases such as cholera, but was perceived to be the responsibility of the government and country (Parker, 1990). Today many psychological, social and emotional factors are acknowledged as being particular influences, with the relationship between individuals and their lifestyle also recognized as potential causes of infection and disease (O'Boyle Williams, 1995).

As a student nurse you will quite possibly be sharing living accommodation, either in a nurses' home or rented flat or house. Such student accommodation is notoriously renowned for being far from hygienically clean! Consider all the practical things (self-induced behaviours) you do within this communal living area that might be putting yourself at risk of contracting an infection.

Self-induced behaviour is an area of concern to infection control teams as particular individuals or groups have an increased risk of disease and infection because of such behaviour or lifestyle. The intravenous drug user sharing needles and the prostitute having unprotected sex, both of whom have an increased risk of contracting HIV and AIDS, may be a first consideration. However, many other groups and individuals also have a particular risk of developing life-threatening diseases and are often ignorant or unaware of them (e.g. people living in communal or shared accommodation).

Such individuals or groups may never become hospital patients through being exposed to infection as their body may be able to cope and fight the invasion of microorganisms or they may respond to treatment given in the community. Nevertheless some people need protecting and so infection control management needs to reach out to the community in a form that is relevant and appropriate to the particular at-risk groups or individuals.

▶ MOTHERS AND BABIES

Mothers of babies and young children need to know and understand the importance of immunizations and be able to attend the clinics. They also need to be listened to when social customs and religious practices conflict with the education that is being put forward by the health visitor.

▶ MENTAL HEALTH

People with mental health problems such as depression may not need hospitalization, but may have poor motivation, self esteem and desire to care for themselves. This can result in food poisoning from being unable or incapable of storing, preparing and cooking food adequately, and fungal and bacterial infections of the skin as a result of poor personal hygiene.

▶ LEARNING DISABILITIES

Reflect upon a placement where you have cared for a person with a learning disability.

How were basic infection control practices such as handwashing before meals and after using the toilet encouraged and carried out?

In what ways did staff teach and encourage such practices?

If basic infection control practices were not carried out, how might you go about implementing them in a similar practice setting?

The carer of a person with a learning disability might need to take extra care and attention to ensure that behaviour and practices do not increase the risk of infection.

▶ CULTURAL BEHAVIOUR

Behaviour adopted by particular ethnic, cultural and religious groups can put them at a greater risk of infection and disease. For example the eating of raw or undercooked foods by some Far East cultures, the prohibition of contraceptives including condoms by religious groups, and the non-seeking of treatment by men because it is considered unmanly or weak (O'Boyle Williams, 1995).

Occupation might also increase the risk of infections and diseases, for example those who have worked in a coal mine or with asbestos have a greatly increased risk of developing chest infections and life-disabling and life-threatening lung diseases in later life.

Smoking as a cultural behaviour has over the years received a great deal of attention in the media and medical and nursing press regarding its effect on the smoker's health as well as on those who are in close contact with the smoker. For example, babies and children who live with parents who smoke have a greater risk of developing respiratory tract infections (Mohler, 1987).

Behaviour, attitudes and practices do change, but this can only happen by influencing individuals and groups. This might be by education in the form of knowledge and understanding, by observation of people, peer groups and organizations, and from outside influences. During the 1980s, mass media education about safe sexual practices resulted in a dramatic reduction of HIV infections among homosexuals, although numbers among heterosexuals did similarly decline.

Certain customs and rituals, despite being considered infection control risks, are still widespread among particular cultural groups. For example, the practice of religious circumcisions on Jewish baby boys in their own homes and female circumcisions of young and teenage girls from certain African, Arabian and Far Eastern countries. Reasons for undertaking such practices include hygienic, psychosexual and cultural (Thompson, 1989). Again the media has highlighted these practices as being dangerous and an infection risk. With regard to the practice of female circumcision, attitudes and behaviour are changing with groups of women fighting for this practice to stop. Yet despite being illegal in Britain since 1985, female circumcision continues. The women argue that only by education and raising the awareness of the inherent dangers of such surgery among their own cultural groups will this surgical practice be eradicated.

▶ EPIDEMIOLOGY

Epidemiology can be defined as the 'study of the incidence and distribution of diseases, and of their control and prevention' (Allen, 1990). Through this the incidence and distribution of disease can be assessed to provide data for the control or eradication of disease. Epidemiological studies can be small (micro) or large (macro) scale. They involve determining the risk or likelihood that a person without a disease (or infection) who comes into contact with certain risk factors will acquire a particular disease (or infection) (Valanis, 1986). Risk factors might be physical, as discussed in the Biological section, for example infective organisms, or psychosocial, for example behavioural, such as smoking or eating raw foods. The risk to an individual is partly determined by estimating the experience of the whole population.

In epidemiology whole populations of individuals are studied to determine the risk of disease occurring. It is possible to identify potential groups or areas that are associated with a high risk for a particular disease or infection by surveillance of the population and gathering facts and data of specific diseases. Epidemiologists provide health care workers with such data to enable planning of the particular health needs and services of a community.

A common infection monitored with the elderly in mind is that due to the influenza virus. By monitoring influenza rates among the population as a whole, it is possible to discern early signs of an outbreak and so offer immunization to the elderly and other high risk groups.

Outbreaks of infection are common in both institutional and community care. However, whereas the outbreak of an infection in a hospital ward or nursing home is usually on a micro scale (i.e. involving relatively few people), outbreaks of infection in the community are usually

The elderly and very young are considered to be two groups that have a particular risk of infections and diseases and are often the specific target groups of immunization programmes. Identify immunizations offered either to the elderly or to the very young.

What social, ethnic or cultural issues might affect a client's decision to accept or refuse the offer of immunization?

on a macro scale, at times involving hundreds of people. The influenza virus is a common cause of a macro scale infection.

▶ HEALTH PROMOTION

Health promotion is an important aspect of infection control. This can be on a small scale, such as teaching a group of ward staff, or large scale, involving large groups or entire communities. Specific groups and individuals have already been noted in this chapter as being at particular risk from infections due to their behaviours, attitudes and beliefs. For these people, health promotion attempts to prevent and control infection either to themselves or to others. The attitudes and behaviours of the health professionals carrying out such health promotion are important. Whether it is meeting a group of drug addicts to discuss the risk of sharing needles or talking to a particular cultural or religious group about child immunizations, health professionals need to be aware of their own personal beliefs, traditions and practices. Often health professionals who are not specifically specialized in infection control nursing are involved. For example, promoting the importance of immunizing babies to prevent and control life-threatening diseases such as tetanus or diphtheria is usually undertaken by health visitors, while community psychiatric nurses usually advise drug addicts about the importance of using sterile needles and not sharing them with others.

Health promotion in the area of infection control is heavily influenced by personal beliefs and attitudes. The health professional needs an understanding of the influences that have an effect on a person or group's behaviour and attitude towards health education. The use of health behavioural models have been cited as theoretical descriptions of interactions that influence health behaviour (O'Boyle Williams, 1995). One such model, the health belief model has had major influences on health education and proposes that four predictors of health exist (O'Boyle Williams, 1995) (Figure 1.3.3). Returning to the earlier example in which a community of elderly is offered an influenza immunization, the use of such a health belief model could be used to help in the health education and promotion of such protection. For example, the nurse could assess an elderly person's perception of the seriousness of influenza and his or her susceptibility to catching it. The nurse could then help the elderly person see the benefits and constraints of the proposed immunization.

The aim of this section has been to enable you to examine and consider some the important biological and psychosocial aspects of infection control. You should by now be more aware of the relevance of the sciences surrounding infection control so that you can apply them to the more practical nursing issues examined in the next section, Practice Knowledge.

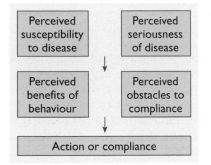

Figure 1.3.3: Four predictors of health belief.

PRACTICE KNOWLEDGE

The prevention and control of infection is largely founded on nursing practice, which in itself must be grounded on sound research-based knowledge. To help the health care professional there are hundreds of articles available from a broad range of journals on the subject of infection control. Many are research studies into particular infection control practices, for example handwashing (Taylor, 1978a), safe disposal of clinical waste (Burns, 1988), and wearing of plastic aprons (Curran, 1991). However, although there are numerous articles on specific nursing practices associated with infection control, such practices are often carried out on an ad hoc basis (Kingsley, 1992). For almost 20 years nurses have used a problem solving approach to the planning and organization of individualized nursing care (Kratz, 1979), the Nursing Process, but few articles appear to have considered the practice of infection control from a similar problem solving approach (Faulkner, 1986; Kingsley, 1992). Yet as infection control is a part of nursing practice, it seems only right that this section, Practice Knowledge, uses the problem solving approach. Therefore the four stages assessment, planning, implementation and evaluation will be used to present the nursing knowledge and practice for infection control.

▶ ASSESSMENT

Part of assessment, as the first stage of the Nursing Process, is to gather information and to analyse it. In the area of infection control, the term 'audit' is becoming almost synonymous with assessment, and as a result of recent NHS reforms it is now a well used term in many health care settings. However, while assessment is usually used in relation to a patient or individual, the term audit is usually concerned with the environment or an institution. The Department of Health (1989) defines it as a 'systematic critical analysis of the quality of clinical care'. With one of its components being quality assurance and because of the strong link between this and infection control (Askew, 1993), audit is fast becoming an essential part of infection control in both hospitals and the community. From such audits nurses are writing standards, protocols and policies to prevent and control infection. Evidence has shown that audits of infection control policies and procedures have an impact on infection rates (Friedman *et al.*, 1984).

For an individual with an infection, an assessment requires an in-depth analysis of both the source of the infection and the individuals and carers at risk. Such assessments need to be routinely and systematically undertaken. By knowing the factors that increase the risk of infection to either the individual or carer, plans can be made to prevent and control the infection and appropriate nursing actions can be undertaken before an infection occurs.

The source of infection may be determined by knowing the site of infection, the organism involved and the mode or route of spread. This allows an assessment of the degree of risk and the planning and immediate initiation of preventive measures such as isolation of the patient or wearing protective clothing (e.g. gloves) before touching the patient or infected site.

The individual and carer may both be at risk from an infection and therefore the degree of risk to both must be assessed. The risk can be considered as high, medium or low. For both the individual and carer there are general and specific risk factors that can indicate the severity of risk (Table 1.3.8). From these, measures can be instigated to prevent and control the infection or cross-infection.

For an institution or a particular environment an audit is often carried out on a regular basis to provide a formal check to ensure that infection control measures are being routinely adhered to in areas involved in patient care. For example, during an audit of a hospital ward all areas would be inspected, both the clinical areas such as the treatment room and more indirect areas such as the ward kitchen. Both areas would be

Consider a client with whom you have been involved in providing care. Reflecting upon this client's specific health problems, assess the general and specific risk factors for infection (see Table 1.3.8) that you think apply. For example, an elderly patient with an infected pressure sore might have general factors such as age, malnutrition (underweight) and immobility, and a specific factor such as diabetes mellitus.

General	Age of patient
	General health
	General hygiene
	Mental state
	Nutrition
	Mobility
	Continence
Specific	Type of invasive procedure
	Present medication
	Surgery
	Pressure sores

Table 1.3.8 General and specific risk factors for infection.

checked for general cleanliness and specific infection control measures would also be looked for. For example, the availability and correct use of a sharps bin would be looked for in the treatment room, while the presence and correct use of a food refrigerator thermometer would be looked for in the kitchen.

▶ PLANNING

Once the risks to the individual and carer have been identified, goals of care and specific nursing measures can be planned. Planning can only commence when the organism, site of infection and mode of spread have all been identified. The goals of care can be divided into those that will control, reduce and prevent self-infection (endogenous) and those that will prevent cross-infection (exogenous). In addition to the planning of nursing practices, this stage might also include the architectural design of the working environment. For example the design of a ward used for the specific care of infectious patients would include individual rooms or cubicles.

Maurer (1985) in her book *Hospital Hygiene*, maintained that many hospitals needed more and better handwashing facilities. She noted that in some areas staff had no handwashing facilities between the lavatory and the ward.

Planning also involves prioritizing goals of care. As the patient's condition improves or deteriorates, priorities may change. Common goals of care include prevention of exposure to an infectious organism, control of the extent of an infection, maintenance of resistance to an infection and understanding of infection control practices (Heath, 1994).

▶ IMPLEMENTATION

Implementation involves the use of appropriate infection control practices to reduce the risk of cross-infection and self-infection. This needs to include all who are at risk from exposure to the infective organism – patient or client, family, friends and all health care personnel.

Safe practice should ensure that the chain of infection is broken, thereby preventing the transmission of pathogens to potential sites of infection. Reservoirs of infection can be eliminated, sites of entry and exit controlled, and modes of spread minimized by actions such as disposal of body fluids, wearing protective garments, effective handwashing and aseptic procedures.

Cross-infection in hospitals is a common problem: one in ten patients have an infection, with one in five of these being acquired while in hospital (Meers *et al.*, 1981). Think back to a particular ward or nursing home that you have been to on clinical placement and reflect upon where the handwashing facilities were situated.

Were they in places that encouraged you to wash your hands?

For example were they near the toilets?

Were there handwashing facilities in each of the resident's bedrooms?

Reflecting upon a recent clinical placement, note down which practices were undertaken to prevent you from becoming infected and which were to prevent the patient from getting an infection.

For example, did you wear a plastic apron to protect yourself or to protect the patient?

Treatment of the infection requires elimination of infectious organisms. Although the doctor might prescribe an antibiotic drug once the causative organism has been identified, the nurse must assess the progress of infection and ensure that complications are prevented. Nursing actions might include prevention of dehydration caused by a fever associated with the infection, ensuring that a drug is given aseptically, and observations for potential drug allergies.

Controlling self- and cross-infection is a complex task involving practices that individually or collectively control the risk of patients or carers infecting themselves or others by direct and indirect contact.

▶ UNIVERSAL PRECAUTIONS

In recent years the concept of a comprehensive approach to infection control that promotes the use of safe practices to ensure protection to everyone from bloodborne infections has been introduced into some hospitals and health authorities (Wilson and Breedon, 1990). Called 'Universal Precautions', it embraces the notion that all blood and certain body fluids are potentially infectious and therefore such practices are to be used with all patients at all times, regardless of whether they are known to have a blood or body fluid infection. The impetus for the introduction of Universal Precautions began in the USA as a result of the problems of identifying individuals with HIV infection.

Universal infection control precautions have been identified as explicit policies for handwashing, broken skin, sharps, protective clothing, spillage, waste and excreta (Wilson and Breedon, 1990). These practices are applied to all patients in all health care settings whenever there is contact with blood and certain body fluids rather than only being introduced when staff consider the patient to be a high risk. One argument for implementing such precautions is that they not only protect staff from known diseases, but also protect against those that are as yet unknown.

However, not all hospitals have taken on board a policy of universal precautions (Wilson and Breedon, 1990; Taylor, 1993). Deterrants to implementing them include a lack of practical workable guidelines, resistance to change by staff, personal prejudices and the financial cost (Taylor, 1993). The financial cost may well have political implications for hospitals and staff, and will be discussed further in the section on Political Issues on p. 92.

It is widely accepted that five specific practices are instrumental in the control of self- and cross-infection and should be undertaken by all health care workers when caring for patient and clients. These are:

▶ handwashing;
▶ safe disposal of clinical material;
▶ wearing of protective clothing;
▶ aseptic technique;
▶ personal hygiene.

▶ HANDWASHING

The important role of handwashing in the transmission of disease was demonstrated most convincingly 150 years ago (Semmelweiss 1847 cited

RESEARCH BASED EVIDENCE

Williams and Buckle (1988) carried out a longitudinal study among staff in a large teaching hospital and discovered that six months after an educational and promotional handwashing campaign involving teaching, posters, videos and leaflets the frequency of handwashing did not increase. Initially there appeared to be an improvement, with more handwashing during the two weeks following the promotional campaign involving posters and videos, but after six months, handwashing had returned to the pre-campaign base line. The conclusion suggested that further studies are needed to address lasting changes in attitude.

DECISION MAKING

When you are next out in clinical practice note down all the times you wash your hands. Also note down what you had done or were about to do that made the handwashing necessary. For example you might decide to wash your hands because you were about to feed a patient. Try to determine whether the handwashing was to protect yourself or to protect the patient.

in Parker, 1990), and today remains 'the most basic as well as the most vital infection control' (Horton, 1996). Laboratory studies and clinical trials on handwashing have repeatedly shown that it is the most important factor in reducing hospital-acquired infections, with most hospital infections being spread via the hands of staff (Reybrouck, 1983). The aim of handwashing is to reduce the number of bacteria to a level below that needed to establish infection when transferred to a susceptible patient. The precise number of bacteria needed is not known, but factors such as the virulence of the bacteria, the health and age of the patient, and any disruption to the body's natural defence to infection (e.g. from catheters, intravenous lines) affect the outcome.

It has been known for over 50 years that there are two categories of bacteria on hands – transient bacteria and resident bacteria (Price, 1938). Thorough handwashing with soap removes the transient bacteria, but the resident bacteria found deep in the crevices of skin and under nails persist and are only removed after prolonged handwashing using an antiseptic (Gould, 1994a). The aim of routine handwashing then is to remove or at least substantially reduce the number of transient bacteria, which are so easily transferrable from one's hand to a patient or client and are the reason for most cases of cross-infection (Gould, 1992). In particular the important role of handwashing after nappy changing and toilet use with young children and babies has been found to reduce the spread of enteric infections in day care nurseries (Worsley *et al.*, 1994). However, despite teaching and reinforcement, McFarlane (1990) suggests that the handwashing message appears to have a limited effect, and this appears to be borne out in health care research.

Handwashing should be carried out every time a health care worker moves from one patient to another, and even between performing different procedures on the same patient.

▶ *Methods of Handwashing*

The method of handwashing is determined by the type of procedure to be undertaken, with the type of handwashing agent, length of handwash and method of hand-drying needing to be selected as appropriate. Table 1.3.9 shows a summary of the three categories of handwashing.

The procedure for handwashing must include a thorough and effective technique, ensuring that all surfaces of the hands come into contact with the washing solution (Fig. 1.3.4)

RESEARCH BASED EVIDENCE

Taylor (1978a) studied the handwashing techniques of all grades of nursing staff using a dye method. The nurses closed their eyes and washed their hands using a dye. The washes were timed and the areas of the hands not covered by the dye marked onto charts. From a total of 129 observed handwashes, 89% of the nurses missed some parts of the hand surface. The mean time spent handwashing was lowest for trained staff.

In a second study by Taylor (1978b), *infection control nurses carried out a survey in seven hospitals observing the handwashing practices of nurses on medical and surgical wards. The results showed that nurses often failed to distinguish between dirty and clean tasks and that the length of time of the handwash was more important than the quality. This study also confirmed that coverage of the skin during the handwash was often inadequate.*

DECISION MAKING

When next out on clinical placement watch and take note of how other nurses are washing their hands.
1. *Consider their technique – is it a quick wash or do they take time and ensure that they wash all the surfaces of their hands?*
2. *Note the handwash solution they use and how they dry their hands.*

3. *A study by Taylor (1978a) observing the handwashing techniques of all grades of nursing staff, highlighted the fact that many failed to ensure that all parts of the hands were washed. This is particularly important when using an alcoholic handrub as alcohol lacks viscosity and slips easily over the skin: it is*

therefore difficult to maintain adequate contact with all the surfaces of the skin. In the light of this study's findings, consider how you might alter your handwashing practice in the future to ensure that your technique is good.

RESEARCH BASED EVIDENCE

Gould et al. (1996) confirm that nurses are still failing to wash their hands when they should. They collected data from two London hospitals and showed that hands were decontaminated only after 28.7% of patient contacts. Performance was considered to be related to nursing workload and the availability of hand decontaminating agents.

Type	Methods	Use
Social (to remove dirt and transient organisms)	Use liquid or bar soap and thoroughly wash with soap and water. Dry with a paper towel	Before starting work, eating and drinking, feeding a patient, leaving work. After visiting the toilet, helping a patient with toiletting, handling patients and bedlinen, cleaning equipment and furniture, between each patient.
Hygienic (to remove or destroy all or most transient organisms)	Use antiseptic soap or detergent (e.g. chlorhexidine) and either wash thoroughly for 15–30 seconds using antiseptic and water and dry with a paper towel (a sterile towel may be required) or apply 5–10 ml of alcohol handrub, ensuring all areas of the hand and fingers are in good contact with the rub, and leave to dry naturally	Before any procedure involving a high-risk patient, all procedures requiring an aseptic technique (e.g. dressing, catheterization). After contact with infected patients, handling contaminated equipment and materials.
Surgical (to remove and destroy transient organisms and reduce detachable resident organisms – a prolonged effect is required)	Antiseptic soap (e.g. chlorhexidine) and water. Brush nails and wash hands and forearms using a defined technique for a minimum of three minutes. Dry with a sterile towel. Alternatively wash hands with soap and water and after drying rub in a minimum of 5 ml of an alcohol handrub (as above).	Before surgery and aseptic techniques for invasive procedures.

Table 1.3.9 Methods of handwashing.

▶ *Length of Handwash*

The ideal duration of a handwash has not been determined. Times of 30 seconds (Bowell, 1992) and 15–20 seconds for the whole procedure (Ayliffe *et al.*, 1982, p. 62) have been put forward. Gould (1994a) suggests a time of 20–30 seconds would be ideal.

▶ *Handwashing Agent*

The type of handwashing agent is important and as Table 1.3.9 shows depends upon the method of handwashing being undertaken. When using soap or a medicated agent the mechanical action of using running water with them appears to be just as important. Although the use of soap and water has been found to be sufficient for removing most transient bacteria, a wet bar soap can itself become a source of infection and become contaminated with gram-negative bacilli (Blackmore, 1987). Some studies show that a prolonged wash using disinfectants such as chlorhexidine and iodine create a bactericidal effect (Nicoletti *et al.*, 1990). However, the type of handwash used might be simply based upon a nurse's preference: a study undertaken by Ojajarvi (1981) found that not all soaps are favourably accepted by nurses.

▶ *Hand Drying*

Hand drying also plays an important part in the control of infection (Gould, 1994b). Wet surfaces transfer microorganisms more effectively

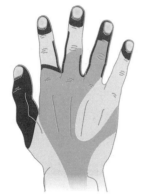

Back

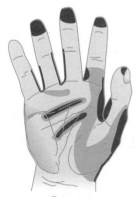

Front

■ Less frequently missed

■ More frequently missed

Figure 1.3.4: Area of hand surface missed during hand washing.

than dry surfaces (Gould, 1994a), and are an important medium for the growth of microorganisms (Gould, 1987). Four methods of hand-drying are commonly available:

▶ hand towels;
▶ roller towels;
▶ paper towels;
▶ warm air hand driers.

Blackmore (1987) recommends the use of paper towels as the most suitable method for hand drying in clinical areas. They have a particularly important role when less effective hand decontamination agents have been used, especially following a less thorough hand wash (Gould, 1994b). Blackmore and Prisk (1984) showed cloth towels to be slightly more efficient at removing bacteria, but overall paper towels were found to be safer to use from a cross-infection angle because they are single-use items. For cloth towels to be as safe as paper towels in the prevention of cross-infection they need to be used as single-use items and laundered after each use. Weiler (1965, cited in Blackmore, 1987) considered warm air driers to be less safe than paper towels because although they initially reduced bacteria the hands quickly became contaminated again by bacteria being fanned around in the current of warm air.

▶ *Recontamination*

Hands can become recontaminated immediately after washing and drying if a dirty surface (such as the waste bin) is touched when throwing the towel away. It is therefore important to have foot pedal-operated bins to dispose of paper towels.

▶ SAFE DISPOSAL OF CLINICAL MATERIAL

Each year hospitals produce thousands of tons of waste (Gibbs, 1990). Some, termed 'household rubbish' can be disposed of at a local council waste or landfill site. However, much is termed 'clinical waste' and must be incinerated. It is imperative that all rubbish is disposed of safely and correctly to ensure that neither health carers nor clients are at risk of causing infection or becoming infected themselves. The disposal of clinical waste is an important issue wherever clients are being cared for. In the community it is becoming an increasing problem as more clients receive nursing care in their own home.

Gibbs (1991) has defined clinical waste as including:

▶ soiled surgical dressings, swabs and instruments;
▶ material other than linen from infectious disease cases;
▶ all human and animal tissue, excretion and blood;
▶ discarded syringes, needles, broken glass and sharp surgical instruments;
▶ pharmaceutical and chemical products;
▶ used disposable bedpan liners, urine containers;
▶ incontinence pads, sanitary pads, tampons;
▶ all items contaminated with human and animal excretion or blood.

In the hospital, clinical material is normally divided into three categories:

▶ rubbish (disposed into a refuse bag);

Think about a placement that has involved you visiting a client's home. Identify the different types of clinical waste that were produced, for example wound dressings.

How were these disposed of?

Were they disposed of by the nurse or the client?

If by the client, were you aware of any special arrangements required for the disposal of clinical disposal?

Some health authorities organize special rubbish collections for clinical-type waste such as colostomy bags.

▶ sharps;
▶ soiled linen.

The first two are actually treated as rubbish, and the soiled linen, although not usually disposed of, must be equally carefully handled to ensure that it does not infect health care workers before being washed.

Following the lifting of crown immunity in 1988, all NHS premises must comply with legislation and regulations regarding waste disposal. Since 1982 Government guidelines (Department of Health and Social Security, 1982) have recommended a colour coding system of rubbish bags for the disposal of all hazardous waste (Gibbs, 1990). It recommended yellow bags for clinical waste and black for domestic (nonclinical) rubbish.

▶ Handling and Disposal of Sharps

For the disposal of sharps the same 1982 Government guidelines (Department of Health and Social Security, 1982) recommend the use of a purpose-made sharps disposal box that conforms to a British standard. However, needlestick injuries are still being reported by staff handling rubbish bags, indicating that health care workers are still disposing of clinical material incorrectly. Domestics and portering staff are two of the most vunerable groups for receiving a sharps injury (Sadler, 1990). Obtaining accurate figures for sharps injuries is difficult because all grades of staff underreport such injuries (The British Medical Association, 1990).

The disposal of all sharps is the personal responsibility of the users. It is imperative that all staff, irrespective of the care setting (e.g. hospital, general practice, nursing home or private home) follow a set policy in the safe handling and disposal of all sharps. Under the *Health and Safety at Work Act* (Department of Health, 1974) all care workers have a responsibility to prevent injury to others, and this must include the safe disposal of sharps. Studies show that many of the injuries taking place could be prevented.

Sadler (1988) reported a 1985 World Health Organization AIDS update that suggested that over 40% of sharps injuries could be prevented if recommended precautions were followed in their use and disposal.

All sharps policies should include guidelines about:

▶ the handling of used needles (e.g. not resheathing);
▶ the care and handling of the sharps box (e.g. not overfilling, correct method of closure);
▶ the disposal of the box;
▶ what to do in the event of a needlestick injury (e.g. encouraging

DECISION MAKING

When next out in clinical practice carry out an audit to help you identify situations where a practice might be improved.

For example, are there places where you consider a sharps box ought to be available or boxes that are overfilled?

If you found an unsafe practice consider who (e.g. ward staff, practice link teacher, personal teacher) might you speak to about it?

bleeding from the puncture site, washing the area, covering with a waterproof dressing, documenting the incident and informing the manager and occupational health).

▶ *Laundry*

The regulations surrounding the handling and washing of laundry are based on Department of Health (1987) guidelines that require a national colour code for laundry bags and standards in the laundry for heat disinfection (Taylor, 1992). Such guidelines should ensure that all workers who handle laundry do not come into contact with it until after it has been heat disinfected. Care in the disposal of linen should be a priority for health carers. However, not only do linen bags carry a risk of cross-contamination from pathogens, but they have also been found to contain more than just linen. Taylor reported a range of material found in linen bags, including surgical instruments, watches, patients' glasses, and cutlery (Taylor, 1992).

▶ PROTECTIVE CLOTHING

Consider any placements where you have cared for children and where they had to be nursed using protective clothing. Were any strategies used to make the children less frightened? For example were teddies and dolls dressed up in similar gowns and hats as those worn by the nurses? Think back to the clothing the children had to wear to go to the operating theatre. Did they wear operating gowns, and if so were they more child friendly, perhaps by being decorated with pictures?

The use of protective clothing, a third specific practice in the control and prevention of infection, must not be used in isolation to other practices, and in particular to handwashing. Under the *Personal Protective Equipment at Work Regulations* (Health and Safety Commission, 1992) all employers must ensure that protective clothing is available, and under the *Health and Safety at Work Act,* such protective clothing should be worn (Department of Health, 1974). Protective clothing may be worn following an assessment of the possibility of direct contact with blood, body fluids or excreta (*Nursing Times,* 1995) or as part of the Universal Precautions. Items of protection include gloves, aprons or gowns, eye protectors, hats, masks, special shoes and overshoes.

Although the use of protective clothing may be important, it must not be forgotten that such protection can be very alarming to the public. Therefore care needs to be taken in explaining the rationale for protective clothing to both the client and their relatives.

Protective clothing is worn by health care workers for a variety of reasons, which include the following:

▶ to prevent the user's clothing or uniform from becoming contaminated (soiled, wet or stained) with pathogenic organisms;
▶ to prevent the transfer of pathogenic organisms to another person or inanimate object;
▶ to prevent the user from acquiring an infection from the patient or client.

The literature has looked at the usefulness of the nurse's uniform as a means of protective clothing. Some argue that personal clothing is acceptable as long as it is practical, clean and washable (Walker and Donaldson, 1993). The results of research into whether nurses' uniforms pose a real risk of transmitting infection is so far inconclusive: Shwarze (1986) found that uniforms were associated with the spread of infection, but Hawkey and Clark (1990) found no difference between swabs taken from uniformed nurses and those out of uniform.

The use of disposable gloves and plastic aprons are the most popular, and possibly the most effective items of protective clothing (Wilson, 1990;

Bowell, 1993). However, if worn incorrectly (e.g. if a plastic apron is not changed between patients) they can become vehicles of infection instead of preventing infection (Bowell, 1993).

▶ *Gloves*

Gloves have been identified as being very important in protecting staff from patient pathogens, in particular from HIV and hepatitis B (Thomas, 1994). They must be worn to prevent infection of both the user and the patient. It is therefore imperative that gloves are worn for:

▶ any aseptic invasive procedure;
▶ any practice that involves the handling of blood and body fluids, including procedures such as the emptying of urinary catheter bags and the handling of dirty linen, soiled dressings, colostomy bags, and incontinence pads.

Gloves are, however, not a substitute for handwashing, which should always be carried out following their removal (Bowell, 1993).

The quality and effectiveness of disposable gloves vary widely. A knowledge of the different types – plastic, latex, vinyl, sterile and unsterile – is important so that the user selects the most appropriate glove according to the level of risk of the contaminant and task being performed.

When wearing gloves Brookes (1994) cites the following six imperatives:

▶ use high quality gloves;
▶ choose the right glove for the job; ·
▶ wash hands after removing one pair and putting on a new pair;
▶ never reuse gloves;
▶ change gloves when noticing a defect;
▶ keep fingernails short to avoid punctures.

> Reflect upon situations where you have observed staff wearing gloves.
>
> *Were you aware of any rationale for the use of specific types of glove such as a hospital or trust protocol or guideline ?*

The actual technique or procedure for putting on sterile gloves is quite complex, but very important, especially before a surgical procedure (e.g. in the operating theatre). If when putting on the gloves the wearer accidentally touches a surface that is not sterile, the outside of the gloves, which will later be in direct contact with sterile instruments and body tissues will have become contaminated, and a vehicle of infection. The scrubbing up procedure, which lasts several minutes, would have become a futile exercise (Brookes, 1994). For this reason gloves are put on in such a way that the outside of the glove never comes into contact with the hand being put inside the glove. For although the hand has been washed using an antiseptic for several minutes it will not be as sterile as the glove itself, which has undergone a very strict sterilizing procedure. In order to fully understand this quite complex procedure, watch a qualified practitioner working in an operating theatre putting on sterile gloves or a video that clearly demonstrates this practice.

> **DECISION MAKING**
>
> Read any 'glove use' policy. Many hospitals now have one to rationalize the use of expensive gloves. Compare this policy with your observations in practice placements to decide whether it is being followed effectively.

▶ *Aprons*

Aprons have been cited as an important and effective item in the prevention of cross-infection (Curran, 1991; Worsley *et al.*, 1994; *Nursing Times*, 1995).The cotton apron, once a common feature of the nurse's uniform, fails to provide an effective barrier to organisms and offers no protection to the user against moisture and wetness (Worsley *et al.*, 1994). Disposable plastic aprons are therefore the apron of choice as they are impervious to both moisture and organisms and cheap to use. However, as

Reflect on your recent clinical placements and identify when you wore an apron.

Was the apron used to protect you or the patient? How often did you change the apron and what was the rationale for using a new one?

Paediatric nurses often wear brightly coloured tabards over their uniform or own clothes. If you are out in a placement where this is the practice, notice whether they wear a plastic apron over it or whether they appear to substitute the tabard for a plastic apron.

with gloves they can become a vehicle of infection if not used correctly. It is therefore imperative that the apron is changed after giving care to one patient that might be capable of causing infection through direct or indirect contact before giving care to another patient.

Curran (1991) recommends that an apron is changed after:

▶ bedmaking;
▶ total patient care;
▶ aseptic technique;
▶ toileting patients;
▶ dirty tasks;
▶ feeding patients and giving meals.

An apron should be used for only one patient and then be disposed of; the nurse's hands should then be washed and a new apron put on before attending to a new patient (Curran, 1991).

It is now recommended that the disposable apron worn during the serving and distributing of food should be a different colour to that worn for other purposes (Bowell, 1993).

▶ Gowns

Gowns are mostly used in the operating theatre and delivery suite where the risk of potential contamination from blood and blood products is very high. Many are still made from cotton, which provides very little protection from infection (Bowell, 1993). If worn, a plastic disposable apron should be worn underneath or they should be replaced by a disposable gown made from a waterproof material. However, increasingly, gowns made from fabrics such as gortex are being used as they provide the necessary waterproof protection, but have the side effect of being uncomfortably warm to wear.

A recent study has proved that plastic aprons are more effective in the prevention of contamination of nurses' uniforms than the traditional cotton gown when caring for a patient with an infection (Wilson, 1990).

▶ Eye Protection

Eye protection should be worn when there is a risk of blood splashing onto mucous membranes or the conjunctiva. Special glasses, goggles or visors may be used in the operating theatre, dentistry and endoscopy. Eye guards also offer protection against splashes of the chemicals that are often used in the sterilization and disinfection of endoscopes and other surgical instruments (Worsley *et al.*, 1994).

Other items of protective clothing have traditionally involved the wearing of masks, hats and overshoes. Studies now consistently show these are of little use in the prevention of infection (Jones and Jakeways, 1988; Lee, 1988; Bowell, 1993; Worsley *et al.*, 1994) and may even assist in spread.

▶ Masks

Masks are rarely worn today outside the operating theatre with research now questioning whether masks need to be worn in many situations, including operating theatres (Worsley *et al.*, 1994). Previously the rationale for wearing a mask was to protect the patient from getting an infection from the staff, but if a member of staff has a cold or sore throat the mask is inappropriate as the member of staff should not be on duty.

Today the rationale for wearing a mask is to protect the user from splashes of blood and body fluids.

▶ *Hats*

Hats seem to be 'something of a white elephant' (Lee, 1988). Nurses have traditionally worn hats, with some still considering them to be linked to hygiene and a method of keeping hair tidy (Lee, 1988). The same study showed that hats are frequently touched during practice and are infrequently changed, leading the author to believe that it is time the old ritual of wearing a hat was forgotten. However, hats are still worn in the operating theatre department where they remain an important infection control measure.

▶ *Overshoes*

Overshoes are similarly considered unnecessary in the prevention of infection. Traditionally all visitors entering operating theatre departments and other units caring for immunocompromised patients put on a pair of paper or plastic overshoes. Jones and Jakeways (1988) reporting on a number of studies undertaken into the usefulness of overshoes concluded that disposable overshoes do not reduce bacterial floor contamination and found no firm evidence to suggest that the wearing of disposable overshoes helped in the control and prevention of infections. They concluded that the use of such overshoes was an expensive practice that ought to be abandoned. Carter (1990) cited hazards associated with the wearing of overshoes, which included the dispersal of bacteria from them when walking and the transfer of bacteria from the person's own shoes to hands when removing the overshoes.

▶ ASEPTIC TECHNIQUE

This is the fourth specific practice that is considered to be instrumental in the prevention of infection. Aseptic means that the procedure or technique 'will be done in such a way as to avoid introducing micro-organisms into a vulnerable site' (Ayliffe *et al.*, 1982, p. 48). Examples of procedures include wound dressings, giving of injections, catheterization, and setting up an intravenous infusion. The method and equipment for a specific procedure varies from hospital to hospital and health authority to health authority, but the principles of asepsis remain, in that the particular procedure will be undertaken in such a way that organisms will not be introduced into the treatment site.

In the past there has been much routine and ritual surrounding an aseptic technique. There continues to be much debate and discussion over issues such as the correct way of setting up a dressing trolley and how many pairs of forceps are needed (Kelso, 1989). However, certain principles must be upheld and it is then arguable whether one method or approach is any better than another. The principles should include:

▶ suitable handwashing;
▶ use of sterile packs, equipment and solutions;
▶ the appropriate use of gloves;
▶ maintenance of asepsis (not introducing infection) and a sterile field throughout the procedure.

In addition to the maintenance of an aseptic technique while carrying

---

DECISION MAKING

Observe a practice that requires the use of an aseptic technique. Consider the principles stated above and how they are upheld. *For example which handwashing procedure is undertaken and what type of glove (if any) is used?*
At the end of your observation decide whether any of the principles were breached in any way?
For example did a nurse touch something that was not sterile such as the trolley?
Consider the possible consequences in relation to infection control.

out the procedure, it is important that the site (e.g. a surgical wound, intravenous cannula or urinary catheter) is cared for to prevent the entry or exit of infection. For example, the use of a clear film occlusive dressing over a surgical wound or intravenous cannula allows examination of the site without removing the dressing (Spencer and Bale, 1990; Keenlyside, 1992), while placing a catheter bag below the level of the patient's bladder ensures there is no backflow of urine and infection that could result from this is avoided (Brown, 1992).

▶ PERSONAL AND GENERAL HYGIENE

Attention to personal health is very important in the prevention of infection. Staff carrying an infection increase the risk to patients who are particularly at risk. Although all patients may be at risk, the very young, the very old and the acutely ill are at particular risk.

Occupational health departments should be available to offer staff advice and support. In particular, staff who have any symptoms of diarrhoea or vomiting must be seen and passed fit and free of infection before returning to work.

Staff may also be symptomless carriers of infection (e.g. methicillin-resistant *Staphylococcus aureus*, HIV or hepatitis virus). If a member of staff has any suspicions that they have been infected or are a carrier it is imperative that they seek medical advice, and again the occupational health department should be able to provide advice and specialist support and help. Under the *Code of Professional Conduct* (UKCC, 1992) every registered nurse is personally accountable to ensure that no action is detrimental to patients (clause 2).

Personal hygiene must also include the care of any uniform worn while caring for patients and clients. Uniforms should never be worn when off duty and ideally staff should remove their uniform before leaving their place of work and wear their own clothes to travel home in. Otherwise the uniform should be completely covered by a coat. Uniforms (dresses, tabards, tunics) should be changed daily and sent to the hospital laundry. Hospital policies may well suggest that a temperature of 60°C is used for washing uniforms.

▶ *Skin Abrasions*

Attention must be paid to any breaks in the skin of staff that may be in direct contact with the patient (e.g. hands). Waterproof dressings should cover all cuts, abrasions and lesions. Staff with dermatological conditions that cause areas of skin to become broken should assess very carefully whether they are putting themselves at risk from contamination with blood and body fluids. Such staff should seek advice from the occupational health department.

Whenever a health care worker suspects or has a needlestick injury, an accident or untoward incident form must be completed. It is important that the manager and occupational health department is informed of the incident so that the worker can be given appropriate care and advice and action can be taken to prevent the incident occurring again. All qualified nurses are personally accountable for their own practice and have a duty to ensure that the health and safety of colleagues is not put at risk (UKCC, 1992, clause 13).

▶ EVALUATION

Evaluation is the fourth stage of the Nursing Process and involves measuring the effectiveness of nursing care. It has been a neglected area of study with the consequence that nurses have not become as familiar with this stage as the other three, and often regard evaluation as difficult (Kratz, 1979). However, without evaluation, Kratz (1979) maintains that the nurse cannot have the information needed to improve quality of care and practice. Methods of evaluation are used by many nurses in their everyday practice and are used to decide whether the nursing care given is assisting patients in their recovery. For example, clinical measurements such as the measurement of temperature can be used to find out whether the nursing care is effective for the patient with a raised temperature caused by an infection.

Like assessment, evaluation also involves the collection of information. However, whereas information collected during assessment is of a general nature, the data collected during the evaluation stage are more specific and often linked to a specific patient goal. Therefore data collected during evaluation can only be collected after the care has been planned and the nursing actions undertaken.

In infection control the process of evaluation, as in other areas of nursing, has to be regular and ongoing. It must be carried out on a regular basis to discern whether a particular practice is effective in the prevention or control of an infection.

Evaluation in the form of a comparison of a patient's response to a treatment with the expected outcomes determines the success of nursing practice. Many areas of care are evaluated every time a nurse attends a patient. For example, a nurse will evaluate the extent of healing when dressing an infected pressure sore by measuring the size and observing the amount, colour and smell of exudate. In this way the nurse is determining and evaluating the success of the treatment and nursing intervention.

Accurate documentation is required at each stage of the Nursing Process. Evaluations of care are particularly important to provide other nurses with a baseline for future comparative evaluations. This way it can be determined whether there is a decrease or increase of infection and the response to treatment and care can be reported.

In the assessment stage audit often provides baseline information about a clinical area or practice that helps determine the risk of infection to a patient or member of staff. However, in evaluation, the information collected during an audit can provide information to help determine the effect and success of infection prevention and control strategies used in the clinical area or area of practice. For example, a patient area such as a ward might have had a regular monthly assessment audit for years, but following an outbreak of a specific infection an audit might be carried out to evaluate whether infection control procedures were effective in containing the infection and preventing its spread.

The issue of hospital-acquired infections, although difficult to quantify accurately, remains an important problem and an area of much concern to infection control nurses. Yet despite the use of many nursing practices to control and prevent infection, there is little formal evaluation of them because of a lack of an identified 'feasible and sensitive method of recording infections' (Glennister, 1990, p. 46).

This section has only outlined the major aspects of nursing knowledge in relation to infection control that ought to be considered when carrying out various nursing practices and procedures. A more in depth understanding of particular nursing practices can be obtained from a range of clinical nursing care books, but to keep up to date with changes in practice specialist nursing journals should be consulted regularly.

PROFESSIONAL KNOWLEDGE

This third section is concerned with issues surrounding personal and professional knowledge in the area of infection control.

▶ PERSONAL AND PROFESSIONAL ISSUES

Personal and professional issues are clearly stated in the *Code of Professional Conduct* (UKCC, 1992). In this it states that every registered nurse, midwife and health visitor is personally accountable for their own practice. When used in the context of infection control several of the clauses in the code show that nurses clearly have several areas of direct responsibility as follows:

▶ to ensure safety of patients and clients (clause 2);
▶ to acknowledge personal limitations of knowledge and competence (clause 4);
▶ to work in cooperation with other health care professionals (clause 6);
▶ to report when the health and safety of colleagues are at risk (clause 13).

In the control of infection nurses have the responsibility to educate and inform others, including both the patient and their family (*Nursing Times*, 1995). Nurses have to demonstrate a wide range of infection control practices (e.g. aseptic techniques in the care of wound dressings, urinary catheters and intravenous cannula sites) as well as the knowledge to enhance a patient's general or specific resistance to infection. Good general hygiene may be required in the form of oral hygiene or adequate diet for patients who are particularly susceptible to infections through a lowered immunity (e.g. patients with HIV infection). Specific resistance might be needed by some to protect against and control a particular infection (e.g. the influenza virus) by giving immunization.

A third area of personal and professional responsibility is to remain up to date with new practices, which are often made clear through guidelines, policies and legislation. The *Professional Code of Conduct* (UKCC, 1992) cites this responsibility (clause 3), with nurses being required to maintain and improve their professional knowledge and competence.

A working knowledge of important and relevant health and safety guidelines is needed to help in the control of infection. For example, legislation laid down in the *Health and Safety at Work Act* (Department of Health, 1974) states that while the employer has responsibility to ensure protective clothing is available for use, all employees have a personal responsibility to use and wear the protective clothing provided.

Wherever patients and clients are receiving care, poor practice might put control of infection in jeopardy, therefore there need to be policies and guidelines. These need to be written, available for referring to, and put into practice by all staff (nursing, medical and ancillary). Such policies and guidelines require regular monitoring by staff and management to ensure that they are current and in line with new national and European legislation and policies.

A further area of personal responsibility is that of self care. All health care workers should ensure that they are self-protected from infections

---

Reflect upon a clinical placement and consider a situation where you felt the nurse failed to uphold clauses 2 and 13 of their code of conduct in relation to infection control.

Why do you think this happened and what might the result have been to the patient's eventual outcome of care?

DECISION MAKING

When out in clinical practice look for the policies and guidelines appropriate to health and safety, and in particular for infection control, for example a policy for emptying a catheter bag. Select a particular policy and notice when it was last updated. If it was more than five years ago, carry out a brief literature search of recent studies into the same subject area. Then try to identify whether in the light of specific research particular changes need to be made to the policy. If you think there should be changes, who might you approach about this?

Consider a practice situation when you were involved in the care of a vulnerable group of patients or clients, for example elderly and confused clients or people with learning disabilities.

In what ways were you able to act as their advocate in the giving of their care and so reduce the risk of them getting an infection?

Were you for example ever able to speak up on their behalf so that they were better understood?

through immunizations and know where they can get advice and guide-lines regarding practice. For example immunization against hepatitis B is widely available from occupational health units, thereby allowing staff who are at risk from contamination with blood to receive protection. A second area of self care results when a member of staff has been in contact with an infection, and although not detrimental to themselves, may be detrimental to other patients who are already ill. For example, staff in contact with methicillin-resistant *Staphylococcus aureus*, may be required to ensure they have not been infected themselves before moving to another ward or area of care.

Acting as an advocate, particularly for vulnerable groups, is an issue that many nurses need to uphold in the area of infection control. Some patients and clients may be particularly vulnerable to infections, but be unaware of the issue themselves. In this situation the nurse or carer must be able to speak up on behalf of their patient or client and ensure that the care being given will not put the individual or group at risk from getting an infection. For example, a child or a person with a learning disability may not recognize the importance of washing hands after using the toilet or before eating a meal. Therefore the carer needs to ensure that this is done, thereby protecting the patient or client from a gastro-intestinal infection.

▶ ETHICAL ISSUES

Personal care by nurses to prevent infection is also an ethical issue. The declaration of personal health status by nurses and other health care workers is an important debatable ethical issue. On the one hand by not declaring a particular illness, a nurse could be putting a patient at risk from an infection. For example, if a nurse is known to be HIV positive and is applying for a job in a critical care unit such as the operating department, it might be argued by some that the nurse is potentially putting patients and staff at risk. Others would argue that as long as the nurse is aware of the importance of the potential causes of cross-conta-mination of blood and blood products and upholds good infection control practices, patients and staff would not be at risk.

Occupational health units have the responsibility to ensure that all staff employed are free from illness and infection, and nurses have an ethical responsibility to provide an honest health declaration. However, this will inevitably mean that for a minority of staff it might be difficult to secure a job because of a specific condition such as HIV infection.

Confidentiality is an ethical issue in infection control for staff and patients. A patient with an infection may wish to keep it confidential and not inform family and friends. However, the ethical debate over whether the patient is putting those they come into close contact with at risk requires examination. As in the previous paragraph, this is commonly seen with HIV infection. Such a patient may demand that their condition is kept confidential, but the potential risk of infecting those they come into close contact with, such as a sexual partner or carers, needs to be assessed.

Nurses have to recognize and accept that patients have the right to confidentiality over their health and professionally uphold clause 10 of their code of practice (UKCC, 1992). However, this same clause also admits that disclosure might be required in the wider public interest. This issue of confidentiality is very difficult to resolve, and in the area

Spend a few moments reflecting upon a situation in clinical practice where there was a dilemma over confidentiality, for example a time when a patient or client's diagnosis was discussed within the hearing of other patients instead of in the privacy of a ward office.

of infection control there will remain many areas requiring ethical and professional debate.

▶ POLITICAL ISSUES

There is a range of political issues associated with infection control and financial implications are often central to them. The government has legislated within the framework of the *Health and Safety at Work Act* (Department of Health, 1974) that health care professionals implement a range of policies and regulations. Central to these are infection control policies, which are often considered expensive to implement. For this reason managers may disregard or only partially implement them. An example of this are the Universal Precautions for controlling and preventing bloodborne infections. In 1990 the government issued guidelines that outlined the factors to be included in universal blood and body fluid precautions (Department of Health, 1990a). However, some hospitals have not implemented them due to their enormous financial implications. From a mandatory view point under the *Health and Safety at Work Act* (Department of Health, 1974), employers are required to provide protective clothing for staff for those involved with cross-infection risks. Such protective clothing includes gloves, aprons, and visors.

Hospitals and other acute nursing service areas are often required to uphold local guidelines and policies to ensure that national legislation on infection control is maintained. For example, the disposal of clinical waste is required to adhere to not only national guidelines regarding the colour coding of bags for clinical waste, but also local policies dealing with the safe handling of rubbish bags and disposal to the incinerator (Gibbs, 1990).

Immunization programmes are another issue often surrounded by political factors. On the one hand government is encouraging the uptake of this important, but expensive infection control measure, both for the elderly and the very young, but the safety of such immunizations (e.g. for measles) has been questioned. Some parents without clear guidelines and understanding about what the safer practice is (i.e. to have the immunization or risk contracting the disease) might simply see the drive for immunizations for all babies as a political weapon.

An example of such a political weapon might be the *Health of the Nation* document (Department of Health, 1992). Since it was published the media have been repeatedly reminded of the important targets for health the government wants to have taken place by the year 2000. Again parents not understanding the importance of immunization might conceivably see the push for more immunizations as such a political target.

Other areas of infection control are also national requirements and are mandatory to ensure the environment is infection controlled. For example, the control of sewage, the provision of clean safe water, and the removal of household rubbish and waste are all central to a clean environment. However, the standard of these services is also determined by finance. They require large financial input by local and national government, but are central to the control of infection for individuals and large populations. The cost of infection if an outbreak of disease occurred due to widespread water contamination would be enormous, therefore it is politically and ethically correct that such control on water is maintained.

In recent years one particular infection that has caused serious financial implications for many hospitals, trusts and health authorities is methicillin-resistant *Staphylococcus aureus* infection. This infection is now considered by some to be of epidemic proportion and has caused an extra financial strain on infection control resources in hospitals and nursing homes. One way of handling it might be to screen all patients admitted to hospital so that infection control precautions can be implemented immediately. A second method would be to use the Universal Precautions principle and treat all patients as if they have the infection, but this would obviously have enormous financial, moral and ethical implications. Yet this is the direction in which some hospitals are moving when deciding to implement Universal Precautions for all situations involving blood and body fluids.

▶ ROLE OF THE INFECTION CONTROL TEAM

Infection control teams are important at district level and within individual hospitals and care units. In England and Wales there are District Health Authorities, each containing at least one general hospital of about 600 beds for acutely ill patients (Ayliffe *et al.*, 1992, p. 12). The district is also responsible for community health and may include specialist hospitals and chronic care settings. The control of infection within the district is managed by the Director of Public Health and the Consultant in Communicable Disease Control (CCDC) (Worsley *et al.*, 1994). The CCDC is the leader for communicable diseases and doctors are legally responsible to notify the CCDC after attending a patient with a notifiable disease.

Many hospital trusts have an infection control team consisting of an infection control doctor, usually a microbiologist, an infection control nurse(s) and other members of staff with a special interest and knowledge of infection control. Some hospitals have ward- and department-based nurses who have a specific interest in infection control and are able to provide a very important link between the ward and infection control team in the education of staff and upholding good practice at clinical level.

▶ ENVIRONMENTAL HEALTH

Infection control is also concerned with 'environmental health', cited by the World Health Organization in 1950 as 'the control of all factors in the environment which exercise a harmful effect on human physical development, health and survival' (Worsley *et al.*, 1994, p. 85). In England the mandatory enforcement of environmental health is a function of local government with qualified environmental health officers and technical support staff. However, as with other areas of infection control, environmental health, as in the notification of communicable diseases, is a role for all health care professionals. While it is the doctor who is legally responsible for notifying particular communicable diseases, much of the surveillance work is undertaken by nurses, for example, the practice nurse in the health centre or a district nurse and health visitor as they visit patients and clients and their families in their own homes. Other places where informal surveillance can take place are in nursing homes, for example staff may report cases of influenza or gastroenteritis so that the situation can be monitored or investigated.

DECISION MAKING

Find out who is in the Infection Control Team while on a placement in a hospital and during a community-based allocation.

Have you been aware of the role of the Infection Control Nurse where you have been in clinical practice?

Find out what happens when an outbreak of infection occurs, both in the hospital and in the community.

Other areas of environmental health work include management of pollutants which have already been addressed as hazards in Chapter 1.1. Air pollution, noise, food hazards, health and safety and housing standards are all aspects subject to environmental control, as are control of infectious diseases, rodent and pest control, hazardous waste disposal and local authority licensing and registration to ensure the health, safety and welfare of the public. Most of the work undertaken by environmental health officers is covered by statute and enables them to have the right of entry to establishments and to prosecute offenders. Their work normally involves both surveillance through routine inspections and targeting to deal with specific issues.

Food safety is one area of specific importance with increasing cases of food poisoning reported in recent years. Routine inspection and surveillance regarding food safety covers people, practices and premises, and is controlled under recent legislation, the *Food Safety Act* (Department of Health, 1990b).

Water used for drinking and leisure use (e.g. swimming pools) is a second important area of environmental infection control. Recent outbreaks of legionnaires' disease have been linked to natural and manmade water systems including air-conditioning systems, cooling towers and extensive plumbing of hotels and office blocks.

A third area is the licensing and registration of various activities, premises and persons to ensure that the health and welfare of the public using them is protected; for example, to ensure that safe practices of hygiene and sterilization are maintained when equipment is used for acupuncture, tattooing, ear piercing and electrolysis.

The environmental health service was introduced in the nineteenth century and despite better health care and improvement in the environment, the challenges facing environmental health officers are as difficult as 100 years ago. This is probably due to the fact that the need for the prevention and control of infection is increasing (Worsley *et al.*, 1994).

This section was aimed at helping you understand the personal and professional responsibility you have to help control infection. As a qualified nurse, midwife or health visitor you have a duty and personal responsibility in this area of nursing practice. It is certainly an enormous task for any one person, but by working together as a team of health care professionals, whether in hospital or the community, it is possible to uphold professional and personal standards that promote the prevention of infection.

This chapter has considered some of the important issues concerning infection control, a fundamental principle that must underpin all nursing practices. Although the prevention and control of infection are commonly perceived as issues that only affects the hospital patient and health care professionals caring for them, this chapter has demonstrated that they are increasingly important aspects of care in the community and issues that affect all, irrespective of age. Failure to prevent or control an infection may seriously affect the health of an individual or fail to ensure the health and safety of the health care worker.

Increasingly nurses are required to educate patients and clients about the control of infection. In order to undertake such a role, it is essential to have a knowledge of the different microorganisms capable of causing infections and their modes of transmission, the environment in which microorganisms thrive, and the body's response to infection.

Today many nurses work in multicultural societies and groups where behaviour and attitude towards infection control are not seen to hold the same level of importance. Therefore an awareness of different behaviours and attitudes, beliefs and practices towards infection is often required in order to understand why individuals take risks or appear not to understand, accept or be influenced by infection control practices. The use of the health belief model described in the Psychosocial section of Subject Knowledge is one way that changes in behaviour and attitude might be implemented by nurses and other healthcare staff.

Nursing practice is considered to be central to the prevention and control of infection for both the indivdual patient or client as well as the nurse. Using a problem solving approach, the Nursing Process, the chapter has provided an overview of five specific practices that are widely accepted by nurses and health care professionals as being instrumental in the control and prevention of infection: these are handwashing, safe disposal of clinical material, wearing of protective clothing, aseptic technique and personal hygiene. Central to these is the principle that such practices are applied to all patients, whether they have an infection or not. Introduced from the USA, such practices are commonly termed Universal Precautions.

The nurse is only just one member of a team working towards the control and prevention of infection. While it might be the nurse who is in most direct and close contact with patients with infections, others have an equally important role to play in the area of infection control, including hospital and community infection control teams and environmental health officers. With increasingly frequent outbreaks of infection such as food poisoning in the community much of the environmental health officer's role and time is spent investigating bad practices and reported infection outbreaks, whereas their role is increasingly required to be educative and preventive. Therefore nurses working in the community also have an important role in this same field of infection control. Such nurses include school nurses, health visitors and district nurses.

Increasingly nurses are being held accountable for the care they give, and infection control is one area where nurses will be expected to uphold such accountability. With the changes in nursing education curriculum, particularly the increased emphasis on theory and the aim to develop qualified nurses who are knowledgeable practitioners (UKCC, 1986), it is hoped that the nurses of the future will be better prepared to understand the issues surrounding infection control and make an impact on the associated nursing practice.

This fourth and final section of this chapter provides you with four case study scenarios, covering the four branches of nursing – adult,

REFLECTIVE KNOWLEDGE

children's, mental health and learning disabilities. Following each are some decision making exercises to enable you to apply the subject matter of this chapter to each scenario.

▶ CASE STUDY: ADULT

Ivy Brookes is 72 years old. She is married to George who is 80 years old. They live in their own two bedroomed house. Their four children live some distance away and are all married and have children of their own. Ten years ago Ivy was diagnosed as having late-onset diabetes mellitus, which is controlled by diet and oral medication. One month ago Ivy fell and cut her left leg. The wound is healing very slowly and is now infected and the district nurse now needs to dress the wound three times a week. Up until his retirement George was employed in a local brick making firm. He always seemed to have good health and was rarely off sick. Last winter, however, he had an episode of acute bronchitis and ever since has been troubled by a cough. Chest radiographs taken three months ago revealed no acute infection, and now George is being treated by his general practitioner for chronic bronchitis.

■ **What microorganisms might be involved with these two infections – one a wound infection, the second a chest infection.**

■ **As a student nurse you are asked by the district nurse to assess Ivy and George. Which of the general and specific risk factors given in Table 1.3.8 are particularly relevant to Ivy and George?**

■ **As part of your community placement you visit Ivy with the district nurse. What specific infection control procedures would you need to consider when dressing the leg wound? How for example would you dispose of the dressings and dressing pack used? What type of protection would you need to take when tending to the wound?**

▶ CASE STUDY: CHILD

Emma Davis is two years old. She has been admitted to hospital with severe diarrhoea and vomiting. According to her mother she has been unwell for two days. She is complaining of abdominal pain and needs rehydration. The nurse admitting Emma decides that for the sake of other children on the ward she must be nursed in a side room. The staff nurse has asked you to be involved with Emma's care. How would you explain to Emma's mother the reason why she must be nursed in a side room?

■ **What is the risk of this infection to yourself, Emma's mother, other staff and other patients?**

■ **Basing your care on the five specific infection control practices discussed in the section Nursing Knowledge, how you would go about assessing, planning and implementing your care for Emma?**

▶ CASE STUDY: MENTAL HEALTH

Richard Crosby is 46 years old. He was divorced eight years ago and his wife cares for their two children aged 14 and 12 years. Over the years Richard has had several episodes of mild depression, but managed to hold down a job. Three years ago he was made redundant from his job as an electrician and since then has only had some casual work. Until recently he has been living in a flat, but was made homeless when a fire destroyed it and all his belongings. At first Richard started to sleep rough on the streets, turning to alcohol as a way of escaping from his financial problems and homelessness. He is now living in a hostel for the homeless. One of the staff members has just discovered that Richard has started to use drugs and some used needles and syringes have been found under his mattress. You are a student on placement with a community psychiatric nurse (CPN) who has been asked to see Richard.

- ■ Taking into account his alcohol ingestion and apparent use of intravenous drugs, consider the specific needs and actual problems Richard has in relation to his health.

- ■ Using Table 1.3.4, consider the ways Richard might be putting himself and others at risk of infections.

- ■ The CPN decides that Richard needs to understand more about the particular risks of infection he and others around him face. Basing this talk upon the modes of spread (airborne, direct and indirect), what are the main infection control measures you think should be included in this talk?

▶ CASE STUDY: LEARNING DISABILITIES

Kevin Roberts is 16 years old and was born with Down's syndrome. He is able to walk with help and requires a lot of help with feeding and washing. For the last ten years he has been attending special schools, but his mental ability has been slow to develop and he requires constant supervision. Kevin lives at home with his mother who is now in need of respite care. She has agreed reluctantly for Kevin to be admitted to a local home that cares for people with learning disabilities. You are a student nurse on placement at this home and are closely involved with Kevin's care.

- ■ Outbreaks of food poisoning are not uncommon in places of communal living. Using the chain of infection shown in Figure 1.3.1 as your framework, what are the different ways in which Kevin might be put at risk of getting such an infection?

- ■ One very important way of preventing infection spreading from client to client is handwashing. What are the particular situations throughout the day when you would need to remember to wash your hands while caring for Kevin?

▶ ANNOTATED FURTHER READING

AYLIFFE, G.A.J., LOWBURY, E.J., GEDDES, A.M., WILLIAMS, J.D. (1992) *Control of Hospital Infection: A Practical Handbook* (3rd edition). London. Chapman and Hall.
This provides a detailed account of the five groups of microorganisms and application of the methods of cleaning, disinfection and sterilization to clinical practice.

HEATH, H. (1994) *Foundations of Nursing Theory and Practice.* London. Mosby. Chapter 28 of this book gives a very good example of how to write a nursing care plan for a patient with an infection.

WORSLEY, M.A., WARD, K.A., PRIVETT, S., PARKER L., ROBERTS, J.M. (eds) (1994) *Infection Control. A Community Perspective.* England. Infection Control Nurses Association.
This provides a very useful discussion of infection control issues in the community. In particular it gives a good overview of some of the principles of infection control, including handwashing and protective clothing.

▶ REFERENCES

ALLEN, R.E. (1990) (ed.) *The Concise Oxford Dictionary of Current English.* p. 394. Oxford. Clarendon Press.

ASKEW, C. (1993) Auditing problems. *Nursing Times* **89(10)**: 68–72.

AYLIFFE, G.A.J., COLLINS, B.J., TAYLOR, L.J. (1982) *Hospital-Acquired Infection.* Bristol. John Wright.

AYLIFFE, G.A.J., LOWBURY, E.J., GEDDES, A.M., WILLIAMS, J.D. (1992) *Control of Hospital Infection: A Practical Handbook* (3rd edition). London. Chapman and Hall.

BLACKMORE, M.A. (1987) Hand-drying methods. *Nursing Times* **83(37)**: 71–74.

BLACKMORE, M.A., PRISK, E.M. (1984) Is hot air hygienic?. *The Home Economist* **4**: 14–15.

BOWELL, B. (1992) Hands up for cleanliness. *Nursing Standard* **6(15)**: 24–25.

BOWELL, B. (1993) Preventing infection and its spread. *Surgical Nurse* **6**: 2, 5–12.

BRITISH MEDICAL ASSOCIATION (1990) *A Code of Practice for the Safe Use and Disposal of Sharps.* London. British Medical Association.

BROOKES, A. (1994) Surgical glove perforation. *Nursing Times* **90(21)**: 60–62.

BROWN, M. (1992) Urinary catheters: patient management. *Nursing Standard* **6(19)**: 29–31.

BURNS, J. (1988) At the sharps end. *Nursing Times* **84(36)**: 75–78.

CARTER, R. (1990) Ritual and risk. *Nursing Times* **86(13)**: 63–64.

CURRAN, E. (1991) Protecting with aprons. *Nursing Times* **87(38)**: 64–68.

DEPARTMENT OF HEALTH (1974) *Health and Safety at Work Act.* London. Her Majesty's Stationery Office.

DEPARTMENT OF HEALTH (1987) *Hospital Laundry Arrangements for Used and Infected Linen.* London. Her Majesty's Stationery Office.

DEPARTMENT OF HEALTH (1989) *Working for Patients – Medical Audit* (Working Paper 6). London. Her Majesty's Stationery Office.

DEPARTMENT OF HEALTH (1990a) *HIV The Causative Agent of AIDS and Related Conditions* (2nd revision). London. Her Majesty's Stationery Office.

DEPARTMENT OF HEALTH (1990b) *Food Safety Act.* London. Her Majesty's Stationery Office.

DEPARTMENT OF HEALTH (1992) *Health of the Nation.* London. Her Majesty's Stationery Office.

DEPARTMENT OF HEALTH AND SOCIAL SECURITY (1982) *The Safe Disposal of Clinical Waste,* HN(82)22. London. Her Majesty's Stationery Office.

FAULKNER, A. (1986) Infection control: an integral part of the nursing process. *Nursing* **3**: 84–86.

FRIEDMAN, C., RICHTER, D., SKYLIS, T., BROWN, D. (1984) Process surveillance: auditing infection control policies and procedures. *American Journal of Infection Control* **12(4)**: 228–232.

GIBBS, J. (1990) Disposing of waste. *Nursing Times* **86(51)**: 34–35.

GIBBS, J. (1991) Clinical waste disposal in the community, *Nursing Times* **87(2)**: 40–41.

GLENNISTER, H. (1990) Investigating infection acquired in hospitals. *Nursing Times* **86(49)**: 46–48.

GOULD, D. (1987) *Infection and Patient Care: A Guide for Nurses.* London. Heinemann.

GOULD, D. (1992) Hygienic hand decontamination. *Nursing Standard* **6(32)**: 33–36.

GOULD, D. (1994a) Making sense of hand hygiene. *Nursing Times* **90(30)**: 63–64.

GOULD, D. (1994b) The significance of hand-drying in the prevention of infection. *Nursing Times* **90(47)**: 30–35.

GOULD, D., WILSON–BARNETT, J., REAM, E. (1996) Nurses' infection-control practice: hand decontamination, the use of gloves and sharp instruments. *International Journal of Nursing Studies* **33(2)**: 143–160.

HAWKEY, B., CLARKE, M. (1990) Dress sense or nonsense. *Nursing Times* **86(3)**: 28–31.

HEALTH AND SAFETY COMMISSION (1992) *Personal Protective Equipment at Work Regulations, Guidance on Regulations.* Leeds. Health and Safety Executive.

HEATH, H. (1994) *Foundations of Nursing Theory and Practice.* London. Mosby.

HORTON, R. (1996) Handwashing, the fundamental infection control principle. *British Journal of Nursing* **4(16)**: 926–933.

JACOBSON, J.T., *et al.* (1983) Injuries to hospital employees from needles and other sharp objects. *Infection Control* **4**: 100–102.

JONES, M., JAKEWAYS, M. (1988) Over-estimating overshoes. *Nursing Times* **84(41)**: 66–70.

KEENLYSIDE, D. (1992) Every little detail counts. *Professional Nurse* **7(4)**: 226–232.

KELSO, H. (1989) Alternative technique, *Nursing Times* **85(23)**: 70–72

KINGSLEY, A. (1992) First step towards a desired outcome. *Professional Nurse* **7(11)**: 725–729.

KRATZ, C. (ed.) (1979) *The Nursing*

Process. London. Baillière Tindall.
LEE, J. (1988) Hats off! *Nursing Times* **84(34)**: 59–61.
MCFARLANE, A. (1990) Why do we forget to remember handwashing? *Professional Nurse* **5(5)**: 250–252.
MAURER, M. (1985) *Hospital Hygiene* 3rd edition. London. Edward Arnold.
MEERS, P.D., AYLIFFE, G.A.J., EMMERSON, A.M. (1981) Report of the National Survey of Infection in Hospitals. *Journal of Hospital Infection* **2**: 23–28.
MOHLER, S.E. (1987) Passive smoking: a danger to children's health. *Journal of Pediatric Health Care* **1(6)**: 298–304.
NIGHTINGALE, F. (1854) *Notes on Nursing* (Reprint). Edinburgh. Churchill Livingstone.
NURSING TIMES (1995) Infection control. The role of the nurse. Professional Development Unit No. 21, Part 2. *Nursing Times* **91(41)**.
O'BOYLE WILLIAMS, C. (1995) The social environment. In Soule, B.M., Larson, E.L., Preston, G.A. (1995) *Infections and Nursing Practice – Prevention and Control.* Baltimore. Mosby Year Book Inc.
OJAJARVI, J. (1981) The importance of soap selection and routine hand hygiene in hospital. *Journal of Hygiene* **86**: 275.

PARKER, L. (1990) From pestilence to asepsis. *Nursing Times* **86(49)**: 63–67.
PATTERSON, B. (1990) Sharps injuries – who is at risk? *Occupational Nurse* **7**: 195–197.
PRICE, P.B. (1938) The classification of transient and resident microbes. *Journal of Infectious Diseases* **63**: 301–308.
REYBROUCK, G. (1983) The role of hands in the spread of nosocomial infections. *Journal of Hospital Infection* **4**: 103–111.
SADLER, C. (1988) Disposing of danger. *Nursing Times* **84(44)**: 48–49.
SCHWARZE, C. (1986) The safe uniform debate. *American Journal of Nursing* **86**: 956–959.
SPENCER, K.E., BALE, S. (1990) A logical approach. *Professional Nurse* **March**: 303–308.
TAYLOR, L. (1978a) An evaluation of handwashing techniques 1. *Nursing Times* **74(2)**: 54–55.
TAYLOR, L. (1978b) An evaluation of handwashing techniques 2. *Nursing Times* **74(3)**: 108–110.
TAYLOR, L. (1992) Infection control policies, *Surgical Nurse* **5**: 6–11.
TAYLOR, M. (1993) Universal precautions in the operating department. *British Journal of Theatre Nursing* **2(10)**: 4–7.

THOMAS, L. (1994) Glove story. *Nursing Times* **90(36)**: 33–35.
THOMPSON, J. (1989) Torture by tradition. *Nursing Times* **85(15)**: 16–17.
UKCC (1986) *Project 2000 – A New Preparation for Practice.* London. UKCC.
UKCC (1992) *Code of Professional Conduct.* London. UKCC.
VALANIS, B. (1986) *Epidemiology in Nursing and Health Care.* Norwalk. Appleton-Century-Crofts.
WALKER, A., DONALDSON, B. (1993) Dressing for protection. *Nursing Times* **89(2)**: 60–62.
WEILER, E. (1965) An investigation into towel hygiene. Cited in Blackmore, A.M. (1987) Hand drying methods. *Nursing Times* **83(37)**: 71–74.
WILLIAMS, E., BUCKLE, A. (1988) A lack of motivation. *Nursing Times* **84(22)**: 60–64.
WILSON, J. (1990) The price of protection. *Nursing Times* **86(26)**: 67–68.
WILSON, J., BREEDON, P. (1990) Universal precautions. *Nursing Times* **86(73)**: 67–70.
WORSLEY, M.A., WARD, K.A., PRIVETT, S., PARKER L., ROBERTS, J.M. (eds) (1994) *Infection Control. A Community Perspective.* England. Infection Control Nurses Association.

1.4 *Medicines*

C. Hall

KEY ISSUES

■ SUBJECT KNOWLEDGE
▶ a nursing definition of 'medicine'
▶ the action of medicine upon the body
▶ potential non-therapeutic action by medicines
▶ calculation of medicine dosages
▶ routes of medicine administration

■ PRACTICE KNOWLEDGE
▶ nursing knowledge for storage and administration of medicines in safety using application of research evidence
▶ assessing clients in relation to medicine administration
▶ planning to administer a medicine
▶ how medication administration can be evaluated

■ PROFESSIONAL KNOWLEDGE
▶ how errors in administration can be effectively managed
▶ the legal acts governing the storage and administration of medicines in the UK
▶ moral and ethical dilemmas that can arise within the practice of medicines' administration.

■ REFLECTIVE KNOWLEDGE
▶ application of principles of medicines administration across all branches of nursing
▶ awareness of personal position in both the giving and the using of medicines

▶ INTRODUCTION

In most nursing settings, medicines need to be administered to some of the client group for which there is responsibility. This chapter aims to introduce you to major issues considered by professional nurses in making decisions about administering medicines to their patients.

It is intended that the broad concept of 'administration' includes many different component parts without which the act of giving a medicine to a client safely and effectively would be impossible. By this definition, there is a need to address issues related to the preparation required to give a medicine and also any follow-up management. This will include knowledge for understanding the way medicines are able to enter the body and the effects that may occur both therapeutically and non-therapeutically as a result of treatment. Although it is not possible to offer comprehensive advice related to all medications in this respect, the more common groups of medicines will be considered and for more detail annotated further reading references are provided. Administration may involve educating other carers to give medicine or educating clients to self-administer medicines. There is also a role in health promotion with regards to the safe handling and storage of medicines both in hospital and community settings. Finally, the nurse can facilitate understanding of the effects of the use of medicines socially, including public use of both 'over the counter' preparations and illegal substances.

Legal and professional issues need to be taken into consideration and the position of the nurse as both a professional and a member of the public is explored.

This chapter aims to help you apply relevant knowledge regarding medicines administration from a range of sources to enable informed decision making in nursing practice. Sources include this book, specialist books and research, as well as your own classroom study and personal experiences in practice-based settings.

▶ OVERVIEW

▶ *Subject Knowledge*

The physical aspects related to treatment with medicines are introduced in the Biological section, with a particular emphasis upon the mechanical and biological bases. Here, classification of medication by type is examined, followed by a consideration of the possible routes of administration, calculation of correct dose and how the body deals with medication. Further reading is offered and viewed as an essential development.

Wider psychosocial aspects of medicine use are included in the Psychosocial section, with a consideration of the potential for abuse of medication and the societal impact of drugs today. You are encouraged to think about societal issues, which must be taken into account by the professional nurse since caring can not and does not take place devoid of such influences.

▶ *Practice Knowledge*

The role of the nurse in the provision of medicines is explored. Based on reader exercises and experiences, the discussion relates specifically to decision making in the assessment, planning, implementing and evaluation of total care for patients. It is intended that the section should lead you to a deeper understanding of your role in the practical setting.

▶ *Professional Knowledge*

In this section, issues related to legality and accountability in particular are highlighted. Again, exercises are used to help you relate the knowledge provided to your particular area of practice. Incidents such as errors in medication are explored and discussed in detail.

▶ *Reflective Knowledge*

You are encouraged to think reflectively over issues related to the care of four different patients by the presentation of case studies with reflective questions. It is anticipated that concepts raised throughout the chapter will be applied by the reader as a knowledge base for nursing practice.

On pp. 123–125 there are four case studies, each one relating to one of the branch programmes. You may find it helpful to read one of them before you start the chapter and use it as a focus for your reflections while reading.

SUBJECT KNOWLEDGE
Biological

▶ THE PHYSICAL BASIS TO MEDICINES ADMINISTRATION

▶ *Defining a Medicine*

When exploring nursing issues related to the medicinal treatment of clients, there is much debate about what constitutes a medicine, especially with regard to legal and illegal substances (Morgan, 1994; Shuttleworth, 1994), and also what constitutes an appropriate role for nurses in treating their clients. Although both these areas are discussed in more detail later in the chapter, they do highlight a need for a clear definition of what a medicine might be. In the booklet *Standards for the Administration of Medicines* issued by the UKCC (1992a), nurses are advised that nursing treatment of a patient with medicines may be for 'therapeutic, diagnostic or preventative purposes. . . .'. This is a simple nurse-orientated definition and will provide a base for discussion.

▶ *Product Licensing*

All medications are issued a licence in the UK that stipulates which routes of administration are considered to be safe for its given strength and constitution. Details of any product licence agreement can be found within the guidance details included in the medicine packaging, and these should be adhered to in order to ensure patients' safety. Additionally, all medications are issued with both a generic and a brand name. The brand name is the one by which the product is marketed, while the generic name is the name used in prescribing.

▶ *Classification of Medicines*

Medicines can be classified two ways. First, there is the legal classification of medicines, which categorizes medicines according to requirements governing their supply to the general public. This type of classification derives from the *Medicines Act* (1968), and will be addressed in more detail in the Professional Knowledge part of this chapter.

Secondly, and less formally, there have been numerous attempts by authors of texts on pharmacology to classify medicines into groups that indicate the effect on a body system, the symptoms relieved or the desired effect of the medication, or a combination of all of these (Clark *et al.*, 1994; Trounce, 1994; Downie *et al.*, 1995; Hopkins, 1995). In fact it probably does not matter, and finding your way around these texts is as much to personal preference as anything else.

A comprehensive list of medicines and their side effects would be inappropriate in a chapter such as this, but it is acknowledged that a clear framework for categorizing drugs for further reference can be useful. The framework in Table 1.4.1 has been devised to assist you when working and studying in practice. Although it must be emphasized that no nurse should give medications they are not familiar with, it is sometimes helpful to jot down notes about medications. By carrying this framework into the practice area, medicines may be noted down as you discover them in use, allowing access for revision and more in-depth study at a later date.

▶ CALCULATING MEDICINE DOSES

Calculation of a therapeutic yet safe dose of any medication is achieved by weighing the patient and determining a safe dose per kilogramme or by calculating the patient's body surface area. In critical care areas a nomogram (Figure 1.4.1) can be used to estimate a dose rapidly.

Medicines prescribed regularly in an adult setting may be appropriate for a wide range of clients and are often prescribed in a form that is held as stock by the pharmacist. For instance, an antibiotic such as ampicillin may be prescribed as a 250 milligram (mg) dose. The pharmacist sends 'stock' capsules, which are 250 mg in strength so that the patient requires one capsule. However, where children are concerned, and in some cases the elderly, or where medication is particularly toxic, the

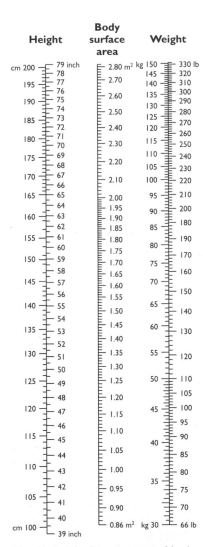

Figure 1.4.1: A nomogram of body surface area for adults. *Directions*: (1) Find height. (2) Find weight. (3) Draw a straight line connecting the height and weight. (4) Where the line intersects on the BSA column is the body surface area (m²). (Reproduced from Geigy Scientific Tables (1990) 8th edn, Vol. 5, p. 105, © Novartis, with permission.)

Type of treatment area	Name of medicine and brief notes for future reference
Infection (continued) Antibiotic (or bacteriocidal/ bacteriostatic/ antiseptic) Antifungal Antiviral	
Immunization	
Cardiovascular	
Respiratory	
Hypersensitivity reaction	
Renal	
Central nervous system Analgesic Hypnotic Psychotropic Anaesthetic	
Blood	
Gastrointestinal tract	
Neoplastic disease	
Vitamin, fluid or electrolyte imbalance	
Hormone or endocrine imbalance	
Topical	

Table 1.4.1 A framework for classifying medicines

dose is usually calculated according to the weight of the patient in mg/kg as recommended by the pharmaceutical company. This may not conveniently fall into a 'stock' dose. Once a dose has been ascertained, it is up to the nurse to decide that the prescription is correct and ensure that it is given. This means a further calculation may be necessary. A formula for calculating medicines is shown in Figure 1.4.2.

Medicine doses are calculated using the metric system and are described in units of this system. When performing any calculation it is important that you ensure that the same unit is used for the stock and the prescribed dose. If the prescribed

DECISION MAKING

1. *In your practice identify one medicine used within each of the classifications in the framework and find out all you can about it using the references for further reading identified at the end of the chapter. If possible, reflect on the exercise with colleagues.*
2. *Use your findings to discuss what factors may influence a nursing decision not to give an identified* medicine to a client.
3. *Although a useful way of identifying individual uses for medications, the above framework categories are not mutually exclusive.*
Looking at your list, can you identify any medication that may fit into more than one of the above categories? What does this tell you about using this drug therapeutically?

$$\frac{\text{What is required (prescribed dose)}}{\text{What is available (stock dose)}} \times \text{Available dilution (stock volume)}$$

So if the dose prescribed is 500 mg of amoxycillin and the stock dose is 250 mg per one tablet (volume), the calculation is:

$$\frac{500}{250} \times 1 = 2, \text{ so two tablets are given}$$

Figure 1.4.2: Calculation formula.

$$\frac{\text{Fluid volume prescribed (ml)} \times \text{Drops per ml (on giving set)}}{\text{Duration of infusion (minutes)}} = \text{Drops per minute}$$

For example, if a man was prescribed 120 ml of medication over 1 hour delivered using an administration set giving 15 drops per ml:

$$\frac{120 \times 15}{60} = 30 \text{ drops per minute}$$

If a child was prescribed 60 ml of medication over 1 hour through a set giving 60 drops per ml then:

$$\frac{60 \times 60}{60} = 60 \text{ drops per minute}$$

Figure 1.4.3: Calculating infusion rate.

dose is in mg and the stock dose is only available in grams (g), then the stock dose needs to be converted into mg before a calculation can take place (see Annotated Further Reading for more information).

Calculating Intravenous Infusion Rate

DECISION MAKING

1. *Mrs Johnston is found to be unwell while taking prescribed digoxin and the dose is reduced from 125 micrograms (µg) to 62.5 µg twice daily. On the ward the stock solution of digoxin is 50 µg/ml.*
Try to decide how much Mrs Johnston should receive at one dose.

2. *Mrs Johnson is later prescribed intravenous antibiotics for a chest infection. She is to receive amikacin sulphate 150 mg infused in 100 ml of dextrose saline over one hour.*
At what rate should the intravenous infusion be set?
(Check your answers with a nurse or nurse teacher to see if you are right.)

Once the correct dose of medicine is calculated, it may be necessary to make a last calculation to ensure the correct rate of delivery to the client, particularly if administration is via infusion, where a flow valve or an infusion pump may be used. If an infusion pump is available, the rate of delivery can be set and the nurse's role is primarily concerned with observing the client and monitoring the equipment. However, if there is no pump available, the rate of infusion may be set manually. To do this, the volume in millilitres (ml) contained in each droplet must be identified. Division of the rate required per hour by the volume of the droplets and then by 60 will enable determination of ml to be administered per minute and this can then be counted out (Figure 1.4.3). Note that administration sets vary in droplet volume and it is extremely important to check details on the packaging of the administration set. Those designed for the administration of clear fluids to children generally either deliver 20 or 60 droplets per ml volume, while those designed for adult use deliver 15 droplets per ml volume.

RESEARCH BASED EVIDENCE

Manley et al. (1994) identified in their work that children with learning difficulties may be at risk of dental caries resulting from the sugary liquid suspension containing anticonvulsants they are frequently prescribed. They interviewed parents, teachers and nurses in their small study and found that most parents (65%) would be happy to give their children either tablets or sugar-free liquids in preference to syrups. The most important point highlighted by the authors concerned the importance of close communication between prescribers and providers of care so that the most appropriate form of medicine can be prescribed for each individual child.

MEDICINES ADMINISTRATION

Routes of Administration

Nurses have a useful contribution to make in their knowledge on what preparations of medication are available and appropriate for their clients, and they are uniquely aware of their clients' needs as a result of client assessment. When selecting a route for administration the nurses and doctors must work with the patient to provide an optimum treatment programme that is safe and acceptable.

There are many different routes that can be selected for administration, as shown in Table 1.4.2. Think about a recent practice experience where a medication was given.

What route was used?

Was this the only possible way to give this medicine or could other routes have been selected?

Route	Notes
Oral (including nasogastric tubes)	Anything swallowed to the stomach
Sublingual/buccal	Allowed to dissolve under the tongue or in the cheek
Topical	Including topical application into eyes, ears, vagina, rectum
Inhalation	Including via masks, nebulizers, breathing tubes
Intravenously/intra-arterially	Administered into a vein or artery by a doctor or nurse with appropriate advanced qualifications
Subcutaneously/intradermally	By injection into the skin layers
Intramuscularly	By injection into the muscle
Intrathecally	Administered by a doctor into the thecal cavity via a lumbar puncture procedure
Intraosseously	Administered by doctor into bone cavity – used for urgent access
Other	It is possible for doctors to use other routes (e.g. into body cavities such as the pleural space or peritoneal cavity in specific circumstances

Table 1.4.2 Routes for administration of medicines.

▶ PHARMACOKINETICS AND PHARMACODYNAMICS

▶ *Pharmacokinetics*

The study of pharmacokinetics considers how a drug is processed as it passes through the body. The main phases of pharmacokinetic action are:

- ▶ absorption;
- ▶ distribution;
- ▶ metabolism;
- ▶ excretion.

▶ Absorption

Medication given is absorbed from the point of administration and into the cardiovascular system. Unless the medication is given by another route (thus bypassing this phase), nurses should be aware of the effects of the medicine in the effectiveness of absorption, but also regarding the potential effect of the medicine at the site where it is being absorbed. With oral medication, consideration must include the effects of gastric secretion upon the efficacy of the drug and the potential effects of the medication upon the client's gastrointestinal tract.

▶ Absorption of topical medications

With the administration of topical medications, there is usually an expectation that the desired effect will predominate at the local site.

DECISION MAKING

When giving six-year-old Ahmed his glucocorticosteroid medication (which is known to irritate the gastric lining causing potential gastric ulceration), the nurse ensured there was a glass of milk for him to drink. Find out the following:
1. *Why did the nurse offer Ahmed milk in this situation?*
2. *Glucocorticosteroids are substances that occur naturally in the body, but synthetically produced glucocorticosteroids can be given therapeutically to produce an anti-inflammatory and immunosuppressive response* (Kee and Hayes, 1993). *What essential knowledge should you remember to help you advise any member of the public who is taking any form of glucocorticosteroid treatment?*
3. *Anabolic steroids are substances that are also produced naturally by the human body and create an increase in body mass and strength* (Kee and Hayes, 1993). *Reflect for a moment and consider why these drugs might be abused? Who might be vulnerable?*

However, modern medicine has begun to recognize the potential for long-acting absorption of medication systemically with the advent of patches, which slowly release medications such as progesterone and oestrogens for hormone replacement therapy. A nursing consideration therefore must also be what effect (if any) may the absorption of topically administered medication have upon a client's wellbeing, especially if the intended action is purely a local one.

▶ Distribution

Once in the cardiovascular circulation, the medication is carried to its site of action. Again, there are areas of nursing knowledge that are important for consideration. It is useful to understand how the treatment is carried in the blood, since many medicines are bound tightly to plasma proteins while others are not (Schwertz, 1991). If a medicine has a high affinity for plasma proteins it may be necessary to give a large dose of the medication to achieve a therapeutic effect since only the proportion of the medicine that is not bound to the plasma proteins can be used effectively (Hopkins, 1995). Commonly used medicines with a high affinity for plasma proteins (more than 80% bound) include the antidepressant amitriptyline, and the anxiolytic diazepam. Other medicines with a high affinity for plasma proteins are propanolol, warfarin, frusemide and the antibiotics erythromycin and rifampicin. A more in-depth review of protein-bound medications is offered by Kee and Hayes (1993).

When planning to administer medicines, a factor that may affect the client's concentration of plasma proteins should be considered. This is because an individual with a reduced albumin concentration may be at risk of toxicity if a dose of medication with a high affinity for plasma protein is given. Increasing age has been shown to reduce the amount of plasma protein by up to 20% (Loi and Vestel, 1988) while malnutrition is also implicated in the reduction of circulating plasma proteins (Schmucker, 1984).

Other issues that should be considered in relation to the distribution of medication via the cardiovascular system include the rate and volume of perfusion to the desired area as any reduction in access to the required site may reduce the impact of the treatment offered. Additionally some areas of the body are protected from receiving many medications as a result of physiological barriers. The brain is one such area as the meninges around the central nervous system create a 'blood – brain' barrier. Another area that selectively reduces the passage of substances is evident during pregnancy when the placenta offers a barrier between mother and baby. However, it should be noted that some substances may pass through these barriers. In nursing, the implications of the effectiveness of such barriers must be addressed when making informed decisions about nursing care. It is critical to assess the possibility of pregnancy in all premenopausal women who require medicinal treatment, with particular awareness of the potentially hazardous effects in causing fetal abnormalities of drugs such as phenytoin and tetracyclines, which can pass the placental barrier (Clark *et al.*, 1994).

Finally, the distribution of medication to infants via maternal breast milk must also be acknowledged. In some cases medication given to the mother may be safe for her, but can have toxic effects on the baby. For more information about the effects of specific medications in breast-feeding please refer to the Annotated Further Reading at the end of the chapter.

DECISION MAKING

Jack Harvey, aged 85 years, is in hospital following a recent diagnosis of congestive cardiac failure. He has been prescribed propanolol, but after a few days his heart rate drops to less than 60 beats/min (compared to a more usual 80 beats/min) and he complains of feeling unwell.

1. **What may be wrong with Jack?**
2. **Within coronary care, there is a variety of medicines that act upon the heart in different ways. Propanolol is a beta blocker. Find out how beta blockers work and compare their action with that of the digitalis group of medicines.**
3. **What special considerations might you need to remember when administering medicines to clients who are elderly?**

Metabolism

Metabolism (or breakdown) of any medication usually occurs in the liver (hepatic system). This may be therapeutic, in aiding the removal of active medication from the body by rendering it to inactive waste metabolites or may hinder the effects of treatment, depending upon when such metabolism takes place. This issue is particularly pertinent when considering medicines that are administered orally, since much absorption via the gastrointestinal tract results in direct passage to the liver through the hepatic portal vein. In this situation the liver metabolizes a proportion of the medication (which varies between medications), before the medication reaches the cardiovascular circulation and is transported to the site of therapeutic benefit. This is known as 'first pass' metabolism, and although sometimes such a metabolism may be beneficial, as the metabolites themselves may have a therapeutic function, often it reduces the available therapeutic dose of medication by inactivating it. 'First pass' metabolism is reduced in individuals with impaired hepatic function, and this is vital knowledge for nursing consideration in order to maintain the safety and wellbeing of the client.

Finally, it is important to understand that it is possible to overload the liver with toxins, resulting from the breakdown of medication as well as other substances such as alcohol, and this leads initially to an inability of the liver to cope effectively. If the liver continues to be overloaded with toxins over a prolonged period or is subjected to recurrent episodes of overload damage may occur. This creates a permanently reduced hepatic function.

When considering administration to infants and young and children, it is essential to recognize that in the young the ability to detoxify medicines is not mature, and therefore extreme caution should be taken when checking for an appropriate dose.

Excretion

After a variable period of time in the body the medication given to the patient will be excreted. This is most often via the kidneys, although other routes of excretion include the lungs, via bile into faeces, and in lactating mothers, breast milk. There may also be some excretion through sweat glands onto the skin surface (Hopkins, 1995; Downie, *et al.*, 1995). Perhaps the most important factor in medicine excretion, however, is the speed at which it is lost from the body, since this varies between individuals and is an issue for consideration by all nurses caring for their clients, especially for those whose clients are at the extremes of the age continuum or have renal impairment. The infant does not develop full renal and urinary tract function until after the first year of life, while the renal function of the elderly (over 80 years of age) deteriorates to about half the capacity of a young adult (Trounce, 1994). A knowledge of the patient's history combined with an awareness of the way in which specific medications may be excreted is vital in providing nursing care in all areas of practice.

DECISION MAKING

Peter, a student, went to a New Year's Eve party where he saw in the New Year with much enthusiasm and a lot of alcohol. Although he was unable to remember much about his night out, he remembered the hangover on New Year's Day. Later, he asked a friend (a nursing student) why he felt so rough and why the tablets he took to reduce the hangover actually seemed to make him feel worse.

1. *How could Peter's friend explain what may have happened to him given that alcohol and paracetomol-based products both require detoxification by the liver.*
2. *How could the nursing student offer health education to Peter, thus allowing him to see the potential dangers of his actions?*
3. *Make a list of common medicines in your field of practice that have a high extraction ratio at 'first pass'.*

DECISION MAKING

Simon is severely learning disabled and has difficulty in maintaining urinary continence due to poor bladder tone causing retention of urine and dribbling incontinence. He is cared for by his mother who maintains that clean intermittent catheterization techniques aid Simon's urinary continence, but he occasionally develops urinary tract infections. Simon's mother, whilst managing his infection, comments to the practice nurse that Simon's urine smells of the current antibiotic treatment and wonders why.

1. *How could you reassure Simon's mother that all is well?*
2. *Find out how antibiotics work and what broad classifications can be identified.*
3. *In a society that does not tolerate ill health, people are inclined to ask for antibiotics for minor infections. Reflect for a few minutes about the impact this may have in the long term.*

▶ The effect of renal impairment on the excretion of medication

Renal impairment can affect the excretion of medicines from the body, resulting in a build-up of metabolites, or in some instances medicines, as in the Decision Making above in the circulation. A knowledge of such possibilities may alert you to making a decision to include specific points for observation related to medication in the client's plan of care.

▶ *Pharmacodynamics*

Once a medicine has reached the site of therapeutic benefit it is able to exert a physiological effect before being excreted by the body. This is identified as pharmacodynamic action, and an in-depth consideration of this action of medicines in the body is comprehensively addressed by Downie *et al.* (1995). It is important to realize, however, that even with today's rapidly advancing understanding of medical science, the exact way in which an agent produces its effect on the body may still not be fully known (Trounce, 1994).

▶ POTENTIAL ADVERSE EFFECTS OF ADMINISTERING MEDICINES TO PATIENTS

Although the aim of using medicinal treatments for clients may be therapeutic, diagnostic or preventive (UKCC, 1992a) it is simplistic to believe that all medicines given are completely therapeutic in all cases. For both nursing and medicine the aim has always been recognized as 'To do the patient no harm' (Nightingale, 1859) or to 'First do no harm', (Hippocrates, cited by Manley *et al.*, 1994). This next section will explore potential threats to such ideals.

▶ *Gaining a Therapeutic Dose*

In order for medicine to be effective, the dose for your client must be sufficient to be effective, but not too much, in which case the client may risk toxicity or poisoning. Factors in achieving a therapeutic dose are related to nursing and medical skill in prescribing and calculating the correct dose of medication and also the pharmacokinetic and pharmacodynamic capacity of the client. This may be related to their age, lifestyle or health condition, as highlighted above. However, even with a therapeutically assessed dose of medication, the response of individual patients can vary significantly, and thus a potentially useful medicine can be harmful. Your nursing decision making may contribute to reducing risks associated with the administration of medicines, and identification of potential adverse effects is helpful. Some potential adverse effects arising when giving a therapeutic medication are identified in Table 1.4.3.

As well as the adverse effects of giving any single medication to an individual, external influences may harm your patient. Your patient may already be taking other medications that could interact with new treatment, causing adverse effects or altering the pharmacokinetic or pharmacodynamic action of either medication. A common outcome is a reduced or halted action (antagonism), which may be useful for use as an antidote, preventing the action of a medication once it has been given, or a potentiated action (synergism). Other reactions are also possible and for a comprehensive listing of such known interactions see the *British National Formulary* (1996).

ADVERSE EFFECT/SIDE EFFECT	NATURE OF REACTION
Idiosyncrasy	Often genetically determined
Hypersensitivity/allergy	May be life-threatening (anaphylaxis)
Skin reactions	Pruritus (itching) Urticaria (nettle rash) Erythematous eruptions (flushing and skin rashes) Skin peeling Eczematous lesions
Blood dyscrasias	Aplastic anaemia (due to bone marrow suppression) Thrombocytopenia (loss of platelets) Agranulocytosis (loss of white blood cells)
Gastrointestinal upset	Diarrhoea Dyspepsia Ulceration Nausea Vomiting Sore or dry mouth Anal pruritus Flatulence Abdominal pain
Central nervous system upset	Drowsiness Headache Dizziness Nausea Vomiting Tinnitus
Photosensitivity	Acute ocular sensitivity to light
Tolerance	The client responds increasingly less effectively to a regular dose of medication
Dependence	The patient may become addicted to the medication

Table 1.4.3 Potential adverse effects of medicines.

▶ *Polypharmacy*

RESEARCH BASED EVIDENCE

Cartwright (1990) studied medicine taking by people aged 65 years or over in Great Britain, and found that in his sample 50% took two or more medications on a regular basis. His data are supported by American literature, which suggests that the average person over 64 of age takes 2–3 prescription medicines, with those over 80 years of age taking even more (LeSage, 1991).

An interaction between different drugs, as described above, may not be restricted to two substances, but may involve a multiplicity of medical treatments. This type of interaction is known as 'polypharmacy', and is documented in the nursing literature, particularly in relation to the elderly (Cartwright, 1990; LeSage, 1991).

Although polypharmacy is more commonly identified in the older population because an increase in medicinal treatment is perhaps more linked to age related problems, it is not exclusive to this age group. There are therefore implications for all nursing personnel involved in taking client histories or in starting a new programme of medicinal treatment. Decisions regarding the likely response to treatment must be made in an informed and reflective way, and in order to do this the nurse's assessment must involve a thorough understanding of the information gained. In the case of the administration of multiple medicines to treat a client, this may mean close collaboration with members of the medical and pharmacy teams as well as using databases such as the *British National Formulary* (1996) in order to become fully informed about the specific risks of polypharmacy to individual clients.

▶ *The Role of the Pharmacist*

The responsibility of the pharmacist both in hospital and in the community is to ensure that any medications dispensed can be taken safely by the individual for whom they are prescribed. Within the hospital setting the pharmacist checks the client's prescription and can observe any possible effects of combining prescribed medications inappropriately. However, this is much more difficult within the community. Pharmacists must ask clients about other medications and point out any specific care that should be taken when using a prescribed medication. Many pharmacies have a computerized database of medicines dispensed for clients, thus allowing them to build up a clearer picture of a client's overall treatment. However, this type of system relies on the client using the same pharmacy outlet to obtain all their prescriptions. Ultimately, the client is responsible for informing those prescibing, dispensing or managing their medicinal treatment about any other medicines already being used.

▶ *The Client's Position*

When caring for individuals requiring treatment with medications there is the possibility that they may not wish to disclose their use of other medicines. This may occur in all branches of nursing and for many different reasons. In childrens' nursing for instance, a teenage girl may not wish her family to know that she is taking oral contraceptives, or another situation may arise if a client is using a substance considered to be illegal. Many issues arise from these scenarios which merit reflection and discussion.

▶ *Teratogenesis and Iatrogenesis*

When considering the possible effects of medicines on the body, it is not just the interaction between the patient and medicine or between two medicines that can cause problems. Additionally there may be occasions when other factors such as the current health state of the client or issues associated with lifestyle may engender hidden dangers when combined with an otherwise acceptable treatment. The outcome of such problems may be described in two ways. First there is teratogenesis, which occurs in the treatment of women during or before pregnancy. The teratogenic outcome would be malformation or death of the unborn child. Perhaps the best-known example of this situation was the treatment of women with the anti-emetic thalidomide in the early 1960s for morning sickness. Although a highly effective anti-emetic, thalidomide was found to cause amelia (absence of limbs) during fetal development, leading to tragedy for many families whose children suffered as a result of this treatment.

A second problem is iatrogenesis, or the causing of sickness or injury as a result of treatment. Any side effect may be considered for inclusion, although usually more serious effects that may cause a need for treatment are highlighted. This situation may seem inconceivable to the nursing student who is advised about the benefits of treatment and assured that they should above all do no harm, but this is a simplistic view of a complex issue and it is probable that a balance of benefits versus harm may be a more reasonable stance to take.

To ensure optimum safety and wellbeing for clients, you have a duty to understand the possible implications of treatment and to advise your clients so that they can make informed choices about proposed interventions.

Ahmed was diagnosed as having leukaemia and his family wished him to receive current medicinal treatment as a potentially life-saving measure, although Ahmed said that he felt 'alright' before his treatment. After his treatment, however, Ahmed was sick and miserable, and his mouth became ulcerated and sore for a while. The Doctors prescribed Ahmed further medicinal treatment to help alleviate his symptoms.

1. *Was it right to offer Ahmed and his family treatment that would make him ill?*

2. *What are your personal beliefs about treatment for Ahmed?*

3. *How could your own personal beliefs affect the support you give Ahmed and his family through this difficult time in his treatment?*

Psychosocial Although nurses generally involve themselves in the use of prescription medicines for therapeutic, diagnostic or preventive benefit, many other substances may be used by clients. In this section, the use of substances that may not be prescribed by a medical practitioner are briefly explored, both in relation to the health of the individual and in relation to you as a nurse and as a member of society.

▶ CLIENT USE OF NON-PRESCRIBED SUBSTANCES – THE NURSE'S POSITION

Within the simple definition of a medicine highlighted at the beginning of this chapter, a number of questions can be raised for discussion. The UKCC (1992a) defines a medicine as something that is 'for therapeutic, diagnostic or preventative purposes'. Here the question must be who decides on such benefits. In relation to nursing in hospital settings this is often simple in that medications are prescribed by medical staff whose qualifications permit

Think back over the past week. How many times have you had;

- *An alcoholic drink.*
- *A cup of coffee or tea.*
- *A cigarette or cigar.*
- *A throat sweet or cough or cold cure*
- *An aspirin or paracetamol tablet.*
- *A vitamin or iron tablet.*
- *An oral contraceptive pill.*
- *Any non-prescription treatments*

Look at the above list. Find out which (if any) items:

1. Would be unsafe if inadvertently ingested by a child?

2. May, if taken in sustained amounts on a regular basis, eventually lead to physical damage to organs in the body.

3. May, if taken in sustained amounts on a regular basis lead to psychological dependence?

For nurses caring for those who have attempted to either seek help by taking an overdose or who have attempted to take their own lives, caring can be emotionally difficult. Consider how you might feel in this situation.

1. Would you feel cross that the person is taking up a bed by making themselves ill?

2. Would you feel confused or unable to understand?

3. Would you simply feel sorry for the person?

4. Could your feelings affect your care for that person?

them to make an accepted decision. For the UKCC, the nurse is primarily concerned with medicines that fall into this category. For nurses who are involved in prescribing medications, extra study is essential following registration. This gives nurse prescribers a forum for consideration of such issues as therapeutic beneficence.

As members of modern society, however, most individuals are involved in the use of many 'unprescribed' yet socially acceptable substances, which may be used for a perceived therapeutic effect. Substances such as tobacco, coffee and alcohol, as well as 'over the counter' preparations such as analgesics, cold cures, antihistamines, or vitamins to name but a few, are used commonly by the public (Clarence, 1990; Plant *et al.*, 1992).

▶ POISONING

In nursing children it is perhaps particularly important to be aware of the presence of these substances in the home, as well as a myriad of other substances such as cleaning agents, especially those containing caustic soda, e.g. dishwasher powder, fertilizers and weedkillers, e.g. Paraquat, which may be extremely dangerous to a child if used inappropriately. Many children are admitted to hospital every year following the inappropriate use of common substances leading to poisoning and the children's nurse has a role in managing their care and in educating parents and families about safety in storage.

▶ OVERDOSE

When considering the issue of overdose, it should be stressed that it may occur either intentionally or accidentally. Accidental overdose may result from the client misreading or misunderstanding the prescription label or failing to realize that more than one medication contains the same drug. Taking medicines containing the same drug concurrently would result in an overdose. This is perhaps most common with over the counter cold cures, many of which contain paracetamol. Accidental overdose may occur by proxy in the form of a medication error if a nurse fails to record that a medication has been given, thus allowing the dose to be unintentionally repeated.

▶ *Intentional Overdose*

An area common to all areas of nursing is the intentional abuse of medicines, whether prescribed or not, with intent to cause injury or death to oneself or another. Nurses in practice may find themselves working with victims of parasuicide or with relatives of those who have committed suicide through overdose. The physical nursing needs of parasuicide patients depend very much upon the type of medication taken and rely on multidisciplinary team working between the nurses, pharmacists and medical team involved in each individual's care. In most parasuicide cases there is an additional referral to a liaison psychiatrist for risk assessment and planning future management. It is likely that the nurse's role would involve monitoring and assessment of the patient. A clear understanding of the substance taken and its likely effects of toxicity is essential. Clients and families involved in such sad situations, will require counselling and support and this will be addressed further in Chapter 3.5.

USE OF ILLEGAL SUBSTANCES

A definition of an illegal substance is one that is classified under the *Misuse of Drugs Act* (1971) and is being manufactured, supplied or possessed by anyone not legally authorized to do so. The use of illegal substances cannot be ignored. Substance abuse is described by Shuttleworth (1994) as 'one of the major social ills in the UK' and can certainly present some very real problems for nurses caring for patients, especially adolescents and young people.

Client Assessment

Although it is not suggested that the use of illicit drugs should be encouraged or condoned by nurses, it is important that you are aware of the nature and use of such substances by all clients in your care. Use must be assessed as part of the individual's lifestyle so that any prescribed medication can be given to best effect, since it is possible for non-prescription substances to interact with prescribed medications with serious consequences.

Client assessment may reveal areas where individuals feel that they need help with managing the consumption of addictive substances, and as a nurse you may have a role in helping a client find appropriate support and advice. However, issues associated with maintaining confidentiality when your client is pursuing an illegal activity are complex. Dimond (1995) explores these issues in more depth in her text *Legal Aspects of Nursing* and you are advised to explore this further.

USE OF ALTERNATIVE OR COMPLEMENTARY THERAPIES

The use of complementary or alternative medicines are within the rights of any patient. However, the nurse caring for that patient must be aware of what is being used and must also be aware of any possible interactions between this and any proposed orthodox treatment. Nurses are able to use complementary therapies with their patients provided that they have successfully undertaken training to do so, take full professional accountability for their actions, and have the consent of the patient who is to receive such treatment (UKCC, 1996).

HEALTH PROMOTION

Nurses have a unique position in society in their capacity to offer appropriate health education to a wide range of clients who receive care. A practice nurse's knowledge about the effects of smoking on the health of unborn children may be an essential contribution in helping a pregnant woman reduce the number of cigarettes she smokes (or better still stop smoking altogether), while the combined skills and knowledge employed by mental health nurses in drug and alcohol dependency units may offer a healthier future for their clients. Many more examples could be cited in relation to all nursing specialities.

RESEARCH BASED EVIDENCE

Shuttleworth (1994) considers the knock-on effect that illegal and black market drugs have in relation to nursing, including caring for those suffering the effects of substance abuse and those whose injuries may be the result of a drugs-related assault.

Morgan (1994) considers the problem of illicit drug use and a range of prevention strategies currently available. Although directed primarily at occupational therapists, this article clearly outlines a summary of the problems faced by carers in the UK today, and addresses strategies that are equally relevant for nurses.

Mr James, aged 62 years, lives in a council-owned flat, but is attended by the local community psychiatric nursing team for treatment of paranoid schizophrenia. A loner, he has no close family and few friends. He resorts to alcohol when he feels unable to cope with his situation.

1. What health promotion role might the community psychiatric nurse have in helping Mr James?

▶ NURSES' USE OF NON-PRESCRIBED MEDICINES

Finally, there is the issue of the use of non-prescribed medicines by nurses themselves. After all, in spite of professional accountability, health carers are human and part of the wider society in which we all live. Social use of 'medicines' and difficulties surrounding abuse of substances are a very real issue, particularly in the stressful occupation of nursing. Plant *et al.* (1992) found in their study of 600 Scottish nurses that stress was associated with an increased alcohol consumption and with the use of illicit drugs, while the UKCC *Professional Conduct Occasional Report on Selected Cases* (UKCC, 1993) heard in the year to 31st March 1992 24 cases where nurses were unfit for duty through drink or drugs, and a further 16 cases where drugs had been misappropriated by nurses. In 1995 it was suggested that the most common reason for referral to the health committee of the UKCC was alcohol and drug dependence (Crabtree, 1995), and yet there is no formal professional support available nationally. For you, awareness of yourself and recognition of personal problems are all important, and for those with whom you are working, you have an obligation within the UKCC (1992b) *Code of Professional Conduct* (paragraph 11) to report to an appropriate person or authority '. . .any circumstances in the environment of care which could jeopardise standards of practice', and this may include colleagues who appear unfit to practice.

PRACTICE KNOWLEDGE

Nurses are accountable for the safe administration of medicines in whatever setting they may be working. To do this effectively they must be able to apply the knowledge discussed above according to the client's individual needs. Nursing skills are required that relate to the assessment of client need, planning of proposed nursing intervention and the implementation and evaluation of any therapy prescribed. Additionally, the role of the nurse extends more broadly in ensuring the safety and wellbeing of patients when considered in relation to the guidance advocated by the UKCC *Standards for the Administration of Medicines* (1992a). This document assumes a much wider role for the nurse both before and after a medicine is actually given. It is useful to explore subject knowledge about medicines and administration above in relation to the organizational context and the intertwined roles of the nurse, multidisciplinary team and the patients themselves.

▶ ORGANIZING MEDICINES ADMINISTRATION

The role of the nurse may vary practically according to the type of nursing delivery mechanism being used in practice. For instance an area where primary nursing takes place with one nurse responsible for his or her own clients will incur a slightly different role in medicines' administration to an area where a team nursing approach is employed, where the nurse may be expected to administer medicines to a larger number of clients with whom he or she is not so familiar. In areas where clients are encouraged to maintain their own independence the nurse may not directly give the medicine prescribed, but rather be involved with administration through education and supervision of the patients or their carers.

Mr James is prescribed fortnightly injections of fluphenazine decanoate (Modecate) as treatment for schizophrenia. As he is not a reliable attender at his local health centre for this injection, the medicine is administered by the community psychiatric nurse. Mr James has the same primary nurse responsible for his medication at all times. Meanwhile another patient, Simon, has constipation resulting from limited mobility. Although the use of oral laxatives are usually effective, recently they have not been controlling his problems. Simon is prescribed a daily enema for a short period of time to resolve his difficulties and Simon's mother (as primary carer) is taught how to administer Simon's enema at home by the community nurse.

1. List the advantages and disadvantages of these different approaches.

2. What is the significance of the nurse's contribution in each of the two approaches?

3. Analyse the knowledge the nurse may need in order to make a competent contribution to each of these approaches.

▶ THE ROLE OF THE NURSE IN THE ADMINISTRATION OF MEDICINES TO CLIENTS

In practice, nurses are accountable for any medication they administer, and to do this safely they must use knowledge gained through education and experience in a personalized way with each of their clients. It is helpful to consider the role of the nurse in relation to a systematic approach, which includes assessing, planning, implementing and evaluating care. This should usually be applied in conjunction with a conceptual model of nursing in accordance with an individual practitioner's philosophy of care. Areas that may be addressed before giving a medicine to a client are revealed by the questions below:

▶ Is the client currently taking any medications? If so, what are they?
▶ Has the client taken this medication before? If so was it tolerated and was it effective?
▶ How does the client prefer to take medication (i.e can they take tablets?)
▶ What is the preferred route for the medication prescribed?
▶ Is the client allergic to any medication?
▶ Do the client and carer understand why the medicine has been prescribed?
▶ Do the client and carer know about any potential side effects that may occur?
▶ Who is going to administer the medicine? Do they know how to do this to gain optimum benefit?
▶ What is the client's weight?
▶ What is the client's past medical history?
▶ Is there any reason why the client should not receive the medicine prescribed?

DECISION MAKING

1. Find out why each of the questions listed opposite can be important.

2. Take one client in your next practice placement and using the points bulletted opposite to analyse how much you can learn about medicine and its administration.

▶ *Planning Nursing Care*

When planning care for a client all the information derived from the medicines assessment by the nurse and other members of the multidisciplinary team needs to be combined to allow the patient to receive their medicine optimally. Nurses should use this information to identify common goals for the administration of the medicine prescribed and outline an individualized plan of care for their patients, which can be followed by implementing patient care and evaluated regularly to determine the effect of such intervention, as illustrated by the following case: *while in hospital for treatment of congestive cardiac failure, Mrs Johnson's needs are individually assessed by her nurses and a specific plan is made to assess the effects of her treatment.* This involves identifying:

▶ The problem – Mrs Johnson has congestive heart failure which requires treatment with digoxin 62.5 µg/day.

▶ The outcome – Mrs Johnson will gain a steady pulse rate of 80–120 beats/min and appear well.

▶ Nursing action – Observe Mrs Johnson for a lowered pulse rate of less than 60 beats/min, coupling of heart beats (felt at the wrist as double beats) or nausea and vomiting. In the event of any of these, contact the medical staff for advice.

In relation to planning, there may be other issues taken into account that are related more to individual preferences, for instance, if a medicine needs to be taken with food, when is the usual meal time for the client? Although in hospital meals may be delivered at set times, meal times can vary widely for individuals in their own homes; and for neonates who are fed on demand, it would be difficult to write up a medication to be taken with food at a set time! With planning and negotiation between the patient, nurse and medical staff, a solution to such problems may be reached that meets the needs of all parties in providing optimum treatment.

Planning also needs to take place within the work organization, and this requires knowledge and skill on behalf of the nurse. If a medicine needs to be given at a specific time, the nurse needs to ensure that both the medicines and the patient are available and prepared. The medication may require retrieving from a locked cupboard, reconstituting (if it is a dry powder to be made into solution) and offered in an acceptable way for the patient, according to the route for which it is prescribed. Procedures need to be followed and the medicine must be given in accordance with the law, local policy and the nurses' *Code of Professional Conduct* (UKCC, 1992b) (see the Professional Knowledge section of this chapter). In the case of the patient, skin may have to be prepared for topical creams or it may simply be necessary to ensure that the patient has a drink ready to swallow tablets.

▶ Safety in Medicines Administration

Reflect upon a recent day in practice.

Can you identify any times when you or your mentor were involved in an activity associated with administering medicines but not actually giving a medicine to a client?

What aspects included assessment and planning for giving medicines to patients?

For the nurse themselves the practice of medicines administration must also be safe. Since all medication is given for the therapeutic or diagnostic effect it is going to have on the client, it is important to remember that carelessness or inappropriate handling of medicine can lead to the nurse and (possibly others) inadvertently receiving treatment. Illustrations of this include the administration of skin creams. If the nurse does not wear gloves to protect the skin, then the cream will be applied to their hand as well as the patient. Where powders are reconstituted by nurses before administration to a patient, carelessness can lead to inhalation during this activity. Many cytotoxic medicines are reconstituted by the pharmacist in laminar air flow cubicles to draw any particles of the medication away.

Finally in the case of liquids, care should be taken to avoid splashing the medicine, which could be absorbed through the skin or inhaled.

With all medicine administration, careful handwashing before and after the procedure is essential in order to avoid cross-infection contamination from the nurse's hand to the patient and potential ingestion of particles of medicine by the nurse. Where medications are particularly toxic the pharmacist may advise extra protective measures when handling, such as safety glasses or a protective gown, and these should be adhered to.

All of the above considerations require planning on the part of the nurse as an outcome of an informed assessment of the situation.

RESEARCH BASED EVIDENCE

Parkin et al. (1976) assessed the actual use of medicines prescribed to take home by 130 patients. They found that 66 patients failed to follow the instructions they were given in hospital, and of these 46 said that they were unable to understand the instructions.

Planning for Client Discharge

There is a considerable role for the nurse in planning a client's discharge from the care setting. He or she has a responsibility to ensure that prescribed medications to take home are available by liaising with the pharmacy department. Additionally there is a responsibility for the nurse to ensure that the client or carer will be able to effectively manage the prescribed treatment once they return home.

The nurse's role may involve advising a patient about the frequency with which tablets should be taken or it could be more complex, involving education and assessment of the ability to perform a skill such as the instillation of eye drops. In either case the nurse must evaluate the ability of those continuing care and be certain that care will continue after discharge. If this cannot be achieved alternative support may need to be planned, for instance a hospital-based nurse discharging a patient to the community may need to plan for intervention by the community nursing staff.

Implementing Nursing Care

In the act of giving a medicine all the assessment, planning and background knowledge comes together to permit safe and accountable action. Additionally, the nurse has to acknowledge and respect the rights of the client in receiving their medication (as discussed in the professional knowledge section of this chapter).

Although delivery systems in nursing may differ, the nurse's responsibility in administering medicines to clients is constant. A useful starting point is identified by Kee and Hayes (1993) in their discussion of the 'six rights' in drug administration (Figure 1.4.4).

Although a useful start, other factors must also be taken into consideration in implementing medicines administration, and the nurse may need to be flexible about how the six rights are achieved. For instance, it cannot be assumed that the nurse will always give a client his or her medicine. Nurses and pharmacists are currently exploring the possibilities of allowing systems of self-medication by clients in hospital.

In children's nursing, there is a drive towards nurses working in partnership with parents and the children, and in the community, nurses may be responsible for overseeing their patients who are self-administering medicines in their own homes.

RESEARCH BASED EVIDENCE

A small study conducted by Sutherland et al. (1995) tried out patient self-medication for one month for some adult patients in a medical ward and a dermatology ward. They reported that 'a self administration scheme would be possible and beneficial in acute medical wards', and a decision has been taken to extend the project hospital-wide to all appropriate areas.

Practical Considerations in Giving Medicines

Some practical issues fall outside the six rights, and must be addressed when implementing the administration of a medicine. Failure to acknowledge these would not perhaps be considered as a medication error, but would make the difference between unacceptable and optimum practice. Such issues are considered elsewhere in this book, but may include for instance the management of infection control (see Chapter 1.3), an issue that is particularly pertinent in relation to the administration of intravenous medication. If a patient becomes septicaemic due to contamination during the administration of an intravenous medication, his or her safety could be as compromised as if they were given the wrong dose of medication.

A final aspect to consider is the nurse's knowledge of resuscitation techniques and equipment in the event of an anaphylactic reaction to a medication (see Chapter 2.2). When any medicine is given, it is the

The nurse must ensure that:

THE RIGHT PATIENT

receives

THE RIGHT MEDICATION

at

THE RIGHT TIME

in

THE RIGHT DOSE

via

THE RIGHT ROUTE

and

THE RIGHT DOCUMENTATION

is completed

Figure 1.4.4: Six rights of medicines administration.

responsibility of the nurse to know what possible side effects may occur and to observe for these once the medication has been administered. This aspect will be addressed further in the evaluation of care.

▶ *Evaluation of Nursing Care*

There is one more fundamental ingredient that is of prime importance in relation to the giving of medicines to clients. This is the use of knowledge about the client, which must be combined with knowledge about the likely impact of any planned therapeutic treatment to create an evaluated stance. The UKCC are concerned that using such knowledge may make the difference between achieving competency in nursing practice or failing to do so, an unacceptable action. In *Standards for Administration of Medicines* (UKCC, 1992a) it is stated that 'The nurse, midwife or health visitor must, in administering any medicines, in assisting with administration or overseeing a self administration of medicines, apply knowledge and skill to the situation that pertains at the time'.

In relation to patients, all treatment with medication requires evaluation regarding its effect (beneficial or otherwise) for the client. The nurse must use both general and clinical skills of observation as well as communication skills, and must be able to record and pass on findings to other members of the multidisciplinary team as appropriate. A major aspect of evaluation is associated with the evaluation and assessment of pain control, an aspect taken up in Chapter 2.3. A fundamental part of the nurse's decision making role with regard to medicine administration is related to identifying whether a medication is effective or sufficient for the patient's needs. If a medicine is prescribed *pro re nata* or PRN, meaning 'as required', then the nurse has an additional role in deciding to select it for use at all. Evaluation of its effect on the patient and assessment of the client's need for the medicine are essential parts of the decision making process. In order to understand what situation currently pertains, the nurse needs to use his or her skills of evaluation. Within this he or she would consider the therapeutic effects of any medication given and any untoward reactions that may have occurred as a result of treatment. Evaluation requires you to use other skills of observation in evaluating outcomes and of communication in reporting findings.

All registered nurses are beholden to administer medicines for therapeutic, diagnostic or preventive benefit, but there are many ways in which client's optimum health and safety can be compromised in spite of the intentions behind the planned treatment with medicines. The qualified nurse therefore plays an important part in promoting the health and safety of clients with regards to the evaluation of the administration of their treatment as well as in the more recognized areas of health and safety already outlined and included in Chapter 1.1.

DECISION MAKING

In your practice placement, try to observe one situation where a nurse ensures that a client receives their medicines. Note in detail what you see, including the nurse's actions and the client's actions.

1. *How did the administration of this medicine integrate with the total care of the patient and with the nurse's total role?*
2. *Brainstorm – what knowledge did the nurse need to have to ensure that the medicine was received safely?*

PROFESSIONAL KNOWLEDGE

In this section the nurse's role in medicine giving is considered in relation to British law currently governing practice, the nurses' *Code of Professional Conduct* (UKCC, 1992b), and the impact of local policy. Clients' rights will be considered regarding their consent to treatment and the right to refuse medicinal treatment will be explored. Finally, the nurse's role in the management of medication error is addressed.

▶ LEGAL CONSIDERATIONS IN THE ADMINISTRATION OF MEDICINES TO CLIENTS

In Britain, the manufacture, prescription, safe handling, storage and custody of medicines are all subject to legislative control arising from two main acts of parliament and a set of guiding regulations as follows:

▶ *Medicines Act* (1968);
▶ *Misuse of Drugs Act* (1971);
▶ *Misuse of Drugs Regulations* (1985).

Each of the Acts determines different legal controls, which must be observed by the nurse in daily practice.

▶ *Legal Classification of Medicines*

Under the *Medicines Act* (1968) drugs are classified into three main groups:

▶ Pharmacy-only products – those only to be sold through a registered pharmacy under the supervision of a pharmacist.
▶ General sales list – medicines that may be sold from a retail outlet without a pharmacist or registration as a pharmacy provided certain conditions relating to the security of the premises are adhered to.
▶ Prescription-only medicines – medicines that are only available on a practitioner's prescription. This group is divided to identify those drugs that are simply to be prescribed by a practitioner and those that are further governed by additional requirements under the *Misuse of Drugs Act* (1971). A clear knowledge of the classification of medications is essential for the nurse who has responsibility for ensuring the safe and legal administration of medicines to patients.

Within the *Misuse of Drugs Act* (1971) and the *Misuse of Drugs Regulations* (1985), controlled drugs are identified and categorized according to requirements governing their import, export supply, possession, prescribing and record keeping (Dimond, 1990). For hospital-based nurses, knowledge regarding these acts is essential in understanding the way controlled drugs are stored and handled in the practice setting. Strict regulations govern where a controlled drug should be kept, how it may be ordered and transported from pharmacy, where it must be kept, who holds the keys to access controlled medicines, and how the prescription checking and use of such drugs must be documented. In non-institutional settings, however, the nurse is not permitted to keep any stock-controlled drugs. Controlled drugs may only be obtained for those who are named on a prescription.

▶ NURSE PRESCRIBING

Following the publication of the Department of Health Report of the Advisory Group on Nurse Prescribing (1989), the *Medicinal Products: Prescriptions by Nurses etc. Act* (1992) has enabled provision in law for district nurses and health visitors to prescribe a number of commonly used medications from a nurses' formulary without recourse to a medical practitioner. This is different from hospital settings where specially trained nurses (usually nurse practitioners) may be able to administer certain medicines by prior agreement with the medical consultant. In

---

DECISION MAKING

You are working as a nurse in charge at a respite home for clients with severe learning disability. One morning, Simon, a short-stay client in the home, develops signs and symptoms of a urinary tract infection. You call Simon's general practitioner, but he is unable to see him until the afternoon. You know that another patient has been prescribed antibiotics for a similar diagnosis. A colleague suggests that if you borrowed some of this client's antibiotics for Simon then he could begin treatment right away.

1. *How should you react to this suggestion?*
2. *What knowledge and legal rationale would influence your response?*

In your practice, find a controlled drug prescription. Try to identify the following:

1. How does a controlled medicine prescription differ from prescriptions that are not for controlled medicines?

2. What is special about the cupboard where controlled medicines are stored? Who has the keys?

3. What governs the administration and storage of controlled medicines?

4. What does the nurse need to know in order to give a controlled drug safely?

5. What is included in the controlled record of administration?

these cases, nurses follow prearranged protocols for the administration of specific medicines (Trigg, 1995). However, this type of medicine administration is subject to local policy and at the time of writing is untested in law. Nurses administering any medication in these circumstances are advised to ensure that their employers sign a legal waiver to formalize the acceptance of such practices (Naish and Garbett, 1996). Within medicines administration, the nurse has to observe more general tenets of law, which should be applied. These include law related to the informed consent of clients and the keeping of records associated with medication administration and outcomes.

▶ Medicines Administration and the Code of Professional Conduct for the Nurse, Midwife and Health Visitor (1992b)

As well as working within the law, the nurse is also accountable to the UKCC, which is the nurses' governing body for professional practice. The *Code of Professional Conduct* (and its supplementary standards paper *Standards for the Administration of Medicines* (UKCC, 1992a) assist the nurse in fulfilling the expectations the UKCC has of them as a professional body. Additional advice can also be gained from the *Scope of Professional Practice* (UKCC, 1992c), especially in relation to the 'extended role' in medicines administration. Although the law will instigate criminal proceedings in the event of a breach, the UKCC's guidance adheres to the general principles of law and to regulations regarding the management of drugs.

The UKCC has the power to remove practitioners who fail to meet professional standards from the professional register, thus removing an individual's right to practice in the UK. The UKCC regulations are more comprehensive and detailed in relation to nursing clients than those required by law, but they also assist the nurse in interpreting the law.

Ms AC, a ward sister, appeared before the professional conduct committee after it was alleged that she increased a dose of diamorphine being administered to a patient via subcutaneous infusion pump from 1 mg/hour to 20 mg/hour without proper authority and also failed to conform to the policies and procedures laid down by her employer (UKCC, 1993).

1. Would this behaviour constitute professional misconduct?

2. What action should be taken in this situation?

3. Although the Professional Conduct Committee decided that the sister's behaviour did constitute misconduct she was not struck off the professional register. What other considerations may the Professional Conduct Committee take into account when judging the above behaviour by the ward sister?

▶ Local Policies for Medicines Storage and Administration

Local policies are established within individual health trusts and care settings and set the expectations of the employer with respect to their employed practitioners. Nurses must be aware of the contents of their local policy, because it is unlikely that an individual nurse who becomes involved in any legal action with a patient would receive support or insurance if the employer's policy is contravened during the incident. This would be irrespective of whether the practice is acceptable to the UKCC or legal standards. This is particularly important in relation to the administration of medicines because there are variations between individual employers in what is deemed to be acceptable practice. This is particularly well illustrated in relation to the checking of medicines

DECISION MAKING

Obtain a copy of the UKCC *Standards for the Administration of Medicines* (1992a) and compare it with your local policy.
1. *Are there any differences in their expectations of you?*
2. *How will local policy guide your practice?*

by individual practitioners. The law holds an individual accountable for medicine administered irrespective of qualification, but the UKCC states that only a qualified practitioner can give medicines, and advocates that 'in the majority of circumstances a first level registered nurse, a midwife or a second level nurse, each of whom has demonstrated the necessary knowledge and competence, should be able to administer medicines without involving a second person'. Local policies, however, vary with regards to how many (one or two) nurses are required to check a medicine, and where a second checker is required, there is variation as to who that person is to be. For nurses who change employment or who participate in agency employment, an awareness of local variations in policy is essential.

▶ *Clients' Rights*

As with any form of treatment all clients have a right to be fully informed about the medicines they receive and most have a right to refuse treatment if it is against their wishes. There are, however, some exceptions to this rule, and for nursing this has moral and ethical implications, which require consideration.

▶ Treatment of children

In the treatment of children, it is beholden to the nurse to ensure that the child patient and their family receive information about their treatment that is appropriate to their understanding. If it is considered that the child client is old enough and mature enough to understand the implications of his or her treatment then his or her decision should be allowed by the health carer. This is supported in law by the precedent set by the Gillick case in which a general practitioner won his case to prescribe a child under the age of 16 years contraceptive medication without recourse to her parents for permission. For a child who is under 16 years of age, however, any decision for treatment is usually made with the joint consent of the parents. This is commonly incorporated into hospital policy as a guideline for health carers. Finally, the *Children Act* (1989) also influences treatment for children in stating that any course of treatment must be in the best interests of the child concerned. In a few cases this may have implications if a parent refuses to consent to treatment for a child where the child is too young to consent for him or herself and where the treatment is unanimously considered by medical professionals to be in the best interests of the child. In this situation the child may be made a ward of court in order to allow treatment to be given without parental consent.

Similar assessments must be made for those with learning disabilities. The administration of medicines for children and those with learning disabilities can cause ethical dilemmas in practice.

Six-year-old Ahmed is undergoing treatment for leukaemia. While you are in practice he is to have oral medication, which he hates intensely. On this particular occasion he refuses to take his medicine, which is a vital part of his treatment.

1. *Does Ahmed have any right to refuse his treatment?*

▶ Treatment of the mentally ill

Most mentally ill clients do have a right to consent to or refuse treatment. In some situations, however, treatment is obliged by law and is involuntary. This is usually because the client's illness indicates a risk to themselves or to the community unless treatment is maintained. Again issues may be raised regarding the rights of the client and the role of the nurse in protecting such rights, especially if the treatment given benefits the community rather than the patient himself, for instance the use of medication to subdue noisy or aggressive clients.

RESEARCH BASED EVIDENCE

Koren et al. (1986) found that calculation errors accounted for 8% of all mistakes made in a children's ward, findings that support similar work completed by Perlstein et al. (1979). Most recently Ridge et al. (1995) used covert observation to look at single-nurse administration in one NHS trust hospital. They observed a 3.5% total error rate and comment that this is too high. There must also be concern that wrong doses accounted for 15% of maladministrations in their study.

RESEARCH BASED EVIDENCE

Arndt (1994) explored nurses' experiences with medication errors using a qualitative approach. She analysed discourse from two group discussions, 12 unstructured interviews and six self-written reports where nurses described their experiences with medication errors.

She concluded that medication errors caused nurses to feel ashamed and humiliated, and they forced situations of conflict, which demanded the nurses to make moral decisions. She also suggested that nurses' ability to cope depends heavily upon the support by colleagues at the time of the incident.

Think about the discussion above.

Ask yourself whether all medication errors are wrong or should the potential severity of outcome be taken into consideration when planning disciplinary action?

Other considerations related to the management of all clients, but especially pertinent to those taking medicines for chronic illness, include the validity of an initial consent if a client changes his or her mind or wishes to stop treatment. Issues that require consideration include what rights a dangerously aggressive client has to stop treatment if the medication is successful. Many medications that affect mood also have side effects, which may be uncomfortable or inconvenient to the client, but if treatment is stopped, will their aggession make them a danger to society? Do such clients have a right to refuse?

Medicines such as fluphenazine decanoate (Modecate) have a long-acting effect, which cannot be reversed quickly. There are also implications for withdrawing treatment, especially where a medicine creates a dependence because it is addictive or it reduces the body's ability to produce a similar substance naturally (e.g. glucocorticosteroids). Rapid withdrawal from such medication could be dangerous and cause discomfort to the patient

▶ *Management of Medication Errors*

Medication errors occur in the event of the nurse failing to ensure that their patient receives the medicine (error of omission) or receives it when there is reason to withhold it or in a manner that is not appropriate (error of commission) (Wolf, 1989). When errors do occur, they may have a devastating effect; at the least they demonstrate the fallibility of individuals, and at worst they can cause discomfort, pain or be potentially fatal for the patients involved. Given the seriousness of such errors, it is perhaps surprising to learn how commonly they occur.

In the event of an error occurring, the nurse concerned must ensure the safety of the patient and staff. This would usually involve immediately contacting members of medical and pharmacy teams and explaining what has happened in the incident so that an appropriate course of action can be taken.

After the practical management of any error, the nurse must complete documentation to record the incident. The nature of further action then depends upon the type of error made and unless the error is in contravention of the *Code of Professional Conduct* (UKCC, 1992b) or the law, or local policy.

Policies vary widely in their attitude and response to error. Some adopt complex means such as the El Dorado Medication Error Tool (EDMET) (Cobb, 1986; Ernst *et al.*, 1991) to determine the severity of disciplinary action in relation to the severity of the error. Others manage all errors in a similar way, while others respond differently according to the numbers of errors made by a nurse.

In conclusion, this chapter has introduced you to many facets of knowledge required to make effective nursing decisions when planning the storage and administration of medicines to patients. The chapter demonstrates the need for a wide range of nursing skills, from understanding the complexities of medicines' law and physiological action to the more practical elements such as perceptual and communication skills required when working with both patients and other members of the nursing and multidisciplinary team. The safe and effective administration of medicines requires nurses to be knowledgeable, and importantly, vigilant in their practice, and as with other areas of practice highlighted in this book, also requires you to be aware of the latest developments in research related to of all the areas addressed. This chapter has introduced research-based evidence in medicines administration supporting rationale for the care to be offered. It is not intended to be a complete record of all applicable research or necessarily the most up to date and relevant to your own specific practice area, but it serves as an illustration of the work that is available and can be used to enhance care in practice.

▶ CASE STUDIES

In summary, case studies are provided to enable the application of concepts presented in this chapter. In each one, issues will be raised that are meaningful to that individual situation, but may also be transferrable to other settings with different clients.

▶ CASE STUDY: ADULT

Julia Hargreaves is 26 years old and lives alone in a flat in the centre of a large city. She moved five years ago from her parents' house in the country to find work after graduating from university. Julia is admitted to hospital after a car knocks her off her bike as she is cycling home one evening. On admission Julia is adamant that she wishes to have no treatment with medicines as she is in early pregnancy and does not wish to hurt her baby. Julia is found to have a compound fracture of her left tibia and is in considerable pain. Without antibiotics she risks seriously complicating her injury by developing osteomyelitis.

■ **What factors would you need to take into account when planning care for Julia?**

■ **Discuss what you consider the nurse's role might be in the above situation?**

■ **If Julia persisted in her request for no medical treatment, what dilemmas may face carers who are looking after her and her unborn child?**

REFLECTIVE KNOWLEDGE

▶ CASE STUDY: MENTAL HEALTH

Mohammed Shah is 20 years old and newly diagnosed as having mental illness, which requires long-term treatment with antipsychotic drugs to prevent deluded, aggressive and occasionally violent behaviour. He has been treated now for six months and feels that he is cured and no longer requires his fortnightly injections. Although Mohammed continues to attend the clinic for these, he is becoming increasingly dissatisfied with the nurses, and is starting to suggest that he may not come any more.

■ **As the practice nurse, how might you respond to Mohammed?**

■ **What would be the dilemmas to be solved in making your response?**

■ **Mohammed was being treated with the antipsychotic fluphenazine decanoate (Modecate). What are the therapeutic benefits and side effects of antipsychotic medications such as this?**

▶ CASE STUDY: CHILD

Cloe Jackson is six years old and lives at home with her mother and father and two-year-old brother Casper. She has had severe eczema since she was a baby and this frequently becomes inflamed with open lesions. At a visit to the surgery Mrs Jackson is advised by her general practitioner to accept a prescription for glucocorticosteroid treatment for Cloe. Mrs Jackson is very anxious about the prospect of this treatment since she has heard that glucocorticosteroids have bad side effects.

■ **What information should be offered to Mrs Jackson about the benefits and effects of glucocorticosteroid treatment?**

■ **What advice should be given if Cloe is to receive glucocorticosteroid treatment for her eczema?**

■ **The glucocorticosteroid treatment is to be administered at home in the form of a topical cream. What education should be included regarding administration and storage?**

■ **Mrs Jackson comments that she has heard that alternative medicine is an effective way of managing eczema. She asks the practice nurse for an opinion. What advice could the practice nurse offer?**

▶ CASE STUDY: LEARNING DISABILITIES

Sam Doppler is a 30-year-old man with mild learning disability. He manages to live alone and works as a kitchen assistant in a small cafe. One day he cuts his hand on an unwashed knife at work. After a few days the cut becomes inflamed and sore and Sam is unable to use his hand and so he attends his general practitioner. Sam is prescribed a course of oral antibiotics and advised not to return to work until his hand has healed.

■ **What advice should Sam receive about taking his antibiotics?**

■ **Given his learning disability, what strategies may be employed to ensure that Sam understands the prescription he is given?**

■ **Sam asks the practice nurse to explain why the doctor has given him tablets when it is his hand that is sore. Discuss the pharmacokinetic action of oral antibiotic treatment from taking the medication to its therapeutic action at the required site.**

▶ ANNOTATED FURTHER READING

BRITISH NATIONAL FORMULARY (1996) No. 30. London. British Medical Association and The Pharmaceutical Society. 1996.
   A useful formulary for identifying types and effects of medication.
ALDERHEY CHILDRENS HOSPITAL (1994) *Alderhey Book of Children's Dosages*. Liverpool. Alder Hey.
   A useful formulary for identifying types and effects of medication.
KEE J.L., HAYES E.R. (1993) *Pharmacology – A Nursing Process Approach*. Chapter 4. Philadelphia. W.B. Saunders Company.
   This chapter offers a clear and comprehensive review of the metric system, calculating medicines and determining body weight and surface area.
DOWNIE, G., MACKENZIE, J., WILLIAMS, A. (1995) *Pharmacology and Drug Management for Nurses*. Edinburgh. Churchill Livingstone.
   Downie *et al.* offer a detailed explanation of current theories regarding pharmacodynamics in a complete chapter on this subject.
PEARSON, A., VAUGHAN, B. (1984) *Nursing Models in Practice*. London. Heinemann.
   This book offers an applied illustration of the use of nursing models and the nursing process in caring for patients.
DIMOND, B. (1990) *Legal Aspects of Nursing*. Chapter 28, pp. 353–361. New York. Prentice Hall.
Issues related to the nurse's duty of care to the patient are found in further detail as applied to medicines storage and administration.

▶ REFERENCES

ARNDT, M. (1994) Nurses medication errors. *Journal of Advanced Nursing* **19**: 519–526.

BRITISH NATIONAL FORMULARY No 30. London. British Medical Association and The Pharmaceutical Society. 1996.

CARTWRIGHT, A. (1990) Medicine taking by people aged 65 or more. *British Medical Bulletin* **46**(1): 63–76.

THE CHILDREN ACT (1989) London. Her Majesty's Stationery Office.

CLARENCE, M. (1990) Over the counter analgesics. *Nursing Standard* **5**: 10.

CLARK, J.B.F., QUEENER, S.F., KARB, V.B. (1994) *Pharmacologic Basis of Nursing Practice.* St Louis. Mosby.

COBB, M.D. (1986) Evaluating medication errors. *The Journal of Nursing Administration* **16**: 4.

CRABTREE, D. (1995) No denying it. *Nursing Times* **91**: 18.

DEPARTMENT OF HEALTH (1989) *Report of the Advisory Group on Nurse Prescribing. The Crown Report.* London. Her Majesty's Stationery Office.

DIMOND, B. (1995) *Legal Aspects of Nursing* (2nd edition). New York. Prentice Hall.

DOWNIE, G., MACKENZIE, J., WILLIAMS, A. (1995) *Pharmacology and Drug Management for Nurses.* Edinburgh. Churchill Livingstone.

ERNST, M.A., BUCHANAN, A., COX, C. (1991) A judgement of errors. *Nursing Times* **3**: 87.

HOPKINS, SJ. (1995) *Drugs and Pharmacology for Nurses* (12th edition). Edinburgh. Churchill Livingstone.

KEE, J.L., HAYES, E.R. (1993) *Pharmacology, A Nursing Process Approach.* Philadelphia. W.B. Saunders Company.

KOREN, G., BARZILAY, Z., MODAN, M. (1986) Errors in Computing Drug Doses. *Canadian Medical Association Journal* **129**: 721–723.

LESAGE, J. (1991) Polypharmacy in geriatric patients. *Nursing Clinics of North America* **26**: 2.

LOI, C–M., VESTEL, R.E. (1988) Drug metabolism in the elderly. *Pharmacology Therapy* **36**: 131–149.

MANLEY, G., SHEIHAM, A., EADSFORTH, W. (1994) Sugar coated care? *Nursing Times* **90**: 7.

MEDICINES ACT (1968) London. Her Majesty's Stationery Office.

MISUSE OF DRUGS ACT (1971) London. Her Majesty's Stationery Office.

MISUSE OF DRUGS REGULATIONS (1985) London. Her Majesty's Stationery Office.

MORGAN, C.A. (1994) Illicit drug use: primary prevention. *British Journal of Occupational Therapy* **57**: 1.

NAISH, J., GARBETT, R. (1996) Don't administer drugs, says union. *Nursing Times* **20**(47): 5.

NIGHTINGALE, F, (1980) *Notes on Nursing: (What It Is and What It Is Not)* (Reprint of 1st edition). Edinburgh. Churchill Livingstone.

PARKIN, D.M., HENNEY, C.R., QUIRK, J., CROOKS, J. (1976) Deviation from prescribed treatment after discharge from hospital. *British Medical Journal* **2**: 686–688.

PERLSTEIN, P.H., CALLISON, C., WHITE, M. (1979) Errors in drug computations during newborn intensive care. *American Journal of Diseases in Childhood* **133**: 376–379.

PLANT, M.L., PLANT, M.A., FOSTER, J. (1992) Stress, alcohol, tobacco and illicit drug use amongst nurses: A Scottish study. *Journal of Advanced Nursing* **17**: 1057–1063.

RIDGE, K.W., JENKINS, D.B., NOYCE, P.R., BARBER, N.D. (1995) Medication errors during hospital drug rounds. *Quality in Health Care* **4**: 240–243.

SCHMUCKER, D.L. (1984) Drug disposition in the elderly: a review of critical factors. *Journal of American Geriatric Society* **32**:144–149.

SCHWERTZ, D.W. (1991) Basic Principles of Drug Action. *Nursing Clinics of North America* **26**: 2.

SHUTTLEWORTH, A. (1994) Time to rethink the strategy on drugs (editorial). *Professional Nurse* **9(10)**: 652.

SUTHERLAND, K., MORGAN, J., SEMPLE, S. (1995) Self administration of drugs: an introduction. *Nursing Times* **91**: 23.

THE MEDICINAL PRODUCTS: PRESCRIPTION BY NURSES ETC. ACT, (1992) London. Her Majesty's Stationery Office.

TRIGG, E. (1995) Promoting innovation, anticipating change. *The Nursing of Children – A Resource Guide.* London. English National Board.

TROUNCE, J, (1994) *Pharmacology for Nurses* (14th edition). Edinburgh. Churchill Livingstone.

UKCC (1993) *Professional Conduct Occasional Report on Selected Cases 1 April 1991 to 31 March.* London. UKCC.

UKCC (1992a) *Standards for the Administration of Medicines.* London. UKCC.

UKCC (1992c) *Code of Professional Conduct.* London. UKCC.

UKCC (1992d) *Scope of Professional Practice,* London, UKCC.

UKCC (1996) *Guidelines for Professional Practice.* London. UKCC.

WOLF, Z.R. (1989) Medication errors: Nursing responsibilities. *Holistic Nurse Practitioner* **4**: 1.

SECTION TWO

Immediate to supportive practice

2.1 Resuscitation

R. Cable and H. Swain

KEY ISSUES

■ SUBJECT KNOWLEDGE

▷ the causes of cardiopulmonary arrest in infants, children and adults
▷ physiology of airway management and chest compressions
▷ coping with sudden death
▷ post-traumatic death syndrome

■ PRACTICE KNOWLEDGE

▷ assessment of the collapsed infant, child and adult
▷ basic life support skills required to resuscitate the infant, child and adult
▷ management of a choking client
▷ individual situations that require adaptation to the normal resuscitation guidelines

▷ drug therapy in the resuscitation situation

■ PROFESSIONAL KNOWLEDGE

▷ the professional role of the nurse in resuscitation within hospitals and the community
▷ legal and professional accountability when undertaking resuscitation
▷ education and skills updating for resuscitation
▷ ethical issues relating to the decision to resuscitate or not

■ REFLECTIVE KNOWLEDGE

▷ assess own personal practice of resuscitation skills and identify strengths and weaknesses
▷ consolidation of knowledge through case studies

▶ INTRODUCTION

Resuscitation encompasses more then just trying to reverse the process of a sudden death. It is a term commonly used to describe active intervention in any emergency situation. This chapter will consider the role of the nurse in undertaking immediate and potentially life saving physical care of the sick and injured both in hospital and the community. The focus of this chapter is on the immediate action at an emergency and in particular, basic life support (BLS).

BLS is the initial action carried out by the rescuer on a person who has collapsed and has no effective cardiopulmonary function while awaiting help from the health care professionals. This action requires no extra equipment and depends on the rescuer assessing and implementing a procedure that includes mouth to mouth and external cardiac compression. Anyone who has undertaken first aid or resuscitation training can carry out BLS.

Advanced life support (ALS) is the second phase of emergency care and requires equipment such as airway adjuncts, drugs and a defibrillator, which are explained later in this chapter. ALS activities are usually undertaken by specially trained paramedics and health care professionals as specialized skills are required.

Immediate physical care is often an issue that is dismissed as the role of the acute hospital nurse and only really within the realm of nurses from the adult or child branches. If potential emergency situations are considered carefully it soon becomes apparent, however, that the nurses most exposed to the problems of emergency care are those working in the mental health and learning disability branches, and especially those nurses working in the community. Community nurses can have a long wait after calling for help from the emergency services and may need to be far more resourceful in their efforts to resuscitate in the emergency situation.

▶ OVERVIEW

▶ *Subject Knowledge*

After initially referring to Resuscitation Guidelines, we review the most common causes of sudden collapse in children and adults, with particular reference to the altered anatomy and physiology. Under psychosocial subject knowledge, reactions to sudden trauma and death by individuals and the public are explored, with particular reference to post-traumatic stress syndrome.

▶ *Practice Knowledge*

In this section we present a systematic and logical approach to assessment and management of resuscitation that can be applied to any emergency situation. We then explain in more detail the 1997 Resuscitation Guidelines for use in the UK (Resuscitation Council (UK), 1997).

▶ *Professional Knowledge*

In this section the role of the professional nurse in the emergency situation and the potential legal issues related to emergency interventions are considered. We also explore ethical dilemmas surrounding resuscitation. The need for education and updating to maintain skills in order to be effective in the emergency situation is discussed.

▶ *Reflective Knowledge*

Throughout this chapter, you will be able to apply theory to practice through reflective and decision-making exercises and to expand your knowledge through identified research-based evidence. The final section of the chapter provides case studies to consolidate your knowledge and suggests how you can assess your own practice through using specifically designed checklists.

On pp. 168–169 there are four case studies, each one relating to one of the branch programmes. You may find it helpful to read one of them before you start the chapter and use it as a focus for your reflections while reading.

SUBJECT KNOWLEDGE *Biological*

▶ RESUSCITATION GUIDELINES

One of the continuing dilemmas in resuscitation relates to the need for a consistent approach to care, that is, the same management by everyone from boy scouts to consultant cardiologists. An approach that is truly international has been a target of the resuscitation training bodies for many years. The European Resuscitation Council (ERC) founded in 1992 has taken this international goal further by integrating the work of many countries. In April 1997, the International Liaison Committee on Resuscitation (ILCOR) presented advisory statements on resuscitation in

Next time you are in the library find out if the Guidelines of the European Resuscitation Council have been recently updated — it is likely that new guidelines will be issued in June 1998. If it is available in your local library, check the journal *Resuscitation*; if not, search the indexing systems *CINAHL* and *MEDLINE* under the topic area 'resuscitation, cardiopulmonary' for commentary on any changes made in the guidelines. Review how the guidelines have changed and the rationale for those changes. Decide whether you need any special training to be able to follow these new guidelines.

order to develop a global approach (ILCOR, 1997). The intention is that the individual resuscitation councils will use these statements as 'blueprints' for guidelines for their own countries. With so many differences in law and provision of emergency care between countries, it is difficult to see how the concept could be further developed. In emergencies, it is obviously helpful if all carers can work together without detailed discussion and this is one of the great benefits of the current resuscitation guidelines. The advantage for this global approach is not only an issue of consistency: it would also provide a much larger research population when it comes to reviewing changes in mortality and morbidity as a result of improvement in the developing techniques of resuscitation. However, a potential difficulty caused by such a global approach is the need for almost continuously updating the guidelines to take into account new research findings. When the pace of change causes concern, it is worth directing individuals to look at the resuscitation methods used in the 1930s to 1950s such as Schafer's and Silvester's methods. These methods describe how to ventilate the collapsed individual by moving the person's arms around. We are not aware of any reported successes using these methods, but you will find them described in old first aid books.

The reason for the term 'guidelines' is to allow for adaptations according to individual circumstances; describing them as 'rules' might discourage 'necessary' variations. Despite differences in the branches of nursing there are only two main approaches to resuscitation and these are based upon the physiological development of individuals across the life span (i.e. the adult and the child). The fact that the individual has a mental health problem or a learning disability makes no difference to the general approach as the guidelines for resuscitation remain the same. However, there may need to be slight variations from the guidelines if for example there is a specific reason for the collapse. Examples would be differences in resuscitation techniques for a client who has taken an overdose of tranquillizers as opposed to an adult who has had a heart attack. It is therefore important to be able to make important instant decisions and to have knowledge of the differences in resuscitation techniques for a child as opposed to an adult.

▶ THE COLLAPSED ADULT

Before considering the 'practicalities' of resuscitation, it is important to have an understanding of the potential mechanism of sudden collapse so that a more logical approach can be made. The Resuscitation Council guidelines have a basic assumption, which is worth mentioning, that is the most common cause of nontraumatic sudden pulseless collapse in adults is cardiac in origin, and more specifically ventricular fibrillation (VF), which will be described further in the next section. 'Collapse' can be defined as 'a potentially reversible, sudden and unexpected loss of normal consciousness'. In infants and children, as we will see later, the situation is usually different, hence the different set of guidelines. The primary cause of infant nontraumatic collapse is classically of respiratory origin.

The aim of the BLS guidelines is to produce an accurate and rapid diagnosis, ensure appropriate help is summoned and limit the effects of hypoxia (lack of oxygen).

DECISION MAKING

The cardiac muscle is supplied with blood from the coronary arteries and it is changes such as narrowing of these vessels which may result in coronary heart disease (CHD).

1. *Review how blood vessels become narrower and the potential causes for this phenomenon occurring.*
2. *How might you use the knowledge of potential causes of CHD to promote a healthy lifestyle?*

▶ THE HEART AND VF

The heart is a four-chambered organ situated centrally and slightly to the left in the chest behind the sternum (Figures 2.1.1 and 2.1.2).

One of the characteristics of cardiac muscle is its ability to contract in the absence of any external stimulation. This independent mechanism is coordinated by a unique electrical system within the heart, which results in a coordinated contraction of the heart muscle.

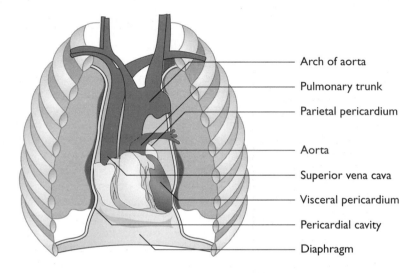

Figure 2.1.1: Location of the heart. (Redrawn from Hinchliff *et al.*, 1996.)

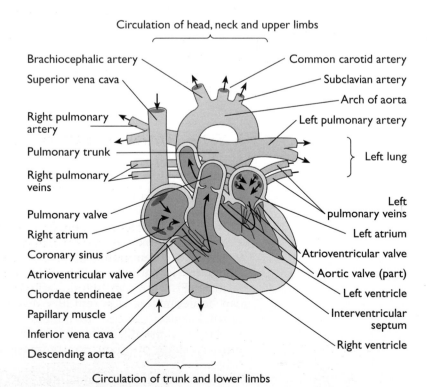

Figure 2.1.2: Structure of the heart and the direction of blood flow. (Redrawn from Hinchliff *et al.*, 1996.)

Figure 2.1.3: Normal sinus rhythm.
(Redrawn from Hinchliff *et al.*, 1996.)

Figure 2.1.4: Asystole.
(Redrawn from Hinchliff *et al.*, 1996.)

Figure 2.1.5: Ventricular fibrillation.
(Redrawn from Hinchliff *et al.*, 1996.)

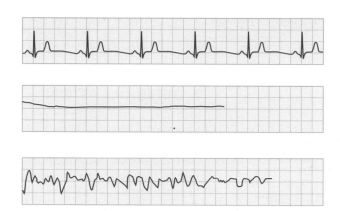

Above is a representation of the normal electrical activity of the heart as measured by skin electrodes and a cardiac monitor (Figure 2.1.3). This is an electrocardiograph or ECG.

Referring to a physiology textbook, explain the above pattern in relation to the way the electrical activity coordinates cardiac muscle contraction. Remember that this is only an indication of electrical activity and it does not necessarily relate directly to mechanical function.

When the normal electric conduction system in the heart fails because of ischaemic heart disease (IHD), instead of stopping 'dead' (known as asystole, Figure 2.1.4), each muscle fibre independently contracts and relaxes giving the heart a shivering appearance: this is ventricular fibrillation (VF, Figure 2.1.5). Although the heart is active there is no effective pumping action, therefore the collapsed individual will have no pulse and will quickly lose consciousness.

During VF there is no coronary circulation and therefore no oxygen supply to the cardiac muscle. As a result VF becomes less 'strong' or 'coarse' with time and eventually decays to asystole.

The significance of VF is the relative simplicity of treatment – passing an electric discharge over the heart, known as defibrillation, will result in a coordinated muscular contraction and (hopefully) a return to a spontaneous rhythm. The key factor in the success of the process of defibrillation is time. The longer the delay between the onset of VF and treatment by defibrillation, the worse the outcome. While the patient is in VF there is no coronary circulation and therefore no myocardial oxygenation, so the patient deteriorates rapidly. It is unlikely that BLS resuscitation is very efficient in maintaining an effective coronary circulation. It does, however, buy the patient time until further help is available.

▶ THE CHAIN OF SURVIVAL

The ideal survival scenario from ventricular fibrillation is described in 'the chain of survival' (Cummins *et al.*, 1991), which indicates the links required (Figure 2.1.6):

▶ early help ensures that defibrillation time is as short as possible;
▶ early BLS slows deterioration;
▶ early defibrillation is the key to reversing the situation;
▶ finally the provision of advanced cardiac life support to stabilize the patient and ALS, which includes improving airway management and the use of drugs.

Figure 2.1.6: The chain of survival concept.

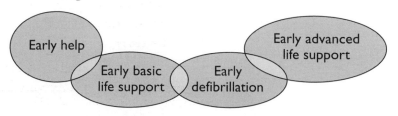

As the VF scenario is potentially so treatable, this is the target of the adult resuscitation guidelines. Conveniently all other medical emergencies are also reasonably managed by these guidelines.

▶ DEFIBRILLATION

Currently, the teaching and practice of defibrillation (Figure 2.1.7) is not widespread among nurses. Current opinion varies, from nurses being worried about the potential legal implications of nurse defibrillation and hence resistance to carrying it out, to widespread implementation across Health Trusts. It is worth pointing out to hesitant nurses that the government used the example of defibrillation by nurses as normal practice for adult branch nurses in their 1997 recruitment campaign advertisement. In order to reduce the mortality from IHD the time from VF cardiac arrest to defibrillation needs to be constantly monitored and audited. Wardrope and Morris (1993) in their review of the resuscitation guidelines stated 'defibrillate as early and as often as possible'.

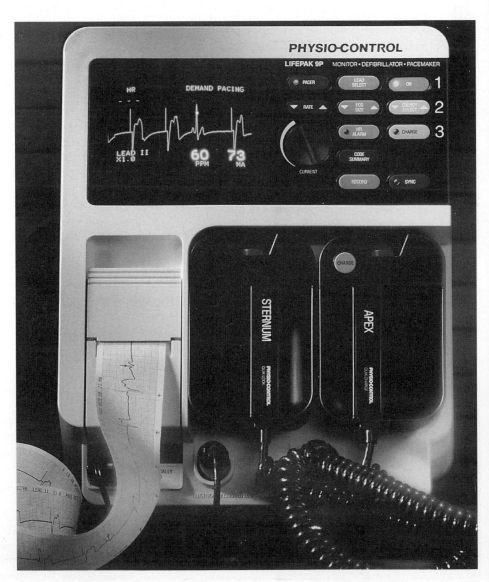

Figure 2.1.7: A typical defibrillator. (Reproduced with kind permission of Physio-Control, Basingstoke, UK Ltd.)

In the hospital setting, nurses are in an ideal position to carry out early defibrillation and make a significant contribution to reducing the death rate from IHD. Nurses should be able to defibrillate in all clinical environments, especially as with improving technology the process is not difficult to learn. In the pre-hospital environment, The American Heart Association argues that early bystander cardiopulmonary resuscitation (CPR) along with rapid defibrillation makes a major contribution to the survival of adults following a sudden cardiac arrest and recommend that we should move towards 'public access defibrillation' as a way of increasing survival rates (Weisfeldt, 1995). Since the mid 1990s, in the UK, the national news has reported on various schemes to promote this activity including defibrillation by transport police and the fire service and cases of some petrol stations with a defibrillator available. Cummins *et al.* (1991) discuss this subject further. An internet site reviews some of the literature on early defibrillation and nurses (see Annotated Further Reading).

One of the most significant recent developments in defibrillator technology is the semi-automatic or advisory external defibrillator (AED). The AED system will analyse a patient's cardiac rhythm and indicate if the patient requires defibrillation or not. In use, it is simply a matter of connecting two large electrodes to the patient and following a '1,2,3' approach in terms of operation where '1' is on, 2 is 'analyse' (determine the rhythm) and 3 is 'fire' (defibrillate).

Although VF is the most common out-of-hospital rhythm in adult nontraumatic cardiac arrest, being the primary rhythm in approximately 80–90% of cases (Colquhoun *et al.*, 1995), there are two other potentially fatal rhythms. These are asystole and electromechanical dissociation (EMD).

Asystole (see Figure. 2.1.4) is the classic 'straight line' on the cardiac monitor that is frequently used in films and TV 'soaps'. The straight line indicates no apparent cardiac electrical activity and commonly occurs as a result of prolonged hypoxia or another significant illness. In practice, apparently well patients do not usually suddenly collapse into asystole as presented by the media.

EMD is the third and least common rhythm associated with cardiac arrest. In this situation, the nurse will see a rhythm on the cardiac monitor that is similar to normal sinus rhythm, but will find no palpable carotid pulse on examining the patient. Essentially, the electrical conduction system within the cardiac muscle is functioning, but there is no associated cardiac output (hence EMD). In the simplest situation, when a patient has lost most of the circulating blood volume, the heart will continue to work while it is still oxygenated, but no significant amount of blood will be circulated. There are several causes of EMD including hypovolaemia (blood loss), pneumothorax (collapsed lung), hypothermia (low body temperature)

During your practice placements review the availability of resuscitation equipment. This is usually a significant part of your orientation to any new practice setting.

1. *Check whether there is a defibrillator available and how it is operated.*
2. *Review the local policies about when, how often and by whom resuscitation equipment is checked.*
3. *Discuss with your practice supervisor which members of the multidisciplinary team are allowed to perform ALS after the initial resuscitation phase (BLS).*
4. *How is resuscitation dealt with in primary health care settings and by individual community nurses.*

The documents *The Health of the Nation* (Department of Health, 1991) and *Targeting Practice, The Contribution of Nurses, Midwives and Health Visitors* (Department of Health, 1993) clearly identify national targets to reduce the death rates from CHD.

1. *Debate the role of the nurse in helping to meet*

The Health of the Nation targets for CHD.

2. *Consider the impact of training sufficient numbers of the public to instigate BLS on the adult mortality figures.*
3. *How could the specialist nurse become involved in training members of the public?*

and electrolyte imbalance in the blood and intracellular fluids. All these situations occur in adults and children so both groups can present with EMD.

▶ THE COLLAPSED CHILD

The causes of collapse in children and infants are usually respiratory problems and resulting hypoxia rather than the cardiac problems found in adults as degenerative heart disease is not common in children (Nadkarni *et al.*, 1997). Innes *et al.* (1993) reviewed 45 resuscitation attempts in hospitalized children, and 21 (47%) were of respiratory origin. Cardiac failure in children and infants rarely occurs as an initial problem and is usually linked to congenital cardiac abnormalities.

The greatest mortality during childhood occurs in the first years of life. Causes include congenital problems, prematurity and infection due to the immature immune system. Sudden infant death syndrome (SIDS) remains the main cause of death in infants aged between one month and one year, although new guidelines on positioning infants have reduced this number considerably (Department of Health, 1992; Coyne, 1996). Over one year of age, trauma is the most frequent cause of death. Those children who have an out-of-hospital cardiac arrest who arrive in accident and emergency departments not breathing and pulseless have a poor outcome due to the brain damage resulting from lack of oxygen (Advanced Life Support Group, 1993).

The respiratory system (Figure 2.1.8) in children continues to develop until approximately eight years of age. Therefore the following points need to be considered in emergency care:

- ▶ infants tend to breathe only through their nose until the age of three months, which adds to the problems of resuscitation, as the nasal passages are small;
- ▶ the tongue is very large and collapses into the oropharynx easily so blocking the airway;
- ▶ the lower mandible is small in comparison to the large tongue, which further exacerbates the problem of airway obstruction;
- ▶ the diameter of the trachea increases threefold by puberty – the trachea is approximately the same size as the child or infant's little finger;
- ▶ the epiglottis is floppy and will easily occlude the airway.

The following additional anatomical characteristics should also be borne in mind, especially when providing ALS:

- ▶ the cartilaginous rings of the trachea are soft and easily compressed;

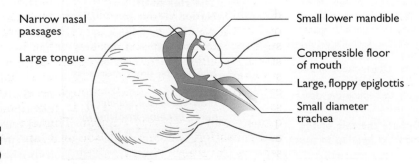

Figure 2.1.8: The upper airway in the infant. (Redrawn from Advanced Life Support Group, 1993.)

In the practice setting when caring for children reflect on the following.

1. *Review how and where the pulse rate may be measured in children of different age groups.*

2. *Note when the pulse is taken for a full minute and when and how an estimate may be taken.*

3. *Check in a paediatric textbook what the different ranges of pulse rate should be in children and find out when it is within the normal adult range.*

- respiration depends upon movement of the diaphragm as the intercostal muscles are not fully developed and therefore abdominal respirations are observed until at least six years of age;
- the left ventricle of the heart does not develop its characteristic thick muscular wall until about six months of age, and this affects how well blood circulates around the body because of the limited power of each contraction;
- the basal metabolic rate and oxygen consumption in infants are much higher than in adults resulting in increased heart and respiratory rates, and therefore they are much more prone to hypoxia and resulting neurological damage.

Because of the above factors of developing anatomy and physiology, the result will be different disease processes, that is, a collapse is likely to be primarily of respiratory rather than of cardiac origin. The BLS guidelines are based on maintaining oxygenation rather than restoring normal cardiac rhythm. However, an infant or child will soon become bradycardic (i.e. have a slow pulse rate) without oxygen and this will quickly progress to pulselessness.

Psychosocial

The main focus in this section is on the impact of sudden collapse and death on individual family members and on society as a whole, particularly in the case of major disasters. The effects of failure to achieve a successful resuscitation on members of the health care team are also considered. Further study in this area of care and decision making is provided in Chapter 3.5 on death and dying and Chapter 4.1 on stress and anxiety.

▶ SITUATIONAL LIFE CRISIS

Whether a resuscitation attempt is successful or not, the individual and their family will have experienced a crisis event in their lives that will lead to either a period of loss and grief or to a period of review and renewal depending on the outcome of the event. According to Wright (1996), situational crises can lead to intensive periods of psychological, behavioural and physical disarray because a person's existing coping mechanisms are challenged by the suddenness and newness of the event. A crisis cannot be tolerated for too long and therefore support in some form is needed. According to Caplan's early work on crisis intervention (Caplan, 1964), the individual or family concerned should be offered the right conditions to deal effectively with the situation in order to prevent later mental health problems.

In early studies on bereavement Parkes (1975) identified six different determinants or predictors of grief (Table 2.1.1, see also Chapter 3.5), and one of the most significant is mode of death. According to Wright (1996) sudden death through trauma is more likely to be thought of as causing suffering to the victim and being unjust. The anger produced in the family suvivors is often directed at themselves for failing to be present or call emergency services quickly enough. Anger may also be directed at those same emergency services if it is perceived that they did not respond quickly and sensitively enough. This anger is compounded if monetary compensation becomes an issue at a later stage, as the deceased is often seen as devalued (Wright, 1996).

Determinant
Mode of death
Nature of the attachment
Who was the person?
Historical antecedents
Personality variables
Social variables

Table 2.1.1 The six determinants of grief (Parkes, 1975).

During and after the time of crisis both the relatives and the health care professionals involved may require support. Support may also be needed by rescuers, particularly if many people have been involved in the resuscitation process, as in major disasters.

▶ THE RELATIVES

The most difficult issue for relatives to grasp is the fact their loved one, who they may have recently seen fit and healthy, is now dead. In a child's sudden death, the parental distress is increased if one or both parents have not been present at the time of death (Renner, 1991). Reactions of relatives can vary from denial to anger. Wright (1991) found relatives identified two emotions when a loved one has died suddenly:

▶ loss of control over their lives;
▶ powerlessness and helplessness to support, prevent or intervene.

In his study Wright also found that relatives had 'needs' that can be met by sensitive health care professionals (Wright, 1991). These include the needs:

▶ for information;
▶ to see their relative;
▶ to have time with their relative:
▶ for time to be spent with them by health professionals;
▶ for time to react and grieve.

Each of these needs will be dealt with in a little more detail.

▶ Need for Clear Information

The relatives may find themselves in one of two situations, either arriving while resuscitation is being attempted or arriving after the attempt. If the resuscitation is still in progress, it is essential that the events are frequently reported to the relatives as a means of 'preparing the ground'. However, in the situation of the relatives arriving after the event, they may become confused if the information is unclear. Therefore, it is important to use the word 'died' and 'death' even if this may appear harsh and blunt. It is particularly important to prevent parents from feeling they have failed their child by making every effort to allow them to be present during and soon after resuscitation (Wright, 1996)

▶ Need to See Their Loved One

To accept the situation, the bereaved usually sees the deceased. The

RESEARCH BASED EVIDENCE

Wright (1996) in his book on sudden death cites a study undertaken by Hanson and Strawser (1992) in which they survey the feelings of 47 family members who were present during the resuscitation of their relatives. Adjustment to the death was found to be easier than if they had not been with the patient according to 76% of respondents, and 64% felt that their presence was valuable to the dying person. Most respondents felt that the dying person had heard them express their love and say their goodbyes.

It has been noted that presence at resuscitation aids the grieving process and it should be an option in as many situations as possible, bearing in mind that it can cause difficulties for the health care professionals who may be undertaking invasive procedures in order to save the loved one (Zoltie et al., 1994).

supporting relatives and friends may try to dissuade the close relative, but seeing does aid the grieving process. There may be some concern if the deceased has received severe injuries and the health care professionals may be required to cover up that particular part of the body. To help the bereaved, it may help for the nurse to be touching the deceased, so letting the relatives know that it is acceptable to do so as well.

Need to Have Time With Their Loved One

Time to say farewell is important and may lead to other information the carer can impart to the family, which will demonstrate a caring approach for the relatives.

Need for Time With the Health Professionals

Sudden death leaves many questions unanswered and time spent by health professionals with the relatives to discuss the deceased's life again emphasizes a caring approach and allows the relatives time to respond to the situation. Chalk (1995) emphasizes the need for a member of staff to look after the relatives exclusively if at all possible.

Need for Time to Respond

Demonstration of emotions by the bereaved can cause concern for the carers. Wright (1991) found that nurses could address responses such as crying, anger, denial, aggression, bargaining, guilt and acceptance. Problems may arise when the relative withdraws and nurses feel there is little to act upon in order to give support. However, Wright (1991) also found that although some of the bereaved showed little response, the presence of the nurse was found to be comforting and reassuring. Inappropriate responses also cause concern to health professionals, but should not be misinterpreted. The relatives have received devastating news and it is difficult to assess what is appropriate and what is not.

THE HEALTH CARE PROFESSIONAL

Wright (1996) states that the cost of caring in crisis situations can physically and emotionally drain staff and suggests several different ways in which staff can support each other. These include debriefing and mutual support, re-education, activities outside work and a change of situation (see also Chapter 4.1 for further discussion on coping with stress).

Debriefing

Feelings of stress and anxiety can easily arise after a 'failed' resuscitation attempt. As long as the attempt has been conducted reasonably, 'failure' as it is often perceived, is more often due to the underlying pathology in the patient then the inadequacies of an effective resuscitation attempt. Debriefing after traumatic events such as a resuscitation are important not just to improve the efficiency of the next attempt, but also to ensure that staff are not left with feelings of self blame. This can be done through a critical incident technique. The important rule to remember for debriefing is that you are there to support each other and that it should be confidential. A traumatic resuscitation attempt is not something you can just walk away from without any follow up.

⫸ *Re-education*

We all become used to our own ways and it is necessary to address our knowledge to develop our skills further. Attending teaching sessions, seminars or conferences can lead to new ways of tackling this stressful situation.

DECISION MAKING

John O'Neill, a 14-year-old boy with a mild learning disability sustained a head injury in a fall from a tree at the day centre he attended. He was rushed to hospital by ambulance and his mother was called at her workplace. There was difficulty in getting information to his father as he was a long-distance lorry driver. John's mother arrived at the accident and emergency (A and E) department just as John began to show difficulty in breathing. The A and E team were beginning the process of intubation and ventilation. John's mother wished to be present and became increasingly agitated and aggressive when denied entrance to the emergency room.

1. *Decide how this crisis situation should be sensitively handled immediately.*
2. *Debate what the particular issues are for each person in the situation including John and what might be the long-term effects on the family.*
3. *What strategies could be developed by the staff of the A and E department to cope with a similar situation should it arise in the future?*

⫸ *Life Outside Work*

Maintaining leisure time away from the area allows the thought processes to rest and to look at life differently. It is also important for the workforce as a team to socialize away from the stressful situations in the clinical areas.

⫸ *Change of Environment*

Many professionals find that a change from a clinical area, even if only temporary, not only relieves the stress, but also allows a development and improvement in skills in other areas.

⫸ POST-TRAUMATIC STRESS DISORDER

Post-traumatic stress disorder (PTSD) was first described in the USA by Durham *et al.* (1985) and involves the long-term distressing emotions that have been experienced by ancillary medical and rescue workers such as the police and firemen in response to a major disaster event. This disorder has been highlighted in recent years after major disasters such as the Hillsborough Fooball Stadium Disaster, the Zeebrugge Ferry Disaster and the mass shooting of children in Dunblane in Scotland in 1996.

According to Wright (1996) sufferers of PTSD may:

⫸ during an initial phase experience denial with a lack of awareness of the severity of the event;

⫸ during an intermediate stage seen as a phase of confrontation and disorder start to experience signs of stress such as sleeplessness, nightmares and hypersensitivity to noise and become more easily angry and irritable.

⫸ during the final phase, readjust and recover and regain control of their life, becoming more hopeful and less dependent on others.

Much has been written about the complex process of helping individuals after traumatic and stressful events. If you undertake a literature search in this area, look under 'post-traumatic stress reaction'. Marion Gibson (1991) in her book *Order from Chaos, Responding to Traumatic Events* has produced a helpful guide to the topic based on her experiences in Belfast, Northern Ireland.

1. *Reflect on how you would react if the rescuers in a traumatic event received more monetary compensation for PTSD than the actual relatives of the victims of the disaster.*
2. *Along with your peer group debate the legal and moral issues involved in the above dilemma.*

Early recognition of the possibility of PTSD now leads to the provision of support in the form of counselling in a major disaster situation in an attempt to prevent the syndrome, while debriefing continues to play an important role for many years after the event. The ongoing difficulties for the victims of the Hillsborough disaster demonstrates this.

PRACTICE KNOWLEDGE

In a chapter devoted to the subject of resuscitation there is a need in this section to give detailed information on how to manage an emergency situation. After initially providing general guidelines on the First Aid Process, the broad framework advocated by the ERC is presented. Permission has been granted by the ERC to reproduce many of their guidelines. However, as these will need regular updating it is important that you use this text in conjunction with a copy of the most up-to-date guidelines available.

▶ GENERAL CONSIDERATIONS AT ANY EMERGENCY SITUATION

The First Aid Process is not unlike the Nursing or Medical Process (Figure 2.1.9). It is perhaps a little more like the medical approach than the current nursing approach because the establishment of a form of diagnosis is important in order to select the most appropriate actions. It is worth noting that although this is a linear process and not cyclical the need to return to the assessment at regular intervals cannot be over emphasized especially when anything changes in the casualty situation. When things appear to go wrong, just start at the beginning again.

A systematic approach is essential as it is easy to get distracted and start to perform 'trivial' tasks before the lifesaving considerations have been completed. An experienced qualified nurse is often asked by newly qualified nurses how to deal with new emergency situations. The usual answer is 'First aid and symptomatic care first, specific care for conditions is always well down the priority list'. This particular approach can be consolidated on courses such as the *Advanced Trauma Nursing Course (ATNC)*, which has been imported into the UK over the last few years from the American College of Surgeons. Each of the phases in the First Aid Process will now be considered in more detail.

▶ ASSESSMENT

Initial assessment involves assessing the situation rather than the individual. In assessing the situation we need to:

▶ consider safety;
▶ consider help required;
▶ establish priorities.

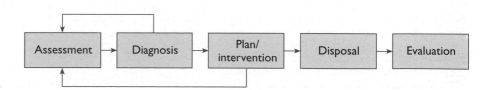

Figure 2.1.9: The first aid process.

▶ Personal Safety of the First Aider

The personal safety of the First Aider is an obvious priority so always look carefully at any situation before you 'dive in'. If you look at experienced staff around you there appear to be two main character types: those who 'dive in head first' without thinking and generally make a mess of things and those who stand and look for a few moments, briefly decide upon a plan of action and then implement it.

There is never a situation when to consider your own safety first is wrong. Potential hazards may include electricity, gas, fire, water and a casualty holding a double barrel shotgun! Some students express concern about the time this might 'waste'; in fact it only takes about the same time as putting on a pair of disposable gloves, which is probably a good thing to be doing while you are thinking if they are available to you in the particular situation. Another health and safety consideration includes infection control. Although there is much concern in this area regarding first aider safety, there is little current evidence that this is a great problem as long as the usual 'Universal Precautions' are followed, for example wearing gloves when handling body fluids (see Chapter 1.3 on infection control for more information).

As far as resuscitation is concerned, there are obvious risks with the spread of airborne organisms. Much concern has been raised about the potential of a rescuer catching the human immunodeficiency virus (HIV) while carrying out mouth to mouth resuscitation. At the time of writing we have heard of no such cases. However, there are other infections that pose a potentially greater risk. Barrier devices for use with mouth to mouth resuscitation need to be considered by the individual rescuer.

> Refer to Chapter 1.3 and other literature on HIV and its mode of spread.
>
> 1. **List the potential airborne infections that might be a risk to rescuers.**
>
> 2. **Review the effectiveness of any methods at present available to reduce risk to the first aider.**
>
> 3. **Review the potential for preventive immunizations from those organisms of high risk.**

▶ Assessing Help Required and Establishing Priorities

Another consideration at this early stage is to ask yourself if you can realistically manage the situation. Do you need help now, help soon or not at all? In the most extreme situation, that of a multiple casualty disaster, you have two basic choices: you either jump in and save a few lives while others are dying or you may choose to obtain a general overview of the situation and then call '999' to ensure the most appropriate response by the emergency services. Evidence from previous disasters shows that this initial stage is crucial to the overall organization of the 'event'. If you look at reports of any of the British disasters you will usually find this area of management of the situation is discussed (Trent Regional Health Authority, 1990a, b; Emergency Planning College, 1993).

The call for help must contain sufficient information to allow the emergency services coordinator to produce a full and adequate response (i.e. it is important to know the number and nature of the injured). If this information is not accurately provided it will be up to the first emergency services vehicle to fulfil this role, resulting in a further delay.

DECISION MAKING

You are the first person to arrive at the scene of a road traffic accident where two cars have hit each other. In the first car the elderly male driver has severe chest pain and a minor head injury. On the back seat of the car is a 30-year-old female with profound learning disabilities who is screaming loudly. In the second car the female driver is bleeding badly from an arm laceration. In the passenger seat of the second car lies an unconscious baby.

1. *How might you initially deal with the situation assuming no help is available?*
2. *What information will it be necessary to give the emergency services when you make your 999 call or direct a passerby to do so?*

In each of your practice placements, it is usually part of your orientation programme to learn about the emergency procedures in each particular placement.

1. *Reflect on how easy or difficult it is to remember the telephone number for emergency calls.*

2. *Find out if there are different teams available for different emergencies, for example a maternity emergency as opposed to a child emergency in a large hospital.*

3. *How do primary health care staff deal with obtaining back up services for emergencies in the home or the general practice setting?*

Most acute hospitals have an emergency team who provide internal emergency support, for example the cardiac arrest team. Some smaller hospitals with limited emergency support may use the 999 system.

▶ *Diagnosis*

A major consideration in the assessment process is making the diagnosis. This activity can be divided into three parts:

- ▶ history taking;
- ▶ signs and symptoms;
- ▶ examination.

When following the medical model, history taking is of great significance. More consideration should be given to history taking in nursing and first aid. It may be as simple as finding out that the individual was simply minding his or her own business and collapsed or alternatively was run over by a bus. Even apparently obvious situations must not be assumed – the collapsed individual on the way to hospital with a knife in his back may also be diabetic and the person run over by the bus might have had a heart attack – so never jump to premature and potentially unfounded conclusions at any stage of an individual's care.

If the situation is not critical, spend time listening to the casualty explain his story and seek clarification when required. This is usually time well spent, both at the early stage when determining what the problems are, and later when you need to determine the causative and exacerbating factors so you can attempt to prevent a recurrence.

Signs and symptoms are what you as a first aider can see and what the patient tells you, for example apparent unresponsiveness, shortness of breath and pain. If you have not reached a diagnosis already, these signs and symptoms will give you a general understanding of the situation.

There are two approaches to the examination: one for the unconscious and obviously seriously ill individual, and one for the non-life-threatening situation. For the unconscious patient, the general approach is described well in the BLS guidelines which follow. The emphasis is on:

- ▶ assessing response;
- ▶ opening the airway (A);
- ▶ checking breathing (B);
- ▶ confirming the presence of a circulation (C).

This is usually known as the ABC approach, which is described in more detail in the next section. After this initial assessment, a more comprehensive assessment can be undertaken.

For the non-life-threatening emergency situation, a systematic top to toe approach is probably most useful. Once it has been determined that the casualty is conscious and not bleeding to death, start at the casualty's head and work your way down (this is a skill that requires practice on a colleague) as follows.

▶ Starting at the head look and feel for any signs of injury, remembering that if you detect a head injury especially if the casualty is unconscious you must assume that there is a significant cervical spine injury until proven otherwise by a radiograph, so find a way to immobilize the neck now. (Some first aid books suggest that you examine the neck of an injured person to detect if the spinal column is in alignment or not, although alignment of the cervical spine is interesting its absence does not actually help you assess the significance of a spinal injury. If the history says there might be a spinal injury, you will need to deal with it.)

▶ Look at the colour of the skin, the movement of the eyes and listen to the respiratory effort.

▶ Now assess the chest. Once you have excluded wounds (and do not forget the back) respiratory movement should be observed. Is the chest fully inflating and is movement equal on the left and right, as only one lung may be damaged?

▶ Checking the back (assuming the patient is on their back) involves turning the casualty and is a risky procedure, especially if you have limited or untrained staff, although on the other hand you do not want to miss anything. Ideally you need a minimum of four people to turn the casualty while you have a look. In practice this may not be possible, so you need to weigh up the possible risks with what you may gain in terms of a more comprehensive assessment.

▶ When looking at limbs a helpful suggestion is to look at the uninjured limb first. Although it sounds a strange idea, a good understanding of the unaffected limb makes it easier to recognize abnormality. The distressed patient might require some reassurance that you know what you are doing, but they will appreciate the reduction in touching and handling of the injured limb that will result. Observe for open wounds, fractures and alterations in sensation or circulation to the limb. If you are concerned about a reduction in circulation, sometimes the capillary refill test can be easier than finding a formal pulse. Light pressure on the nail bed (fingers or toes) will result in a white blanch because you have emptied the blood vessels by the external pressure. On releasing the pressure the capillary bed should refill in 2–3 seconds; if it does not refill, be concerned about the circulation.

Try the capillary refill test on yourself. How long does it take for the capillary bed to refill?

As you systematically examine the casualty do not be distracted in your mission unless the situation requires immediate remedial action because something quite important may yet be discovered. If you do need to stop do not forget to continue your examination as soon as possible.

▶ INTERVENTION

When assessing responsiveness regardless of the age of the victim, there should be a response whether it is eye opening, a vocal response or movement. The unresponsive casualty may not breathe unless he or she has a patent airway (Figure 2.1.10). Although it is not possible to swallow the tongue, this phrase is often used to describe the relaxed tongue dropping into and blocking the posterior oropharynx. The manoeuvres described in the guidelines aim to relieve this obstruction. When opening the airway, the position of the lower jaw is at least as important as the head tilt (Figure 2.1.11), especially the need to realign it into its normal functional position with the upper and lower teeth on the same plane.

Figure 2.1.10: Normal anatomy of the upper airway. NMI (Nuclear Magnetic Image) of individual, conscious. Reproduced with the permission of The University of Nottingham.

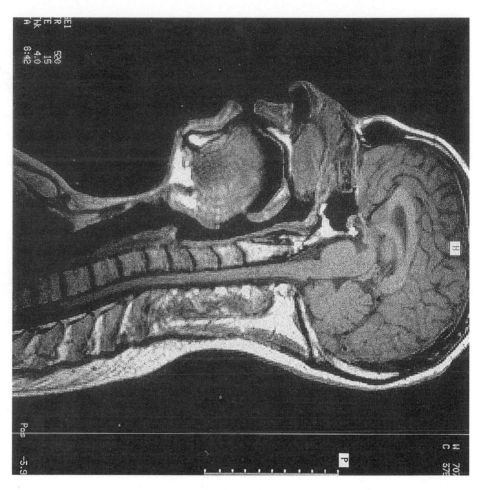

Identify the normal anatomical structures on Figure 2.1.10.

An additional manoeuvre is the jaw thrust (see Figure 2.1.12). The idea for this is to bring the lower jaw forwards – along with the jaw will come the attached tongue, hence clearing it from the airway. This is an especially important manoeuvre if the casualty has a potential neck injury, in which case it can be used alone without the head tilt manoeuver (Figure 2.1.11), which could cause further damage.

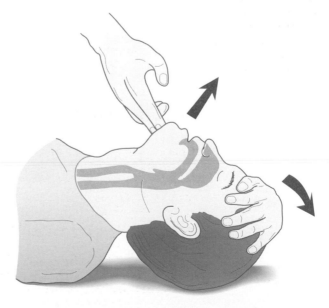

Figure 2.1.11: Head tilt.

Figure 2.1.12: Jaw thrust.

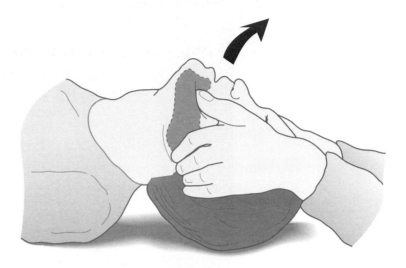

▶ *Checking the Circulation*

When checking the circulation, the only appropriate pulse to check is the carotid or femoral as the peripheral pulses are unreliable indicators in the collapsed patient. The femoral pulse is more difficult to find even if the casualty is suitably dressed (or undressed). In order to prevent uncertainty when the rescuer is anxious and adrenaline levels are high, the carotid pulse is best felt via anatomical landmarks rather then by guess work. On the casualty's neck palpate the trachea and the sternomastoid muscle. Place your fingers in the trough between these two structures in the midneck region and press down with the tips of the fingers until they reach the bottom of the trough (Figure 2.1.13). Preferably do this on the side nearest you to avoid occluding the trachea. Especially when practising this exercise, press on one side only, or you might cause fainting as a result of reducing blood flow to the brain. Handley *et al.* (1997) comments that the practice of the pulse check may be a less than reli-

Position of trachea

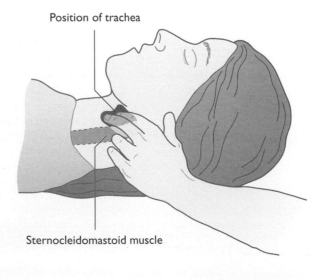

Sternocleidomastoid muscle

Figure 2.1.13: Locating the carotid pulse.

List the possible signs of a circulation, other than a pulse check.

able technique, especially by lay First Aiders, and perhaps the expression 'look for signs of a circulation', which includes a more general assessment of circulation as well as a pulse check is more appropriate.

▶ *Mouth to Mouth Ventilation*

Once ready to ventilate the casualty's lungs, one of the key words is 'slowly'. In the unconscious casualty, the oesophagus is relatively flat because it is not held open by cartilaginous rings as is the trachea, so slow (and low pressure) ventilations will tend to go into the lungs rather then the stomach. The harder and faster you blow, the more air will enter the stomach and the process becomes less efficient.

Unconscious people are unable to vomit. However, they can passively regurgitate their stomach contents into the upper airway, so ventilating too hard is also to the detriment of the rescuers! As far as ventilation volumes are concerned, judgement of these is a subjective art based on chest movement. According to Baskett *et al.* (1996) 400–600 ml is needed for adults, and one tenth of this volume (i.e. 40–60 ml) is needed for infants. Note that some adult resuscitation training mannikins may be calibrated to a larger volume.

Barrier devices are easily obtainable if you are concerned about the spread of any infection, although such spread is unlikely. The Ambu Company produce a 'LifeKey', which is a shield on a key ring, while the Laerdal Company produce both a shield and a pocket mask. If you want to make use of such devices make sure you are well practised with their use on a mannikin first as there is little point in having an emergency device with which you are unfamiliar. The pocket mask is especially useful as an oxygen supply can be added to the mask, increasing the percentage of oxygen delivered to the casualty from less then 20% to up to 50%, so making the whole process much more efficient.

▶ *Chest Compressions*

The two major theories regarding chest compressions are the cardiac theory and the thoracic pump theory. Robertson and Holmberg (1992) consider that neither of these are actually proven. It is likely that chest compression moves blood by a combination of:

▶ directly squeezing the heart between the sternum and the spine (cardiac pump theory);
▶ generally increasing the intrathoracic pressure (thoracic pump theory).

This forces blood out of the heart and chest, with the venous valve system ensuring a unidirectional flow.

As with ventilations, efficiency is related to rate and timing. Theoretically the faster the rate the greater the output, assuming a constant stroke volume (the volume of blood filling the ventricles). In practice as the compression rate increases, the stroke volume may be falling because the venous return to the chest and heart is reduced, therefore the actual rate is a compromise between these factors. To make the best use of the rate remember that the relaxation phase is at least as important as the compression phase, so leave adequate time between compressions to allow thoracic and ventricular refilling before the next compression.

A relatively new innovation in this area is the concept of active compression–decompression. Several pieces of research have now been

RESEARCH BASED EVIDENCE

Lack of oxygen (hypoxia) caused by a static circulation to vital organs takes various lengths of time to take effect. Lungs can withstand long periods of hypoxia, the liver 1–2 hours, the heart and kidney 30 minutes, and the brain 4–6 minutes (Newbold, 1987). Therefore the effect and efficiency of compressions is very important.

The blood flow that occurs as a result of chest compressions is only about 25% of normal, and cerebral blood flow only 15% of normal, and this is assuming good quality chest compressions (Mackenzie, 1964; Jackson, 1984).

Therefore delaying cardiac chest compressions for up to five minutes can result in no cerebral blood flow because of the pathological changes such as stasis of deoxygenated blood in the large veins (Lee, 1984).

An area currently undergoing vigorous research is the use of thrombolysis ('clot busting') to improve the recovery of stroke patients with the return of cerebral circulation. If the recovery is dramatic it may be evidence that the need to consider cardiac oxygenation is much greater than brain oxygenation in the early phases of resuscitation.

undertaken into the idea of actively sucking the chest up on the relaxation phase to increase refill and efficiency. Tucker and Idris (1994) undertook a review of the current research and found that the idea is derived from a resuscitation incident using a sink plunger to undertake the chest compressions. Although the evidence for this device is as yet inconclusive, it seems likely that it will be adapted as an adjunct to resuscitation in the future, either alone or incorporating other techniques such as the hydraulic 'thumper'. This device is a machine operated by compressed oxygen that will perform chest compression and ventilate the patient automatically (Fisher and Handley, 1995).

▶ Combining Ventilations and Compressions

During presentations by the ILCOR working groups at the 1997 CPR conference in Brighton, it was pointed out that there is little evidence to indicate what combinations of ventilations and compressions are the most effective in adults, and hence it is difficult to recommend changes for any valid reason. Current ratio guidelines have been in operation since closed chest compressions were first introduced. Table 2.1.2 gives an

> Review the timings exercise applying the most recent resuscitation guidelines.

Time	Event	'Running' time (s)
First minute	Two ventilations	10
	15 compressions	25
	Two ventilations	35
	15 compressions	50
	Two ventilations	60
Second minute	15 compressions	15
	Two ventilations	25
	15 compressions	40
	Two ventilations	50
	10 compressions	60

Table 2.1.2 Approximate timings for combined ventilations and compressions, based on the 1992 ERC Guidelines.

DECISION MAKING

John, the community psychiatric nurse, has been visiting 50-year-old Mohan Khan in his home weekly for the past three months. Mohan had become very depressed after he had been forced to take an early retirement offer when the company he was working for cut staff costs. Mohan's wife and two children and the local Seikh community had given him as much support as possible, but despite this and medication and counselling, Mohan has become steadily more withdrawn. On his regular Monday visit John could not get into the house and had to call Mohan's wife at the factory where she worked. On gaining entry as advised by Mohan's wife, John found Mohan collapsed in the bathroom with obvious signs of having slashed his wrists.

1. **Decide on the immediate steps that** John should take to provide BLS.
2. **When Mohan's wife arrives, how should John direct her activities?**
3. **How might this family react to the immediate situation?**
4. **Decide what strategies John may have to use to support Mohan and his family if he survives this suicide attempt (see also Chapter 4.1 on stress and anxiety).**

indication of the very approximate timings for the current situation. Therefore in any given minute the casualty is receiving 4–6 ventilations and 30–40 compressions. Even with the most competent rescuer, survival is not good without advanced help arriving rapidly.

▶ RESUSCITATING INFANTS AND CHILDREN

In the Subject Knowledge section of this chapter it was pointed out that there are major differences between children and adults in both the causes of sudden collapse and also in some of the anatomical features, and these have an impact on resuscitation techniques. Again the ERC guidelines (1997) act as the framework for directing decision making when reviving the collapsed child (Table 2.1.3). The ERC guidelines for adults assume that the collapse is of cardiac origin while those for infants and children assume that the collapse is of respiratory origin. The ERC guidelines for infants and children are divided into two age groups – 0–1 year and over one year of age – to take account of developmental changes. Note the differences as you read the table.

Action	Rationale
Assess response by gentle shake and speak loudly	Voice and physical stimulation may cause a response in a deeply asleep infant or child
Call for help	Someone may be nearby
Open airway	Place hand on forehead and lift chin; do not overextend the head as this can close the airway
A 'sniffing' or neutral position for infants	This action may also stimulate breathing
Look, listen and feel for breathing	Allow 10 seconds, and watch the abdomen as infants and children depend on their diaphragm as the main respiratory muscle.
Give two to five expired air respirations if not breathing. If no chest expansion, commence obstructed airway procedure	Watch the chest rise and fall between breaths to assess how deep you, the rescuer, needs to exhale. Breaths should be delivered over 1 to 1.5 seconds to reduce abdominal distension
Palpate the pulse – the brachial in infants, the carotid in children – and look for movement	Allow 10 seconds to ensure the pulse is 60 beats or less if an infant or absent in a child
Commence chest compressions if the pulse is less than 60 in infants or absent in children	Position of chest compressions for infants and children differs because of size: • in infants, draw a line from nipple to nipple, place one finger below this line, and two fingers on the sternum, and aim for a third of the diameter of the chest at a rate of 100/minute • in children, find the point where the bottom rib joins the sternum, place two fingers above this point, then place the heel of one hand on the sternum and aim for a third of the diameter of the chest at a rate of 100/minute
Continue at a ratio of one breath to five compressions until help arrives OR 15:2 if a larger child/adolescent	Always use a ratio of 1:5 on the principle of maintaining some oxygenation with some circulation

Table 2.1.3 ERC BLS guidelines for infants and children. Based on ILCOR guidelines 1997.

You will need access to an infant and junior resuscitation mannikin for this exercise. Using the marking grids available in the ERC Guidelines (1997) (see pp. 166 and 167) test your skills in BLS for infants and children following the guide lines. Ideally, ask another student to assess your skills, and remember the real situation may last a long time, so demonstrate your skills over at least 5 minutes.

The technique is important, hence the advice regarding chest compressions and airway positioning. Infants also have a large round occiput (back of head), therefore they may need repositioning after each sequence of chest compressions. The pulse site in infants and children differs in location because infants have a short neck and the brachial pulse is the easier to palpate. This is found midway between the elbow and armpit on the underside of the arm. Remember that children can be different sizes at the same age; if you feel that the action you are carrying out has little effect, you may need to change the technique, for example from the heel of one hand to two hands for compressions.

▶ VARIATIONS TO THE RESUSCITATION SITUATION

So far the assumption has been that the collapse has been due to a single and relatively simple cause. Obviously in reality other factors may need to be considered in the management. In general terms, it does not matter which speciality of nursing you are working in as the same principles apply to adult, child, mental health or learning disability nursing. The key to success is the systematic assessment of 'the case at hand' using the simple ABC system, which has already been described. Other specific factors that need to be considered include:

- ▶ collapse due to trauma;
- ▶ collapse in pregnancy;
- ▶ collapse of an individual with altered anatomical airways;
- ▶ collapse due to choking in the adult;
- ▶ collapse due to choking in the infant or child.

Each of these situations will be dealt with briefly.

▶ *Collapse Due to Trauma*

Spinal injury has already been mentioned in the section on adult BLS and airway control.

Remember that you will never definitively find out about the spinal injury in a casualty with an obstructed airway and you must assume it is present if the history indicates its potential existence. However, professional nurses are expected to give a higher standard of care than that given by the general public, if the casualty has a possible cervical spine injury great care should be taken while dealing with the airway. Ideally the neck should be properly immobilized (Figure 2.1.14), that is a hard collar, sandbags or equivalent should be used to increase lateral stabilization and tape over the forehead and upper chest to hold the whole thing together. A good example of this is given in the film *Days of Thunder* when Tom Cruise crashes his racing car; alternatively the television series *ER* usually demonstrates good practice. The whole procedure can be combined with the jaw thrust to maintain an open airway (see Figure 2.1.11). In class, when teaching these principles to students, someone always says 'get real' at this point. We hope that any court of law would take into consideration the reality of the situation because of the difficulties with such complex interventions in an emergency.

▶ *Collapse During Pregnancy*

The additional requirements of the woman in late pregnancy have some significance, but are not really widely highlighted. Cardiac arrest in late pregnancy is relatively rare, but potentially treatable. Physiologically the

A potential controversy is the issue of priorities. Pause and reviewing information given previously in this chapter decide which of the following is more important: the patent airway or immobilization of a potential fracture of the cervical spine. Think for a few moments about how you might open the airway of a patient who has suffered a neck injury?

Figure 2.1.14: Cervical spine immobilization.

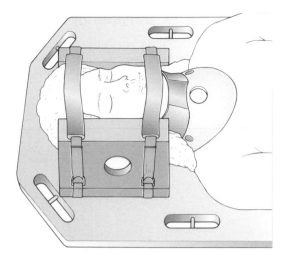

pregnant woman has higher oxygen requirements, an increased risk of regurgitation of stomach contents, and increased pressure on the diaphragm due to the pregnant uterus. Probably the most significant factor that needs to be remembered is the effect of the pregnant uterus on the unconscious casualty lying on her back (Figure 2.1.15). A pregnant uterus can easily weigh 5 kg, and when it lies directly over and pressing down on the inferior vena cava there are significant sequelae. The first few chest compressions have the same effect as usual, but there will be no venous return from the legs and pelvis due to the compression on the abdominal blood vessels, so the cardiac output will quickly fall to zero.

The management of this situation is relatively simple – either the uterus is manually displaced to the left by an assistant or the casualty's pelvis is inclined in the same direction at an angle of approximately 30°, either by pillows or by a device known as The Cardiff Wedge, which you will find in most labour suites. Either of these techniques will remove the compression from the vena cava and allow normal venous return to the chest from the lower body.

Figure 2.1.15: Cross-section of pregnant abdomen in late pregnancy. (a) Lying flat. (b) Lying in the left lateral position (i.e. inclined to the left using a Cardiff resuscitation wedge), demonstrating relief of vena caval and aortic compression.

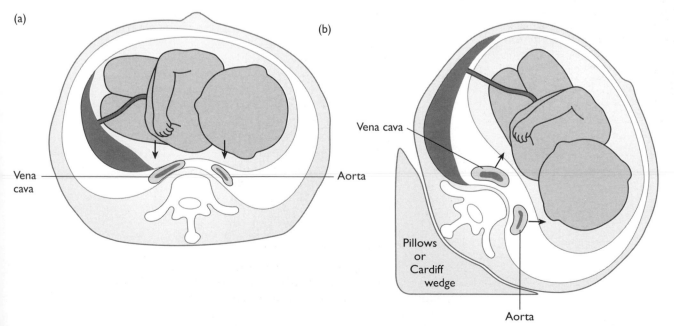

(a)

Vena
cava

Aorta

(b)

Vena cava

Pillows
or
Cardiff
wedge

Aorta

❯ *Collapse of an Individual with Altered Anatomical Airways*

This is currently a relatively uncommon situation, but is ever increasing as a result of reconstructive surgery following treatment for neoplasms (cancers) in the region of the throat. It is therefore probably good practice to ensure that you inspect the casualty's throat down to the

Figure 2.1.16: Altered anatomical upper airway. (a) Temporary artificial airway. (b) Permanent artificial airway (laryngostomy).

(a)

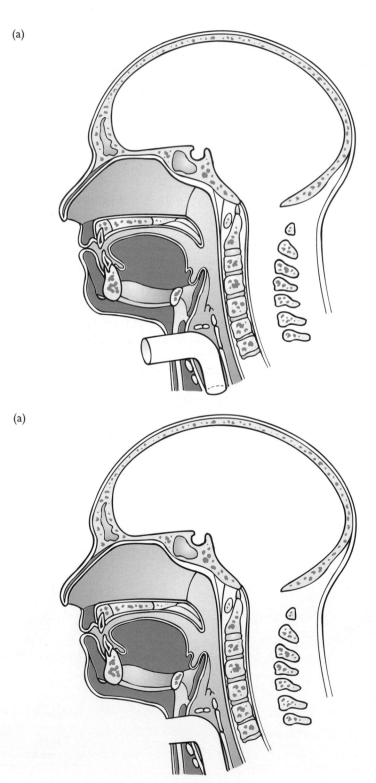

(a)

suprasternal notch, and definitely if you experience any difficulty in ventilating the casualty. The management of the situation is exceptionally easy – just ventilate down the alternative hole (Figure 2.1.16).

▶ *Collapse Due to Choking in the Adult*

A possible additional complication that might occur during the resuscitation process is choking. If the individual still has some respiratory effort, just helping the casualty empty the mouth may prevent the situation deteriorating further. This may be especially important for individuals with swallowing difficulties such as the elderly stroke patient or the young physically disabled. Figure 2.1.17 shows the current recom-

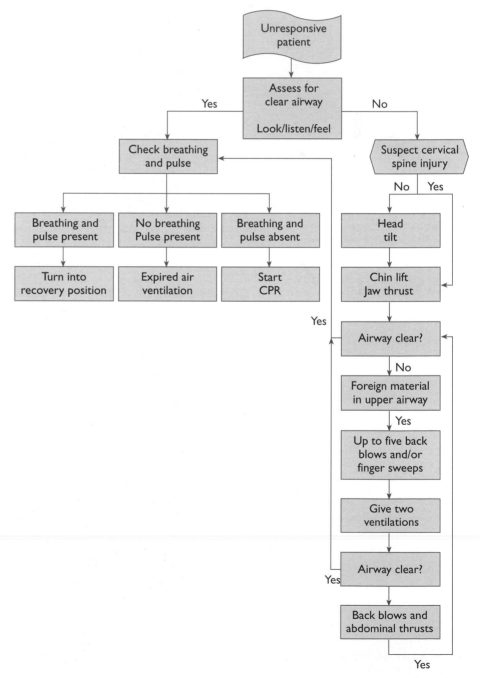

Figure 2.1.17: Basic airway management of choking in the adult. Adapted from ERC Airway Management Guidelines (1996).

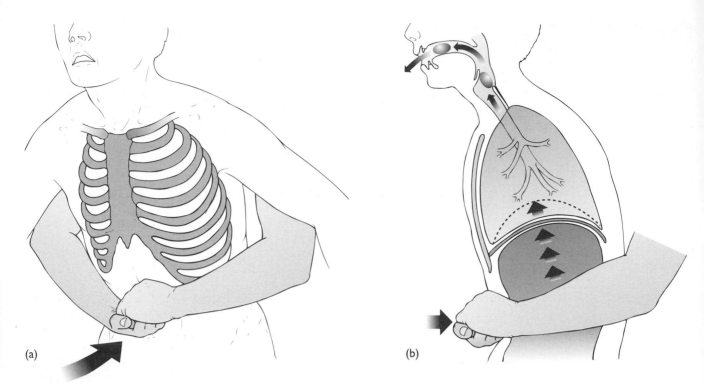

(a)

(b)

Figure 2.1.18: The Heimlich manoeuvre used if a patient is choking. (a) Stand behind the patient and clasp your hands over their mid-abdomen. (b) Apply a sharp movement to compress the abdomen. Repeat as necessary. (Reproduced by the kind permission of Nottingham Health Authority, 1985.)

mendations for the management of choking in the adult (European Resuscitation Council, 1996)

The Heimlich manoeuvre or abdominal thrust (Figure 2.1.18) aims to push the diaphragm upwards to increase the pressure in the chest cavity and so push or squeeze the object out of the trachea, If successful, the object will be ejected with some force.

▶ *Collapse Due to Choking in the Infant or Child*

The risk of choking is higher in infants and children than in adults because the airway is narrower and the swallowing reflex is not as well coordinated. The upper airway should be observed carefully during the initial assessment. Obstruction of the airway is not anticipated until the chest will not inflate. Only then is the choking procedure commenced. However, if choking is witnessed initially, the choking procedure should be started immediately.

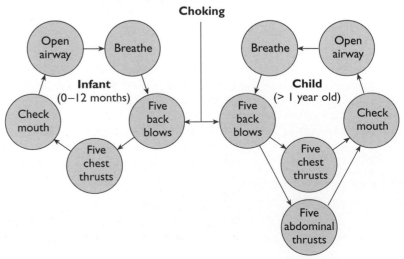

Figure 2.1.19: Dealing with choking in the infant or child.

The European Resuscitation Council (1994) has produced guidelines for the management of choking in infants and children (see Figure 2.1.19). The differences between the two age groups is linked to the immaturity of the liver and disconnection of the spleen from the back of the abdomen in the younger age group when the Heimlich manoeuvre (abdominal thrust) is used. Therefore this manoeuvre should be avoided at all costs in babies and replaced by the chest thrust as indicated. Chest thrusts are performed in the same manner and place as chest compressions but are carried out more rapidly.

▶ FURTHER RESUSCITATION SKILLS FOR NURSES

Although the relative efficiency of BLS is not good, it is a significant part of 'the chain of survival' as it 'buys time' and should not be forgotten, especially in high technology settings. We have already identified the significance of defibrillation in adults and airway care in children, so what are the other interventions of resuscitation?

With a patent airway, one of the early considerations is the addition of supplementary oxygen. All suddenly collapsed patients will benefit from the administration of additional oxygen. It is likely that either the patient's respiratory or cardiac function will be reduced, therefore increasing the oxygen saturation of the available circulation will be in the best interests of the patient. There are, however, two commonly expressed concerns by nurses regarding oxygen delivery.

▶ Firstly oxygen is a prescription medication and therefore a physician's signature is required before administration. Read your local oxygen administration policy carefully and you will always find a clause that relates to emergency administration. When a patient is suffering from acute hypoxia, as in sudden chest pain, shortness of breath and blood loss they will always benefit from high-flow oxygen administration during the acute phase.

▶ The second concern expressed by nurses relates to administering oxygen to patients with chronic obstructive airways disease. Very rarely a patient with hypoxic respiratory drive will stop breathing when given high concentrations of oxygen. All acutely ill patients on emergency oxygen are closely observed and this will therefore be noticed immediately. Even patients who are normally hypoxic will suffer adverse effects with further hypoxia. Nancy Caroline, a well-respected American paramedic trainer summarizes the situation well: 'Never, never, never withhold oxygen therapy from any patient in respiratory distress, even (or especially) a patient with chronic obstructive pulmonary disease' (Caroline, 1995a).

Many devices are available to increase the patency of the patient's airway during the resuscitation process. Baskett (1993a) identifies the various airway adjuncts (equipment) that can help to maintain an airway. The most useful for nurses is the Guedal airway, but this requires correct measurements to ensure the correct size is selected. These are obtained by measuring the Guedal airway alongside the jaw, the flange of the airway level with the incisor teeth and the distal part of the airway level with the corner of the jaw. In children over five years of age and in older age groups, the airway is inserted upside down and turned over in the mouth to hook over the back of the tongue. If the child is under five years of age, the tongue should be pushed down with a tongue depressor and the airway is then inserted the correct way up.

Administration of oxygen when an airway is being used can be by a self-inflating bag. These bags are available in differing sizes according to whether the victim is an infant, child or adult. This piece of equipment has useful features such as a pop off valve to prevent overinflation and can be used without a continual gas flow. It is important to select a face mask that covers the nose and mouth comfortably and creates a good seal so that the victim can receive adequate ventilation. However, self-inflating bags will refill with air and oxygen when not being squeezed and do not allow air and oxygen to reach the victim unless being compressed by the nurse.

▶ ADVANCED CARDIAC LIFE SUPPORT

The procedures for advanced cardiac life support in adults and children are shown as separate flow charts and these charts act as guidelines for a team approach to resuscitation (Figures 2.1.20 and 2.1.21).

▶ DRUGS AND RESUSCITATION

The use of drugs during the resuscitation process has been a controversial topic over the years and it is only recently that objective research studies have started. Although there are potentially many drugs that might be required during a cardiac arrest, the two most commonly used drugs are adrenaline (Epinephrine) and atropine.

Spend some time going through the flow charts shown in Figures 2.1.20 and 2.1.21 which explain ACLS in the adult and child.

1. *Note the differences between the two flow charts.*

2. *During your practice placements, if you witness a situation where a patient (whether adult or child) has collapsed and needs resuscitation by a cardiac arrest team reflect afterwards on how the situation was managed.*

3. *Review the guidelines and compare your experience with the recommendations.*

4. *Discuss any differences that occur between the theory and the practice with an experienced nurse who was present at the resuscitation in order to understand the reasons behind them.*

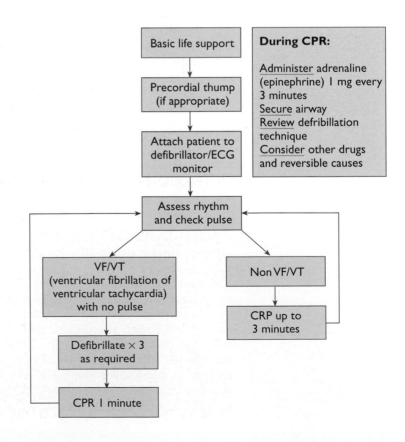

Figure 2.1.20: Core flow chart from the adult advanced life support guidelines—abridged version. (1997 Guidelines for use in the UK.)

Figure 2.1.21: Paediatric advanced life support guidelines. (Reproduced from Nadkarni *et al.*, 1997.)

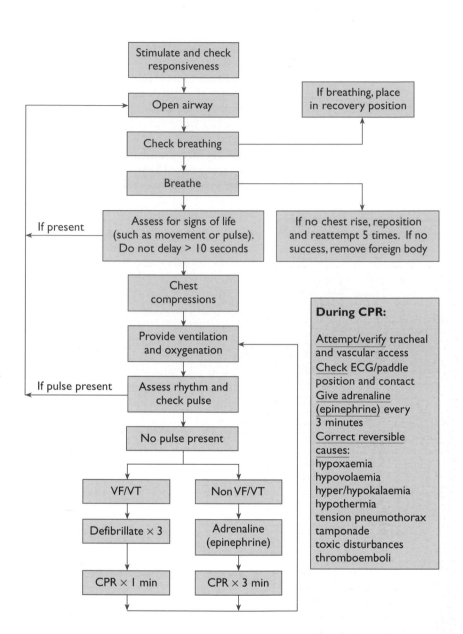

RESEARCH BASED EVIDENCE

Adrenaline has become the drug of choice in resuscitation due to research conducted by Geotting and Paradis (1991). They found through animal studies and retrospective examination of adrenaline administration during cardiac arrest in children that restoration of the circulation and neurological outcome was improved.

For both adrenaline and atropine identify the following.

1. **The indications for their use.**
2. **Their actions.**
3. **Their potential side effects.**
4. **The normal adult and child doses.**
5. **The potential routes of administration.**

Flowchart boxes:
- Stimulate and check responsiveness
- Open airway
- Check breathing → If breathing, place in recovery position
- Breathe → If no chest rise, reposition and reattempt 5 times. If no success, remove foreign body
- Assess for signs of life (such as movement or pulse). Do not delay > 10 seconds → If present
- Chest compressions
- Provide ventilation and oxygenation
- Assess rhythm and check pulse → If pulse present
- No pulse present
- VF/VT | Non VF/VT
- Defibrillate × 3 | Adrenaline (epinephrine)
- CPR × 1 min | CPR × 3 min

During CPR:

Attempt/verify tracheal and vascular access
Check ECG/paddle position and contact
Give adrenaline (epinephrine) every 3 minutes
Correct reversible causes:
hypoxaemia
hypovolaemia
hyper/hypokalaemia
hypothermia
tension pneumothorax
tamponade
toxic disturbances
thromboemboli

▶ HANDING OVER RESPONSIBILITY FOR CARE

The final stage in the resuscitation process is the handing over of responsibility for care from the first aider to health care professionals, who will then become responsible for the collapsed individual's welfare. This final 'disposal' of the casualty is as fraught with legal risk as any part of nursing. The same consideration should be applied when discharging the casualty into the hands of professional health carers. The easiest option is to dial 999. In this situation, continuity of care is assured, as long as you hand over effectively, so your responsibility for subsequent care is minimized. Although the 999 system is often abused by the public, do not be afraid of using it. If you are outside the acute hospital situation (or even sometimes in it) and consider the situation warrants an emergency ambulance then call for one.

There is one misconception about the ambulance service commonly held by the public and that is the issue of charges. Generally in the UK emergency treatment is free and there are no charges, but the *Road Traffic Act* (Department of Transport, 1972) has a provision for an emergency treatment fee. This emergency treatment fee will be claimed by whichever service treats the casualty first. If an ambulance is called, the ambulance service claims it, if the casualty walks to an A and E department the hospital will claim it, and if you visit your general practitioner several days later, your general practitioner is allowed to claim it. Any accident involving a motor vehicle on a public highway constitutes a road traffic accident (RTA) and includes the full spectrum of trauma from being run over by a lorry to breaking your little fingernail in a parked car door if the car is parked on a public highway.

The second 'disposal' option is to take the injured person to hospital in your own vehicle. Do consider carefully the risk of the casualty collapsing or even just fainting in your vehicle while travelling. It is worthwhile where possible to ensure someone else is also in your car to assist if the casualty deteriorates and to allow you to concentrate on driving rather then the casualty. If you decide that the casualty does not require hospital treatment consider the situation very carefully before you leave them. Are you sure that this casualty does not need to visit their general practitioner? What else could go wrong? Are there any possible complications?

If you are sure the treatment is within your realm of expertise, give the patient full instructions (preferably written) about what to look out for, how to care for the injury now, and when to seek help. As when discharging a patient, always leave them with a help option and tell them where to go if they are concerned. This is not only of benefit to the patient, but is also a useful defensive tactic for the nurse.

PROFESSIONAL KNOWLEDGE

Within this section, the nurse's professional accountability is examined by focusing on:

▶ the role of the nurse in both BLS and ALS situations;
▶ the nurse's responsibility to maintain her resuscitation skills;
▶ the importance of the nurse evaluating her own level of competence.

The expectations of society will be reviewed and ethicolegal issues surrounding resuscitation will be discussed.

▶ THE ROLE OF THE NURSE IN BLS AND ALS

Within the community environment, the nurse acts as a first aider when undertaking BLS resuscitation. However, the nurse is not expected to be an expert, but should ensure a call for competent help has been made. The UKCC (1996) states in reference to an off duty nurse coming across an RTA that '. . . in this situation it could be reasonable to expect the nurse to do no more than comfort and support the injured person'. The word 'support' still leaves the discussion fairly open as it may mean anything from holding the injured person's hand, to undertaking ALS.

Within the hospital setting, the role of the nurse in resuscitation changes in the sense that he or she is an integral part of the health care team. Initially, the nurse is often the locater of the incident, having found the collapsed individual. At this point, after the assessment, the nurse raises the alarm and commences BLS. A colleague will summon the arrest

In a previous exercise, you reviewed who might be involved in the resuscitation process within a hospital-based team (ALS). From a professional role perspective:

1. *Discover their individual roles and responsibilities.*

2. *Reflect on the training needs for each member of the team.*

3. *Discover if there are any mechanisms for auditing the process and outcomes of resuscitation events within the practice unit.*

team and begins to collect equipment for ALS, such as a defibrillator. When the team arrives, the nurse will still have a role as he or she:

▶ has knowledge of the event;
▶ knows the ward;
▶ knows the individual and their relatives.

It is not unusual for the cardiac arrest team to be led by a nurse, either from the ward or in the role of resuscitation officer or clinical nurse manager for a 'floor' or a clinical unit. Within the trauma resuscitation protocols described by The American College of Surgeons, the nurse has a significant role. Hadfield-Law and Kent (1996) describe this role and how the the resuscitation event may be managed.

▶ EDUCATION AND TRAINING FOR RESUSCITATION

As developing resuscitation skills 'on the job' is inappropriate, a number of nationally recognized courses have been developed to provide these skills. St John Ambulance and The British Red Cross undertake excellent first aid training that develops individual skills in BLS. For more advanced training in adult cardiac collapse there is the Advanced Cardiac Life Support (ACLS) course and for dealing with children there is the Paediatric Advanced Life Support (PALS) course. Finally, for those more interested in the trauma approach, there is the Advanced Trauma Nursing Course (ATNC). All of these courses are usually residential as they last 2–4 days and are regularly advertised in the nursing press.

All first aid and resuscitation skills require regular practice. Under local regulations, yearly updates may be mandatory in your areas of practice. Simulations set up in your work area can either be practical or 'talk through' and can be completed on a regular basis to keep your skills fresh and up to date. Working as a team is especially important, so undertake these exercises with as many members of the regular team as possible.

RESEARCH BASED EVIDENCE

Training and maintenance of competence levels for resuscitation skills is poor among hospital personnel (Crouch, 1993). Poor skill retention is linked to a lack of competence, and skills can deteriorate after six weeks without practice (Cavanagh, 1990; Wynne et al., 1990). A survey of hospital resuscitation statistics found that only 14.6% of collapsed patients survived resuscitation, but where hospital personnel are trained and competent in CPR skills 50% of collapsed patients survived (Casey, 1984; Wynne et al., 1990).

Crouch (1993) surveyed nurses' theoretical knowledge of resuscitation and found that less than half the sample group (62 in total) had heard of The Resuscitation Council UK. Many respondents answered questions poorly regarding the drug of choice and when the precordial thump was indicated. However, he also found that 24% had received a CPR update in the previous year, while 6.5% had never received a CPR update. Regular updating is recommended, including role play and team practice for the resuscitation team.

▶ THE PUBLIC'S EXPECTATIONS OF THE NURSE AS A FIRST AIDER

Society expects nurses to help in all emergency situations. When the new student nurse is first identified as 'a nurse' by her home community everyone appears to make a mental note of this fact so that when an emergency occurs friends and relatives know where to turn for help. This general principle appears to apply equally to nurses who have specialized in diverse areas of practice because many members of the public only recognize the 'traditional' general nurse, and all nurses are expected to fill this role. How 'the nurse' fulfils her role in the resuscitation situation when called to help as 'a nurse' has legal implications.

A crowd gathers around a motorcyclist who has fallen off his motorbike as it skidded on ice.

1. *Consider what factors you need to take into consideration when you as a member of the public decide whether or not to assist at an incident.*

2. *How would these factors change if it became known that you were a nurse or stated you were a nurse before you started to help this motocyclist.*

▶ THE 'DUTY OF CARE' TO A NEIGHBOUR AS A MEMBER OF THE PUBLIC

In the UK there is no legal duty of care to a 'neighbour', who maybe anyone you meet and not just your physical neighbour. In practice this means you can walk past an accident or step over a collapsed person in the street. Although a legal duty of care does not exist, we must, however, also consider our moral duty to fellow human beings. When talking to other nurses I often feel that they would have less dilemma in caring for an injured bird than for another human being because of their concerns over being 'sued'.

In the British legal system the two major divisions are criminal law and civil law. If you enter a patient's house without consent it may be trespass which is a civil offence, though may in some cases be criminal. If you touch a patient without consent it might be assault. If you treat a patient inappropriately you might find yourself accused of actual bodily harm.

One of the major considerations in criminal law is the 'intent' and 'motive' that is associated with the act. Both 'intent' and 'motive' are very complex legal issues and it would be advisable to consult a legal text to investigate these further. The courts will consider the situation where the intent when aiding an individual is to do harm in a very different light to a situation where the rescuer is trying to help. It is generally more likely that the first aider would be involved in a case related to civil law, and most probably that of negligence where the patient has suffered additional harm due to the actions of a first aider.

John Tingle (1991) undertook a review of the situation regarding first aid and the law. One of his major considerations was that 'legal action against good samaritan acts is a remote possibility'. The good samaritan act is simply that as described in the Bible (Bible Society, 1976), where a stranger comes to the assistance of a fellow human being to relieve suffering. In our opinion, the principle of the good samaritan is one which our culture needs to encourage and support. Tingle (1991) considers this to be of significance in British courts. If 'resuscitation' cases were brought to court and first aiders found guilty, it may lead to the same state that is now found in the USA where members of the public and professionals are hesitant to assist their neighbours. Because of these legal considerations some American states have introduced so called 'good samaritan' acts to promote first aid and to some extent protect the rescuer from the nightmare of litigation.

Caroline (1995b) cites one of these laws from Florida State: 'Any person, including those licensed to practice medicine, who gratuitously and in good faith renders emergency care or treatment at the scene of an emergency outside of a hospital, doctor's office or other place having proper medical equipment, without objection of the injured victim or victims thereof, shall not be held liable for any civil damages as a result of any act or failure to act in providing or arranging further medical treatment where the person acts as an ordinary reasonable prudent man would have acted under the same circumstances'.

The statement of particular significance is 'ordinary reasonable prudent man'. This level is difficult to determine and really left to the judgement of the court; however, the word 'man' would be replaced by 'nurse' if one were involved and an expert witness would be called in an attempt to determine what this level is. Although the current situation in the UK is not one that really requires this legislation, such an act might be reassuring and encourage the act of first aid by professional carers.

▶ THE 'DUTY OF CARE' TO A NEIGHBOUR AS A PROFESSIONAL NURSE

It is important to remember that although there is no duty to care for everyone, if an injured person is already 'under the care' of the potential first aider's employer, the first aider then has a duty to care for him or her. As Tingle (1991) says 'a nurse could not leave a fallen patient but could leave a witnessed accident'. Although there is no immediate legal duty of care to the witnessed accident, once the nurse has presented herself as a nurse to help, ' a duty of care' exists.

If a case were to be taken to court it would probably be in the area of negligence. The crucial factor in negligence cases is the issue of 'reasonable care' where the standard of care is expected to be that of the reasonable and ordinary nurse or first aider considering the individual circumstances in question. In our opinion, as long as a first aider continually asks him or herself why he or she is doing each action and ensuring that their actions are always for the benefit of the injured person, we consider that litigation would be unlikely. However, this is no guarantee. Barber (1993) applies a more cautionary approach to first aid and points out that 'a nurse acting on her own initiative, under no instruction from an employer and other than in the course of her own duties, is clearly responsible and liable for her own acts and omissions'.

When undertaking emergency care for individuals 'in the care' of an employer, for example a National Health Service Trust, if anything goes wrong it is more likely that the individual will sue the employer than the employee. This is likely to be the case for a nurse who is the 'designated' first aider as described in the first aid regulations of the *Health and Safety at Work Act* (Health and Safety Commission, 1991). Outside this situation the first aider is 'on their own' and it seems reasonable that every nurse should have some personal indemnity insurance to cover them in such circumstances. Personal indemnity insurance is often part of a 'package' a nurse receives if they join a union or professional organization. Such a move appears to be sensible.

Barber (1993) also points out the importance of obtaining consent for all interventions and only undertaking those interventions that are 'necessary' to save life and prevent further deterioration. As a nurse there is a significant additional consideration in this debate. This is the professional consideration. We have seen that as a member of the public there is no legal duty to help a stranger. However the UKCC (1992) puts this responsibility on all nurses in its *Code of Professional Conduct*. The code starts by stating: 'Each registered nurse, midwife and health visitor shall act, at all times, in such a manner as to: safeguard the interests of society; serve the interests of society; justify public trust and confidence and uphold and enhance the good standing and reputation of the professions'. The wording of the *Code of Professional Conduct* provides a clear mandate for all nurses that goes beyond the legal responsibilities and indicates that nurses must always and in all circumstances act in the manner of the 'good samaritan'.

Castledine (1993) cites a case from the UKCC's professional conduct hearings where a district nurse passed by an RTA because she feared that she did not know what to do. A member of the public reported this action and the nurse was found guilty of misconduct. Although the nurse was not removed from the register, this is a clear signal from the professional body that nurses must help in all emergency situations, even if they lie out of their direct realm of responsibility. The extent of this 'required' help is unclear. We would expect the minimum would be no

DECISION MAKING

Review the *Code of Professional Conduct* (UKCC, 1992).
1. *Identify which of the specific clauses need to be considered in the emergency situation.*
2. *Review the situation of the motorcyclist in the previous exercise (see p. 160) and decide, based on your own knowledge and skills and the requirements of the Code of Professional Conduct, how you would act in that particular scenario.*

more then ensuring competent help is on its way (i.e. someone has summoned the emergency services) and undertaking simple supportive action.

▶ ETHICAL ISSUES SURROUNDING RESUSCITATION

Much has been written about the ethics of resuscitation and the Royal College of Nursing (1992) has identified three major concerns:

▶ bringing about the best consequences and outcomes;
▶ respecting the wishes of individuals directly affected;
▶ valuing and respecting human life.

The issue of whether to actively resuscitate an indivudal or not is a difficult situation to address. However, it must be remembered that the final decision should be in the patient's interest, respect the individual's desires as far as possible, and consider the value of human life.

Baskett (1993b) states 'in the absence of a patient's precise previous instructions to the contrary, consent to attempt CPR, as with other emergency procedures, is presumed since the patient is incapable of communicating his or her wishes at the moment of arrest and failure to render care immediately is certain to result in death'.

The Royal College of Nursing (1992) has produced guidelines addressing the dilemmas of resuscitation and they indicate that 'do not resuscitate' orders are at times appropriate. It is, however, important that in this situation appropriate discussions take place between the patient, the patient's relatives and friends, and health care professionals. Discussion is important especially for those who are regarded as vulnerable, that is children, the mentally handicapped and those debilitated by mental illness. When resuscitation would have no effect on the process of dying or the patient does not wish to have their life extended then the decision not to resuscitate should be formally documented. We do not think there is a place for 'blanket orders', for example in elderly care units, where it is decided without individual consents not to resuscitate simply because all the residents are old.

Living wills are not recognized by British law, therefore adding to the dilemma of whether health professionals follow medical instructions or the patient's wishes. This may result in failure by the nurse to comply with a patient's request that might have been expressed in a 'living will'. Patients can refuse treatment if of sound mind, but this cannot happen in the situation where the patient requires immediate resuscitation. The health professional should act in the best interests to save life, ensure improvement or prevent deterioration (Royal College of Nursing, 1992).

DECISION MAKING

You have been involved in the resuscitation of Mr James, who is 55 years old, after a severe myocardial infarction (heart attack). This gentleman was very ill before the arrest. The resuscitation continued for 30 minutes with no cardiac activity as a result. Mrs James was present when Mr James collapsed and has requested that her husband is allowed to die. The medical staff want to insert an artificial pacing device, which they feel will save Mr James's life.

1. *Decide on what the legal issues are for all those involved in Mr James's care.*

2. *Using a model for ethical decision making (see Seedhouse, 1988; Curtin and Flaherty, 1989) review* *the possible decisions that could be made that might take into consideration Mrs James's request that her husband be allowed to die.*

3. *What should the role of the nurse be as part of the team involved in the resuscitation process?*

▶ AGE OF CONSENT AND INCOMPETENCY

Specifically in relation to emergency care investigate the issue of informed consent for:

1. *Children.*
2. *The unconscious adult.*
3. *The individual with learning difficulties.*
4. *Those with mental health problems.*

(Cross refer to Chapter 3.5 on death and dying and your ethicolegal textbooks.)

Although our discussions have just been addressing the issue of emergency care it is important to remember the concept of consent. All nursing interventions require informed consent by the patient. In an emergency situation when the patient is unconscious it is generally accepted that the nurse may undertake what intervention is 'necessary' to save life and prevent further deterioration. Patients who are conscious need to be informed of what is 'going on' and what treatment is proposed so that they have the opportunity to accept or refuse the treatment. A witness can be very helpful, especially in the emergency situation, in case of any difficulties at a later date. The same rules apply for those under the age of consent (i.e. 16 years) and a parent or legal guardian must be sought for their permission if at all possible. There is currently considerable discussion about the role of the child in the process of consent, which requires further study – see for example *The Children Act* (Department of Health, 1989). The same considerations also apply for those with significant mental health problems and learning disabilities.

REFLECTIVE KNOWLEDGE

The public appear to expect nurses to help in emergency situations and therefore we consider that nurses should be able to deal with the initial management of any physical emergency until more specialist staff are available. The practice of first aid and resuscitation carries legal risks. A basic understanding of the legal and professional basis of nursing practice will help you decide how to practice safely. Nurses should not be overworried when helping out at the scene of an emergency as long as they proceed with caution according to a well-tested plan and only undertake those interventions that are 'necessary'. It appears to be reasonable that nurses ensure that they have some form of personal indemnity insurance cover.

Resuscitation is primarily a practical skill that requires a fairly wide knowledge base. As a practical skill the ability to use it decays with lack of use. Simulation exercises need to be a common feature of the updating process. Nurses are obliged to become involved in emergency care, if not

---

Checklist For Single Rescuer Basic Life Support For Adults

Ref: 1997 Adult CPR Guidelines for use in the UK (Resuscitation Council UK)
This assumes the patient is Adult, has suddenly collapsed without apparent reason, is unconscious, is not breathing and has no pulse.
You are alone as the rescuer.
(Replies for the 'tester' are in **bold**)

CRITERIA	LEVEL REACHED	INCORRECT 0	READJUSTED 1	CORRECT 2	MAXIMUM SCORE
Assess safety	**SAFE**				2
Assess responsiveness (shout, gentle shake)	**UNCONSCIOUS**				2
Shout for help					2
Open airway (head tilt, chin lift)					2
Assess breathing (look, listen and feel) check for up to 10 seconds	**ABSENT**				2
Call for definitive help					2
Reassess on return					2
Maintain open airway					2
Make up to 5 attempts to perform 2 slow, effective ventilations					2
Assess for signs of circulation, including pulse check for up to 10 seconds	**ABSENT**				2
Give 15 chest compressions. Rate=100/min. Depth=4–5 cm					2
Continue at ratio of 2 ventilations to 15 compressions					2
Continue to practice for 5 minutes at a minimum of 4 cycles per minute					2
TOTAL					26

Name: ....

Tested by: .... 'Safe'/Requires further practice   Date: ....

Figure 2.1.22: Self-assessment for single-rescuer BLS for adults using an adult mannikin. May also be used for assessment by peers or a nurse teacher. Acceptable minimum score is 24 (allowing for adjustment in head position to open up airway).

Checklist For Two Rescuer Basic Life Support For Adults

Ref: 1997 Adult CPR Guidelines for use in the UK (Resuscitation Council UK)
This assumes the patient is Adult, has suddenly collapsed without apparent reason, is unconscious, is not breathing and has no pulse.
You have a second rescuer.
(Replies for the 'tester' are in **bold**)

CRITERIA	LEVEL REACHED	INCORRECT 0	READJUSTED 1	CORRECT 2	MAXIMUM SCORE
Assess safety	**SAFE**				2
Assess responsiveness (shout, gentle shake)	**UNCONSCIOUS**				2
Second rescuer, call ambulance or equivalent					2
Open airway (head tilt, chin lift)					2
Assess breathing for up to 10 seconds (look, listen and feel)	**ABSENT**				2
Maintain open airway					2
Make up to 5 attempts to perform 2 slow, effective ventilations					2
Assess for signs of circulation, including pulse check for up to 10 seconds	**ABSENT**				2
Give 15 chest compressions. Rate = 100/min. Depth = 4–5 cm					2
Continue at ratio of 2 ventilations to 15 compressions					2
On return of second rescuer, take over chest compressions					2
Rescuer 2: Give 5 chest compressions (as above)					2
Rescuer 1: Give one slow, effective ventilation					2
Continue one ventilation to 5 compressions					2
Continue to practice for 5 minutes at a minimum of 10 cycles per minute					2
TOTAL					30

Name: ....

Tested by: .... 'Safe'/Requires further practice   Date: ....

Figure 2.1.23: Self-assessment for two-rescuer BLS for adults. Ideal acceptable minimum score is 24 (allowing for adjustment in head position to open up airway).

by law then by the UKCC. It is necessary that all nurses receive instruction and updating in emergency care to fulfil this role.

Overall we would like to encourage cautious intervention by nurses in emergency situations. The well-tested plan of action at any emergency is that described in the *First Aid Manual* of the voluntary first aid organizations by Webb *et al.* (1997). The ERC reviews and updates it guidelines based on evidence gathered from the increasing number of research

Self Assessment For Basic Life Support With Babies

Ref: 1997 Paediatric CPR Guidelines for use in the UK (Resuscitation Council UK)
This assumes no respiratory effort, a profound bradycardia.
You are alone as the rescuer.
(Replies for the 'tester' are in **bold**)

CRITERIA	LEVEL REACHED	INCORRECT 0	READJUSTED 1	CORRECT 2	MAXIMUM SCORE
Assess safety	**SAFE**				2
Assess responsiveness (shout, very gentle shake)	**UNCONSCIOUS**				2
Shout for help					2
Open airway (face parallel with chest)					2
Assess breathing for up to 10 seconds (look, listen, feel)					2
Give 2–5 ventilations (minimum of two being effective)					2
Look for potential airway obstruction if no chest expansion					2
Assess for signs of circulation for up to 10 seconds (brachial pulse and movement) **(Assessor states that rate is less than 60/min)**					2
Compressions: (indicated if pulse less than 60/min and/or no movement) 1 finger below nipple line, lower sternum					2
Rate = 100/minute					2
Depth = 1/3 of chest diameter					2
Continue resuscitation 5 compressions to 1 ventilation					2
After 1 minute call for definitive help					2
Continue at a minimum of 10 cycles/minute					2
TOTAL					28

MAXIMUM POINTS GAINED 28, MINIMUM ACCEPTED 26
(ALLOWING FOR ADJUSTMENT IN POSITION TO OPEN UP AIRWAY).

Tested by: .... PASS/REFER   Date: ....

Figure 2.1.24: Self-assessment for basic life support for infants. Minimum acceptable score is 26 (allowing for adjustment in head position to open up airway).

studies in the field of resuscitation. These should be adhered to by all health care personnel in any team involved in the resuscitation process.

Throughout the chapter there are many reflective exercises for you to complete. In the practice setting, it is important that you learn from critical events such as those we have described. Get into the habit of thinking about your actions and identifying both the positive points and those that you could improve next time.

During your nursing education and training programme, you will receive practical BLS training. Use the checklists supplied through the ERC training manuals when you are updating yourself (European Resus-

Self Assessment For Basic Life Support With Children

Ref: 1997 Paediatric Guidelines for use in the UK (Resuscitation Council UK)
This assumes that there is no respiratory effort, no pulse will be found.
You are alone as the rescuer.
(Replies for the 'tester' are in **bold**)

CRITERIA	LEVEL REACHED	INCORRECT 0	READJUSTED 1	CORRECT 2	MAXIMUM SCORE
Assess safety	**SAFE**				2
Assess responsiveness (shout, gentle shake)	**UNCONSCIOUS**				2
Shout for help					2
Open airway (minimal head tilt)					2
Assess breathing for up to 10 seconds (look, listen and feel)	**ABSENT**				2
Give 2–5 ventilations (minimum of two effective)					2
Assess for potential airway obstruction if no chest expansion					2
Assess circulation for up to 10 seconds (carotid pulse and movement) Chest compressions only if NO pulse and/or no movement					2
Chest compressions: Use one hand Position: 1 finger breadth above base of sternum					2
Rate = 100/minute					2
Depth = 1/3 of chest diameter					2
Continue resuscitation 5 compressions to 1 ventilation or 15:2 if an older child					2
After 1 minute call for definitive help					2
Continue at a minimum of 12 cycles/minute					2
TOTAL					28

MAXIMUM POINTS GAINED 28, MINIMUM ACCEPTED 26
(ALLOWING FOR ADJUSTMENT IN POSITION TO OPEN UP AIRWAY).

Tested by: .... PASS/REFER   Date: ....

Figure 2.1.25: Self-assessment for BLS for children. Minimum acceptable score is 26 (allowing for adjustment in head position to open up airway).

citation Council, 1992). These are specially designed for adult, infant and child resuscitation situations and also include checklists for single-rescuer BLS as well as two-rescuer situations (Figures 2.1.22–2.1.25).

If you have undertaken a public first aid course or belong to one of the voluntary first aid organizations you will be aware that training in two-person BLS does not always take place. It has been found that the public have difficulty learning both methods and often therefore only one method is taught. In practice, efficient two-person BLS is more effective, but it is more difficult to acquire and maintain the skills as well as depending on the presence of a second rescuer.

▶ CASE HISTORIES

The following case histories should take you back into the content of the chapter and reflect situations you may have to deal with in your particular field of nursing in the future. Completing them will help you consolidate your learning so far.

▶ CASE STUDY: LEARNING DISABILITIES

Remember the 30-year-old woman (Linda) with profound learning disabilities who was a passenger in one of the two cars involved in a crash (see Decision Making exercise on p. 142 in Practice Knowledge). Linda was the back seat passenger in one of the cars and when you came on the scene she was screaming loudly. This lady needs to come to terms with such a traumatic event and coping strategies need to be developed to help her in the future. Obviously, Linda needs to understand how the events happened and, in some ways, most importantly of all, realise that it was an accident and no-one's fault.

- **Reflect on and identify some of the feelings Linda may have experienced immediately following and subsequent to the accident.**

- **Review again how you would have prioritized her particular care within the 'life-threatening' scenario of the car crash.**

- **Linda's father recovered from his chest and head injuries, but is concerned that his daughter's needs were ignored by the rescuers. He intends to sue for negligence. Decide on the type of defence you will have in law should there be a civil case for damages.**

▶ CASE STUDY: CHILD

You are on a practice placement in a local school for children with special needs. Jennifer, a four-year-old child with cerebral palsy is found collapsed by the dinner table at school. As the only 'nurse' present you are immediately called upon by the teacher in charge to help.

- **What is your first action?**

- **Your attempts at expired air respiration fail. What should you assume?**

- **After several cycles of the choking procedure a piece of meat is retrieved from Jennifer's mouth, but she is still not breathing. What should you do now?**

- **Rehearse practically what you have decided to do using a mannikin and self-assess your performance using the ERC checklist for resuscitation of children.**

▶ CASE STUDY: MENTAL HEALTH

James is a 17-year-old client who has been admitted to an acute mental health ward with manic depression. He tells you that he has taken 50 of his lithium carbonate and haloperidol tablets over the last ten minutes and states that he wants to die. He makes it very clear that he does not want to be treated.

■ **Consider whether you would undertake active resuscitation should he collapse in your presence.**

■ **What immediate actions would you take if he did collapse?**

■ **Reflect on and debate with your peers the ethical and legal issues involved in this particular situation.**

▶ CASE STUDY: ADULT

You are having an evening out with a friend. While walking home you have come across a middle-aged man slumped against a wall, who has been vomiting profusely. He smells strongly of alcohol and is barely rousable.

■ **Consider how you might approach this situation.**

■ **Should his condition deteriorate, how would you carry out mouth to mouth ventilations and still protect your own safety?**

■ **It is later discovered that this gentleman has hepatitis B. What additional actions might you now have to take to protect yourself in the long term.**

▶ ANNOTATED FURTHER READING

BASKETT, P. (1993) *Resuscitation Handbook* (2nd edition). London. Wolfe.
  This book discusses the guidelines in more detail and offers clear diagrams of the techniques required for basic life support and also the equipment used in advanced life support.

CAROLINE, N. (1995) *Emergency Care In The Streets* (5th edition). Boston, USA. Little, Brown & Co.
  This book was written for paramedics in the USA. It offers good insight into the skills and knowledge required of the paramedic with clear explanations and pictorial evidence. It is a text commonly used in UK paramedic training schemes.

COLQUHOUN, M.C., HANDLEY, A.J., EVANS, T.R. (1995) *ABC of Resuscitation* (3rd edition). London. British Medical Journal.
  Further insight to the guidelines with further pictorial support. The chapters on special considerations such as drowning and pregnancy are worth reading. It is also a British perspective on ethical problems relating to resuscitation.

INTERNATIONAL LIAISON COMMITTEE ON RESUSCITATION (1997) The ILCOR advisory statements. *Resuscitation* **34(2)**: 97–149.
  A series of articles reviewing resuscitation from an international perspective. Do note that these are not the current guidelines, but advisory statements for resuscitation councils.

TINGLE, J. (1991) First aid law. *Nursing Times* **87(35)**: 48–49.
  A common sense review of British law as it relates to the nurse as a first aider.

WEBB, M., SCOTT, R., BEALE, P. (1997) *First Aid Manual* (7th edition). London. Dorling Kindersley.
  The authorized manual of the voluntary aid societies.

WRIGHT, B. (1996) *Sudden Death – A Research Base for Practice* (2nd edition). Edinburgh. Churchill Livingstone.
This is an excellent book on the psychological impact of sudden death of a loved one (adult or child) on families, based on the research and experience of its author as a clinical nurse specialist in crisis care. The book also deals with the effects of crisis managment on health care staff and makes very useful suggestions for staff support and training

▶ *Videos*

BBC EDUCATION (1995) *999 Lifesaver Video Pack*. London. BBC Education.
A 90-minute video consisting of short dramatic sequences explaining the first aid for common situations. Very well produced by the BBC.
BRITISH HEART FOUNDATION (1995) *Advanced Life Support*. Plymouth. Two Four Productions.
A video that explains and demonstrates hospital based resuscitation. It reviews both the 1992 basic life support and the advanced life support guidelines.

▶ **Computer Web Sites**

http://www.arto.org
This site was set up for the Association of Resuscitation Training Officers. It is a valuable site to access for updates on guidelines, training aids and details of advanced life support courses. There is also a links page to other international sites of specific interest.
http://www.amhrt.org:80/index.html
The web site of the American Heart Association.
http://www.nda.ox.ac.uk/rc-uk/
The web site of The Resuscitation Council (UK).

▶ REFERENCES

ADVANCED LIFE SUPPORT GROUP (1993) *Advanced Paediatric Life Support*. London. British Medical Journal.

BARBER, J. (1993) Legal aspects of first aid and emergency care. *British Journal of Nursing* 2(12): 641–642.

BASIC LIFE SUPPORT WORKING PARTY OF THE EUROPEAN RESUSCITATION COUNCIL (1992) Guidelines for basic life support. *Resuscitation* 24(2): 103–110.

BASKETT, P. (1993a) *Resuscitation Handbook* (2nd edition). Wolfe. London.

BASKETT, P. (1993b) Ethics in cardiopulmonary resuscitation. *Resuscitation* 25(1): 1–8.

BASKETT, P., NOLAN J., PARR, M. (1996) Tidal volumes which are perceived to be adequate for resuscitation, *Resuscitation* 31(3): 231–234.

BIBLE SOCIETY (1976) *Good News Bible*. Luke 10 vs 25–37. Collins. Glasgow.

CAPLAN, G. (1964) *Principles of Preventative Psychiatry*. New York. Basic Books.

CAROLINE, N. (1995a) *Emergency Care In The Streets* (5th edition). p. 459. Boston, USA. Little, Brown & Co.

CAROLINE, N. (1995b) *Emergency Care In The Streets* (5th edition). p. 23. Boston, USA. Little, Brown & Co.

CASEY, W.F. (1984) Cardiopulmonary resuscitation: A survey of standards among junior hospital doctors. *Journal of the Royal Society of Medicine* 7(11): 921–924.

CASTLEDINE, G. (1993) Ethical implications of first aid. *British Journal of Nursing* 2(4): 239–241.

CAVANAGH, S.J. (1990) Educational aspects of cardiopulmonary training. *Intensive Care Nursing* 6(1): 38–44.

CHALK, A. (1995) Should relatives be present in the resuscitation room. *Journal of Accident and Emergency Nursing* 3(2): 58–61.

COLQUHOUN, M.C., HANDLEY, A.J., EVANS, T.R. (1995) *ABC of Resuscitation* (3rd edition). London. British Medical Journal.

COYNE, I. (1996) Sudden infant death syndrome and baby care practices. *Paediatric Nursing* 8(10): 16–18.

CROUCH, R. (1993) Nurses' skills in basic life support: A survey. *Nursing Standard* 7(20): 28–31.

CUMMINS, R.O., EISENBERG, M.S., HORWOOD, B.T. *ET AL.* (1990) Cardiac arrest and resuscitation: A tale of 29 cities. *Annals of Emergency Medicine*. February: 19(2) 179–186.

CUMMINS, R.O., ORNATO, J.P., THIES, W.H., PEPE P.E. (1991) Improving survival from sudden cardiac arrest: The "chain of survival" concept.

Circulation 83(5): 1832–1847.

CURTIN, L., FLAHERTY, M.J. (1989) *Nursing Ethics: Theories and Pragmatics* (2nd edition). Bowie, MD. Brady.

DEPARTMENT OF HEALTH (1989) *The Children Act*. London. Her Majesty's Stationery Office.

DEPARTMENT OF HEALTH (1991) *The Health of The Nation*. London. Her Majesty's Stationery Office.

DEPARTMENT OF HEALTH (1992) *Back to Sleep: Reducing the Risk of Cot Death*. London. Her Majesty's Stationery Office.

DEPARTMENT OF HEALTH (1993) *Targeting Practice: The Contribution of Nurses, Midwives and Health Visitors*. London. Her Majesty's Stationery Office.

DEPARTMENT OF TRANSPORT (1972) *Road Traffic Act*. London. Her Majesty's Stationery Office.

DURHAM, T.W., MCCAMMON, S.L., ALLISON, E.J. (1985) The psychological impact of disaster on personnel. *Annals of Emergency Medicine* 14: 7.

EMERGENCY PLANNING COLLEGE, 1993 (Video) *The Clapham Railway Disaster*. Easingwold, Hull. Emergency Planning College.

EUROPEAN RESUSCITATION COUNCIL (1994) *Basic Life Support* (Video). Antwerp, Belgium. European Resuscitation Council.

EUROPEAN RESUSCITATION COUNCIL AIRWAY AND VENTILATION WORKING GROUP (1996) Guidelines for the basic management of the airway and ventilation during resuscitation. *Resuscitation* **31(3)**: 187–200.

FISHER, J.M., HANDLEY, A.J. (1995) Basic life support. In Colquhoun, M.C., Handley, A.J., Evans, T.R. (eds) *ABC of Resuscitation*. London. BMJ Publishing Group.

FRASER, S., ATKINS, J. (1990) Survivors' recollections of helpful and unhelpful emergency nurses activities surrounding the sudden death of a loved one. *Journal of Emergency Nursing* **16(1)**: 13–16.

GIBSON, M. (1991) *Order From Chaos, Responding To Traumatic Events.* Birmingham. Venture Press.

GOETTING, M.G., PARADIS, N.A. (1991) High dose epinephrine improves outcome from paediatric cardiac arrest. *Annals of Emergency Medicine* **20(1)**: 22–26.

HADFIELD-LAW, L., KENT, A. (1996) Role of the trauma nurse. In Skinner, D., Driscoll, P., Earlam, R. *ABC of Major Trauma* (2nd edition). London. BMJ Publishing Group.

HANSON, C., STRAWSER, D. (1992) Family presence during cardio-pulmonary resuscitation – Foote Hospital's 9 year perspective. *Journal of Emergency Nursing* **18(2)**: 104–106.

HEALTH AND SAFETY COMMISSION (1991) *First Aid at Work, Approved Code of Practice*. London. Her Majesty's Stationery Office.

HINCHLIFF, S., MONTAGUE, S., WATSON, S. (1996) *Physiology For Nursing Practice* (2nd edition). London. Baillière Tindall.

ILCOR (1997) The ILCOR Advisory Statements. *Resuscitation* **34(2)**: 97–149.

INNES, P.A., SUMMERS, C.A., BOYD, I.M., MOLYNEUX, E.M. (1993) Audit of paediatric cardio-pulmonary resuscitation. *Archives of Disease In Childhood* **68**: 487–491.

JACKSON, R.J. (1984) Blood flow in the cerebral cortex during CPR with dogs. *Annals of Emergency Medicine* **13**: 657.

LEE, S.K. (1984) Eeffect of cardiac arrest time on the cortical cerebral blood flow generated by subsequent standard CPR in rabbits. *Annals of Emergency Medicine* **13**: 385.

MACKENZIE, G. (1964) Haemodynamic effects of external cardiac compression. *Lancet* **1**: 1342.

MARSDEN, A., MOFFAT, C., SCOTT, R. (1992) *First Aid Manual* (6th edition). London. Dorling Kindersley.

McKEE, D.R., WYNNE, G., EVANS, T.R. (1994) Student nurses can defibrillate within 90 seconds. *Resuscitation* **27(1)**: 35–37.

NADKARNI, V., HAZINSIKI, M.F., ZIDEMAN, D. et al. (1997) Paediatric life support. *Resuscitation* **34(2)**: 115–127.

NEWBOLD, D. (1987) Critical care: The physiology of cardiac massage. *Nursing Times* **83(25)**: 59–62.

PARKES, C.M. (1975) *Bereavement – studies of grief in adult life* (2nd edition). Harmondsworth. Penguin.

RESUSCITATION COUNCIL (UK) (1997) CPR '97. Annual Scientific Symposium, Brighton, England, April 1997.

RESUSCITATION COUNCIL (UK) (1997) The 1997 Resuscitation Guidelines for Use in the United Kingdom. London, Resuscitation Council (UK).

ROYAL COLLEGE OF NURSING (1992) *Resuscitation: Right or Wrong? The Moral and Legal Issues Faced By Health Care Professionals*. London. Royal College of Nursing.

RENNER, S. (1991) I desperately needed to see my son. *British Medical Journal* **302**: 356.

ROBERTSON, C., HOLMBERG, S. (1992) Compression techniques and blood flow during cardiopulmonary resuscitation. *Resuscitation* **24(2)**: 123–132.

SEEDHOUSE, D. (1988) *Ethics the Heart of Health Care*. Chichester. Wiley Medical Prod.

TINGLE, J, (1991) First aid law. *Nursing Times* **87(35)**: 48–49.

TRENT REGIONAL HEALTH AUTHORITY, (1990a) *Major Accident Procedures, Code of Good Practice*. Sheffield. Trent RHA.

TRENT REGIONAL HEALTH AUTHORITY, (1990b) Report: Aircraft Accident BD092, M1 Motorway East Midlands Airport. Sheffield. Trent RHA.

TUCKER, K.J., IDRIS, A. (1994) Clinical and laboratory investigations of active compression–decompression cardiopulmonary resuscitation. *Resuscitation* **28(1)**: 1–7.

UKCC (1992) *Code of Professional Conduct*. London. UKCC.

UKCC (1996) *Guidelines for Professional Practice*. p. 11. London. UKCC.

WARDROPE, J., MORRIS, F. (1993) European guidelines on resuscitation. *British Medical Journal* **306**: 1555–1556.

WEISFELDT, M.L., KERBER, R.E., McGOLDRICK, R.P. et al. (1995) Public Access Defibrillation—AHA Medical/Scientific Statement. (Internet reference: http://www.amhrt.org:80/pubs/scipub/statements/1995/21952222html). Published also in: *Circulation* (1995) **92**: 2763.

WOODRUFF, I. (1989) A report on staff reaction at Mayday University Hospital following the major incident of the Purley train crash. *British Journal of Accident and Emergency Medicine* **4**: 2.

WRIGHT, B. (1991) *Sudden Death*. Edinburgh. Churchill Livingstone.

WRIGHT, B. (1996) *Sudden Death – A Research Base for Practice* (2nd edition). Edinburgh. Churchill Livingstone.

WYNNE, G., KIRBY, S., CORDINGLY, A. (1990) No breathing. . .no pulse. What shall we do? *Professional Nurse* **5(10)**: 510–513.

ZOLTIE, N., SLOAN, J., WRIGHT, B. (1994) Observed resuscitation may affect a doctor's performance. *British Medical Journal* **309**: 404.

H. Dobbins and G. Adams

KEY ISSUES

■ SUBJECT KNOWLEDGE

▷ mechanism of feedback loops in maintaining homeostasis

▷ biological basis of thermoregulation, blood pressure maintenance and respiratory homeostasis

▷ behavioural, cultural and environmental factors that affect health

▷ approaches to health promotion in maintaining homeostasis

■ PRACTICE KNOWLEDGE

▷ assessment of thermoregulation and problems in maintaining homeostasis

▷ blood pressure measurement

▷ respiratory assessment and common problems

■ PROFESSIONAL KNOWLEDGE

▷ skill mix debates related to monitoring homeostasis

▷ ritualistic practices

▷ educational issues

■ REFLECTIVE KNOWLEDGE

▷ skills laboratory learning

▷ case study consolidation

▶ INTRODUCTION

Being healthy implies a feeling of general wellbeing. Although originally focused primarily on physical wellbeing, it is now recognized that there are multiple dimensions to feeling healthy, including psychosocial, spiritual and emotional dimensions. To maintain personal health individuals need to constantly adapt to changes within their own internal environment and to the changing external environment. An individual becomes 'unhealthy' or 'unwell' when any of the dimensions of his or her health are affected by internal or external forces to which he or she is unable to adapt. The nurse, through multiple roles involving health promotion and observation and therapeutic skills, is an important decision maker in supporting the individual patient or client's ability to adapt.

The central focus of this chapter is on how we maintain the balance and adaptability of our internal environment in order to remain healthy. This chapter will explore the ways in which the body acts as a finely tuned engine in establishing and maintaining a stable internal environment. The human body is subjected to many physical and social assaults from the external environment as well as from the self in the form of changes in emotional and mental states. In order to remain stable, we possess a rapid response mechanism that allows us to meet the changing demands placed on us as a result of day to day encounters. This balance of the system is known as homeostasis. The word homeostasis is derived from the Greek words 'homeo' (same) and 'stasis' (staying). However, things are never static within ourselves and in the outside world; growth is change and there is constant change around us. The brain therefore helps us to adapt to change and remain stable but not static in a changing world (Orstein and Sobel, 1988).

This chapter will help you examine the fundamental bases of homeostasis and the ways in which the body responds in an attempt to meet the specific demands placed upon it by a changing blood pressure, a changing body temperature and a changing respiratory rate. As the content of this chapter focuses on these three specific areas of homeostasis, it is expected that you will cross-reference with many other chapters for other complementary aspects of homeostasis, for example Chapter 1.1 on environmental safety, Chapter 2.1 on resuscitation, Chapter 2.4 on skin integrity, Chapter 3.2 on nutrition and Chapter 4.1 on stress and anxiety.

▶ OVERVIEW

▶ *Subject Knowledge*

In the Biological section of Subject Knowledge, we explore the mechanism of feedback loops, which are essential to maintaining homeostasis, and then concentrate on how the normal temperature, blood pressure and respirations are maintained and controlled by the body.

Individual behavioural, environmental, social and emotional factors also have an effect on how we maintain internal body balance. These factors are explored under Psychosocial Subject Knowledge. How we behave to maintain our health and how environmental factors can affect our behaviour are also examined.

▶ *Practice Knowledge*

The knowledge needed by the nurse for making a comprehensive assessment of elements of homeostasis such as a person's temperature, blood pressure and respirations is explored. The nursing management of certain situations that threaten homeostasis is also covered in this section.

▶ *Professional Knowledge*

Professional issues which influence the role of the nurse in the assessment of homeostasis are identified. The discussion includes an exploration of the impact of changing role boundaries and the skills mix of the healthcare team, the effects of ritualistic practice, the benefit of audit and the need for ongoing education to ensure competent practice.

▶ *Reflective Knowledge*

Suggestions are made for experiential exercises in which assessment of homeostasis can be practiced in a safe environment. Consolidation of knowledge gained from the chapter and through your practice experience is facilitated through case study work.

On pp. 207–208 there are four case studies, each one relating to one of the branch programmes. You may find it helpful to read one of them before you start the chapter and use it as a focus for your reflections while reading.

SUBJECT KNOWLEDGE
Biological

Before outlining the specific knowledge needed for decision making regarding body temperature, blood pressure maintenance and respiratory control, it is important to understand the mechanisms involved in maintaining balance in all body systems. Most of the control systems of the body are based on the principle of negative feedback, that is, any deviation from the desired normal range results in the body correcting the

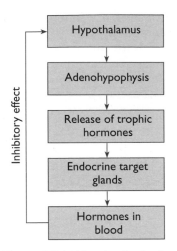

Figure 2.2.1: Negative feedback loop.

Inhibitory effect

Hypothalamus

Adenohypophysis

Release of trophic hormones

Endocrine target glands

Hormones in blood

high or low value and reestablishing a state of equilibrium. Within the process of negative feedback, there is an inhibitory component which prevents the body from becoming too cold or too hot. For example, when the body is too hot, vasodilatation (peripheral) occurs and heat is lost under the direction of the heat-losing centre in the preoptic area of the hypothalamus. As a consequence, body temperature drops. A further reduction in temperature is prevented by thermoreceptors in the skin sending messages to the hypothalamus to inhibit vasodilatation. Thus the inhibitory message 'kicks in' (Figure 2.2.1).

The hypothalamus is the 'brain of the brain' and is part of the limbic system, which helps to maintain homeostasis. The hypothalamus regulates eating and drinking, sleeping and waking, body temperature, hormone balances, heart rate, sex drive and emotions. It also directs the master gland of the brain – the pituitary gland – which is responsible for regulating hormonal balance within the body. The brain is therefore the major organ of adaption and can respond to changes in the external and internal environment quickly and flexibly to maintain health.

▶ HOMEOSTASIS – THE BALANCE OF BODY TEMPERATURE

The main organ for maintaining normal body temperature is the skin. The skin has many vital functions. However, in this particular section, thermoregulation and its homeostatic control will be the main focus (see Chapter 2.4 for other functions of the skin).

Humans, like other mammals, are homeothermic and can only maintain core temperature within a narrow range of 36–38°C despite the day to day fluctuations encountered as a consequence of environmental temperatures and our own metabolic activities. Homeothermy is dependent upon continual thermoregulation (Case and Waterhouse, 1994) with the scales finely balanced between metabolic heat production and heat loss.

Four major physical processes are involved in the loss of heat from the skin to the environment and are:

- ▶ evaporation;
- ▶ conduction;
- ▶ radiation;
- ▶ convection.

Each of these processes is important in your decision making about managing patients with altered body temperature.

▶ *Evaporation (22% of Heat Loss)*

The process of evaporation requires energy. If you wet the back of your hand and then blow on the area you will experience the process of evaporation. The body loses heat through the use of sweat glands present in the skin. Sweat is composed mainly of water and as it evaporates the energy used in the process of evaporation cools the body.

Water is constantly being lost from the body even when the surrounding temperature is relatively low. Insensible (i.e. too small or gradual to be perceived) water loss is approximately 500 ml/day as a result of evaporative loss from the skin and the respiratory passages. This loss can be increased as a result of exercise or sweating in a hot environment. The rate at which heat is lost by evaporation depends upon the relative humidity of the air. That is to say:

RESEARCH BASED EVIDENCE

Case and Waterhouse (1994) indicate that homeothermy is dependent upon continual thermoregulation. Environmental temperature variation studies demonstrate that these may be circadian (diurnal), circannual or geographic. Diurnal ranges of 35°C are commonly recorded in continental hot deserts. The largest circannual temperature variations occur in the centre of large land masses where winter temperatures can fall to −65°C and summers have a mean of +20°C. Geographically, individual populations live in environmental temperatures ranging from −65°C to 50°C.

> ● high concentration of water in air = low evaporation = low heat loss;
> ● low concentration of water in air = high evaporation = high heat loss.

▶ Conduction (3% of Heat Loss)

In conduction, heat loss or gain is brought about by contact between the surface of the skin and some other object. For example, if the skin temperature is higher than the temperature of the clothes you wear, then heat will be lost to the clothes. This is particularly relevant when discussing heat loss and gain in the elderly and children for whom it is important to wear additional clothing in low environmental temperatures. The additional clothing provides insulation from the cold and therefore heat is lost much more slowly.

▶ Radiation (60% of Heat Loss)

Radiation is a process whereby heat is transferred from one heat source to another. For example, a cold individual who wants to become warmer can gain heat by standing next to something that is giving off heat. The sun gives off heat and if you are subjected to its heat long enough both your superficial and core temperatures increase. Our bodies also lose heat via radiation. This factor can be life-saving as it enables the emergency services to use heat sensitive cameras to locate victims buried in building rubble or lost underground.

▶ Convection (15% of Heat Loss)

In convection heat is lost to the movement of air surrounding the skin surface. When the skin is surrounded by air that does not move the air forms an insulating barrier and as a result reduces the amount of heat lost. However, when movement of this insulating barrier increases the heat lost to the environment also increases.

▶ Homeostatic Control of Body Temperature

Body temperature is regulated by a feedback loop. Heat is constantly being produced by metabolic activity. In order for this heat production to become and remain homeostatically balanced, there has to be a heat loss of the same proportion. This is obtained by balancing the scales between heat input and heat output (Figure 2.2.2).

▶ Physiological Response to Low Temperatures

Thermoreceptors located in the periphery and central nervous system respond to a lowering of temperature and transmit impulses to the preoptic area located in the hypothalamus, stimulating the heat promoting centre. As a consequence, there is sympathetic nervous system stimulation resulting in vasoconstriction, increased metabolism and shivering (Figure 2.2.3).

Sympathetic stimulation resulting in the release of the adrenaline and noradrenaline increases the basal metabolic rate by mobilizing the fat stores from adipose tissue and as a consequence generating heat. This process is known as chemical thermogenesis or non-shivering thermogenesis and its function is vital in the newborn because their heat loss is large due to their large surface area. This adipose tissue is called 'brown fat' and humans have only a small quantity and can therefore only raise their body heat production by 10–15%.

In your practice placements you may encounter many ways of managing heat loss or gain in both children and adults. Reflect on and decide which of the four processes opposite is primarily involved in each of the following methods used in practice.

- *A baby placed in an incubator.*
- *A child wrapped in a foil blanket or 'space blanket'.*
- *Fan therapy in the room of a person with a high temperature.*
- *Tepid sponging of an adult with a high temperature.*

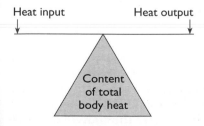

Figure 2.2.2: Balancing the scales of body heat.

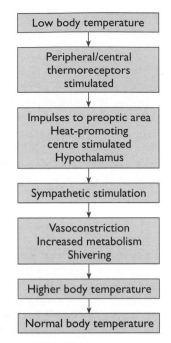

Low body temperature

↓

Peripheral/central thermoreceptors stimulated

↓

Impulses to preoptic area Heat-promoting centre stimulated Hypothalamus

↓

Sympathetic stimulation

↓

Vasoconstriction Increased metabolism Shivering

↓

Higher body temperature

↓

Normal body temperature

Figure 2.2.3: Thermoregulatory mechanism when the body temperature is low.

Physiological Response to High Temperatures

A rise in temperature is recognized by peripheral and central thermo-receptors, which relay this information to the preoptic area of the hypothalamus and the heat losing centre is stimulated. As a result, there is parasympathetic stimulation; cutaneous vasodilatation, diaphoresis (sweating) and decreased metabolism ensue and heat loss is increased. Shivering is inhibited.

Physical Factors that Affect Thermoregulation

These include:

- exercise;
- hormones;
- drugs;
- food intake;
- circadian rhythms;
- age.

Exercise produces extra heat, which must be expelled in some way. In the initial stages of exercise, the core temperature begins to fall because of the increase in cooler venous blood returning from the cooler limbs. However, as the exercise increases in duration, sweating begins and heat is lost via the respiratory tract and the exercising limbs. If the exercise increases in duration and intensity, the body tries to compensate, even to the extent of organ failure. Cardiac ouput and integumentary blood flow increase. As a result of this intensified exercising there is extensive loss through diaphoresis of water, potassium and sodium ions.

Thermoregulation Failure

Under certain conditions the normal thermoregulatory mechanisms can be compromised. These include:

- fever(pyrexia);
- heat stroke;
- heat exhaustion;
- hypothermia.

RESEARCH BASED EVIDENCE

According to Timms-Hagen (1984) brown fat, which is found in the newborn, has a rich supply of blood and nerves. When the body is exposed to cold, brown fat can be rapidly hydrolysed and oxidized in a reaction that produces a large quantity of heat. During the first ten years of life the human brown fat is widely distributed; thereafter, it disappears gradually, although it does persist into old age around the kidneys, suprarenals and aorta. The reason for this gradual loss of brown fat is unknown, but is probably something to do with the fact that temperature can be controlled much better as we get older.

- **Review the relative effects of circadian rhythms on temperature.**
- **In your practice placements, note the times of day when temperature is recorded.**
- **Discuss with your practice supervisor how you would differentiate the effects of time of day on temperature from possible upsets in thermoregulation.**

Fever

Fever (pyrexia) is an elevation in body temperature up to 41°C and can be caused by inflammation as a result of pyrogen/interleukin-1 release. (Pyrogens are classified as either endogenous or exogenous depending on whether they operate inside or outside the hypothalamic thermoregulatory centre. Interleukin-1, which is an exogenous pyrogen, promotes the release of prostaglandins, endogenous pyrogens, from preoptic neurons.) This initiates an upward displacement of the hypothalamic 'set point' for temperature control. As the 'set point' has been reset the individual feels the need to increase body temperature to this new level. A rise in temperature is said to help the body's immune responses eliminate the pathogens.

▶ Heat Stroke

Heat stroke occurs as a consequence of thermoregulatory failure when the ambient temperature is higher than the body's ability to maintain homeothermy. The condition manifests itself with a loss of energy and irritability followed by more serious neurological and mental disturbances. There is a large reduction in sweating and coma ensues as the core body temperature approaches 42°C. This very high temperature results in protein coagulation and cellular damage. Treatment is aimed at cooling the vital organs such as the brain, liver and the heart. Heat stroke is not common in the UK, but children and the elderly can be at risk, especially if taking holidays abroad in countries where the air temperature can be very high.

▶ Heat Exhaustion

The precipitative factors of heat exhaustion fall into two categories:

▶ salt deficiency;
▶ water deficiency.

Salt deficiency results when salts lost through sweating are inadequately replaced. This leads to cramps in the legs, arms or back with associated fatigue and dizziness. Water deficiency is due to inadequate replacement of lost water. This results in dehydration with fatigue and dizziness as the loss approaches 5–8%. Further losses precipitate cellular damage.

Appropriate rehydration is the answer for both types of deficiency. Nutritionists advocate that 1200–1600 ml a day are sufficient to maintain hydration, but exclude caffeinated and alcoholic drinks, which precipitate diuresis and therefore increase the need for fluid intake. Athletes are now advised to consume a drink called Gatorade (Goldman *et al.*, 1994). When water intake is supplemented with sodium, dehydrated individuals rehydrate much more readily as sodium has the effect of replenishing plasma volume and retaining water in the blood.

▶ Hypothermia

A fall of body temperature to 33°C causes mental confusion and sluggishness and further reductions result in dysfunction of the central nervous system's thermoregulatory ability. Shivering in an attempt to gain heat ceases and loss of consciousness results. Muscle rigidity follows with associated cardiac dysrhythmias and eventual death. The elderly and the very young in particular can be at risk during the winter months in the UK, especially during periods of prolonged cold weather – the elderly may not respond quickly enough in an appropriate way to maintain body heat due to their decreased ability to perceive that the ambient temperature is falling.

Children have a protective mechanism which is triggered if they fall into cold water. This response is referred to as the dive reflex, and results in a decreased heart rate and an increased cerebral and cardiac blood flow. As

Age (years)	Blood pressure (mmHg) Systolic	Diastolic
Newborn	80	46
10	103	70
20	120	80
40	126	84
60	135	89

Table 2.2.1 Some average blood pressure values, taken from 250 000 healthy individuals (from Durkin, 1979)

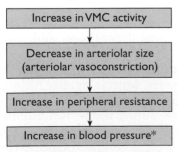

*There will be a rise in blood pressure provided the cardiac output stays constant

Figure 2.2.4: Increase in vasomotor activity.

children are small in size they have a relatively smaller circulating blood volume, which means that the cold water in the lungs rapidly chills the blood in the pulmonary circulation which then results in brain cooling and a reduction in the brain's oxygen (O_2) requirements. Consequently, a child may survive immersion in cold water for longer periods of time.

▶ HAEMODYNAMIC HOMEOSTASIS

Blood pressure is the pressure that is exerted on the walls of the blood vessels in which blood is contained. Its level is dependent upon the interaction of three components:

- ▶ the volume of blood in the circulatory system;
- ▶ the heart rate (velocity);
- ▶ the resistance offered by constricted blood vessels (peripheral resistance).

Normotension (i.e. normal blood pressure) is the pressure of the blood within the systemic circulation and the range varies according to age (Table 2.2.1). Systolic blood pressure (upper value) indicates the maximum pressure produced by the left ventricle during contraction or systole. Diastolic blood pressure (lower value) represents the pressure in the artery at the end of the diastole or relaxation of the left ventricle.

▶ Factors Contributing to a Change in Blood Pressure

If the needs of the body increase then the delivery of blood to those areas will also have to increase to meet the needs. The speed with which the heart contracts each minute (heart rate) multiplied by the amount of blood it expels (stroke volume) is referred to as the cardiac output (i.e. cardiac output = heart rate × stroke volume) and should this increase a corresponding increase in blood pressure will be observed.

Another factor that must be borne in mind is the degree of friction created when blood travels rapidly through the blood vessels. This is referred to as peripheral resistance. The widening (vasodilatation) or narrowing (vasoconstriction) of a blood vessel will result in either a reduction or increase in this friction of blood against the walls of the blood vessels and, as a consequence, a decrease or increase in the blood pressure. The size of blood vessels is regulated by a division of the autonomic nervous system called the sympathetic nervous system. The middle layer in the arteriolar wall called the tunica media is in a state of partial contraction as a result of continual activity by the sympathetic division of the autonomic nervous system. This is referred to as sympathetic tone and the tone derives from a group of cells in the vasomotor centre within the medulla oblongata in the brain. An increase or decrease in vasomotor centre activity will lead to a corresponding increase or decrease in blood pressure (Figure 2.2.4).

▶ Hypertension (High Blood Pressure)

Hypertension is the chronic elevation of blood pressure above a normal value which is acceptable for the patient's age. This is usually accepted as 100 plus the chronological age of the patient for systolic pressure, and for the diastolic pressure it is usually above 90 mmHg. Hypertension may be mainly systolic, or a combination of systolic and diastolic (Thomas *et al.*, 1992). Hypertension can be separated into two categories:

Using your biological sciences textbook review the effects on the homeostatic control of blood pressure of:

- *The baroreceptor control system.*
- *The chemoreceptor control system.*

Review the relative effects of each of these mechanisms when:

- *You get patients up suddenly from a lying position to a standing position and they complain of feeling dizzy and faint.*
- *You start to get a headache in a smoke-filled room.*

RESEARCH BASED EVIDENCE

McGee et al. (1992) state that the distribution of blood pressure in human populations is unimodal, suggesting a polygenic inheritance (i.e. a combined action of a number of genes). This fact has been confirmed by twin studies and comparing the blood pressures of adopted and natural children with the same parents. With regards to race, hypertensive black Afrocaribbean men have a death rate about six times that of hypertensive white men. Essential hypertension is more common and has a better prognosis in women.

The prevalence of hypertension in a population correlates with salt intake. Cigarette smoking increases the risk of malignant hypertension (i.e. blood pressure rises very rapidly causing serious damage to organs) and urban populations have higher blood pressures than rural ones.

- primary hypertension;
- secondary hypertension.

Primary hypertension

This is commonly referred to as essential hypertension and usually occurs in people who are 35–45 years of age. It is not caused by any specific disease but is associated with a combination of factors. The effects are insidious and develop over many years. Hypertension is frequently discovered by chance at routine health checks. Factors known to predispose individuals to primary hypertension include:

- Genetic factors.
- Racial factors.
- Age and sex.
- Diet.
- Smoking.
- Environmental factors.
- Stress.

Secondary hypertension

This develops as a consequence of an underlying disease, and occurs in approximately 5–10% of patients with hypertension and is more common in young patients. The primary causes for secondary hypertension are:

- renal in origin;
- stenosis of the aorta, commonly called coarctation;
- arteriosclerosis, which causes a narrowing of the lumen of blood vessels leading to increased peripheral resistance.

Hypotension

Hypotension is usually a condition in which the systolic blood pressure falls below 100 mm Hg in the adult. Remember that a child's normal blood pressure is age related (see Table 2.2.1). A hypotensive state can be precipitated by either a loss of blood or a fluid shift from one physiological fluid compartment to another. Children are particularly vulnerable as they have a relatively low circulating blood volume and can develop hypovolaemic shock very rapidly. A fall in blood pressure initiates a cyclical chain of events, which initially brings about hypoxia (i.e. a reduction of O_2 to the tissues). Hypoxia leads to cell and tissue damage, resulting in the release of vasodilator substances and a further fall in blood pressure.

The Pulse

Contraction of the left ventricle forces blood into the aorta and as a result creates distension and elongation in the arterial wall. As a consequence of this distension, the wave passing along an artery can be felt whenever it is pressed carefully against a bone in places such as the wrist (radial and ulnar pulses), ankles (posterior tibial pulse), neck (carotid pulse) and groin (femoral pulse) areas (Figure 2.2.5). In babies of less than one year of age, heart rate is measured by listening with a stethoscope to the apex beat. This is defined as the heart beat which is heard at the apex or lower tip of the heart. The nurse listens for the characteristic lub-dub sounds and counts each full cardiac cycle for one minute to determine the apical rate (Lewis and Timby, 1993). In young children the brachial pulse is the

Blood pressure is constantly adapting to meet the changing needs of the body. Review the list below and decide whether blood pressure will be increased or decreased and explain why in each case.

- *Exercise.*
- *Stress.*
- *Sleep.*
- *Digestion.*
- *Time of the day.*

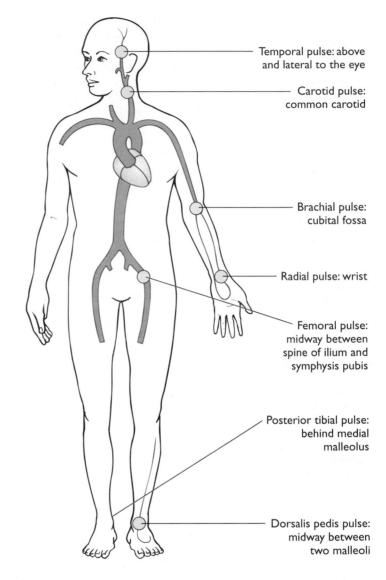

Temporal pulse: above and lateral to the eye

Carotid pulse: common carotid

Brachial pulse: cubital fossa

Radial pulse: wrist

Femoral pulse: midway between spine of ilium and symphysis pubis

Posterior tibial pulse: behind medial malleolus

Dorsalis pedis pulse: midway between two malleoli

Figure 2.2.5: Common sites in the body where pulses can be felt. (Redrawn from Hinchliffe *et al.*, 1996.)

most common site for measurement. When trying to establish information about a patient's pulse, it is important to consider three factors:

▶ rate;
▶ rhythm;
▶ strength of the pulse wave.

▶ Pulse rate (Table 2.2.2)

Age	Approximate range	Approximate average
Newborn	120–160	140
1 month to 12 months	80–140	120
2 years	80–130	110
2 years to 6 years	75–120	100
6 years to 12 years	75–110	95
Adolescence	60–100	80
Adulthood	60–100	80

Table 2.2.2 Normal pulse rates per minute at various ages

Pulse rate indicates the speed with which the heart is beating and varies with age. An abnormally rapid pulse is indicative of excitement, exertion, haemorrhage or fever, and is referred to as sinus tachycardia. Conversely, an abnormally slow pulse is referred to as sinus bradycardia. Bradycardia can be indicative of a well-trained athlete, stimulation of the parasympathetic nervous system, increased intracranial pressure, and heart problems.

▶ Pulse rhythm

The normal pulse is regular and the time between each beat is constant. If the normal rhythm of ventricular contraction alters, the interval between beats is interrupted. This can be due to a heart beat occurring earlier (premature) or later or a missed beat. An irregular pulse pattern is called an arrhythmia or dysrhythmia and can be either continuous or intermittent. Sinus arryhthmia is a change in rhythm more commonly found in children and is associated with an increase in heart rate on inspiration and a decrease on expiration (Hinchliff *et al.*, 1996). Other changes are often associated with cardiovascular disease and can be life-threatening if cardiac output is seriously affected (see Chapter 2.1 on resuscitation).

▶ Pulse strength

Pulse strength can be separated into two important factors:

▶ volume;
▶ tension.

Pulse volume is the degree of distension felt in the arterial wall in response to the pressure wave exerted on ventricular contraction. It usually relates to the amount of blood pumped out with each contraction.
An altered pulse volume is often described as being:

▶ weak and thready, here the pulse is difficult to feel and disappears if slight pressure is exerted;
▶ bounding and full, here the pulse is easy to feel, it is pronounced and strong and does not disappear with moderate pressure (Lewis and Timby, 1993).

Tension is specifically related to blood pressure. More force is needed when compressing the artery to feel for a pulse when the blood pressure is high. Conversely, less force is required when the blood pressure is low.

▶ RESPIRATORY HOMEOSTASIS

The respiratory and circulatory systems work synergistically in an attempt to establish and maintain a homeostatic balance and any disruption in this mechanism will result in dysfunction. This subsection is concerned with the physiology of respiration from the level of the organism. Cellular respiration involves a process known as oxidative phosphorylation, that is the production of ATP when glucose is completely oxidized to carbon dioxide (CO_2) and water (H_2O). (For further information about this process see Chapter 3.2 on nutrition.)

In the practice laboratory:

• *Measure and comment on the rate, rhythm and strength of the pulse rate of your peer group.*

• *Note any differences related to age and other factors such as recent exercise.*

In your practice placements:

• *Observe the different sites for taking the pulse in different client groups.*

• *Under supervision practice taking the pulse of individual clients and note any changes and the reason for those changes in rate, rhythm and strength.*

Physiology of Respiration

The primary purpose of respiration is to supply the cells of the body with O_2 and remove CO_2. The three basic processes involved include:

- pulmonary ventilation, otherwise known as breathing, which is concerned with air passing into (inspiration) and out of (expiration) the respiratory passageways in an exchange with the atmosphere;
- external respiration, which refers to the exchange of respiratory gases between the lungs and the blood;
- internal respiration, which is the exchange of respiratory gases between the blood and the cells of the body.

In the processes of pulmonary ventilation, there is an exchange of respiratory gases as a result of a pressure gradient, which exists between the atmosphere and the alveoli of the lungs. Through the action of the diaphragm and the intercostal muscles the chest cavity and the lungs expand. This creates a pressure within the alveoli lower than that of the atmosphere, leading to a movement of air from the atmosphere to the lungs during inspiration. However, on expiration when the diaphragm and the intercostal muscles return to their normal position, the pressure gradient is reversed and air moves out of the lungs.

Once the tissues of the body have used the O_2 it is essential that not only is the waste product CO_2 removed, but that O_2 concentrations are replenished. External respiration is the process whereby there is an exchange of O_2 inward and CO_2 outward between the pulmonary blood capillaries and the lung alveoli. This is achieved by the pressures exerted by the O_2 and CO_2. Figure 2.2.6 refers to the partial pressure of O_2 (pO_2). This is the pressure exerted in its particular location and is proportional to its concentration and can be measured in mm Hg or kPa. Because the pO_2 in the alveoli is greater than in the pulmonary blood vessels, O_2 moves down the concentration gradient. The diffusion of O_2 from alveoli to blood capillaries allows deoxygenated blood to be converted to oxygenated blood.

The diffusion of CO_2 from the blood capillary to the alveoli works on exactly the same principle as O_2 diffusion. Due to the relatively high partial pressure of CO_2 (pCO_2) in the pulmonary blood capillary and the low pCO_2 in the alveoli, CO_2 diffuses down its concentration gradient (see Figure 2.2.6).

On completion of external respiration, oxygenated blood is transported back to the left atrium via the pulmonary veins, and thence to the circulation and tissue cells via the aorta. Exchange of gases between the blood capillaries of the tissues and the tissue cells themselves is referred to as internal respiration and works on the same principles as external respiration (see Figure 2.2.6).

Oxygen Transport

Because of its reduced solubility in water, the majority of O_2 is carried in chemical combination with haemoglobin in the erythrocytes (red blood cells). Haemoglobin (Hb) is a protein in which the haem portion contains four atoms of iron, each of which is capable of attaching itself to a molecule of O_2. Therefore, four molecules of O_2 can combine with one molecule of Hb (Figure 2.2.7). When the Hb is fully saturated with O_2 (oxyhaemoglobin) it is bright red, while a gradual diminution in the O_2 content results in a dark red coloration (deoxyhaemoglobin).

Hb is so important in the carriage of O_2 that a reduction in Hb concentration from whatever cause will be a threat to the patient or client. In maintaining or restoring homeostasis the patient or client may need to have a blood transfusion. During your practice placements :

- *Find out where, how and from whom blood is obtained for transfusion.*

- *How soon after obtaining blood from a donor should it be transfused into the recipient and what changes can occur to donor blood during storage?*

- *Are there any other intravenous fluids that can be given as a replacement for blood? What are the problems with these fluids in relation to restoring O_2 homeostasis?*

Figure 2.2.6: The process of respiration. (Redrawn from Hinchliffe *et al.*, 1996.)

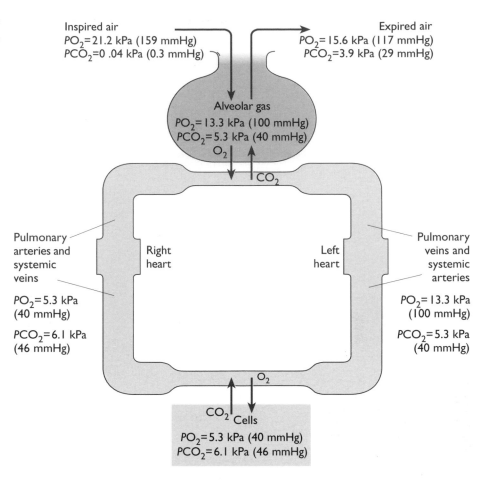

Figure 2.2.7: The association of oxygen with haemoglobin. This is a reversible reaction as denoted by the two-way arrow.

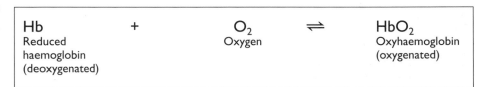

❱ Control of the Respiratory System

The control of the respiratory system is an interrelated one between neural and chemical stimuli, which regulate the rate of respiration in order to meet the metabolic requirements of the body. Many factors affect respiratory rate and are summarized in Figure 2.2.8.

Chemical control is related specifically to levels of CO_2 in the blood, the primary stimulus to breathe being the response of the respiratory centre in the brain to an increase in CO_2 concentration in the blood passing over central chemoreceptors in the medulla (Mateika and Duffin, 1990) and peripheral chemoreceptors in the arch of the aorta. A high level of CO_2 stimulates a feedback loop through the respiratory centre that will result in an increase in the rate and depth of breathing in order to return the blood CO_2 concentration to normal and therefore maintain homeostasis.

Neural control is via areas within the respiratory centre, which have the ability to stimulate and inhibit respiration. These areas include the medullary rhythmicity area (MRA), pneumotaxic area and the apneustic area.

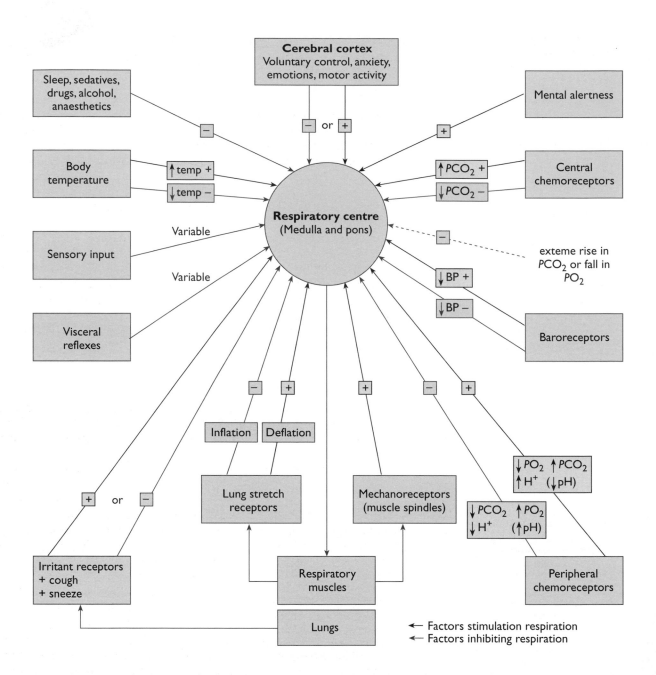

Figure 2.2.8: Factors that affect respiratory homeostasis. (Redrawn from Hinchliffe *et al.*, 1996.)

▶ MRA

The MRA is located in the medulla oblongata and is responsible for controlling the rhythm of respiration. During normal resting state breathing, inspiration and expiration continue for approximately five seconds. As it is essential that the basic rhythm of respiration has a control mechanism for inspiration and expiration, the MRA possesses both an inspiratory and expiratory neuronal network.

▶ Pneumotaxic area

The pneumotaxic area is situated in the upper portion of the pons varolii and is responsible for effective physiological communication between inspiration and expiration so that one phase leads smoothly into the other without errors. The pneumotaxic area is responsible for inhibiting inspiration. As a consequence of this action, the lungs do not have the ability to overinflate and the act of expiration is promoted.

Apneustic area

As with the pneumotaxic area, the apneustic area, which is located in the mid section of the pons varolii, is also responsible for the smooth interchange of inspiration and expiration. In order to achieve this effectively, the apneustic area transmits stimulatory messages to the inspiratory area. As a result, the act of inspiration is activated and prolonged. In addition, the act of expiration is inhibited. In principle, the apneustic area works in the opposite way to the pneumotaxic area and by doing so achieves balance in the system.

An understanding of the neural and chemical control of respiration is helpful when assessing respiration. The voluntary control of breathing is achieved through descending pathways from the cerebral cortex to the medullary respiratory centre. Voluntary control is limited in duration, it is demonstrated during hyperventilation, breath holding, singing, speech and deep breathing for relaxation. Enhancing voluntary control through teaching patients how to adapt their breathing can be useful in managing respiratory problems.

> Although most of the time we are not conscious of our breathing as we go about our daily lives, attention will be drawn to how we breathe in certain situations. Reflect on whether control of our breathing is voluntary or involuntary in each of the following situations and explain why.
>
> - **When singing in an opera.**
> - **In a panic when breathing shallowly and at a very fast rate.**
> - **When swimming.**
> - **When breathing is very shallow and slow after drinking many pints of beer.**

Psychosocial

When learning about homeostasis and the mechanisms in place to sustain a balance of body systems, it is also important to explore how changes in the social world and in individual emotional and mental states can affect our health.

Although the focus of this chapter is on measuring physiological status through taking and recording vital signs, which are very important when an individual is acutely ill, measuring health status overall can be undertaken more broadly by using many other indicators of health, which also include psychosocial factors. The Nottingham Health Profile (Hunt *et al.*, 1986) is a well-known example of a subjective health assessment tool that places equal emphasis on mental and physical health. It is also important to be aware that our beliefs about health will influence how we behave in maintaining our health.

> Orstein and Sobel (1988) in their book *The Healing Brain* ask the following questions:
>
> Why does your blood pressure drop when you touch your pet?
>
> Why should hostility bring about heart attacks and why not anger?
>
> Why do people who lose their jobs have increased rates of heart and lung disorders no matter what their occupation?
>
> - **Reflect on your own lifestyle and review any personal and social factors that may have an effect, however temporary, on your body homeostasis.**
> - **Identify any other health problems that you know have a significant relationship with psychosocial factors.**

▶ INDIVIDUAL BEHAVIOUR AND HEALTH

According to Tones (1993) an individual's lifestyle and the physical, social, cultural and economic environment will all have an effect on health. Many of these factors are integrated within our learned social behaviour and our personal beliefs about our health (Bright, 1997). Influences on the way we behave are individual to each person, but are usually strongly associated with the family and school in childhood, peers in early adolescence and our social groupings, religious affiliations, the media and multiple other sources during our adult lives.

Health promotion strategies (Table 2.2.3) have been developed to explore with people their learned behaviour in relation to maintaining health with the aim of changing that behaviour if it is seen as detrimental. The target populations for these strategies are all age groups, with a particular focus in recent years on health promotion within schools (Department of Health, 1992), especially as it has become recognized that children are adopting unhealthy behaviours such as smoking and drug misuse at an earlier age (While, 1989; Department of Health, 1994).

According to Lee (1997) just giving information and advice to an individual on risk factors for diseases such as coronary heart disease may have little effect on their lifestyle. Stress and worry are perceived to be important factors in causing high blood pressure. Such factors may be the result of tension over job security or job loss, which is often outside the control of the individual. However, learning how to cope with experiencing such tensions can be addressed (see Chapter 4.1 on stress and anxiety). Despite the limitations of indivualistic approaches, there is an increased awareness of risk factors and the public in general are motivated to change unhealthy lifestyles (Backett, 1990; Dawson, 1994).

The public are becoming more interested in alternative methods for coping with changes in their health. Yoga techniques perfected over many years have allowed the yogi to control involuntary body functions. More recently these controls have been achieved using hypnosis, autogenic training and biofeedback (Schwartz, 1987; Bray, 1995). A complementary therapy that can be used specifically in relation to maintaining physical homeostasis is biofeedback. Measuring instruments are needed initially to teach the individual the technique. Biofeedback techniques are particularly useful because they give the control back to the client experiencing the difficulties and fit within the self-empowerment approach to health promotion (see Table 2.2.3).

Approach	Activity
Educational	Give information so that individual can make choices
Preventive	Encourage the individual to modify their behaviour in order to prevent disease
Radical	Influence the social, economic and political factors that are detrimental to health
Self-empowerment	Encourage individual self-esteem and assertiveness in order to affect change

Table 2.2.3 Health promotion approaches (Tones, 1993)

▶ SOCIAL AND CULTURAL INFLUENCES ON HEALTH

We are all strongly influenced by the beliefs of society around us and how we become ill or remain healthy is affected by cultural beliefs on what is good and bad 'healthy' behaviour. Many sociologists have commented on the 'lay' perceptions of health as opposed to how professionals describe, label and classify 'ill-health' (Kleinman, 1980; Mishler, 1981; Helman, 1994).

Lay beliefs are important in examining the concept of homeostasis as a balance or harmony between two or more elements or forces within the body, this is an important cultural component of health. An example of a lay theory is the humoral theory, which has its origins in China

Explore in more detail
The Health Belief Model developed by Becker (1974).

- *Reflect on your own behaviour in relation to health and identify who has influenced your behaviour in the past and who and what influences your present behaviour.*

- *Join with a group of your peers and compare notes.*

- *Discuss who and what might have a strong influence on you changing your behaviour.*

- *How do your findings fit with The Health Belief Model (Becker, 1974).*

(Yin and Yang) and India and was prominent in Europe during the middle ages. It forms the basis of the 'hot' and 'cold' theory of health much favoured in Latin American folk medicine. This theory is also a prominent part of Islamic beliefs and the Ayurvedic system of medicine practiced in India (Helman, 1994). In a multicultural society, it is important that cultural beliefs about maintaining body balance and health are integrated into any decision making about restoring or maintaining health. Food, herbs and medicines are classified as either 'hot' or 'cold' as are all mental states and physical illnesses. To remain healthy or restore health, the body's internal 'temperature' balance must be maintained, which means exposing oneself or ingesting items of the opposite quality to those believed to be responsible for the disease (Helman, 1994). Elements of these beliefs are also evident in Western culture through the belief that 'warm' drinks, a 'warm' bed and 'feeding a cold and starving a fever' will help to restore body balance.

Besides cultural beliefs, which are part of a large ethnic specific belief system, there are also lay beliefs that arise out of the labelling of an illness, which can be misinterpreted by people. An example would be the association of high blood pressure with stress and anxiety (i.e. causing 'too much tension' or 'hyper tense') (Blumhagen, 1980). There may also be regional, social class and gender differences in how people perceive health. All these differences can be important in deciding how to approach individuals and groups when involved in health promotion activities. Cultural beliefs can also lead to misunderstandings and may even be a threat to health. An example would be using a hot water bottle during the shivering phase of a fever for a young child aged between six months and three years. Besides the danger of burning the skin, the child's temperature may rise rapidly, leading to an increased risk of fitting.

▶ ENVIRONMENTAL FACTORS

Environmental factors, which include political and economic factors over which individuals have limited control, have often been underestimated in the past as a source of ill-health (Townsend and Davidson, 1982; Blackburn, 1991). More recognition has been given in recent years to the issues of equity and equality (Department of Health, 1994), although there is still much to be done to correct the imbalances (Parish, 1991). Government legislation and policy are important in controlling situations that have a detrimental affect on health (see Chapter 1.1 on environmental safety). In the context of this chapter, the most significant policy is in relation to smoking and health. The ability of the government to curtail cigarette smoking through national policies should not be underestimated. However, to date there has been only limited non-directive action taken by government because of the revenue generated by taxation on cigarettes (Lee, 1997).

Government economic policy has also had a direct impact on individuals in society who are at risk of hypothermia. It could be argued that imposing a tax on fuel and limiting extra payments to the elderly and disabled until certain low temperatures have been reached over consecutive days has little impact overall on reducing morbidity and mortality due to hypothermia during the winter months. Research in this area is fraught with difficulties as hypothermia is often not the main recorded cause of death (Watson, 1996). Although health promotion may be addressed at behaviour and lifestyle, it may still be the cost factor

DECISION MAKING

In your practice placements you may observe many different approaches to health promotion depending on the circumstances of the patient or client and the philosophy of the health professionals involved. Decide on which health promotion strategy might be the most effective for each of the following situations:

- *A middle aged business man who developed chest pain when rushing to catch a plane has become very frightened about having a heart attack. He is seeking help from the general practitioner and practice nurse.*
- *A 13-year-old schoolgirl describes how much she enjoys smoking cigarettes when out of school at lunchtime with her mates. She discloses this in a group session with the school nurse.*
- *An elderly, slightly confused widow who lives on her own has been admitted to hospital with hypothermia. After recovering from the subsequent chest complications, her discharge is being planned by her primary nurse.*

that predominates in an individual's ability to keep warm in winter.

Both Tannahill (1985) and Tones (1993) recognize the interrelationship between individual behaviours and environmental factors in relation to health promotion and recommend a mixture of political action, creating supportive and strong community action groups, changing the approach of health services and professionals, and developing the individual's personal esteem and ability to make informed choices.

PRACTICE KNOWLEDGE

A fundamental component of a nurse's role is the thorough and accurate physiological assessment of children and adults. The information gained for each patient provides the foundation for nursing decisions and often contributes towards the decisions of other health professionals involved in the patient's care. It is vital that changes in homeostasis are detected promptly and monitored as they can indicate serious alterations in health due to disease, injury, treatments and therapies. Monitoring changes that occur slowly over time is also important within the context of health promotion and the prevention of ill health.

Physiological assessment involves the collection of both objective and subjective data, the most common of which are the measurement or observation of:

- blood pressure;
- pulse;
- temperature;
- respiration;
- fluid balance;
- skin condition and pallor.

These objective measurements and observations are often referred to by nurses as 'doing the observations' or 'checking vital signs'.

Subjective data also plays an important role, for example you may become concerned about a person whose physical measurements are within acceptable limits but whose behaviour has become restless, confused and aggressive. These changes indicate a problem developing with homeostasis such as shock or respiratory failure. The converse situation can also arise as you may detect a low blood pressure in a patient who is perfectly healthy. It is also extremely important to listen to what patients say about how they feel as changes can occur before any physiological alterations are measurable or observable.

Single measurements are not generally acted upon in isolation as temporary changes can occur in response to emotional, physical and environmental factors such as pain, anxiety and a cold environment. A change in any one aspect of homeostasis has an effect on the other homeostatic mechanisms, therefore the nurse needs to interpret a combination of observations, consider any trends and where possible eliminate any extraneous factors influencing the measurements. As a consequence a composite picture emerges and contributes to an overall understanding of a patient's physiological status. Many health promotion and treatment decisions by members of the multidisciplinary team depend upon accurate observations of homeostasis in the child and adult.

▶ GENERAL PRINCIPLES FOR ACCURATE ASSESSMENT OF HOMEOSTASIS

When carrying out a physiological assessment the nurse must ensure that the privacy, dignity, safety and comfort of individual patients or clients are maintained and that throughout any procedures the patient or client is kept fully informed. Other general principles are as follows:

- ▶ Correct measurement equipment must be used for the different age groups and be in good working order.
- ▶ Correct techniques must be used and should follow local guidelines and be research based.
- ▶ Measurements must be accurate, clearly documented and communicated to others when necessary – deviation from the normal or age-adjusted values or significant changes from the individual's normal value warrants reporting to the patient's doctor.
- ▶ The nurse should consider if the measurements obtained are reasonable, account for any extraneous factors and when in doubt seek further clarification.
- ▶ Measurements should be performed when there is a rational patient-centred reason to do so.
- ▶ Identified problems or needs should be reflected in the subsequent recording of decisions taken and any therapies implemented should be evaluated;
- ▶ Measurements should be performed by appropriately trained competent health care staff or carers.

▶ THERMOREGULATION

A thorough knowledge of thermoregulation and the factors that influence it provides a valuable contribution to decision making in many aspects of nursing practice. This knowledge can be applied to health education, for example when advising an elderly person on how to prevent hypothermia during cold weather. It influences decisions about the environment of care, such as ensuring a warm draught-free environment when bathing an infant to minimize heat loss. Importantly, this knowledge also forms the basis for the rational assessment, planning, implementation and evaluation of care of those individuals who have the potential for or an altered body temperature. Those most at risk of thermoregulatory disturbance are the very young, the elderly and people with chronic or acute illness (Childs, 1994). The effects of limited mobility and an inadequate nutritional intake are particularly important as they limit heat-gaining mechanisms. Alterations in body temperature from the normal range may indicate a health problem, as occurs when temperature is raised due to an infection. Behavioural problems in an individual can also influence body temperature, such as when a client suffering from schizophrenia does not dress appropriately on a very cold day and consequently develops hypothermia.

Nurses need to consider a wide range of factors that can influence thermoregulation. In addition to the physical and psychosocial factors oulined under Subject Knowledge, other factors which are important are:

- psychological factors – emotional states such as excitement and anxiety can generate heat;
- sociocultural factors – dressing codes may differ, behaviours in response to temperature change may be established;
- environmental factors – ambient temperature, humidity, wind, rain, housing, place of work (some jobs are carried out in environments where it is difficult for the worker to sustain normal thermoregulation due to extremes of temperature or humidity, e.g. in a foundry or at sea);
- economic factors – may affect heating expenditure, food intake and housing.

ASSESSMENT OF THERMOREGULATION

The assessment of thermoregulation initially involves gathering subjective information through touching and observing the client's skin, noting any change in behaviour, and listening to how the client reports feeling (Woollons, 1996). Specific aspects to consider are:

- Is the skin excessively warm or cool, dry or moist? (Use the back of your fingers as they are more sensitive to temperature.)
- Are the extremities pale, mottled or flushed?
- Is the client shivering, restless, lethargic, drowsy, delirious, convulsing? Shivering can occur when a person is cold or during the heat-gaining phase of pyrexia. It causes discomfort in the short term, however, prolonged uncontrolled shivering can lead to exhaustion, pain and helplessness (Holtzclaw, 1990). It is also important to remember that when caring for young infants (under one year of age) that they do not shiver but use their store of brown fat.
- Does the client's behaviour indicate that they are trying to gain or lose heat, e.g. adjusting their clothing?
- How does the client report his or her feelings, both verbally, and especially in the child, non-verbally?

It is important both in the home and in institutional settings to assess the physical environment, particularly air temperature, heating and ventilation, dampness and draughts, and if appropriate clothing and bedding are available. Other relevant areas to consider are nutritional intake, mobility, the potential for or any signs of infection, and the potential for or any signs of hypothermia (e.g. an elderly patient with hypothyroidism who is immobile is at risk of hypothermia).

Nurses are responsible for providing a safe and comfortable environment of care; where a deficit is identified, they must take appropriate action, for example, reporting to the heating engineers a problem with the heating system.

TEMPERATURE MEASUREMENT

The aim of temperature measurement is to provide an objective approximation of core body temperature. This information together with the subjective data and the other vital signs makes a significant contribution

In your practice placements:

- **Review the types of devices used to monitor body temperature.**
- **Note the differences in devices in relation to the safety of the particular client group.**
- **If mercury thermometers are still in use, find out about your local guidelines for the safe disposal of mercury spillage.**

to clinical decisions. Measurements must therefore be accurate, comparable, timely, reproducible and reliable. All measurement techniques must also be safe and acceptable to the individual patient.

Safety is particularly relevant when considering the use of glass and mercury thermometers, which are frequently encountered in the UK. Broken glass is a potential hazard to both patients and nurses. Mercury is a highly toxic substance and is extremely hazardous. If a thermometer breaks, mercury vapour is emitted into the atmosphere and may be inhaled or absorbed through the skin, and if not correctly disposed of, mercury remains in the environment for years (Cutter, 1994). The handling and disposal of mercury is controlled by the 1989 *Control of Substances Hazardous to Health* (COSHH) regulations (HSC, 1988). However, these regulations have to be enforced in the practice environment to be effective. The average life expectancy for an NHS thermometer is only 80 days (Board, 1995), which suggests the potential for a large amount of mercury to build up in the health care environment. Sweden banned the use of mercury thermometers in 1992 and the UK could soon pursue the same policy (Blumenthal, 1991; Woollons, 1996).

Patient acceptability often relates to the site used for monitoring temperature. The use of the rectal site for measuring temperature is an example of how a practice may be unacceptable to an adult or the parents of a child. This can vary between cultures and will depend on the context of care.

Thermometry (measurement of temperature) has been widely researched in nursing, yet practice still seems to be governed by ritual rather than research and the literature available reveals many bewildering inconsistencies. Recent technical developments have challenged the status quo and introduced to nurses a much wider choice of temperature-measuring devices such as tympanic thermometry, and electronic and disposable thermometers. Although some research into these newer techniques exists, considerably more is required to confirm their benefits to nursing practice.

The nurse needs to consider the three main variables that influence the accuracy of temperature measurement (Woollons, 1996). These are:

- the site;
- the measuring device;
- the technique.

▶ *Choosing a Site*

The best sites for core temperature measurement are those that are in close proximity to major arteries and organs in the central core of the body and are well insulated from external factors. The pulmonary artery is considered the optimal core site, but this measurement requires the insertion of a pulmonary artery catheter and thermistor, which are only suitable for use in high-dependency or critical care areas (Fulbrook, 1993). For everyday measurement, the key factors to consider when choosing a site are the individual's:

- age and health status;
- the degree of accuracy required;
- accessibility and acceptability;
- degree of cooperation (Erickson and Yount, 1991).

The most commonly used sites are the mouth, rectum and axilla, however, all have relative advantages and disadvantages which require consideration. More recently the tympanic membrane site has been gaining popularity. Tympanic thermometry measures the infrared emissions from the surface of the tympanic membrane of the ear, which is in close proximity to the hypothalamus and cerebral arteries. Information is processed by the thermometer to provide an accurate measurement of core temperature. A number of studies report a good correlation between pulmonary artery temperature and tympanic membrane measurements (Ferra-Love, 1991; Edge and Morgan, 1993). Table 2.2.4 lists the relative advantages and disadvantages of each measurement site.

▶ *Choice of Temperature Measurement Device*

An increasing number of devices are available for practice as new technology is applied to measuring body temperature. Although well established in practice, the traditional glass and mercury thermometer has many documented disadvantages (Cutter, 1994; Board, 1995; Woollons, 1996; Buswell, 1997). The benefits of newer devices have been particularly attractive to nurses in paediatrics and in health care of the elderly as they tend to be safer and have a shorter response time.

The devices available are:

▶ glass and mercury thermometer;
▶ electronic – probe and digital display – thermometers (Figure 2.2.9);
▶ liquid crystal thermometer;
▶ tempadot – a disposable strip impregnated with heat-sensitive chemicals, which change colour as temperature alters:
▶ tympanic membrane thermometers;
▶ thermistors – pulmonary artery, oesophagus, bladder, skin.

There are numerous criteria for choosing a device, these include accuracy, reliability, adaptability across sites and age group, safety, ease of use, low risk of cross-infection, cost-effectiveness, full range of temperature measurements, durability, maintainability and anti-theft properties.

A considerable amount of research is available comparing the use of different devices. Tympanic thermometry (Figure 2.2.10) has generated much research interest as it seeks to establish a foothold in practice (Flo and Brown, 1995; Board, 1995).

DECISION MAKING

Woollons (1996) provides a good overview of some of the products currently available in the UK. Find out which devices are used in your area and ask why they have been chosen. Decide which devices and sites would be suitable when measuring the temperature of:
• **An infant with an ear infection.**
• **A drunken young adult in the accident and emergency department.**
• **An adult with a mild learning disability who is a planned admission to an acute unit for routine surgery that afternoon.**
• **A hypothermic elderly confused adult in the community.**

Site	Advantages	Disadvantages
Oral	• Close proximity to the lingual and sublingual arteries provides good correlation with core temperature if the correct technique is used. • Responds rapidly to changes in core temperature. • Suitable for use with most adults and older children. • Very accessible and acceptable and a variety of suitable devices are available for use (e.g. glass and mercury, electronic and disposable thermometers)	• Accuracy of measurement influenced by external factors (e.g. eating, drinking, smoking, talking, mouth breathing), poor lip seal, incorrect positioning in the sublingual pocket and inadequate recording time. • Potential for cross-infection. • Not suitable for infants, young children and some adults (e.g. confused patients).
Rectal	• Well insulated from external environment. • Accurately reflects core temperature due to proximity of haemorrhoidal artery. • Can be used with most adults and children. • Variety of suitable devices available: glass and mercury, electronic and disposable.	• Potential discomfort, trauma and embarrassment. • Not easily accessible. • Rectal temperature is higher than the core temperature and has a lagged response to changes in the core. • Recording influenced by the presence of stool. • Unsuitable for very restless adults or children. • Potential for cross-infection.
Axilla	• Safe, accessible and acceptable to all age groups. • Possible to achieve good correlation with other sites in most individuals if correct technique used.	• Accuracy of measurement very dependent upon recording time and positioning of thermometer in axilla. • Site not well insulated from the environment. • Need to disrupt clothing and bedding. • Thermometer can easily become displaced or forgotton about as hidden from view. • Not appropriate to use in shock or hypothermia.
Tympanic membrane	• Good correlation with core temperature due to proximity of carotid artery and hypothalamus. • Rapid response to temperature change. • Easily accessible and acceptable to the patient. • Very rapid response time. • Suitable for children and adults. • Not influenced by external factors such as room temperature.	• Inaccuracy or discomfort may occur if the equipment is not used correctly. • Should not be used with clients who have a discharging ear or who have had surgery or trauma to the ear. • Devices available are relatively expensive.
Skin	• Useful as a guide for parents at home where children are pyrexial but non-cooperative. • Comparison between skin and core temperature useful in critical care situations. • Head strips are simple and of minimal cost. • Electronic skin probes available.	• Inaccurate readings. • Influenced by room temperature.

Table 2.2.4 Advantages and disadvantages of different thermometry sites.

Figure 2.2.9: An electronic thermometer. Photograph courtesy of IVAC.

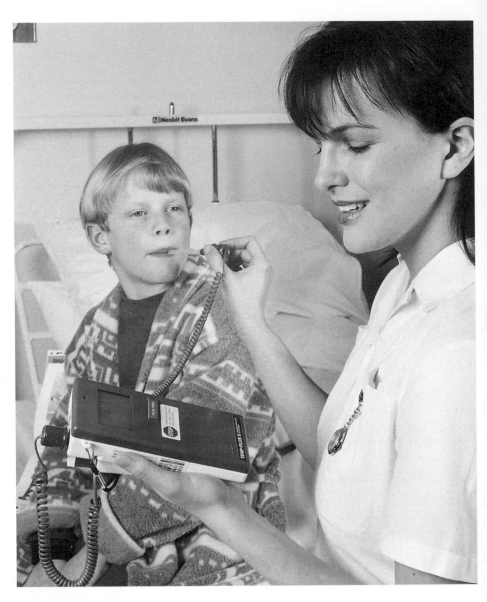

▶ *Technique*

Using the correct technique should ensure a safe and accurate temperature measurement. This involves having knowledge of both the site and the device being used and minimizing extraneous variables such as drinking before an oral measurement. Newer devices have manufacturer's guidelines provided; however there are many inconsistencies in practice and in the literature regarding the time required to record temperatures at all sites when using a glass and mercury thermometer (Closs, 1987; Cutter, 1994). It is generally accepted that in most situations a clinically significant measurement can be achieved by taking the oral temperature for three minutes (Pugh Davies *et al.*, 1986).

▶ PYREXIA

Pyrexia is defined as a core temperature raised above 38°C, this commonly occurs in response to an infection or tissue damage. Decisions

Figure 2.2.10: A tympanic thermometer. Photograph courtesy of IVAC.

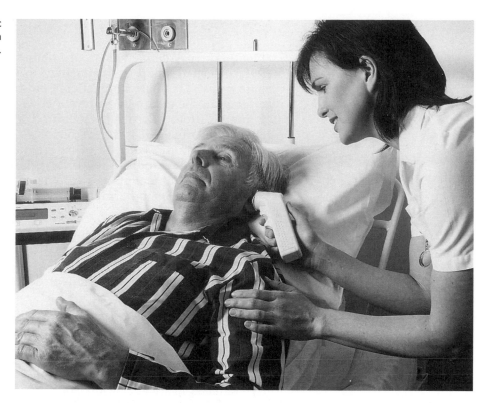

DECISION MAKING

Oliver is three years old and has been generally unwell for the past two days with a temperature fluctuating between 38°C and 39°C. The general practitioner diagnoses an ear infection and prescribes antibiotics and paracetamol.

- *Decide on what advice you would give Oliver's parents on how to manage the pyrexia*
- *What is the likely cause of the pyrexia?*
- *Find out how paracetamol reduces temperature and review the advice you would give Oliver's parents about its use in this case.*

about nursing care are determined by the stage of the pyrexia (Table 2.2.5). If the rise in temperature is slight, symptoms may not be observable (Faulkner, 1990).

If the temperature rises above 40°C it can affect cerebral function and cause restlessness, delirium and convulsions due to nerve cell irritability. This is a particular risk in infants and young children because their thermoregulation mechanisms are immature.

Stage	Features	Nursing management
Stage 1: heat gaining	• Patient complains of feeling cold and shivery • If a child, looks pale and feels cold to the touch peripherally	• Promote rest and comfort in a warm draught-free environment and adjust bedding to maintain comfort • Administer antipyretics prescribed
Stage 2: heat dissipation	• Patient looks flushed and complains of feeling hot • Diaphoresis (sweating) • Thirst and dry mouth • Headache • Reduced appetite • Disorientation • Lethargy • Aching • Weakness • Pulse and respiratory rate increase	• Promote rest • Adjust environment and bedding to increase the circulation of cool air – use a fan, but do not direct at the patient as this causes vaso-constriction • Encourage fluids • Reassure and explain what is happening • Administer prescribed antipyretics
Stage 3	• Return to normal	

Table 2.2.5 Stages in pyrexia with nursing management.

▶ HYPOTHERMIA

Hypothermia is defined as a core temperature below 35°C (Roper *et al.*, 1993). It can develop gradually over a period of time or have a sudden acute onset. The main aims of care are to reduce further loss of heat and to promote the return of a normal body temperature with the minimum of complications, if possible by natural warming. The temperature should return to normal at a rate of no more than 0.5°C/hour. Rapid uncontrolled rewarming will lead to peripheral vasodilation, this causes a fall in blood pressure and the return of cold acidotic peripheral blood to the heart. This may precipitate a cardiac arrest.

Early signs of hypothermia (i.e. when the core temperature is between 35°C and 33°C) are:

▶ patient looks and feels cold;
▶ puffy face and husky voice;
▶ pale, cool and waxy skin;
▶ shivering (the ability to shiver decreases as temperature falls below 34°C);
▶ fatigue and impaired cognitive function;
▶ drowsiness.

Later signs of hypothermia (i.e. when the core temperature is lower than 32°C) are:

▶ reduced heart and respiratory rate and blood pressure;
▶ cyanosis and mottled peripheries;
▶ cardiac arrhythmias;
▶ reduced responsiveness leading to loss of consciousness.

Prevention is central to caring for individuals who are at risk of hypothermia and this is best achieved by educating such individuals and their family and friends about their personal vulnerability and how to minimize their risk (Webster, 1995).

Slow, natural rewarming can be achieved by caring for the patient in bed, with lightweight blankets and maintaining a warm environment (26–29°C). Warm drinks and food can commence as the patient's condition improves. Active strategies are usually decided upon by the doctor and include the use of a warming mattress, administering warm IV fluids, warm peritoneal lavage and respiratory gases.

▶ BLOOD PRESSURE MEASUREMENT

Blood pressure measurement is one of the most frequently undertaken procedures in the assessment of an adult's physical health. In the child the blood pressure is recorded only if there is a specific indication. Measurement of blood pressure is required in many diverse situations, involving all client groups in primary care, community care institutions and hospitals.

This section does not aim to provide a 'how to do it' approach to blood pressure measurement, but to explore the knowledge required to understand the practice of blood pressure measurement (see Mallett and Bailey, 1996, for an overview of 'how to do it').

Blood pressure may be measured either directly or indirectly.

▶ Direct Measurement

Blood pressure can be measured directly when a catheter is inserted into an artery and the external end is attached to a pressure-sensitive transducer, this senses the pressure in the artery and displays an electronic reading of the blood pressure either digitally or as a waveform. This method is mainly used in high-dependency areas such as theatres or intensive care (Mallett and Bailey, 1996).

▶ Indirect Measurement

The indirect method for measuring blood pressure is noninvasive and the most common method involves using a compressive cuff with either auscultation or palpation of the blood flow in an artery, usually the brachial artery. This requires the use of a sphygmomanometer and stethoscope.

Automatic blood pressure devices (e.g. Dinamap) measure blood pressure in adults and children using the oscillatory (vibration) principle. The cuff is automatically inflated and then deflated and as the blood pulsates, the walls of the artery vibrate. These vibrations and the cuff pressure are detected by the cuff and this information is calculated by the machine to determine the blood pressure. Dinamap monitors have been shown to have a strong correlation with intra-arterial pressure in both adults and children (Bolling, 1994). These machines have been developed to include measurement of pulse and O_2 saturation (pulse oximetry) and are particularly useful in assessing infants and young children under five years of age (Petrie *et al.*, 1990). Assessing the blood pressure in infants and young children can be difficult because the child may be restless and various errors can be made in the use of measuring equipment (National Heart, Lung and Blood Institute, 1987).

▶ Accurate Measurement of Blood Pressure

Research suggests that blood pressure measurement is a poorly understood nursing and medical procedure that can result in inaccurate measurement. The potential consequences of inaccuracies for the patient is that blood pressure problems go undetected or inappropriate treatment and care are given. The majority of errors reported are associated with:

▶ poor technique;
▶ use of the wrong or defective equipment;
▶ a preference for rounding off the measurement to the nearest 5 mmHg (e.g. 120/75 mmHg instead of 122/74 mmHg);
▶ inadequate preparation of the patient.

It is suggested by the American and British hypertension societies that standardization of technique is important to avoid inaccuracies and discrepancies in measurement. These experts produce guidelines, which are regularly updated and tested. The American Society of Hypertension (ASH) recommend that all extraneous variables be minimized and where possible blood pressure is measured in ordinary and reproducible circumstances. Many studies have found that the accuracy of the measurement obtained is influenced by the technique and equipment used, in particular the size and location of the cuff and the arm position (American Society of Hypertension, 1992).

It is recommended that the width of the cuff is 40% of the patient's arm circumference and the length, 80%. Using a cuff that is too large

During your practice placements:

- *Observe any differences in the way the blood pressure is measured and recorded for different client groups, especially infants and children.*
- *Find out if there are local standards for accurately measuring the blood pressure and note how often these standards are audited.*

RESEARCH BASED EVIDENCE

Webster et al. (1984) found a mean difference of 11–12 mmHg between the arm in a dependent position and the arm held at heart level. Croft and Cruikshank (1990) found that for most adults using the large size adult cuff provided a satisfactory degree of accuracy in blood pressure measurement.

results in a false low reading and too small a cuff, a false high reading (Hill and Grim, 1991). The centre of the cuff's bladder is placed over the brachial artery and the bottom of the cuff should be 2–3 cm above the bend in the elbow. It is important that the arm is positioned at heart level, slightly flexed and well supported. Frolich *et al.* (1988) states that for every centimetre the cuff sits above or below the heart the blood pressure varies by 0.8 mmHg. The blood pressure of children under five years of age cannot be measured with a conventional sphygmomanometer and in older children errors of 10–15 mmHg can occur. The use of the correct cuff size is very important in the child to ensure accuracy, and measurements should only be undertaken when clinically indicated. At least three different cuff sizes will be needed for children between 0–14 years of age (Petrie *et al.*, 1990).

Another potential source of error is the position of the sphygmomanometer. It should be vertical and the centre of the manometer at eye level in order to view the mercury meniscus accurately against the calibrated tube.

It is possible for a nurse to not hear the first systolic sound as about 5% of patients have an auscultatory gap (recognized by Korotkoff sounds stopping and starting again), therefore systolic pressure should be estimated initially by palpating the radial or brachial pulse during cuff deflation. This will also provide an indication of how high to inflate the cuff in the subsequent measurement – no more than 30 mmHg above the estimated pressure is recommended.

Both sides of a dual-headed stethoscope can be used, but the bell side provides greater amplification of low frequency sounds such as Korotkoff sounds, which facilitates a more accurate measurement (Hill and Grim, 1991). Care must be taken to maintain good skin contact and to exert minimal pressure over the brachial artery with the stethoscope as this can distort the Korotkoff sounds.

Some confusion exists in practice about which sound correlates to diastolic pressure. It is usually accepted that in adults this occurs at phase V of the Korotkoff sounds (Figure 2.2.11), which is the point at which the sounds completely disappear. Continuation of sounds to 0

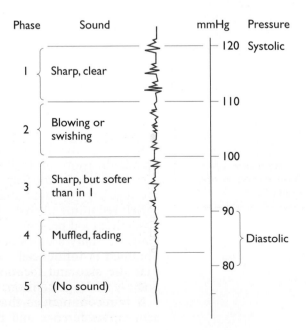

Figure 2.2.11: Korotkoff phases. (Redrawn from Hinchliffe *et al.*, 1996.)

DECISION MAKING

Any of the individual client variables may affect the clients you will meet during your practice placements.

- *Decide what effect on the blood pressure you would anticipate for each of the client variables and explain why these occur.*
- *Decide how you could minimize the effects of these variables when planning to take a patient's blood pressure?*

With reference to *The Health of the Nation* (Department of Health, 1992):

- *Review the targets the government has set that relate to respiratory disease.*
- *Make a list of the possible opportunities nurses have to promote healthier living that could reduce the incidence and symptoms of respiratory disease.*

(absent phase V) is frequently seen in pregnant women, the elderly and children (Petrie *et al.*, 1986). In these instances, phase IV should be taken as the diastolic pressure and this fact should be clearly documented.

Some of the individual client factors influencing blood pressure were identified in the Biological section of Subject Knowledge. These must be considered when measuring blood pressure along with the effects of:

- position – supine, standing, sitting;
- full bladder;
- smoking;
- caffeine;
- talking during the procedure;
- environmental temperature;
- anxiety;
- stress;
- exercise.

RESPIRATIONS

Nurses require a sound knowledge of normal respiration together with an understanding of how and why respiratory homeostasis can be disrupted. The factors that influence respiration are complex, often inter-relate and can be broadly described as being physical, psychological, social and environmental. In fact very few health problems do not affect respiration in some way.

Knowledge of factors affecting respiration can be effectively used by nurses to:

- promote health and provide health education;
- detect respiratory problems through screening;
- assess and monitor respiratory status;
- provide competent care for individuals with respiratory problems.

Many of the frequently encountered respiratory diseases such as asthma, chronic obstructive airways disease and lung cancer have been closely linked to environmental factors and individual lifestyle and are considered by health professionals to be largely preventable. The government has focused specifically on this issue in *The Health of the Nation* white paper (Department of Health, 1992).

ASSESSING RESPIRATIONS

It is relatively simple for a nurse to assess breathing directly by observing the rate, depth and rhythm of respiration. These observations provide a good basic indicator of respiratory function. Impaired gas exchange during external and internal respiration is more difficult to monitor. If more detailed information is required additional assessment tools can be used such as:

- an oximeter, which measures the O_2 saturation level in the blood;
- laboratory equipment to measure arterial blood gases;
- apnoea monitors, which alarm if an infant has an episode of apnoea.

The use of technology supplements the information gained through observation and measurement and allows the nurse to note both subtle and rapid change in a patient's condition and the patient's responses to interventions. In children where there can be a rapid deterioration in condition and for whom respiratory problems such as asthma and bronchiolitis are common, the oximeter and apnoea monitors are essential.

Observation of Breathing

At rest, normal respiration is passive and quiet, and the chest wall and abdomen gently rise and fall with each breath. In more active breathing there is an increase in the use of the intercostal and accessory muscles, which allows greater lung expansion. This increase in depth of respirations can be observed by the rise and fall of the shoulders, increased movement of the rib cage and the contraction of the accessory muscles in the neck during inspiration. It is important to assess the symmetry of chest movement and the type of breath, while noting the amount of effort required to breathe at rest and during activity. Prolonged, laboured breathing at rest is a cause for concern and indicates serious respiratory dysfunction. It can be difficult to assess breathing during sleep, especially with children – placing a hand gently on the upper abdominal area allows you to feel respiratory movement. It is important to observe for the use of the accessory muscles in breathing should the adult or child have difficulties. Observe for nasal flaring and rib recession breathing in the young child as these indicate problems that can lead to a rapid deterioration in the child's condition (see Chapter 2.1 on resuscitation).

Respiratory Rate

The respiratory rate is simply assessed by counting each full breath over either 30 seconds or one minute depending on the patient's condition. Limiting extraneous variables such as talking and the effects of activity need to be considered. An awareness of being observed may alter respiratory rate and depth and this can be minimized by counting respirations while appearing to take the patient's pulse. The rate of pulse and breathing tends to maintain a ratio of approximately 5:1 (Faulkner, 1985). The respiratory rate of the newborn is approximately 35 breaths per minute (BPM) and the range in young children varies between 30 and 20 BPM (Wong, 1996). The respiratory rate decreases as the child's size and age increases (Table 2.2.6).

Tachypnoea is a respiratory rate above age-adjusted normal values. Tachypnoea is a normal response to increased activity, but can also be an indication of hypoxia (low O_2), hypercarbia (high CO_2), acidosis, raised temperature, pain, stress and anxiety.

Bradypnoea is a respiratory rate lower than the normal age-adjusted values. It is less commonly seen than tachypnoea and can be an indication of severe hypothermia, narcotic drug overdose, acid–base imbalance and neurological dysfunction.

Apnoea is the absence of breathing for at least ten seconds. It can be transitory as in 'sleep apnoea', which is associated with a brief obstruction of the upper airway and causes snoring or it may be life-threatening as in sudden infant death syndrome in the young infant.

Age	Rate (breaths/min)
Newborn	35
I to II months	30
2 years	25
4 years	23
6 years	21
8 years	20
10 years	19
12 years	19
14 years	18
16 years	17
18 years	16–18

Table 2.2.6 Respiratory rates and volumes for infant, child and adult. (From Wong, 1993, with permission.)

Respiratory Depth

The depth of respiration is dependent upon the amount of air inhaled, which is known as the tidal volume. For an average adult at rest it is about 500 ml of expired air. Depth is assessed by observing the degree of movement of the chest wall during inspiration. However, a more objective way is to measure the amount of air exhaled with a spirometer or peak flow meter (Figure 2.2.12). This method is particularly beneficial when caring for individuals with respiratory problems such as asthma and chronic obstructive airways disease.

Posture can affect the depth of respiration achieved as slumped, supine and lateral positions can limit chest expansion. This can also be observed when the movement of the diaphragm is restricted by obesity, pregnancy and ascites. Orthopnoea is the term used to describe difficulty in breathing when lying down. Patients with respiratory disease tend to feel more comfortable sitting well up and leaning slightly forward or standing as gravity enhances lung expansion. Before making decisions it may be valuable to assess which position if any provides relief from symptoms.

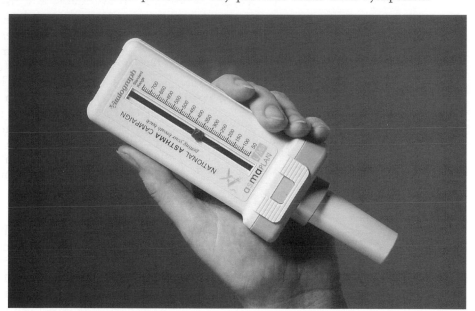

Figure 2.2.12: Photograph of a peak flow monitor. Photograph courtesy of Vitalograph Ltd.

▶ *Respiratory Rhythm*

Normal breathing in adults is regular and uninterrupted except for the occasional sigh, but infants and young children can have a less regular pattern. The rhythm is maintained by the carefully controlled timing of the respiratory cycle. Many of the abnormal patterns in breathing occur as the result of brain injury or disease that affects the respiratory centres in the brain such as the apneustic or pneumotaxic centres mentioned in the Biological section of Subject Knowledge in this chapter.

Cheyne–Stokes respiration may occur as death approaches and is characterized by a gradual increase in the rate and depth of respiration followed by a gradual decrease over 30–45 seconds in the depth and rate of respiration. This cycle may be followed by a period of apnoea for up to 20 seconds (Faulkner, 1985). It can be distressing to observe and families need an explanation and reassurance.

▶ *Breath Sounds*

Further information can be gained by assessing the sounds of breathing. Normal respiration is almost silent, therefore any respiratory sound requires investigation. Noisy respiration is referred to as stertorous breathing and can be caused by:

> secretions in the trachea and bronchi, which make a gurgling type of noise;

> obstruction to air flow, which sounds like a wheeze or a harsh crowing sound (e.g. stridor in children).

> ### *Observation of Skin Colour*

Cyanosis occurs when the Hb in the blood is not carrying sufficient O_2 to the tissues and is demonstrated by a bluish pallor. Peripheral cyanosis occurs when the circulation is poor or closed down in the hands and feet, as in cold weather. Central cyanosis is more serious and indicates hypoxia. It is most clearly seen in the tissues of the lips, tongue, cheeks, ear lobes and nail beds, but it can be difficult to assess in dark-skinned people. Cyanosis is an unreliable and late sign of hypoxia so you should be alert to alterations in the rate and depth of breathing and any behavioural changes in the individual. The use of an oximeter to monitor oxygen saturation levels is strongly indicated in the assessment and monitoring of patients who are at risk of hypoxia.

> ### *Behavioural Changes*

Common responses to inadequate respiratory function include restlessness, confusion, anxiety, fatigue, agitation and loss of concentration. There can be an altered level of consciousness, which will depend upon the degree of cerebral hypoxia and acidosis.

> ### *Cough and Sputum*

Coughing is a normal protective mechanism; however, if the nature and frequency of a cough change there may be a respiratory problem. Sputum coughed up from the lungs also provides valuable information and the amount, consistency, colour and odour need to be assessed. Blood-stained sputum is referred to as haemoptysis.

> ### *Pain and Dyspnoea (Difficulty in Breathing)*

Pain on breathing needs to be assessed to determine its cause and can indicate infection, inflammation or trauma. Dyspnoea describes the feelings experienced by a patient of difficult and laboured breathing. Gift (1990) describes dyspnoea as a subjective sensation that is often associated with chronic lung disease and stresses that the intensity of the dyspnoea is not always reflected in the findings when respiratory function is assessed. Gift also provides a useful model based upon three dimensions of dyspnoea: physical, psychological and social. This model is very important for nurses to consider as it reminds us of the holistic needs of our patients and focuses our attention on the effects of living with dyspnoea.

PROFESSIONAL KNOWLEDGE

Physiological measurements were originally the responsibility of the medical profession, but these skills have been devolved to nurses to perform and are now a well-established part of a nurse's role. A number of professional issues emerge in relation to the nurse's role in the assessment of homeostasis. These include:

> the theory/practice gap;

> the skills mix, delegation and role boundaries;

Learning to use a stethoscope to listen to particular breath sounds is a skill you may have an opportunity to observe if you are involved in specialist nursing of patients with respiratory difficulties or if you work with a specialist nurse practitioner, in a general practitioner practice or alongside a physiotherapist who is also caring for clients with respiratory problems.

- *In appropriate practice placements listen to breath sounds that are normal and abnormal under the guidance of the experienced health professional.*

- *Note and record in your reflective diary your experiences and continue to develop your skills as you gain further experience.*

▶ ritualistic practice;
▶ education.

▶ THEORY/PRACTICE GAP

The mechanics of physical assessment are relatively simple – it is the interpretation of information and its use in decision making that is the real challenge for nurses. Assessment of homeostasis involves considerably more than just measuring vital signs – it is an integral component of nursing assessment and leads to the development of rational individualized care. Keen (1994) states that 'Focusing on the task only results in neglecting the role of the nurse in preventative care, assessment and decision making'.

Nursing currently finds itself in the conflicting situation of being on the one hand professionally committed to the delivery of individualized research-based care and on the other functioning within a context of well-established traditional practices, increasing clinical demands, redefined roles, reduced resources and technological developments. All these factors can lead to fragmented care for patients, particularly in institutional settings when many differing grades of professional health care staff may be involved in the assessment and evaluation of their health status. All can potentially affect the accuracy of homeostatic observations and the subsequent decision making.

▶ SKILL MIX DEBATES

Measuring vital signs has traditionally been organized in a task-centred way and often delegated to student nurses and health care assistants (Walsh and Ford, 1989, pp. 50–51). Task-centred nursing operates within a hierarchy of skills and unqualified health care staff may undertake a variety of skills under the supervision of a qualified nurse (Keen, 1994). It has been argued that continuing with this approach devalues and limits the nurse's role in patient assessment and that it encourages ritualistic and non research-based practice, which results in less effective care (Carr–Hill *et al.*, 1992). The assumption behind involving less skilled staff in the measurement of vital signs is that qualified nurses should not spend costly time carrying out activities that can be delegated to less skilled and cheaper staff (Keen, 1995). At a time when resources are under strain it becomes an attractive proposition to redefine the boundaries between qualified and unqualified roles in order to become more cost-effective. In some situations it may be appropriate to delegate; however, it must always be under supervision and the nurse must ensure that the individual to whom the task has been delegated is competent.

Recent developments in the 1990s have led to the introduction of 'Patient Focused Care' into some UK hospitals. The aims of Patient Focused Care are to:

▶ improve the quality of care and service provision;
▶ increase patient satisfaction and staff job satisfaction;
▶ promote efficiency (Buchan, 1995).

A feature of this innovation is the redefining of health care roles and multiskilling. There is a positive argument for all grades of staff within a particular field to have the skills needed by the patient or client within that particular environment. Such developments lead specific professional groups to argue over the boundaries of their role and have implications for deciding on the appropriate skill mix in a particular setting. Patient Focused Care can create the opportunity for nurses to either further delegate aspects of their role such as measuring vital signs or to reaffirm professional boundaries (Royal College of Nursing, 1994).

Sophisticated monitoring of homeostasis in the acute setting or in clients with particular problems such as the child with recurrent asthma may need a different skill mix than that required in a long-stay health care of the elderly ward or a short-stay surgical ward for children. The development of the clinical nurse specialist has resulted in advanced nursing knowledge and practice to meet the needs of individuals with specific problems, for example the respiratory nurse specialist. Nurse-led clinics in primary health care also acknowledge a level of decision making that goes beyond the simple mastering of assessment skills.

▶ OBSERVATION RITUALS

Ritualistic practice evolves when an activity is seen as a task, a job to be done. Walsh and Ford (1989, p. ix) state that 'Ritual action implies carrying out a task without thinking it through in a problem solving, logical way'.

DECISION MAKING

You are allocated to a practice setting that involves caring for adults who have been admitted for surgery that requires a hospital admission for 1–5 days. Your practice supervisor has requested you to take the 'four-hourly observations' of the group of patients allocated to your joint care. As you get to know your patients you note the following: patient A is five days post surgery and is about to be discharged this afternoon; patient B is 24 hours post surgery and still feels weak and uncomfortable; patient C was admitted yesterday evening, but has just had surgery cancelled due to emergencies; patient D is three days post surgery, is ambulant and is feeling well.

- **Decide on which patients need to have their observations checked four-hourly and explain the reasons for your decision.**
- **Decide on how you might deal with your relationship with your practice supervisor if he or she insists that all patients should have their observations completed.**

There is plenty of evidence that measuring vital signs is strongly influenced by ritualistic practice, for example the frequency with which observations are performed. The routine measurement of observations every four hours is an established practice, which in many cases is not necessary. A ritualistic approach limits the opportunity to develop practice through the application of research. It is evident that a considerable theory/practice gap exists, particularly in relation to ensuring the accuracy of measurements and their frequency.

▶ EDUCATIONAL NEEDS

Education is a key factor both at pre and post registration level. Nursing students need to develop a sound knowledge base about homeostasis together with competency in measuring vital signs and patient assessment. The significance of information must be understood and applied in planning and evaluating patient care. The increasing use of new technology to measure vital signs means that staff need updating on a regular basis. The accuracy with which observations are taken also needs auditing to ensure decisions are based on accurate ongoing assessment of patients' conditions. Studies that have audited both medical and nursing staff in taking blood pressure have highlighted deficits in knowledge and skills of both groups (McKay *et al.*, 1992; Kemp *et al.*, 1993; Nolan and Nolan, 1993; Hutchinson *et al.*, 1994). A small survey by Cutter (1994) using a

RESEARCH BASED EVIDENCE

McBride (1994) studied the attitudes, beliefs and health promotion practices of hospital nurses in acute adult wards and found that the nurses in general had a positive attitude to health promotion activities and that other health professionals acknowledged that nurses had an important role to play in this domain of practice.

Wilson-Barnett and Latter (1993)

found that the health promotion activities of nurses in acute hospital wards were focused on giving health advice and information to patients and was seen as a separate activity rather than integrated with other nursing activities. Lack of time and knowledge were recognized as major constraints in carrying out the health promotion role effectively.

sample of 150 nurses and midwives found disturbing variations in temperature measurement and a lack of knowledge about established guidelines.

The context in which health status is being measured is also important because all nurses will have the opportunity to promote health as a consequence of being involved in any measurement of homeostasis. The health promotion role of the nurse is a relatively recent phenomenon (Naidoo and Wills, 1994; Bright, 1997) and the opportunities that exist to integrate this role into everyday practice should not be neglected.

REFLECTIVE KNOWLEDGE

The primary focus within this chapter has been on how we maintain body homeostasis. Internal body mechanisms that come into play as a result of changes or alterations both internally and externally have been outlined. The environmental and cultural influences that affect our abilities to remain stable and healthy have been explored briefly.

The chapter emphasizes the key role of the nurse in monitoring and maintaining thermoregulation and haemodynamic and respiratory homeostasis in many health care contexts. Children's nurses must develop a high level of competence in assessing homeostasis and an in-depth knowledge, as changes in homeostasis occur so rapidly in infants and children. Nurses also have an increasing role to play in health promotion, which should be integrated into all aspects of their practice. Debates on skill mix and the ritualization of practice are particularly pertinent to the nurse's role in relation to the assessment of homeostasis in the future health case system.

▶ EXPERIENTIAL EXERCISES

Undertaking homeostatic assessment of clients and patients involves learning and understanding a considerable amount of theoretical knowledge as well as mastering certain manual skills. This chapter has alerted you broadly to the scope of knowledge and skills needed, but this knowledge should be supplemented by other more specialized texts and consolidated through reflection and discussion of learning in your practice placements. Many of the exercises throughout the chapter will have encouraged you to reflect on your experiences and the decisions you have seen being made or those you have made yourself. Keeping a record and reviewing these experiences will help in building up your particular body of knowledge and repertoire of skills.

Students are involved in undertaking skills in the practice setting and being confident and secure in your abilities is important in terms of quality of care being delivered to clients. Being able to practice certain measurement skills in the safety of a learning laboratory is an important precursor before undertaking assessments on clients and patients (Neary, 1997). This is very important when early detection of problems is necessary and decisions to remedy any problems need to be taken urgently and quickly. Recent research by Torrance and Serginson (1996a and 1996b) into the knowledge and skills of a group of student nurses who had completed the Common Foundation Programme (first 18 months of course) indicated deficits in the assessment of blood pressure that would lead to inaccuracies in clinical practice.

When learning how to assess temperature, pulse, respirations and blood pressure on your peers take note of any differences you observe, especially if through classroom experiential exercises the circumstances in

Spend some time in the 'skills laboratory' learning how to take and record a blood pressure accurately. Undertake a peer and tutor audit of your knowledge and skills before going into practice.

During your practice placements:

• *Note the differences and possible difficulties in measur-* *ing the blood pressure of clients rather than of your peer group in the classroom or skills laboratory setting.*

• *Record in your reflective diary how and why you have improved in this particular nursing skill.*

which measurements are made are altered. Experiential exercises could include testing the effects of appropriate factors such as exercise, rest, noise and ambient room temperature on 'vital signs'.

▶ CASE STUDIES

The following case studies are included so that you can consolidate knowledge gained from this chapter and your practice experience. These can be completed on your own or along with your peers. Tutorial support and discussion with an experienced nurse may help.

▶ CASE STUDY: ADULT

Pauline Scott is 56 years old and has had progressive multiple sclerosis for 30 years. She is unable to mobilize and is confined to a wheelchair for most of her day. She lives with her husband, John, who is a retired farmer and her main carer. They live in a rural area in an old farm house. The living area is comfortable and warm, but Pauline finds the bathroom and bedroom very cold in the winter and as a result is now washing and dressing in the kitchen, which she finds unsatisfactory.

■ **What factors would you need to consider when assessing Pauline's ability to maintain her body temperature?**

■ **What advice would you give to Mr and Mrs Scott about minimizing the risk of hypothermia?**

■ **Find out which other agencies or members of the primary care team that could help with this problem.**

▶ CASE STUDY: LEARNING DISABILITIES

Malvika Singh is an eight-year-old girl with mild learning disability and profound physical disability. She attends a special needs school in a wheelchair, which has been made to accommodate her needs. Malvika's posture is severely affected by scoliosis of her spine and her trunk deviates to the right; she is unable to sit upright. Malvika experiences swallowing difficulties if she eats or drinks too quickly. Over the last year she has had repeated chest infections, which have required antibiotic therapy, and this is worrying Malvika's family as they are not keen on their child taking drugs so often and would prefer to use alternative methods to help Malvika overcome her episodes of illness

■ **What are the factors that make Malvika at risk of recurrent chest infections?**

■ **Decide on what observations you should take when Malvika has a chest infection and why?**

■ What could the team caring for Malvika do to minimize her risk of developing a chest infection?

■ Discuss how you would explore and deal with the family's concerns about the use of antibiotic therapy.

▶ CASE STUDY: MENTAL HEALTH

Paul Grey is a 47-year-old recently-divorced man with three school-aged children who live with his wife. He is a senior lecturer in business studies at the local university and is under constant pressure to publish and has a heavy teaching load. Paul has become increasingly anxious and unable to deal with his daily workload. The head of his department, who is aware of the stresses in Paul's personal life, has asked him to seek help through the university's occupational health unit. The occupational health nurse finds that Paul's blood pressure is elevated for his age at 160/100 mmHg and he is 10 kg over-weight. Paul and the nurse discuss his lifestyle and problems.

■ Review the factors that might have led to the increase in Paul's blood pressure.

■ Revise the physiological mechanisms that control blood pressure and explore how lifestyle and life events can lead to hypertension (see also Chapter 4.1 on stress and anxiety).

■ Decide on what health promotion approach might be the most useful for Paul in order to help him with his long-term needs.

▶ CASE STUDY: CHILD

Mandy, a nine-month-old infant, has been admitted to the children's ward along with her 18-year-old single mother, Jean, who lives at home with her mum and dad. Mandy looks flushed, has been crying and irritable, and is not taking her feeds. Jean is very tearful, upset and worried about her baby.

■ Decide on which 'vital signs' you need to assess and how often.

■ What techniques would you use to assess these 'vital signs' in Mandy.

■ Decide on the advice and information that should be given to Jean before discharge should Mandy develop similar symptoms again.

▶ ANNOTATED FURTHER READING

CHILDS, C. (1994) Temperature control. In Alexander, M., Fawcett, J., Runciman, P. (eds) *Nursing Practice: Hospital and Home, The Adult.* Chapter 22, pp. 679–695. Edinburgh. Churchill Livingstone.
A very good overview of thermoregulation in adults with the biological basis covered in more detail.
FULBROOK, P. (1993) Core temperature measurement in adults: A literature review. *Journal of Advanced Nursing* **18**: 1451–1460
A good summary of the literature on temperature measurement up to the early

1990s. A critical appraisal and summary of research completed. Again the focus is on the adult.

HELMAN, C.G. (1994) *Culture, Health and Illness* (3rd edition). Chapter 2 on cultural definitions of anatomy and physiology. Oxford. Butterworth Heinemann Ltd.

This is a good comprehensive text on cultural influences on health, which is now in its third edition. Although only referred to briefly in this chapter there is much information that is useful to support other chapters in this textbook.

HINCHLIFF, S., MONTAGUE, S., WATSON, R. (1996) *Physiology for Nursing Practice*. Chapter 6.1. pp. 640–646 on temperature regulation; Chapter 4.2 on cardiovascular function; Chapter 5.3 on respiration. London. Baillière Tindall.

This excellent physiology textbook, and particularly the chapters outlined above, provides good back-up information in relation to the biological basis of the elements of homeostasis covered in this chapter. There are also useful sections that relate theory to the practice of nursing.

MALLETT, J., BAILEY, C. (1996) *The Royal Marsden NHS Trust Manual of Clinical Nursing Procedures* (4th edition). Oxford. Blackwell Science.

A good reference book about how to carry out the skills of measuring homeostasis. The rationale for each of the activities is provided.

PETRIE, J., O'BRIAN, E., LITTLER, W., DE SWEIT, M., DILLON, J. (1990) *Blood Pressure Measurement*. British Medical Journal Pamphlet. London. British Medical Association.

Arising from an original publication in the *British Medical Journal* (1986), this pamphlet book provides the 'gold standard' for accurate blood pressure measurement for adults. The authors write on behalf of The British Hypertension Society.

TORRANCE, C., SERGINSON, E. (1996) An observational study of student nurses' measurement of arterial blood pressure by sphygmomanometry and auscultation. *Nurse Education Today* **16**: 282–286.

This is a very instructive piece of research because of the use of observation of accuracy in the application of skills in blood pressure measurement. It highlights the need for students to be taught and supervised in skills acquisition in nursing.

WALSH, M., FORD, P. (1989) *Nursing Rituals: Research and Rational Actions*. Chapter 5 on making observations. Heinemann. Oxford.

This book, and particularly the chapter on observations, is particularly helpful in presenting the culture of rituals in nursing and helps to explain why the ritualization of 'taking vital signs' may still exist in some areas of practice.

WONG, D. L. (1996) *Whaley and Wong's Nursing Care of Infants and Children* (4th edition). Chapter 1 on assessment of the child. St Louis. Mosby.

For students who wish to specialize in children's nursing, this book is a very comprehensive resource book for all aspects of infant, child and teenage care. Maintaining homeostasis in infants and children differs from that in adults and requires specialist knowledge and skills.

▶ REFERENCES

AMERICAN SOCIETY OF HYPERTENSION (1992) Recommendations for routine blood pressure measurement by indirect cuff sphygmomanometry. *American Journal of Hypertension* **5**: 207–209.

BACKETT, K. (1990) Image and reality: health enhancing behaviours in middle class families. *Health Education Journal* **49**: 61–63.

BECKER, M.H. (1974) *The Health Belief Model of Personal Health Behaviour*. New York. Slack.

BLACKBURN, C. (1991) *Poverty and Health, Working with Families*. Milton Keynes. Open University Press.

BLUMENTHAL, I. (1992) Should we ban the mercury thermometer? Discussion paper. *Journal of the Royal Society of Medicine* **85(9)**: 553–555.

BLUMHAGEN, D. (1980) Hyper–tension: a folk illness with a medical name. *Culture, Medicine and Psychiatry* **4**: 197–222.

BOARD, M. (1995) Comparison of disposable and glass mercury thermometers. *Nursing Times* **91(33)**: 36–37.

BOLLING, K. (1994) *The Dinamap 8100 Calibration Study: A Survey Carried out by the Social Survey Division of OPCS for the Department of Health*. London. Her Majesty's Stationery Office.

BRAY, D. (1995) Biofeedback. In Rankin-Box, D. *Complementary Therapies*. Chapter 9. Edinburgh. Churchill Livingstone.

BRIGHT, J. (1997) Health promotion in nursing practice. In Bright, J. (ed.) *Health Promotion in Clinical Practice – Targeting the Health of the Nation*. London. Baillière Tindall, London.

BUCHAN, J. (1995) Are patient focused hospitals working? *Nursing Standard* **10(8)**: 30.

BUSWELL, C. (1997) Comparing mercury and disposable thermometers. *Professional Nurse* **12(5)**: 359–362.

CALNAN, M., JOHNSON, B. (1985) Health, health risks and inequalities: an exploratory study of women's perceptions. *Sociology of Health and Illness* **14(2)**: 233–254.

CARR–HILL, R., DIXON, P., GIBBS, I., GRIFFITHS, M., MCCAUGHAN, D., WRIGHT, K. (1992) *Skill Mix and the Effectiveness of Nursing Care*. York. Centre for Health Economics, University of York. Department of Health.

CASE, R.M., WATERHOUSE, J.M. (eds) (1994) *Human Physiology: Age, Stress and the Environment* (2nd edition). Oxford. Oxford Science Publications.

CHILDS, C. (1994), Temperature control. In Alexander, M., Fawcett, J., Runciman, P. (eds) *Nursing Practice: Hospital and Home, The Adult*. pp. 679–695. Edinburgh. Churchill Livingstone.

CLOSS, J. (1987) Oral temperature measurement. *Nursing Times* **83(1)**: 36–39.

CROFT, P., CRUIKSHANK, J. (1990) Blood pressure measurement in adults: large cuffs for all. *Journal of Epidemiology and Community Health* **44**: 107–173.

CUTTER, J. (1994) Recording patient temperature are we getting it right? *Professional Nurse* **9(9)**: 608–616.

DAWSON, J. (1994) Health and lifestyle surveys: beyond health status indicators. *Health Education Journal* **53**: 300–308.

DEPARTMENT OF HEALTH (1992) *The Health of the Nation. A Strategy for Health in England*. London. Her Majesty's Stationery Office.

DEPARTMENT OF HEALTH (1994) *On the State of the Public Health*. London. Her Majesty's Stationery Office.

EDGE, G., MORGAN, M. (1993) The Genius infrared tympanic thermometer. *Anaesthesia* **48(7)**: 604–607.

ERICKSON, R., YOUNT, S. (1991) Comparison of tympanic and oral temperatures in surgical patients. *Nursing Research* **40(2)**: 90–93.

FAULKNER, A. (1985) *Nursing: A Creative Approach*. London. Baillière Tindall.

FERRA-LOVE, R. (1991) A comparison of tympanic and pulmonary artery measures of core temperature. *Journal of Post Anaesthetic Nursing* **6(3)**: 161–164.

FLO, G., BROWN, M. (1995) Comparing three methods of temperature taking: oral mercury in glass, oral Diatek and tympanic first temp. *Nursing Research* **44(2)**: 120–122.

FROLICH, E., GRIM, C., LABARTHE, D.,

MAXWELL, M., PERLOFF, D., WEIDMAN, W. (1988) Recommendations for human blood pressure determination by sphygmomanometer. *Circulation* **77**: 501A–514A.

FULBROOK, P. (1993) Core temperature measurement in adults: A literature review. *Journal of Advanced Nursing* **18**: 1451–1460.

GIFT, A. (1990) Dyspnoea. *Nursing Clinics of North America* **25(4)**: 955–965.

GOLDMAN, M.B., NASH, M., PETKOVIC, M.S. (1994) Do electrolyte-containing beverages improve water balance in hyponatraemic schizophrenics. *Journal of Clinical Psychiatry* **55(4)**: 151–153.

HALLE, A., REPASY, A. (1987) Classic heatstroke: A serious challenge for the elderly. *Hospital Practice* **22(5)**: 26.

HEALTH AND SAFETY COMMISSION (1988) *The Control of Substances Hazardous to Health, Regulations*. London. Her Majesty's Stationery Office.

HELMAN, C.G. (1994) *Culture, Health and Illness* (3rd edition). Oxford. Butterworth Heinemann Ltd.

HILL, M., GRIM, C. (1991) How to take a precise blood pressure. *American Journal of Nursing* **2**:38–42.

HINCHLIFF, S., MONTAGUE, S., WATSON, R. (1996) *Physiology for Nursing Practice*. London. Baillière Tindall.

HOLTZCLAW, B. (1990) Shivering: A clinical nursing problem. *Nursing Clinics of North America* **25(4)**: 977–985.

HUNT, S., McKENNA, S.P., McEWAN, J. et al. (1986) *Measuring Health Status*. London. Croom Helm.

HUTCHINSON, P.J.A., TRILL, A., TURNER, P. et al. (1994) Views of hospital staff on the management of hypertension. *Postgraduate Medical Journal* **70(823)**: 355–358.

KEEN, A. (1994) Political influences in nursing. In Jolley, M., Brykczynska, G. (eds) *Nursing: Beyond Tradition and Conflict*. pp. 111–128. London. Mosby.

KEMP, F., FOSTER, C., McKINLAY, S. (1994) How effective is training for blood pressure measurement. *Professional Nurse* **9(8)**: 521–524.

KLEINMAN, A. (1980) *Patients and Healers in the Context of Culture*. Berkely, CA. University of Calfornia Press.

LEE, P. (1997) Health of the nation – targets for coronary heart disease and stroke. In Bright, J. (ed.) *Health Promotion in Clinical Practice – Targeting the Health of the Nation*. London. Baillière Tindall.

LEWIS, L.W., TIMBY, B. (1993) *Fundamental Skills and Concepts in Patient Care*. London. Chapman and Hall.

MALLETT, J., BAILEY, C. (1996) *The Royal Marsden NHS Trust Manual of Clinical Nursing Procedures* (4th edition). Oxford. Blackwell Science.

MATEIKA, J.H., DUFFIN, J. (1995) A review of the control of breathing during exercise. *European Journal of Applied Physiology and Occupational Physiology* **71(1)**: 1–27.

McBRIDE, A. (1994) Health promotion in hospitals: the attitudes, beliefs and practices of hospital nurses. *Journal of Advanced Nursing* **20**: 92–100.

McGEE, J., ISAACSON, P.G., WRIGHT, N.A. (1992) *Oxford Textbook of Pathology: Principles of Pathology* (1st edition). Oxford. Oxford Medical Publications.

McKAY, D.W., RAJU, M.K., CAMPBELL, N.R.C. (1992) Assessment of blood pressure measuring techniques. *Medical Education* **26**: 208–212.

MISHLER, J. (1981) *Social Contexts of Health, Illness and Patient Care*. Cambridge. Cambridge University Press.

NAIDOO, J., WILLS, J. (1994) *Health Promotion – Foundations for Practice*. London. Baillière Tindall.

NATIONAL HEART, LUNG AND BLOOD INSTITUTE (1987) Report of the second task force on blood pressure control in children – 1987. *Paediatrics* **79(1)**: 1–11.

NEARY, M. (1997) Project 2000 students survival kit: a return to the practical room (nursing skills laboratory). *Nurse Education Today* **17(1)**: 46–52.

NOLAN, J., NOLAN, M. (1993) Can nurses take an accurate blood pressure? *British Journal of Nursing* **2(14)**: 724–729.

NYHOLM, B., JEPPENSEN, L., MORTENSEN, B., KJAERGAARD, B., GLAVIND, K. (1994) The superiority of rectal thermometry to oral thermometry with regard to accuracy. *Journal of Advanced Nursing* **20**: 660–665.

ORSTEIN, R., SOBEL, D. (1988) Bodyguards. In Orstein, R., Sobel, D. (eds) *The Healing Brain*. pp. 35–54. New York. Touchstone.

PARISH, R. (1991) Policy or public procrastination? Part 11: The implications of *The Health of the Nation*. *Health Education Journal* **50(3)**: 141–145.

PETRIE, J., O'BRIEN, E., LITTLER, W., DE SWIET, M. (BRITISH HYPERTENSIVE SOCIETY) (1986) Recommendations on blood pressure measurement. *British Medical Journal* **293**: 611–615.

PETRIE, J., O'BRIAN, E., LITTLER, W., DE SWEIT, M., DILLON, J. (1990) Blood pressure measurement. (British Medical Journal Pamphlet). London. BMJ Publishing.

PUGH DAVIES, S., KASSAB, J., THRUSH, A., SMITH, P. (1986) A comparison of mercury and digital thermometers. *Journal of Advanced Nursing* **11**: 535–543.

ROPER, N., LOGAN, W., TIERNEY, A. (1993) *The Elements of Nursing* (3rd edition). Edinburgh. Longman.

ROYAL COLLEGE OF NURSING (1994) *Guidance on Patient Focused Care, Issues in Nursing and Health No. 29*. London. Royal College of Nursing.

SCHWARTZ, M.S. (1987) *Biofeedback – A Practitioners Guide*. New York. Guildford Press.

TANNAHILL, A. (1985) What is health promotion? *Health Education Journal* **44(4)**: 167–168.

THOMAS, C., GEBERT, G., HAMBACH, V. (1992) *Textbook and Colour Atlas of the Cardiovascular System*. London. Chapman and Hall.

TIMMS-HAGEN, J. (1984) Thermogenesis in brown adipose tissue as an energy buffer. *New England Journal of Medicine* **311**: 1549.

TONES, K. (1993) The theory of health promotion: implications for nursing. In Wilson-Barnett, J., Macleod Clark, J. (eds) *Research in Health Promotion and Nursing*. London. Macmillan.

TORRANCE, C., SERGINSON, E. (1996a) An observational study of student nurses' measurement of arterial blood pressure by sphygmomanometry and auscultation. *Nurse Education Today* **16(4)**: 282–286.

TORRANCE, C., SERGINSON, E. (1996b) Student nurses' knowledge in relation to blood pressure measurement by sphygmomanometry and auscultation. Nurse Education Today **16(6)**: 397–402.

TOWNSEND, P., DAVIDSON, N. (1982) *Inequalities in Health – The Black Report*. Harmondsworth. Penguin.

WALSH, M., FORD, P. (1989) *Nursing Rituals: Research and Rational Actions*. Heinemann.

WATSON, R. (1996) Hypothermia. *Elderly Care* **8(6)**: 25–28.

WEBSTER, C. (1995) Health and physical assessment. In Heath, H. (ed.) *Foundations in Nursing Practice*. pp 71–102. London. Mosby.

WEBSTER, J., NEWNHAM, D., PETRIE, J., LOVELL, H. (1984) Influence of arm position on measurement of blood pressure. *British Medical Journal* **288**: 1574–1575.

WOOLLONS, S. (1996) Temperature measurement devices. *Professional Nurse* **11(8)**: 541–547.

WHILE, A. (1989) *Health in the Inner City*. Oxford. Heinemann Medical.

WILSON-BARNETT, J., LATTER, S. (1993) Factors influencing health education and health promotion practice in acute ward settings. In Wilson–Barnett, J., Macleod Clark, J. (eds) *Research in Health Promotion and Nursing*. London. Macmillan.

WONG, D.L. (1993) *Whaley and Wong's Essentials of Pediatric Nursing*. St Louis. Mosby.

WONG, D.L. (1996) *Whaley and Wong's Nursing Care of Infants and Children* (4th edition). St Louis. Mosby.

2.3 *Pain*

K. Jackson

KEY ISSUES

■ SUBJECT KNOWLEDGE
▶ theories of pain
▶ how pain is transmitted within the individual
▶ the physiological signs of acute pain
▶ an exploration of the psychosocial elements of the pain experience

■ PRACTICE KNOWLEDGE
▶ decision making in relation to pain management
▶ the use of pain assessment tools in practice

▶ different ways of reducing pain in an individual

■ PROFESSIONAL KNOWLEDGE
▶ the professional role of the nurse in pain management
▶ the team approach to pain management

■ REFLECTIVE KNOWLEDGE
▶ application of knowledge gained from this chapter and other sources in practice situations

▶ INTRODUCTION

Ideas that pain is healthy and expected and that in small amounts will not harm are outdated. It is now considered unacceptable for patients to suffer pain unnecessarily (Carroll and Bowsher, 1993). This chapter will explore the experience of pain. Although most people can readily identify with the concept of physical pain, other areas such as the emotional and psychological elements of pain are often overlooked. This chapter is designed to further your knowledge in this region and to encourage you to continue to explore this area beyond the activities incorporated here. Pain is now accepted as a key responsibility for the nurse as a member of a multidisciplinary team and therefore up-to-date knowledge of pain is essential throughout your nursing career. Pain is a problem in its own right, but may be associated with other areas of care. Pain is also a symptom common to many illnesses and therefore nursing knowledge in this field is vital. It has, however, been found that nurses often lack this knowledge as well as an awareness of the resources available for the effective management of pain. Such nurses are therefore unable to perform their role effectively. This chapter seeks to inform you of some of the fundamental issues involved and to encourage you to develop your knowledge further in order to make effective decisions in practice.

This chapter will help you explore the issues involved in the pain experience from a broad perspective. The approaches will encourage you to use other resources, including your personal experience and practical experience in various settings, as well as the usual library resources and interactions with your peers. Additional reading is suggested to enable you to develop your knowledge and skills further.

▶ OVERVIEW

This chapter is divided into four parts, each with a specific focus in relation to pain.

▌ *Subject Knowledge*

This section considers the physiology of pain, pain transmission, physiological signs of pain, theories of pain, and psychosocial elements of pain.

▌ *Practice Knowledge*

Practice knowledge considers the assessment of pain in adults and children. Related symptoms relevant to pain assessment, the use of pain assessment tools, and the use of carers and parents to aid assessment are also considered. Effective pain management, pharmacological interventions and modes of delivery, and non-pharmacological interventions are explored.

▌ *Professional Knowledge*

This section explores the nurse's role in effective pain care in relation to adults and children in a plural society. The nurse's specialist role and multidisciplinary team role in pain management are also considered.

▌ *Reflective Knowledge*

In this section you are able to bring together the issues covered by the previous three sections as well as your existing knowledge and experiences to explore the care of four individuals related to the specialist branches of nursing. You therefore have the opportunity to apply existing knowledge in the area of effective decision making and to increase your knowledge by a wider investigation of the issues involved in the nursing care of these individuals.

On pp. 241–244 there are four case studies, each one relating to one of the branch programmes. You may find it helpful to read one of them before you start the chapter and use it as a focus for your reflections while reading.

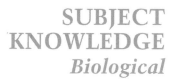

SUBJECT
KNOWLEDGE
Biological

This section explores the physiology of pain. Theories of pain transmission are discussed and you are encouraged to apply these to your own experiences.

▌ **THE PHYSIOLOGY OF PAIN**

The theoretical understanding of pain cannot proceed unless the relationships between the major components have some quantification and qualification (Stevens *et al.*, 1987). Pain theories (Stevens *et al.*, 1987) are often classified as:

- ▌ sensory–discriminatory;
- ▌ affective–motivational;
- ▌ evaluative–cognitive.

Merskey (1970) offers the following definition of pain as 'an unpleasant experience which we primarily associate with tissue damage or describe in terms of such damage or both'. This definition allows for the concept of pain to be invoked even if there is no direct indication of tissue damage, and seems to agree with the everyday definition of pain. The exact mechanism for the transmission of pain is unknown, but several theories have been put forward. However, it must be borne in mind that a theory does not necessarily represent an actual fact, but forms the basis for research and provokes thought (McCaffery and Beebe, 1994).

Pain transmission theories include:

▶ that pain is an emotion rather than a sensation;
▶ that pain is a specific entity;
▶ that pain is produced by stimulation of nonspecific receptors given a nerve impulse pattern (McCready *et al.*, 1991).

Several theories of pain have evolved and guide the conceptualization of pain (Table 2.3.1).

Theory	Theorist	Major contribution
Specificity	Descartes (1664/1972)	Pain is a distinct sensation mediated by nerves designed for nociceptive processing with physiological specialization
Intensity	Darwin (1794)	Pain is the result of intense stimulation of nerve fibres in any sensory organ
Pattern theories		Several conceptualizations of pain stimulus intensity and central summation are key concepts
a) Central summation	Livingstone (1943)	Central mechanisms for summating peripheral pain impulses and pathological stimulation of sensory nerves initiates activity in reverberating circuits between central and peripheral processes
b) Sensory interaction	Bishop (1946, 1959) Nordenbos (1959)	Rapidly conducting fibre system excite and inhibit synaptic transmission in the slowly conducting system for pain. From this evolved the theories of myelinated and unmyelinated fibre systems, functions of nerve fibres, and the multisynaptic afferent system
Affect	Marshall (1894)	Emotional quality of pain distorts all sensory events
	Melzack and Wall (1965, 1973, 1982, 1988)	Global theory accounting for the sensory, affective and cognitive dimensions of pain – pain processing not rigid, but flexible

Table 2.3.1 The evolution and major contributions of pain theories. (Adapted from Stevens and Johnston.)

▶ THE EVOLUTION AND MAJOR CONTRIBUTIONS OF PAIN THEORIES

Although pain theories enable some understanding of pain an examination of how pain messages may be transmitted is necessary to develop understanding and further conceptualization.

▶ *Pain Transmission*

Nociceptors (noxious sensation receptors) are specialized neurones located throughout the body, particularly in the skin. These specialized nerve endings recognize tissue damage. Pain results when the impulses from these nerves reach consciousness. The nerve endings are stimulated by a chemical substance that is released or formed as a result of cell disruption. When the peripheral nerve fibres carrying impulses generated by the painful stimuli enter the spinal cord, they enter the dorsal horn of the spinal grey matter, passing through the dorsal root of the spinal nerve. When a nerve fibre ends it is involved in a synapse where the nerve message is chemically transmitted to the next nerve cell and its fibre. Many different chemicals are involved in transmission at different synapses and no one transmitter substance is confined to a single functional system. For example, substance P is found in many peripheral nerve fibres, but is also found in the central nervous system in certain fibre systems that have nothing to do with pain. The major neurotransmitter responsible for the transmission of pain messages at spinal cord level is substance P. Angiotensin II, 5 hydroxytryptamine, noradrenaline, cholecystokinin, somatostatin, enkephalins and endorphins of endogenous opioid peptides are also involved. The primary actions and functions of some of these neurotransmitters are listed in Table 2.3.2.

Neurotransmitter	Action
Substance P	Is thought to be the neurotransmitter substance released that results in increasing pain perception
Enkephalins	Produce analgesia, euphoria and nausea
5-Hydroxytryptamine	Enhances pain transmission at local level, but inhibits pain when acting on central nervous system structures such as the dorsal horn
β-Endorphins	Probably responsible for dulling pain perception from injuries

Table 2.3.2 Functional relationships of neurotransmitters.

▶ *Functional Relationships of Neurotransmitters*

Conduction speed is dependent upon the diameter of the axon and whether it is myelinated: large axons conduct more rapidly than smaller axons, while the myelin forms an electrical insulator that enhances the speed of transmission. Neurones are known as presynaptic or postsynaptic. The presynaptic neurone travels from the nociceptor to the spinal cord and the postsynaptic neurones send the impulses on towards the brain.

Three types of nerves are associated with the transmission of pain:

▶ A beta fibres, which have a large diameter and are myelinated;
▶ A delta fibres, which have a small diameter and tend to be myelinated;
▶ C fibres, which have a small diameter, a slow conduction rate and are generally not myelinated.

A delta fibres are associated with the transmission of sharp pin prick pain and conduct impulses rapidly. C fibres are associated with the transmission of dull aching sensations. Once the impulses are in the spinal cord, the messages usually pass through several synapses within a short distance in the grey matter. They are then transmitted from the superficial layers to the deeper layers of the grey matter in the spinal cord on the same side. From here long nerve fibres cross over to the other side of the cord and run up to the brain in the funiculus of the spinal white matter. When the anterolateral funiculus of the spinal cord reaches the brain the long nerve fibres undergo further synaptic relays. Thus the impulses are eventually dispersed to most of the cerebral cortex where they become consciously perceived (Figure 2.3.1).

- Reflect and try to describe in your own words how you as an individual are able to perceive pain.
- Given this description consider factors that would affect your perception of pain. It may be helpful here to compare the differing perceptions of pain when 'banging your thumb' or having a headache or having a toothache.

Figure 2.3.1: The central nervous system, pathways and structures.

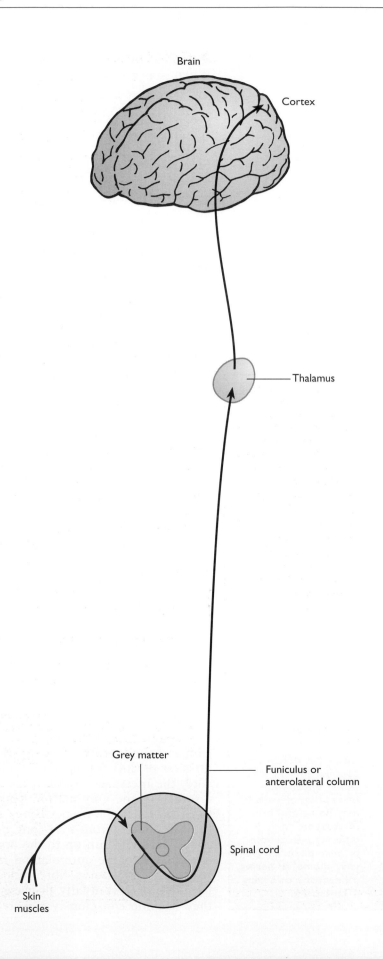

Brain

Cortex

Thalamus

Grey matter

Funiculus or
anterolateral column

Spinal cord

Skin
muscles

▶ Gate Theory

One of the most widely accepted theory of pain is the gate theory, which speculates that pain is determined by interactions between three spinal cord systems (Puntillo, 1988). It suggests that pain impulses arrive at a gate, thought to be the substantia gelatinosa. When open the impulses easily pass through, if partially open only some pain impulses can pass through, and if closed none can pass through. It further suggests that the gate position depends on the degree of small or large fibre firing. Accordingly, when large fibre firing predominates, the gate closes, and when small fibre firing predominates the pain message is transmitted (Figure 2.3.2).

Gate theory revolves around two key concepts. The first is that it is possible to alter the transmission of pain messages to the brain by deliberately activating another type of sensory receptor. In this instance rubbing or vibration of the skin causes a sensory message to be carried along type A beta fibres along pathways similar to those carrying pain signals. Thus the type A beta fibres stimulate the secondary neurones in the dorsal horn to carry touch and vibration messages to the brain. These type A beta fibres are larger than the type A delta or the type C fibres and electrical impulses travel at high speed along them, so beating the pain stimuli travelling along the type A delta or type C fibres to the secondary neurones. Therefore if the touch or vibration signals are emanating from the site of pain, they will always operate the secondary neurones first and block the pain signals.

The second concept infers that the transmission of pain messages can be modulated within the spinal cord, by descending messages from the brain itself. Messages are transmitted from the periaqueductal grey area in the midbrain and upper part of the pons to the raphe magnus nucleus in the lower pons and the upper medulla, and on into the spinal cord. Two neurotransmitters are involved: serotonin in the transmission between the raphe magnus nucleus and the cord, and enkephalin, which is released at the synapses within the raphe magnus nucleus and the spinal cord. Enkephalin release inhibits the uptake of calcium ions by the spinal cord neurones. The neurotransmitters involved in the transmission of pain signals to the brain need this calcium for their release and therefore pain messages to the brain are blocked. This theory finds that pain is both sensory and emotional.

▶ Endorphins and Non-opioid Pathways

Endorphin means morphine within. Theorists believe that endorphins are released when a brain impulse triggered and that they lock onto narcotic

> • Consider in everyday life an experience where it may be possible to consciously or subconsciously close the gate on pain (e.g. what might be your immediate reaction on 'banging your thumb')?
>
> • Now consider where and when these mechanisms may be used in the practice of pain control in health care.

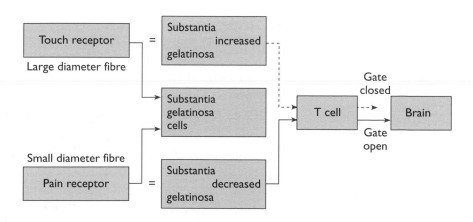

Figure 2.3.2: Gate theory. (Adapted from Melzack and Wall, 1965.)

receptors at nerve endings in the brain and spinal cord to block the transmission of pain signals, thereby preventing the impulses from reaching the brain and consciousness. Differences in the levels of endorphins found in individuals helps explain the individuality in the perception of pain (Janal *et al.*, 1984).

▶ *Multiple Opioid Receptor Theory*

One of the most current pain theories is the multiopioid receptor theory, which suggests that narcotics bind to or occupy multiple opioid receptor sites at the end of nerves (McCaffery and Beebe, 1989). Three receptor sites are thought to be relevant in relation to the effective use of narcotics in pain relief: mu (μ), kappa (κ) and sigma (σ). Drugs bind to the opioid receptor sites either very tightly (pure) or less tightly (partial). When a drug binds to the receptor site the action may be pure or partial agonist (turns activity on) or antagonist (blocks or turns off the activity). Table 2.3.3 lists the activities at the receptor sites.

Receptor site	Activity
Mu (μ)	Analgesia, respiratory depression, physical dependence, tolerance, constipation and euphoria
Kappa (κ)	Analgesia, sedation, no physical dependence, no respiratory depression
Sigma (σ)	Vasomotor stimulation, psychomimetic effects such as paranoia and hallucinations

Table 2.3.3 Drug activity at opioid receptor sites.

▶ *Drug Activities at Opioid Receptor Sites*

Binding of an agonist drug such as morphine to a μ or κ receptor site results in pain relief. An antagonist at these sites, however, will block or displace an attached agonist drug, reversing the analgesic and other effects. If proven, this theory has implications for giving pain medications and current pain management (McCready *et al.*, 1991).

▶ PHYSIOLOGICAL SIGNS OF PAIN

In sudden episodes of acute pain certain physiological signs of pain may exist (Table 2.3.4). These signs are linked to the 'fight and flight' mechanism of the adrenaline and noradrenaline functions as an initial response to the experience of pain. However, over time the body seeks equilibrium physiologically as these responses cannot be maintained without

- *Consider some drugs that you have seen in use in practice placements for the relief of pain.*
- *Identify which of these are morphine derivatives.*
- *Consider why the decision was made to give this drug rather than a non-morphine-based analgesic.*

Physiological response to acute pain	Adaptation over time (chronic pain)
Increased blood pressure	Normal blood pressure
Increased pulse rate	Normal pulse rate
Increased respiration rate	Normal respiration rate
Dilated pupils	Normal pupil size
Perspiration	Dry skin

Table 2.3.4 Physiological manifestations of acute pain and adaptations.

DECISION MAKING

Through further reading, explore the definitions of acute and chronic pain.

- *How and to what extent might the labelling of pain as either 'acute' or 'chronic' be used in the decision-making processes involved in pain management?*
- *Reflect on these differences in management in relation to pain you have observed in others or you have personally experienced. It could be helpful to consider how you would self-manage a chronic backache compared with a sudden acute toothache.*

causing physical harm. The major problem with physiological indicators of pain is that they may be due to other factors such as stress. Also these physiological responses to pain are short-lived and return to near normal limits as the body's systems acclimatize (Hawley, 1984). Therefore although they may be indicators of acute and sudden pain, they are of little use as indicators of chronic pain.

▶ *Physiological Manifestation of Acute Pain and Adaptation*

There are therefore some differences between acute and chronic pain. This has an impact on the individual experiencing pain, in that not only the physiological responses, but also the psychological and social consequences differ. Melzac (1981) stated that acute pain is associated with a well-defined cause, has a characteristic time course, and vanishes after healing. Chronic pain continues long after an injury has healed and may spread to adjacent and distant parts of the body (Melzac, 1981).

Psychosocial

In this section definitions and ideologies are explored along with misconceptions of the experience of pain for the individual.

▶ PSYCHOSOCIAL ELEMENTS OF PAIN

Pain is a difficult concept to understand. The assumption that there is a simple and direct relationship between a noxious stimulus and subsequent pain has been disputed by the realization that many environmental and internal factors modify pain perception (McGrath, 1989).

There are numerous causes of pain. The threshold (level at which pain is felt) varies between individuals, and can vary within the same person at different times (Gillies, 1993). This is further complicated by factors such as emotion, culture and previous experience, the end result being a unique experience for that individual. Therefore, pain should be regarded as a subjective phenomenon (Devine, 1990). It is important then that the nurse working with a person experiencing pain is able to accept that pain is both physical and psychological. McCaffery (1983) stated that some health care professionals mistakenly believe that if emotions cause or perpetuate pain then it is imaginary. She further stipulates that no pain sensation is truly imaginary particularly to the patient. Thus pain is both biologically and phenomenologically embodied. Moreover culture intercedes in the pain experience and therefore transcends the mind–body divide.

Some of the recognized behavioural responses to both acute and chronic pain are listed in Table 2.3.5. These may be used as cues by nurses in their quest to determine the pain experience of the patient.

- *In your own words try to define the term pain.*
- *Looking at this definition, explore how you view pain and from this try to consider on what your views are based. For example you may have had a particularly painful experience that colours your views of pain or you may never have experienced pain.*
- *Consider if these views influence your beliefs about other people in pain and in what way?*
- *Reflect on how your personal beliefs could affect your decision making when a patient or client requests pain relief.*

▶ BEHAVIOURAL RESPONSES TO ACUTE PAIN AND ADAPTATION

Pain has been defined as whatever the person experiencing it says it is, existing whenever the person says it does (McCaffery, 1972). This

Behavioural response	Adaptation over time
Observable signs of discomfort	Decrease in observable signs, though pain intensity unchanged
Focuses on pain	Turns attention to things other than pain
Reports pain	No report of pain unless questioned
Cries and moans	Quiet, sleeps or rests
Rubs painful part	Physical inactivity or immobility
Frowns and grimaces	Blank or normal facial expression
Increased muscle tension	

Table 2.3.5 Behavioural responses to acute pain and adaptations.

RESEARCH BASED EVIDENCE

Mather and Mackie J (1983) investigated the administration of analgesics to children after an operation. Nurses administered non-narcotic analgesia more frequently than narcotics and appeared to interpret the 'as required' (i.e. pro re nata or PRN) prescription as meaning 'give as little as possible'. Of the children studied who described moderate to severe pain 16% (170) did not receive pain medication. Conclusions were drawn that both medical and nursing staff would benefit from education on pain and its management to increase knowledge and practice in this area.

In 1990 Stevens looked at the use of a multidimensional pain assessment and management sheet, the Chedoke–McMaster Pediatric Pain Measurement Sheet (CMPPMS) for children between 18 months and 12 years of age. A control and experimental group were set up. Results showed that the patients of the nurses who used the CMPPMS were in less pain, assessed more frequently, and received more analgesic drugs. The control group had more pain and received fewer and less potent pain medications. The researcher concluded that such tools provide health care professionals with an intervention that can improve the child's experience of pain.

- *Think about a painful experience you have had and try to write a description about it.*
- *Include thoughts about how it made you feel and how people close to you responded to your pain*
- *Try to remember if the pain altered your lifestyle. Were there some activities, for example, that you felt unable to take part in?*
- *Does your description fit with any of the categories outlined by Fordham and Dunn (1994) (e.g. non-verbal behaviour, appearance)*

definition allows for the complexity of pain, but in some ways limits its understanding. The literature indicates that the definition of pain depends upon the one person defining it. The International Association for the Study of Pain has attempted to recognize the problem in multiple definitions of pain-related terms. It seeks to establish a universal definition of pain as 'an unpleasant sensory and emotional experience associated with actual or potential tissue damage, or described in terms of such damage' (Bonica, 1979). These definitions may not, however, be appropriate or useful for young children who are often unable to describe or say what or where the pain is, people with communication difficulties, or sedated patients. It has been established that pain causes powerful emotions in its sufferers, and fear, anxiety, anger and depression are frequently cited. These emotions have a great impact on the individual's understanding and control of the pain. The person in pain encounters an elaborate array of internal and external environmental signals (Wachter-Shikora, 1981).

Pain in any individual has to be judged by indirect evidence, and the appearance, nonverbal behaviour, physiological status and circumstance of the pain need to be interpreted (Fordham and Dunn, 1994).

Many misconceptions can be problematic in the interpretation of pain. The amount of tissue damage is not an exact prediction of the intensity of pain. It is easy to suppose that individuals receiving the same surgery, appendicectomy for example, will experience the same pain. The evidence, however, is that the pain experience is individual and varies from both person to person and situation to situation. Both McCready *et al.* (1991) and McGrath (1989) suggest that an individual's reaction to pain is determined by past experiences, state of health and level of growth and development.

It is also necessary to explore some of the myths and assumptions that prevail regarding children's pain. These unproved assumptions exist as a consequence of the limited knowledge about children's experience of pain (Price, 1990). These assumptions (Beyer and Byers, 1985; Stevens *et al.*,

1987; Broome and Slack, 1990; Lloyd-Thomas, 1990; McCready *et al.*, 1991; McConnan, 1992; Stevens and Johnston, 1992) are:

◗ children do not feel as much pain as adults;
◗ children tolerate pain better than adults;
◗ the neural system of infants is different from that of adults, so they do not experience or perceive pain as acutely or as meaningfully as adults;
◗ children do not have past experiences of pain so do not experience or perceive it in the same negative way as adults.

It has been stated that there is evidence that erroneous beliefs have been used to justify regrettable clinical practices (Craig, 1992). Furthermore health care professionals have acted as if they believed claims about the insensitivity of infants to pain (Craig, 1992). Children may not have past experience of pain, but they learn quickly. Ethological theory supports this: an expression of emotion that is helpful to the survival of the organism is likely to emerge (Charlesworth, 1982). Therefore an expression of distress in relation to tissue damage is of extreme importance to the infant's survival. Pain would logically become one of the first emotions to emerge. It has been found that tolerance to pain increases with age, so the child is more likely to have an intense pain experience. In relation to the neural system of infants, it is now believed that the process of myelination occurs *in utero* and by birth myelination of the sensory roots has begun. Therefore the ability to experience and perceive pain has been established.

Many factors influence the way pain is perceived by the individual. Past experience of pain, the personality of the individual experiencing the pain, anxiety related to the pain experience and cultural influences all affect the pain sensation. Most of us grow up thinking in certain ways that cause us to erroneously doubt others who indicate they have pain (McCaffery and Beebe, 1994). We need to be aware of this and by this awareness prevent ourselves from acting on these misconceptions.

Any past experience of pain or pain relief can affect the intensity of the pain (Wells, 1984). Pain can be influenced by the meaning it has to the individual. For example, the headache that you previously have dismissed as nothing may with a limited knowledge of medical theory be interpreted as being due to a brain tumour. This associated meaning will influence the way you perceive the pain. Anxiety, fear and depression can all increase pain sensation. Pain is reported to be more intense when an individual is anxious and reduced when anxiety levels are reduced (Akinsanya, 1985).

DECISION MAKING

During a child placement experience you are observing a physical education session. Peter Smith is known to dislike physical exercise. He appears to slip down a climbing rope, landing heavily on his right foot. He immediately begins to cry and crumples to the floor clutching his ankle. The teacher in charge asks him what is wrong. "I've hurt my foot" he says, "It really hurts, I don't think I can walk on it".

• *What are your first thoughts about Peter's pain?*

• *Note the questions that are going through your mind about the situation. What other facts do you need to know here? You may quite naturally assume that Peter is trying to get out of the exercise or you might feel genuine concern for his welfare, but it is likely that some of that concern will be coloured by your perception of Peter not enjoying the class.*

• *You may be shocked to see a boy cry. Depending on your own personal beliefs and value systems, you may find it acceptable or unacceptable for a boy to cry. You also have no idea how old Peter is and this could be a consideration for you here.*

• *You may find yourself wondering what Peter's background is. Has he had previous experience with pain, what are his cultural norms and his perception of the situation?*

• *You will probably come to some decision about Peter and his pain. Make some brief notes of the points that influence your decision.*

RESEARCH BASED EVIDENCE

Wakefield (1995) examined how nurses talk about patients' pain and pain management. She conducted a series of in-depth unstructured group interviews with nurses during which they were encouraged to discuss postoperative pain management and its effectiveness. This talk revealed that nurses tended to categorize patients according to their symptoms or overt pain behaviours. Essentially this led to patients not being believed when they signalled that pain was becoming a distressing symptom.

▶ CULTURAL AND SPIRITUAL INFLUENCES ON PAIN

The cultures within the profession of nursing or the institution of a hospital affect the way that pain is assessed, the way that decisions are made about the possible treatments, and the way that pain is managed.

Ethnicity in pain management is of particular significance in a multi-cultural country, such as the UK. Each individual has intrinsic associations with culture: it socializes us to know what is expected of us and of others. Culture shapes beliefs and constrains behaviours. In such an environment the nurse must constantly be aware of professional issues in providing culturally appropriate care, and also of constraints on other practitioners due to their cultural beliefs and values. The process of the nurse–patient interaction occurs within the context of the demands and culture of the workplace (Walker *et al.*, 1995).

There are theological overtones in the pain experience as pain plays a central part in religious thought. The Christian concept is of pain as a paradox: Christ healed others in pain, but allowed himself to be crucified and endured agonizing pain. Pain is viewed as a challenge to be overcome. Buddha has been cited as a warrior, a saint and a victim. Examples of pain control can be found in many cultures, for example, the Indian fakir who controls pain while lying on a bed of nails and the African tribes that practice lip or cheek piercing as ritualistic ceremonies do not appear to experience pain. Where stoicism is a cultural value, the behavioural expression of distress is generally less acceptable. Older people may view pain as a preliminary to death. Each culture has its own set of beliefs and attitudes with respect to the way people react to pain. These are passed on through the generations and acquired by socialization (Parsons, 1992). Chinese, Arabic-speaking and southern European patients are more likely to tell their families or their doctor how they feel, rather than report their pain to their nurse, unless the nurse has become credible to them (Meinhart and McCaffery, 1983; Kanitsaki, 1993). Therefore the relative may need to act as an intermediary between the patient and the nurse. However, care must be taken not to stereotype people, remembering that there is variability within cultures as well as between cultures. These misleading effects of cultural stereotypes, and the belief by nurses and doctors that they are the experts regarding the patient's pain, lead to problems in assessing the patient's pain. Also the ethnicity of both the individual in pain, and those attempting to assess the pain, cloud the perceptions of health professionals (Walker *et al.*, 1995). Many of the early works investigating the sociocultural dimensions of pain have been criticized for reinforcing ethnic stereotypes, for example Zola's study into the reactions of Italian–Americans and Irish–Americans to illness (Zola, 1966) or the Zborowski study into the cultural components of experiencing pain among Italian–Americans and Jewish–Americans (Zborowski,1952).

Helman (1990) suggests that:

- ▶ not all cultural or social groups respond to pain in the same way;
- ▶ cultural background can influence how people perceive and respond to pain, both in themselves and others;
- ▶ cultural factors can influence how and whether people reveal their pain to health professionals and others.

Gender is also an issue in the pain experience. Both male and female subjects believe that females have an innate ability to cope with pain and this is generally linked to reproduction (Bendelow, 1993). In the available literature the views are that gender is of no significance or that

---

RESEARCH BASED EVIDENCE

Lipton and Marbach (1984) found differences between ethnic groups in their expressiveness in response to pain and in the individual's tolerance of pain. Their study examined interethnic differences and similarities in the reported pain experience of Black, Irish, Jewish and Puerto Rican patients with facial pain. A 35-item scale was used to measure the patients' pain experience. No significant interethnic differences were found for 23 of the items.

The majority of items where interethnic differences were found concerned the patients' emotionality in response to pain and the interference in their daily functioning attributed to the pain. The five ethnic groups were generally found to be similar in their reported responses to pain, but the factors that influenced the responses differed. For example for Irish patients, the degree of social assimilation was most influential, such as belonging to a close long-standing

friendship group composed of people from an Irish background, though for Puerto Rican patients, the level of distress, social assimilation and duration of pain were found to be most influential in predicting the pain response. Thus they concluded that given the multiplicity of sociocultural, psychological and clinical factors which seem to influence intraethnic response to pain, it is inappropriate to base expected behaviour and attitudes for ethnic groups on stereotypes.

---

females have lower pain thresholds than males. Gender differences in the pain experience are usually recorded in terms of sensitivity to experimentally-induced pain (Bendelow and Williams, 1995).

PRACTICE KNOWLEDGE

DECISION MAKING

Rituals in nursing practice can become entrenched, and in many health care institutions drugs are still administered via a 'drug round'.

- *During your practice placements compare the experiences of patients on the unit or ward that links pain relief to 'drug rounds' and those where self-administration of drugs is the norm.*
- *To what extent do 'drug round' practices need to be modified to suit individual needs for pain relief?*
- *How might ritualistic practices affect your decision making in relation to pain management?*

In order to make the most of decision-making skills in practice, the nurse must access appropriate knowledge to support and rationalize these actions. This section applies knowledge about the areas of pain assessment and relief of pain to the practice of nursing. You are encouraged to examine and apply this knowledge to exercises that will help you develop decision-making skills.

The prescribing of analgesia by physicians on an 'as required' basis leaves the responsibility for the decision to give analgesia firmly with the nurse (McCaffery, 1977; Craig, 1992). Nurses are the gatekeepers of medication usage and as such have a responsibility to increase their knowledge in pharmacological as well as non-pharmacological techniques for pain management. Nurses can therefore be instrumental in pain management in all settings. Many writers have stressed the need for nurses to assess an individual's beliefs and attitudes about pain and pain management accurately (McCaffery and Beebe, 1989; Bonica, 1990). Because of its subjective nature, the individual in pain is the only one who can assess the pain accurately.

The routine and traditional practices of many care institutions can pose difficulties in the assessment of pain. The use of 'drug rounds' may cause patients to comply, accepting analgesia at this time and feeling unable to ask for it at a more appropriate time for them. Skilful assessment techniques will limit this problem, identifying both the individual nature of the pain and its recurrence at more frequent intervals than the 'drug round' timing. An awareness of pain should therefore be a routine matter in caring for patients.

▶ ASSESSMENT OF PAIN

▶ *Pain Expression*

Assessment is a process by which a conclusion is reached about the nature of a problem. Planning effective pain management is a crucial part of the nurse's role. In order to achieve this it is necessary to assess the level of the individual's discomfort in an attempt to identify a potential course of action. Thus the cycle of the nursing process becomes part of the equation. The nurse needs to be able to draw conclusions about the individual's pain to 'assess' the level and intensity of the pain based on information from the patient. Once this has been achieved it is then possible to 'plan' a course of action to alleviate the pain, 'implement' this and 'evaluate' the action. Although this is possible without the patient's cooperation, it is better to involve the individual in the assessment of their pain. Otherwise nurses are simply applying their own beliefs and values to the situation and making assumptions about patients' pain levels. The nurse must therefore be proactive and skilled in recognizing potentially painful situations, particularly in those instances where the patient may not be able to communicate verbally. To achieve this we need to ascertain whether pain assessment is an appropriate action, believe that the person has pain, and be committed to assessing the pain. This should lead to a clarification of the extent of pain and its treatment. In some circumstances, this assessment will need to be not only accurate, but also swift, for example when dealing with a patient suffering the pain of a myocardial infarction (heart attack), where the need for immediate and effective pain relief is a priority.

Although the nurse's role in this area is paramount, the only individual who is truly able to assess the pain is the person who is suffering it. So wherever possible the patient should be assessing the pain and not the nursing staff. In circumstances where the patient is unconscious, has a communication difficulty or is a child the nurse must use their observational skills and make an informed decision based on the evidence presented by the patient, bearing in mind that the family and other carers can be asked for further clarification.

The accurate assessment of an individual's pain is an inherently difficult process. The nurse must be able to establish a trusting relationship with the patient and his or her family or carers. The nurse must also be aware of his or her own beliefs and prejudices about pain. Timing of the pain assessment is very important and dependent upon many factors, not least of which is the desire of the patient to participate in the assessment, the severity of the pain and the potential pain treatment. Such assessment involves the skills of observation so that the nonverbal pain behaviours can be seen and recognized (Table 2.3.6). It must be remembered that these behaviours are influenced by the individual's social and cultural norms. Your interpretation will also be influenced by these factors. Therefore it is not possible to make assumptions based on the absence of a recognized nonverbal pain behaviour since each pain experience for the individual is unique.

The nurse may conclude that someone is in pain if:

- an individual states that this is the case;
- an individual's behaviour is indicative of pain;
- an individual has undergone some experience that we would consider to be painful.

DECISION MAKING

Mrs Singh is an elderly widow living in a maisonette. Her family live close by and have very regular contact with her. She is receiving treatment for glaucoma and the community nurse has been asked by her general practitioner to assess her needs as her family are unable to instil her eye drops at lunch time. She speaks very little English and has limited mobility. When the nurse arrives Mrs Singh is accompanied by her niece who says she has just arrived and is worried about her aunt who does not appear to be herself today. On meeting Mrs Singh she is sitting hunched in a chair and is moaning and rocking back and forth slightly.

- *Consider the appropriate nursing actions in this instance.*
- *Using the list of aspects related to pain assessment in Table 2.3.6 and with the help of Mrs Singh's niece complete an assessment of her pain.*
- *What more do you need to know that might help you in effective decision making about Mrs Singh's care?*

Pain	Nature, intensity and site
	Likely cause
	Precipitating factors and circumstances (e.g. time of day, movement, eating)
Examples of non-verbal pain behaviours	Facial expression
	Change in mood
	Crying, screaming, wailing, weeping
	Lack of appetite
	Nausea, vomiting
	Pale or flushed skin colour
	Reluctance to move
	Increased activity
	Unusual behaviour
	Unusual posture
	Holding, pressing on the part that hurts
Related symptoms	Nausea, anxiety, breathlessness
Resources	Patient's coping strategies
	Nursing knowledge and skills in using and teaching non-pharmacological methods of pain relief
	Medical and pharmacological knowledge and skills in both pharmacological and non-pharmacological methods of pain relief
	Availability of resources such as time, equipment, privacy and so on
Meaning and significance to patient	Purpose and consequences

Table 2.3.6 Aspects of pain assessment.

▶ *Related Symptoms*

An initial assessment should include some information about the history of the pain as follows.

- ▶ Information about the initial onset of the pain. This includes a comparison of the medical history with the patient's own version and allows similarities and discrepancies to be addressed. This may be linked to surgery, illness, trauma or an unknown cause. The patient may believe that something totally unrelated to the identified clinical cause of the pain is responsible.
- ▶ Position of the pain. A body outline may be used for this purpose and then used as a baseline to chart any improvement or deterioration in the pain.
- ▶ A description of the pain. The patient should be encouraged to use his or her own words for this exercise. Children have a limited vocabulary and may well use words that an adult would not normally use, such as 'owie', 'sgwidgy' or a 'headache in my tummy'.
- ▶ Elements affecting the pain. These can include position, eating, activity, and time of day.
- ▶ Previous treatment. The success or otherwise of past treatments helps the nurse plan effectively in this pain experience.
- ▶ Any other medical history.
- ▶ Psychological aspects. The possibility of stress, changes in lifestyle, depression or behavioural disorders in the individual and their relevance to the pain experience need to be considered, and specialist referral may be necessary.
- ▶ Social aspects. Information about the family, housing, employment and other interests are relevant in a pain assessment as often these positively or negatively influence a pain problem.

▶ Observation. The most natural reactions are seen when observation is informal and carried out when the patient is unaware of being observed. Formal observation usually involves the use of some form of documentation or pain chart.

▶ *Use of Pain Assessment Tools*

There are many formal pain assessment tools to aid in assessing the patient's pain, from a simple visual analogue scale to the more complex. When using the visual analogue scale the patient is asked to rate the pain along a line between no pain and the worst pain imaginable (Figure 2.3.3). An intensity rating can also be used, in which case the patient picks the description that most closely relates to the pain they are experiencing (Figure 2.3.4). Other pain tools use a variety of other ways in an attempt to clarify the patient's pain (Figure 2.3.5).

Figure 2.3.3: A visual analogue scale.

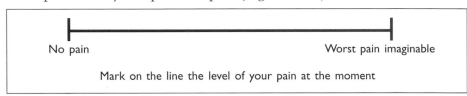

For clients other than inpatients the use of a personal pain diary has been recommended. The patient records the pain, describes it and includes comments about how it has changed, if at all, how it affects their daily lifestyle and any effective pain relief. The patient needs to get into a routine of recording in this diary since it is likely that more accurate information is achieved with the recent experience of pain. The patient therefore records the information as it occurs, if possible, within their normal lifestyle.

The method of pain measurement should be bias-free and there must be a particular focus on practicality and versatility (McGrath, 1989). However, although these are desirable aims they may be difficult to achieve. An array of pain assessment tools have been developed for adults, but most rely on communication and cognitive abilities not mastered by young children (Stevens *et al.*, 1987). This also restricts their use for people with some learning disabilities or those who are unable to communicate verbally.

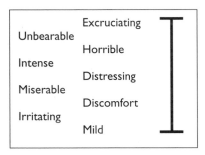

Figure 2.3.4: An intensity rating scale.

▶ ASSESSMENT OF PAIN IN CHILDREN

DECISION MAKING

Mrs Singh, whom you met in an earlier Decision Making has now been assessed. There is nothing physically wrong with her. It transpires that she had received bad news from her family in India and a very dear nephew has been killed in a road traffic accident.

- *Does this information make a difference to your initial thoughts about your nursing actions?*

- *Would the use of any of the pain assessment tools discussed above have been helpful in this case?*
From information already covered in Psychosocial Subject Knowledge what might be the most important part of a pain managment strategy for Mrs Singh.

The literature has shown that there is inadequate knowledge in the area of the pain experience for children. Beyer and Byers (1985) stated that current knowledge of paediatric pain was limited and did not provide sufficient information to assess and manage patients thoroughly and effectively. This was reiterated in a later paper by Price (1990). The criteria for a pain measure for children are the same as for any reliable measuring instrument

DECISION MAKING

Pain assessment tools are becoming increasingly popular in the practice situation and vary in use according to the client group and the evidence about their reliability and validity. In relation to specific client groups or specific health care situations that you have experienced during your practice placements:

- *Find out what pain assessment tools are available for use and review how they are used.*
- *Have any of these tools been tested as valid and reliable? You may have to look at the research literature to find this out.*
- *Using these practice experiences and the case studies at the end of this chapter decide which pain tool is appropriate for each patient. Try to justify your choice.*

1. Where pain is WORST, please shade area(s) heavily ▆

2. Where pain is LESS SEVERE, please shade area(s) lightly ▢

3. Show shooting pain(s) with arrow(s)

4. Write "DEEP pain" or "SURFACE pain" where appropriate

NO PAIN ——————————————————— SEVERE PAIN

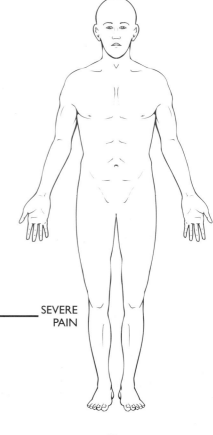

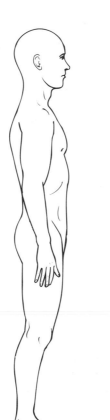
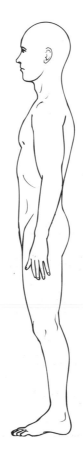
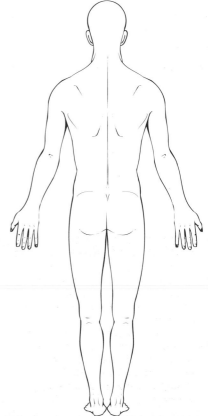

Figure 2.3.5: A pain tool with combination outline and verbal descriptors of pain. (Source Derbyshire Royal Infirmary NHS Trust).

RESEARCH BASED EVIDENCE

In one study analgesic doses received by 18 adults were compared to those received by 18 children who had identical surgical procedures. The adults received 372 doses of narcotics and the children 11 doses. In respect of non-narcotics, the adults received 299 doses and the children 13 doses (Eland and Anderson, 1977).

In a more recent study, Gilles et al. (1995) found that young children's pain after surgery is often poorly recognized and consequently poorly treated. This study also found that staff required more focused training in the accurate assessment and management of children's pain. The study looked at 40 children under five years of age who had received surgery. Parents and staff also participated and the study further concluded that mother's had an important role in assessing and managing their child's pain.

(McGrath, 1989). Few reliable and valid tools are available for assessing pain in children. Most tools require the child's participation, relying on their understanding of numbers, colours or drawings and their ability to communicate verbally and to be able to see and assume that they are alert enough to respond (Buckingham, 1993). Eland and Anderson (1977) in their study found that the word pain is meaningless to children below the age of six years. Assessment scales have a limited use in children under four years of age (McCready *et al.*, 1991; Buckingham, 1993). There has been some success with older children, and children that can count to four can probably help nurses assess their pain (Ellis, 1988). There is strong evidence that pain assessment in children must be multidimensional. Verbal reports and behavioural and physiological observations must be considered (McConnan, 1992). Behavioural observation methods circumvent the possible difficulties of comprehension that are inherent in any paediatric self-reporting scale (Lloyd-Thomas, 1990). They can therefore be said to be more objective since they are discreet and unconstrained by verbal skills, and reflect the social milieu. Pain measurement is based on three components: behavioural indicators, physiological parameters, and the child's report of his pain (Ellis, 1988).

Although the assessment of a child's pain is an important issue, the effective relief of that pain must be achieved to ensure that the experience causes minimal damage to the child and the child's family or other carers. In relation to the nurse's role in pain relief, however, there does not appear to be a formal accountability in this area, but if we are working in an ethos of providing holistic care, then pain assessment and relief must form an important part of the children's nurse's function. Nurses should be enabled to anticipate pain in the child and manage this based on obvious alterations in anatomical or physiological integrity (Broome and Slack, 1990). For example, it would seem inevitable that pain will occur following a surgical procedure, therefore pain relief should be provided in anticipation of this pain.

▶ *Parents and Others as Aids in Assessing Children's Pain*

Children and their parents or carers can provide cues, such as a previously seen behaviour that has been found to indicate pain, to the level of suffering a child may be experiencing (Buckingham, 1993). Behaviour assessment is used by the nurse to infer whether the child is in pain, whether to medicate and whether some other intervention may be appropriate (Broome and Slack, 1990). Pain behaviours in children can be misinterpreted as separation anxiety, fear, and distress due to immobilization. In 1977 McBride stated that behaviours are more reliable pain indicators than verbalizations in children. Nurses have reported that they rely on nonverbal cues in paediatric pain assessment. Although this is appropriate, assumptions made by nurses about behaviour should be validated with the child if possible, or the parents or carers. Children who are withdrawn or asleep may be interpreted inaccurately as having no pain (Broome and Slack, 1990). Some sources have cast doubt on the reliability of behavioural data for assessing paediatric pain. For example McCaffery in 1977 stated that children may suffer in silence because of their view that pain and illness are a punishment for being 'bad'.

Children identify their parents and carers as the most important source of comfort when in pain. However, nurses do not appear to use the parents and carers as a source of information or an active intervener in pain management (Broome and Lillis, 1989). It must be a consideration that the parents and carers themselves are in a stressful situation and may need to be enabled to perform this role. Usually parents are reliable sources of information about their child's behaviour during hospitalization. They are effective corroborators in the decision about whether the child is in pain or responding to other events in the environment (Broome and Slack, 1990). They can also give an indication of the child's experience of pain and ways of coping with it, thus providing baseline information on which the nursing staff can build. Parents should be adequately prepared to meet the challenges of their child's pain (McCready *et al.*, 1991). This is a further role of the children's nurse who needs to ensure that the parents are as informed as possible so that they can help their child manage the pain (Douthit, 1990).

▶ PLANNING EFFECTIVE PAIN MANAGEMENT

It has been suggested that the management of pain should be diverse enough to take account of the various dimensions of the pain experience. The management of pain then must be an important issue for nurses in their professional role. Nurses are responsible for the administration of drugs to patients. They are also responsible for educating patients and their families or carers, as appropriate, in the management of their prescribed medications (see also Chapter 1.4 on medicines). The nurse can be instrumental in ensuring a more personalized approach to the individual's pain management, but to achieve this the nurse needs a sound knowledge of the various methods of managing pain. Such actions are usually considered in terms of pharmacological and non-pharmacological interventions.

▶ *Pharmocological Interventions*

The correct use of medication is essential for effective pain management, but has been shown to be an area where nurses often fail to excel. Most commonly problems occur due to inaccurate assessment of pain as the presenting problem and a lack of insight into which drugs to use in the treatment of different types of pain (Latham, 1991). Nurses are unable to prescribe drugs, but need knowledge of the methods of administration and how they are applicable to the patient's pain experience. For example children have been shown to consider the pain from an injection as the worst pain ever experienced (Eland and Anderson, 1977). It is therefore unsatisfactory to administer an analgesic intended to relieve pain using this route. Equally some medicines have been found to be more effective for certain types of pain. The nurse interacts with both the patient and the doctor responsible for prescribing analgesia and is therefore in an ideal position to influence appropriate prescribing. This will result in an individualized and consequently more effective regimen to aid the patient's pain management. A sound knowledge base and experience will enhance the recognition of the implications of the information yielded by the assessment (Fordham and Dunn, 1994).

DECISION MAKING

Mr Phil O'Reilly has been admitted suffering from chest pain. This is thought to be due to a severe angina attack. He is grey, sweating profusely and is complaining of chest and left arm pain. He is obviously frightened and has asked you to contact a priest as he is convinced that he is about to die. His partner has been contacted and is on the way to the hospital from work. Accurate and quick assessment is required in this case of acute pain.

- *What areas of pain assessment would take priority in this case?*

- *Consider the additional information you would require from Mr O'Reilly's partner to enable you to liaise effectively between the patient and the doctor managing Mr O'Reilly's pain.*

- *Once adequate pain relief has been achieved what health promotion strategy would be necessary from the nurse to help Mr O'Reilly prevent or reduce the frequency of recurrence of the chest pain in the future?*

▶ Types of analgesia

A variety of issues are relevant in considering appropriate analgesic therapy. There are three categories of analgesics: opioid drugs, non-opioid drugs and co-analgesic drugs and their usage is generally based upon their method of action.

▶ Opioid drugs (e.g. morphine, pethidine, codeine) mainly work in the brain and spinal cord to inhibit the transmission of pain. They are generally used to relieve severe pain and associated effects include a sense of wellbeing in the individual. They are therefore linked with a tendency to produce mental and physical dependence. They are subject to the *Misuse of Drugs Act* (Department of Health, 1971) and have to be prescribed by a medical or dental practitioner.

▶ Non-opioid drugs (e.g. aspirin, paracetamol, ibuprofen, indomethacin) mainly work in the peripheral tissues by interfering with chemicals that stimulate pain endings. Useful in the relief of musculoskeletal pain and mild to moderate pain.

▶ Co-analgesic drugs have a variety of actions, for example muscle relaxant or sedation (diazepam), antidepressant (amitriptyline), or suppress inflammatory reactions (corticosteroids).

These drugs can be used alone or in combination to produce pain relief. The intensity of pain should influence the type of analgesic prescribed. The effective dose varies for each individual and therefore the effect of the drug given should be carefully monitored. There is a ceiling with non-opioid drugs so that beyond a certain dose there will be no increased analgesic effect, but with opioid drugs the limitations of dosage appear to be the associated side effects. Repeated administration of narcotic (opioid) drugs have been shown to cause tolerance and dependence. This is no deterrent, however, in the control of pain in terminal disease. Recommended practice is to adjust both the dose and the frequency of administration so that the patient never suffers pain.

Ideally the carers try to achieve an optimum level of pain control by using analgesic agents. This may take time to achieve, and because of the uniqueness of the individual pain experience, should be constantly evaluated and updated. The duration of action of the analgesic is an important issue since the ideal is to maintain an acceptable level of pain relief for the patient. The nurse therefore needs an awareness of both the effectiveness of the drug and its duration. In this way the nurse will be able to limit the delay between the time when the patient needs pain relief and the time when the administered drug becomes effective. Analgesic ladders are frequently used in practice situations to achieve this aim (Figure 2.3.6).

DECISION MAKING

- Consider the drugs that may be given to an individual in mild, moderate or severe pain.
- Investigate the use of each of the following analgesic drugs – paracetamol, ibuprofen, dihydrocodeine tartrate, morphine – from your textbooks and reflect on how you have seen them used in practice. Establish how each drug works and its common side effects.
- How will side effects affect your decision making in the choice of drugs to administer to a particular client group (e.g. children, adults or the elderly)?
- How will side effects affect your decision making in the choice of drugs to administer in a particular pain context (e.g. postoperative pain, cancer pain, chronic pain)?
- Will the client's locality make a difference to your decision making (e.g. whether at home or in hospital)?

(You may need to refer to information given in Chapter 1.4 to complete this exercise.)

▶ Modes of delivery

Many routes are available for the administration of medicines (see also Chapter 1.4) and it is now necessary to explore some of these routes in relation to the administration of analgesics. Opioid and non-opioid

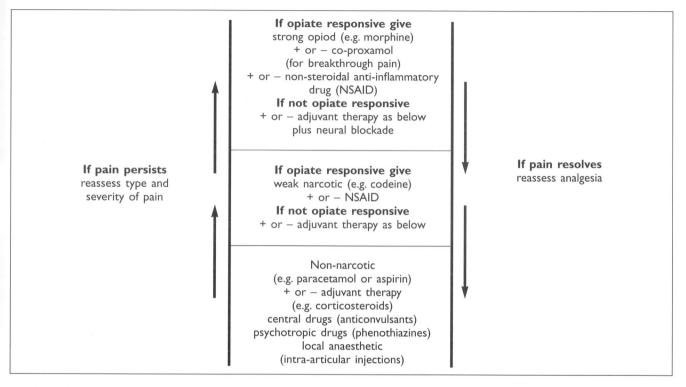

Figure 2.3.6: An analgesic ladder.

RESEARCH BASED EVIDENCE

Knapp-Spooner et al. (1995) examined the differences in pain intensity, sleep disturbance, sleep effectiveness, fatigue and vigour in cholecystectomy patients who received either PCA or intramuscular injections of narcotics for postoperative pain. Data were collected on the first two postoperative days from the sample of 16 women (aged 22–58 years) who received PCA and ten women (aged 22–60 years) who received intramuscular injections. Results indicated that patients receiving PCA reported less pain on day 1 and less fatigue on day 2 than the other group of patients.

DECISION MAKING

Using the example of Mr Phil O'Reilly from the Decision Making on p. 229 who was admitted with acute chest pain caused by angina:

- *Explore the potential analgesia that may be used to help relieve his acute pain.*
- *Decide on an appropriate method of delivery for this choice and justify your decision.*

analgesics can be given by various routes including orally, intramuscularly, intravenously, rectally, and subcutaneously.

Infusion pumps are often used for the administration of analgesics and can be:

- intravenous (commonly used for acute postoperative pain);
- subcutaneous (commonly used for palliative care);
- epidural, that is, a nerve block (commonly used for labour pain).

Pumps can also be operated by the patient to provide 'patient controlled analgesia' (PCA). The analgesic is prescribed as for the infusion pump and the nurse sets up the system as required. The patient is then able to take control of their pain in a positive way. There is usually a button control and when the patient depresses the button he or she receives a bolus dose of the analgesic to limit the pain. Each PCA pump has a 'lock out' time between doses so that the patient cannot overdose. There are also security features such as a key to lock the pump to limit the risk of interference once the prescribed rate has been set.

Whatever the mode of delivery a careful explanation is required for the patient and their family or carers as appropriate so that they can take an active part in the pain control.

Non-pharmocological Interventions

There are many strategies that do not involve drugs that can be used to help relieve pain. These non-pharmacological interventions can be used successfully with most client groups and include distraction, cutaneous stimulation and relaxation techniques (May, 1992). For the infant, distraction can include holding and cuddling or using a dummy or comforter. Older children may be encouraged to count or talk about other more pleasant experiences to help distract them. Play therapy can also be useful in taking the child's mind away from the pain. Cutaneous stimulation includes gentle massage or rubbing of the skin, which may be used for all age groups. Relaxation techniques can be used effectively with older children who have the cognitive skills to understand instructions as well as with adults. Deep breathing and counting can be used to take the focus off the pain and can result in a lessening of the pain experience.

▶ Transcutaneous electric nerve stimulation (TENS)

TENS can be used for the relief of chronic and acute pain. The precise mechanism of pain relief using TENS is unknown, but it may act by stimulating the production of endorphins or by blocking the primary afferent nerve fibres. The system consists of a battery-powered electrical pulse generator that is connected via some leads to electrodes placed on the skin over the area of a peripheral nerve innervating the painful site. The stimulation is usually felt as a tingling or buzzing sensation. TENS has been found to be useful for labour pain and postoperative and chronic pain. One of the advantages of TENS is that it can be used by the patient independently of the nursing staff and is therefore useful in the home environment as a method of pain control.

▶ Massage

Massage is a therapeutic manipulation of the soft tissue of the body. It is believed that it limits the pain experience by stimulation that 'closes the gate' on the pain or alternatively stimulation of the skin may result in the release of endorphins (McCaffery and Beebe, 1989). It can also be viewed as a form of relaxation or distraction, drawing attention from the pain and altering the perception of pain.

The massage is usually carried out over and around the site of the pain. Care should be taken with this therapy, however, since it is a form of communication and may be open to various interpretations. Culturally the intimacy involved in this technique must be handled sensitively, and an acceptable approach must be sought. Sometimes a foot massage may be more acceptable than a body massage.

▶ *Complementary Therapies*

Over recent years interest in alternative therapies has grown. Complementary therapies are holistic natural therapies that may be used in conjunction with conventional medical or nursing treatments to enhance the physical and psychological wellbeing of the patient. The use of such therapy demands the practitioner to be autonomous in their practices. The practitioner in this instance need not necessarily be a nurse. The nurse in this situation will be answerable for the choices made in the treatment delivered and will be accountable under the *Code of Professional Conduct* (UKCC, 1992a) for such actions. The therapies require a hands-on approach by the practitioner and the therapies need time as well as privacy in which the practitioner and patient can communicate. These approaches need careful handling, since some nurses may believe that they can learn all there is to learn about a complementary therapy in a half day's study. They may then go on to put the patient at risk because of a lack of competence. Complementary therapies could offer the patient benefits by focusing on the process of promoting health and healing (Armstrong and Waldron, 1991). In 1991 Armstrong and

---

DECISION MAKING

Using the case study for Jordan Simpson, a 13-year-old boy admitted in acute pain due to a sickle cell crisis (see Reflective Knowledge, Child Case Study):

- *Consider the non-pharmacological methods of pain relief that you might use to help Jordan deal with his pain.*
- *As Jordan's condition is long term, examine how these strategies can be developed to help him cope with future pain experiences.*
- *Explore how you would involve him in identifying the strategies that may help him cope with future pain experiences, and why certain non-pharmacological approaches may be more suitable than others for Jordan.*

- *Consider how your professional role as a nurse may enable you to work together with the patient in the use of complementary treatments as part of conventional treatment.*
- *Make notes of the various aspects of your role and how these may benefit patients in their choice of therapy.*

Waldron suggested criteria for the practice of complementary therapies in their strategy for the use of such therapies. These include:

▶ consent from the patient, relative or carer before treatment;
▶ consultation with a relevant medical practitioner;
▶ authorization agreed between the nurse and nurse manager;
▶ documentation with a record of the treatment in the patient care plan.

The UKCC have included a section about complementary and alternative therapies in the 1996 *Guidelines for Professional Practice*. They recommend that nurses ensure that the introduction of these therapies is always in the best interests and safety of the patient or client. Further they suggest a team approach where it should be part of professional team work to discuss the use of complementary therapies with medical and other members of the health care team. Furthermore practitioners are reminded that we can be called to account for any activities carried out outside conventional practice.

▶ Aromatherapy

Aromatherapy is the use of essential oils in the treatment of medical conditions or as relaxing agents, and has been in use over many centuries. Essential oils are extracted from different parts of plants and are usually absorbed through the skin in a lotion. They may also be absorbed into the lungs as steam inhalations or with vaporizers. The exact way aromatherapy works is unknown, but it has been found to be effective for enhancing wellbeing, relieving stress and rejuvenating and regenerating the body. Aromatherapy has been particularly used in the treatment of:

▶ stress-related conditions (e.g. anxiety, depression, insomnia);
▶ digestive disorders (e.g. colic and constipation);
▶ skin conditions (e.g. acne and eczema);
▶ minor infections (e.g. cystitis).

Treatment usually involves massage and can take several hours. Essential oils are powerful chemicals and practitioners must know exactly what they are using. Some oils are toxic, some are irritants, and some cause problems if used in pregnancy, so a sound knowledge base is essential. The use of aromatherapy appears to have many benefits for some patients.

DECISION MAKING

- *Make a list of the areas of pain management where you feel aromatherapy may be useful and how it could be used.*
- *Find a research-based study on the use of aromatherapy in nursing practice (e.g. Stevensen, 1994). Analyse the paper and summarize the conclusions with the ascribed benefits of aromatherapy and methods of use.*

▶ Acupuncture

Acupuncture was developed by the ancient Chinese. Fine needles are used that pierce the skin at points on the body where particular effects can be obtained. These needles may then be rotated or stimulated. The theory is based on the belief that life force (ch'i) flows around certain lines on the body (meridians). The needles are thought to correct an abnormal flow of life forces. Traditional acupuncture points may be used or 'trigger' points. These therapies are able to produce localized analgesia. Certain types of acupuncture are thought to promote endogenous opiate (endorphins and enkephalins) release (Wall and Melzack, 1989). Other theories are that nerve fibres carry and transmit the acupuncture effect (Melzack, 1978) or that the meridians are electrically distinct and that changes within them are responsible for triggering the neural and hormonal responses (Jessel-Kenyon *et al.*, 1992).

Acupressure

Acupressure has evolved from the same Oriental roots as acupuncture. Acupressure uses finger pressure on the acupuncture points to manipulate the energy imbalances. The treatment works on the recipients Qi by pressing the fingers and thumbs on specific points that are located along channels (meridians) of Qi, in a similar way to acupuncture. Oriental medicine seeks to identify the underlying cause of the disease concentrating on the flow and level of Qi in the body. From this a treatment plan is developed. Acupressure is a versatile treatment that can be given wherever and whenever it is convenient. Acupressure should not be used around an open wound or where there is inflammation or swelling.

Reflexology

Reflexology is based on the belief that the body's natural healing mechanisms can be enhanced by the application of pressure to certain areas of the feet and hands. The areas are connected to different parts of the body by a flow of energy. The body is divided into ten vertical zones with five closely associated zones on each arm. Within these zones the structures are connected by a flow of energy and the five zone areas on each foot and hand are linked to five zones on each side of the body, so applying pressure on a reflex point will affect different organs that lie within the zone. Applying local pressure also stimulates blood supply to the area. Reflexology is an attempt to restore the body's natural balance by correcting problems of circulation, allowing the body to heal itself.

Treatment usually involves the patient sitting with their legs raised, while the feet are examined. Pressure is then applied to all areas on both feet. The therapist uses the feel of certain areas to establish which areas need attention. It is usual for a treatment to last between 30 and 60 minutes. Transient effects may be noticed as the body heals itself, where unresolved health problems may flare up temporarily. There have been attempts to relate the mode of action of reflexology to neurology, where the nerve supplies appear to be related in several areas of the body. Therefore stimulation of the body's surface can affect the functioning of internal organs. However, there is limited evidence of this to link the identified areas of the feet and all other parts of the body.

Homeopathy

Homeopathy is a treatment based on the belief that a substance that produces the symptoms of a health problem may also cure it (i.e. treating like with like). According to homeopaths, symptoms are a manifestation of the body's efforts to fight the process of disease. There is therefore no point in suppressing the symptoms. The aim is to establish the cause of the symptoms and to treat the whole person, allowing the body's natural defences to restore health. It is claimed that homeopathy can be used for any reversible illness and that it has other benefits including a preventive role and a strengthening role. By helping the body's natural defences homeopathy may complement the action of other medicines.

Homeopathy has been found to be particularly effective when used with:

- allergic conditions such as hayfever;
- stress-related conditions such as eczema or migraine.

RESEARCH BASED EVIDENCE

In 1995 Rogers, a mental health nurse, found that homeopathy proved useful for alcohol-dependent patients during detoxification when distress and mental 'pain' can be very acute. In a small scale pilot study he worked with the assumption that successful homeopathic treatment would reduce the frequency and length of relapses and help the patients maintain abstinence or control consumption. Of the seven clients that received treatment all reported benefits. In the case studies included, the benefits to the individual of the homeopathic treatments are clearly outlined. One of the major benefits was an improvement of sleep patterns: a disturbed sleep pattern is often the most intractable problem after detoxification.

An example of homeopathic treatment of eczema is the use of petroleum, despite the knowledge that petrol and oil can cause cracks and itchiness in a person with sensitive skin exposed to them.

Hypnotherapy

Hypnosis appears to be a relatively recent phenomenon dating back to the late eighteenth century. Rhythmic dancing and drumming that induce similar state have a long history in Africa and North America and something closely resembling hypnosis can be traced back to ancient Egypt, Greece and the Druids in the UK. Hypnotherapy is the use of hypnotic techniques in the treatment of certain conditions. The trance-like state allows the individual to become more compliant, relaxed and open to suggestion. Suggestions are implanted that can be triggered after the individual has come out of the trance, but it is probably impossible to make anyone do something against their will. The individual is usually induced into a hypnotic state by the therapist. People can be taught to induce the state themselves to help with relaxation, and tapes can be used to aid this process.

There is no adequate explanation of how hypnotherapy works. It is thought that on hypnosis the individual enters a mental state between wakefulness and unconsciousness, and electroencephalograms (EEGs) taken on hypnotized subjects support this. Hypnotherapy can be particularly useful in the treatment of physical conditions where there may be a large psychological element such as eczema, psoriasis, migraine and colitis. Insomnia and phobias, obsessions, some addictions and compulsions, for example smoking, eating disorders, compulsive gambling, can benefit from hypnotherapy. Care is needed, however, for those with severe psychological health problems such as depression or psychosis as hypnosis can lead to further disturbance.

Therapeutic touch

Therapeutic touch dates from the 1960s. It works on the principle that imbalances and breaks in the flow of a vital energy can be corrected by a trained practitioner who is able to sense where there is depletion. Drawing energy from the environment through their body or from other areas in the patient where there is congestion, the therapist directs it into the area where it is lacking. Therapeutic touch postulates that in a healthy person there is an equilibrium between inward and outward energy flow. Health is a manifestation of the free flow of this energy through the body and ill health results when there are problems with this energy flow. Therapeutic touch practitioners claim to be able to attune themselves to this energy and to be able to help alter the flow to restore health.

The practice has four basic steps:

- centering, which is a form of meditation, finding inner peace;
- assessment to sense differences in energy flow – the hands are held apart, one each side of the patient's face and concentrating on the patient the practitioner scans the patient's energy field, moving the hands slowly towards their feet;
- treatment or rebalancing, in which the goal is to restore balance to the patient's energy field;
- evaluation to reassess the field for balance.

There are no known contraindications for therapeutic touch on

---

RESEARCH BASED EVIDENCE

A study conducted in 1995 found that hypnotherapy should be considered as a complementary treatment in dermatology (Stewart and Thomas, 1995). The participants, 18 adults and 20 children with extensive atopic dermatitis that had proved resistant to conventional therapy, were given hypnotherapy and their conditions were monitored for up to 18 months. All except one showed an immediate improvement after the first treatment and this was maintained at the following two clinic appointments.

A further study investigated the antiemetic effect of hypnosis for children receiving chemotherapy (Coanch et al., 1995). Children in the experimental group who were taught a self hypnosis technique reported a significant decrease in the frequency, severity, amount and duration of nausea.

DECISION MAKING

John, a 50-year-old community psychiatric nurse (CPN) was involved in a road traffic accident five years ago in which he sustained a 'whip-lash' injury to the neck. He had seemed to recover quickly from the acute injury, but was now suffering from chronic neck pain at night and after driving all day. Conventional analgesic drugs did not appear to help and John now considered the use of non-pharmaceu-

tical means of controlling his pain and discomfort. Using the information given in the above section and any further reading you may have done:
- *How would you advise John in his choice of the most suitable form of therapy for his particular problem?*
- *Identify other sources of advice that he may be able to access in order to make his choice.*

physiological grounds, but the apparent similarities between this and spiritual or psychic healing may offend people with deeply held beliefs. One of the first responses to therapeutic touch is relaxation, and it has been suggested that it affects the autonomic nervous system by reducing the sympathetic response (Mackey, 1995).

PROFESSIONAL KNOWLEDGE

This section explores the areas of decision making in relation to your future professional role in practice, specifically in relation to team work and the specialist role of the nurse. Legal and ethical areas are highlighted, but these are not exclusive and you should explore the multifaceted professional role further.

▶ ROLE OF THE NURSE IN RELATION TO PAIN

The UKCC's *Code of Professional Conduct* requires the nurse to 'act in such a way as to promote and safeguard the well-being and interests of patients and clients' (1992a). The nurse therefore has a responsibility to his or her patients and clients to increase their knowledge of pain and to use this knowledge in the implementation of pain care. A conceptual framework is necessary if the complexity of pain is to be understood. The basis for assessment and management of pain is provided when a theoretical position is taken, and this unlocks some of the mysteries of individual response (Stevens and Johnston, 1993).

The concept of the named nurse introduced in *The Patient's Charter* (Department of Health, 1991), has led to improved documentation and improved coordination of each patient's care (Davies and Davis, 1992; Royal College of Nursing, 1992). These are key areas in the pursuit of effective pain management.

Pain is a complex phenomenon involving physical, psychological, emotional and spiritual components. It is therefore vital that the nurse views each individual's situation holistically. The nurse's sphere of responsibility may be within a hospital or other establishment or more widely in the community. The role includes teaching the patient, administering medications and using non-pharmacological pain relief methods (McCaffery and Beebe, 1994). Nurses should also take into account their own views about pain as these influence the way we interact with others. It is difficult to look at our own fears, myths and prejudices honestly, but without this we risk misinterpreting the experience of others (Fordham and Dunn, 1994). It is therefore necessary to attempt to have a positive attitude to the person in pain and to accept overall what he or she is able to tell you about their pain.

In summary each individual nurse has many roles in the care of patients in pain. Figure 2.3.7 illustrates this multifaceted role and conceptualizes the discussion that has taken place.

RESEARCH BASED EVIDENCE

Experience seems to influence the nurse's approach to pain control. In one study it was identified that less experienced nurses infer greater pain and are therefore more likely to administer the prescribed analgesia (Mason, 1981).

A further problem identified by Walsh and Ford in 1989 is that nursing staff having preconceived ideas of how painful certain injuries should be and therefore how much analgesia they will allow the patient to have.

Another study has commented on the fact that nurses give less priority to the relief of pain than other nursing duties (Baillie, 1993).

Figure 2.3.7: The role of the nurse in pain management.

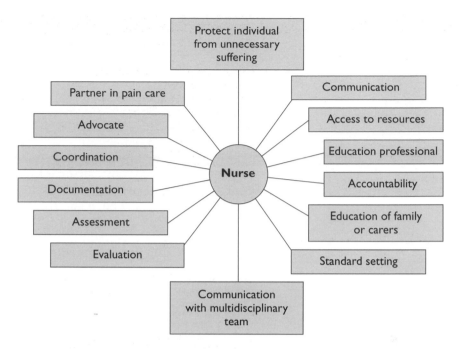

◗ THE MULTIDISCIPLINARY TEAM IN PAIN MANAGEMENT

The nurse works as part of a team. Usually this team is working towards a common goal for the promotion of the ultimate good of the patient or client. In pain control many team members may be involved. Commonly these include:

- the patient or client and their family, carers, or significant others;
- nurses – perhaps a specialist nurse with specific responsibility for pain management;
- doctors – anaesthetists with their specialized skills in relation to local and regional block analgesia;
- physiotherapists.

Frequently other individuals are involved in the pain care, particularly in cases of chronic or uncontrolled pain, for example:

- an occupational therapist;
- a pharmacist;
- a radiotherapist;
- a psychologist.

A complementary therapist, who may or may not be a nurse, may also be involved in the individual's pain care. Since the environment of care is commonly a hospital or the patient's home, the nurse is in the ideal position to act as the coordinator of the team approach to pain control. Thus the importance of effective communication is further highlighted.

The patient and their family or carers have a greater responsibility and control of the pain plan when the patient is cared for in the community. The patient and their family or carers must therefore be adequately prepared to carry out this responsibility. While in hospital patients adopt a routine that is part of the hospital environment, but in their own home they need the support to facilitate their abilities to deal effectively with their pain. The teaching role of the nurse is a major factor in ensuring the patient is able to manage at home.

All nurses have a role in health promotion in relation to the use and abuse of analgesic drugs by the public. Mild analgesics can be obtained without a medical prescription and can be overused for minor ailments. Prolonged and continued use can be detrimental to the long-term health of the individual. The public are often not aware of the 'hidden drug' element when advertising promotes a product under a user friendly name such as 'Night Nurse'. The actual content of analgesia within the drug may not be noticed. People have inadvertently overdosed themselves because of this problem.

Easy to obtain analgesics are often the most readily at hand when someone wishes to take an overdose, as in attempted suicide or deliberate self-harm (Davenport, 1993; Carrigan, 1994). The most dangerous drug in overdosage and also ironically one of the safest in its usual prescribed dose is paracetamol (Panadol). Because of its delayed effects on the liver a relatively small ingestion of this drug can have fatal consequences (see Chapter 1.4 for further information).

▶ THE ROLE OF THE SPECIALIST NURSE IN RELATION TO PAIN MANAGEMENT

The growth of the clinical nurse specialist role and specialist practitioners is a relatively recent phenomenon in the UK. Essentially this came about as a result of the UKCC's papers considering the future and scope of professional practice (UKCC, 1992b, 1994). The suggestion of these papers is to promote autonomous practice sensitive to changing health care needs. The development of the clinical nurse specialist stimulates the individual to become more involved in one area of nursing, applying their skills to identify problems and seek answers (McSharry, 1995). A study undertaken in England in 1996 showed that pain was one of the most common areas of specialist nursing practice (McGee *et al.*, 1996). This pain specialist nursing role within a hospital or community unit has often been instigated within a multidisciplinary team. The pain specialist nurse gives advice to both health care professionals and the public on the effective management of pain. Thus health education and research are primary functions of such a team. The specialist nurse is a key member of the team and advises nurses, carers and the public, often through a system of links with individual representatives of a ward or unit or patient representative group. Through 'link nurse' schemes difficult individual cases can be referred directly to the specialist nurse for advice. Such schemes also allow for updating of all health professionals on recent research-based evidence of practice (Elliott, 1995), such as pain management.

With the advanced nurse practitioner roles (Elliott, 1995) there is scope for further development of the nursing role to enhance the continuity of patient care (Gee, 1995). This could include activities such as defibrillation in resuscitation, intravenous cannulation or the prescribing of some analgesic drugs. Primary health care nurses have been able to give advice to patients in relation to pain relief for many years, but actually being able to legally prescribe a certain list of drugs is a new role for nurse practitioners in the UK. In 1986 the Cumberledge Report investigated the nursing services provided outside the hospital environment and the subsequent report highlighted how community care could be enhanced to produce improved client services. These findings were published in a report to the Secretary of State (Department of Health and Social Security,

Nurse prescribing in the UK is still being developed and remains a controversial issue for the nursing and medical profession.

- *Review the list of drugs related to pain relief that can be legally prescribed by the nurse practitioner and reflect on the additional educational needs of the nurse who is allowed to prescribe.*
- *Review the possible interprofessional issues that can arise as nurses become more involved in this 'extended' role.*
- *Decide whether this developing role of the nurse will be of benefit to the patient or client.*

1987). A suggestion was made that some nurses should be permitted to use their own judgement in matters of timing and dosage of drugs administered for the relief of pain. It was also suggested that a limited list of items and simple agents that could be prescribed by nurses as part of a programme of nursing care was established with detailed protocols and guidelines to control drug dosage in well-defined circumstances. Other government papers supported these recommendations (Department of Health, 1987; Social Security Services Committee, 1987). In 1989 *The Report of the Advisors Group on Nurse Prescribing* (Department of Health, 1989a) was published, which concluded that suitably qualified community nurses should be allowed to prescribe from a limited list of items and simple agents. A private member's bill was introduced to make legislative provision for the limited list and in 1992 it received royal assent. Nurses must receive appropriate training under the legislation to become a prescriber, the basis of which is safe and effective prescribing. Presently this role is limited to health visitors and some district nurses, but it seems likely that this will be expanded to include other nurse specialists and practitioners, depending upon the results of the pilot schemes that have been set up in eight sites throughout the UK. Changes in the health care environment are certain, but the nursing profession needs to be clear in its aims to produce an environment of care that is patient focused (Gee, 1995).

ETHICOLEGAL ISSUES IN PAIN MANAGEMENT

Thompson *et al.* (1988) suggest three models that the nurse may adopt in terms of professional role:

- code based ethics – related to a code of conduct under which most nurses operate;
- contractual ethics – usually apply where the patient or client approaches the carer before the start of treatment;
- covenantal ethics – apply to long-term situations such as palliative care.

Moral thinking is primarily a matter of reflecting on past experiences and predicting future consequences (Kenworthy *et al.*, 1992). The main moral dilemmas in pain management are often focused around the care of the dying (see Chapter 3.5, Professional Knowledge) and in the day to day decision making about adequate levels of analgesia.

Providing prompt and adequate management of pain relief for adults is now a widely accepted philosophy, but there are still misconceptions when it comes to managing a child's pain. Misconceptions about the effects of analgesia on children can seriously affect the care of children in pain. Controversies exist over the safety of pharmacological interventions (Stevens and Johnson, 1992). Specific reasons given for the undermedication of infants include the fear of addiction and respiratory depression and lack of knowledge concerning the physiological effects of opiates in the pain relief of infants (Craig, 1992; Stevens and Johnson, 1992).

The nurse must have a clear understanding of the ways in which children can experience and exhibit pain. Despite the child's limited ability to communicate we must recognize them as an authority about the nature and existence of their pain (McCaffery, 1977). A major role of the nurse must be to alleviate the child's pain. This complex task requires developmental, societal and professional knowledge and skills. From childhood

---

DECISION MAKING

Charles is a 60-year-old retired miner who has been diagnosed with lung cancer, has had surgery but now has symptoms of spread of the cancer to the spine. He has been discharged home to the care of the primary health care team. The district nurse has noted that Charles's pain, despite regular doses of morphine, is not being controlled adequately. The general practitioner has been reluctant to increase the drug dosage any further and stated that he 'considered the dosage adequate for the stage of the disease'.

- *Decide on how the district nurse should approach this situation if she is to remain accountable for providing Charles with adequate pain relief.*
- *Review the moral dilemma for the nurse if the general practitioner refuses to increase the dosage and review Charles's case in order to provide pain relief at this stage of his illness.*

---

we have experienced pain, located the source, avoided it and learned socially acceptable ways of expressing and reacting to it (Eland, 1985). A further factor that influences the nurses' medication practice is their ability to assess the level and intensity of a child's pain and then to intervene to manage that pain. Ideally the child should receive pain relief before they develop severe pain. The management of pain relief in children could and should be improved. The nurse has this responsibility in her professional role. With the arrival of *The Children Act* (Department of Health, 1989b), and the quality mechanisms of clinical areas that provide children's charters to improve the wellbeing and increase the rights of children in hospital, freedom from pain should become a priority.

The rights of all patients, adult or child, are for high quality care in all aspects of pain management. Nurses are accountable for their own individual level of knowledge, skills and attitudes. They will also, because of their position in the health care team, have a significant role in patient advocacy in relation to pain management (Mallik, 1994; Royal College of Nursing, 1995).

To make effective decisions in relation to the patient in pain the nurse requires knowledge and skills in the area of pain management. An understanding of the theories of pain and pain transmission is necessary to help conceptualize the experience for the patient. Nurses have an important part to play in pain management by individualizing the assessment of pain and acting as advocates for their patients. They should be proactive and anticipatory in the care and assessment of their patients' pain. Involving the individual, if possible, and his or her family or carers, in the assessment, management and evaluation of pain, and using a partnership approach will provide holistic and theory-based nursing care. To provide optimum care for your patient you must be aware of influences such as your own beliefs and values about pain, cultural norms, behaviours and stereotyping. This awareness should enable you to be less biased and lead to effective treatment of the patient's pain. Nurses have a responsibility to constantly improve and update their knowledge and skills in all areas of pain management.

▶ REFLECTION AND CONSOLIDATION

The experience you gain in practice placements is of vital importance to your learning about pain management. Keeping a reflective diary will help you isolate those experiences that are relevant to the knowledge base provided by this chapter and the further reading necessary to solve specific problems you have encountered. Reflective and decision-making exercises throughout the chapter should prompt you to take a reflective and questioning approach to your practice experience.

The following case studies will help you consolidate the knowledge gained from the chapter and further your reading and practice experience.

▶ CASE STUDY: ADULT

Miss Prudence Allison has been admitted for rehabilitative treatment after a fall at home. She has sustained a fractured right femur and a dislocation of her right shoulder. She has osteoporosis of the spine that has recently deteriorated. She has a great deal of pain and distress from this condition and she has frequently stated that she feels its time her life came to an end. She has been prescribed analgesia of dihydrocodeine (DF118) on a pro re nata (PRN) basis. She has now been hospitalized for four weeks and has developed a chest infection.

The nurse is not in a position to address Miss Allison's request to end her life, but should seek to interpret the reason why this request may have been made. Miss Allison is in continual pain and lately her injuries and now her chest infection have combined to cause her added distress and discomfort.

'Decisions about beginning or ending treatment should be based upon a consideration of the patients' rights and welfare' (Beauchamp and Childress, 1994). Social, educational, racial, gender, religious and family circumstances can impact upon the behaviour and attitudes of the patient. The nurse should be

aware of and able to judge the effect of these factors in assessing the patient and formulating the best approach to treatment. (See also the debates in Chapter 3.5, Professional Knowledge, to help you with this exercise.)

■ There are many areas within Miss Allison's care for an ethical debate. In the light of the information you have about Miss Allison, consider the request that she has made.

■ What might be the reason for this request?

■ How is your role as a nurse affected by the ethical and legal issues that surround this request?

■ What might be considered the difference between effective pain relief for Miss Allison and her request to end her suffering?

■ Miss Allison is suffering with her long-term condition. Consider the actions the nurse may be able to take to help Miss Allison cope more effectively with it?

■ What advice and resources may be available to Miss Allison to limit her pain?

▶ CASE STUDY: MENTAL HEALTH

Malique King is a 45-year-old man, of no fixed address with an itinerant lifestyle. He suffers from schizophrenia and is also an alcoholic. He has been brought into the accident and emergency department on several occasions in the last few weeks. He has usually been found collapsed in a drunken state in the street or park. Previously, despite attempts to refer Malique for appropriate mental health and medical consultation, he has disappeared from the department after a couple of hours. He has come into the department this evening of his own accord, smelling strongly of alcohol. He is dirty and unkempt and is complaining of 'bellyache'. His baseline observations of pulse and respiration are slightly elevated. The doctors have been informed, but they appear to believe that Malique is looking for a bed for the night. Malique has never complained of pain before when he has been brought into the department; in fact he has always appeared very unhappy at being in the department and has not been very communicative.

■ Consider the reasons why the doctors do not believe Malique's complaints of pain.

■ Consider the appropriate action that the nurse should take to assess Malique and to ensure his needs are met.

■ What are the grounds for these actions?

■ What are the responsibilities of the nurse?

■ Write a short account of your actions in relation to the theory that supports the accountability role of the nurse in this instance. This will help you to rationalize the decisions you have made in relation to Malique's needs.

▶ CASE STUDY: LEARNING DISABILITIES

Louise Freeman is 29 years old. She has cerebral palsy that arose as the result of trauma during her birth. She is quadriplegic with developmental delay and has very little communication, though is usually able to vocalize whether she is happy or sad. She has some difficulty swallowing and eating has always been difficult. She has been cared for at home by her elderly parents. Recently Louise has developed pressure sores on her buttocks and elbows and her parents are finding it increasingly difficult to maintain her normal eating pattern. She has been admitted to hospital to give some support to her parents and to assess the difficulty with feeding. She has recently lost weight and on admission she weighs 30 kg. Mrs Freeman tells you that she thinks Louise is not comfortable.

■ You need to be able to assess the level of Louise's pain so that you can make decisions to carry out appropriate nursing care. Find out what tools are available to you and if they are suitable to assess Louise's pain.

■ Consider the factors involved here so that the pain can be accurately assessed.

■ What members of the multidisciplinary team may be involved in Louise's pain care and why would they be included?

■ Louise is now able to return home. She has been prescribed pentazocine (Fortral) suppositories to help control her pain. Consider the information her parents will need about her analgesia to keep her pain under control.

■ Louise's mother is reluctant to give her the analgesic as she does not want her to be sleepy in the daytime. How would you explain to her the way that the drug works and its effects?

▶ CASE STUDY: CHILD

Jordan Simpson is 13 years old. He has sickle cell anaemia and has been admitted to the ward in crisis. Jordan is the eldest of five children and his mother Joan, who is a single parent, relies on him to help with the care of his brothers and sisters. Joan works in a local public house and in the evenings Jordan babysits. Joan has had trouble paying the bills and Jordan has been very worried about this. It is felt that this stress has brought on the current crisis.

On admission Jordan is in severe pain. He is quiet and uncommunicative. His facial expression is a grimace. His mother has accompanied him, but she needs to return home very shortly to collect her other children from school. PCA has been commenced with a morphine infusion.

■ **Consider the care decisions that have to be made to achieve optimum pain relief for Jordan.**

■ **Find out about sickle cell disease and the precipitating factors.**

■ **Are there any special observations to be made when Jordan is receiving morphine.**

■ **Make a decision about how you may be able to help Jordan and his family prevent further crises.**

■ **Consider the various roles of the nurse here to provide Jordan with appropriate care and support.**

▶ ANNOTATED FURTHER READING

CLUETT, E. (1994) Analgesia in labour: a review of the TENS method *Professional Care of Mother and Child* **4**(2): 50–52.
This article considers the use of TENS and potential theories of how it works in pain relief. Research studies are reviewed in relation to its effectiveness and why women like it. The findings appear to support the effectiveness of TENS for pain relief.

JARMEY, C., TINDALL, J. (1991) *Acupressure for common ailments.* London. Gaia Books Ltd.
A manual providing clear and concise information of acupressure for common ailments. The first part gives an overview of the concepts involved with simple techniques of acupressure. The second part gives clear instructions of which point to treat for some common ailments.

MACKEY, R.B. (1995) Discovering the healing power of therapeutic touch. *American Journal of Nursing* **95**(4): 27–32.
This useful article is written by a nurse educator who comments on her experience with therapeutic touch. There is a research section that corroborates its analgesic and healing attributes. This is written as a continuing education tool.

WATERS. J., THOMAS, V. (1995) Pain from sickle cell crisis. *Nursing Times* **91**(16): 29–31.
This article presents a qualitative study that explored perceptions and expectations of pain management of patients with sickle cell disease and nurses. The nurses contributed to poor pain control of sickle cell patients because of misconceptions about narcotic addiction, inadequate formal pain assessment and neglect of the psychosocial implications of this disease.

▶ REFERENCES

AKINSANYA, C.Y. (1985) The use of knowledge in the management of pain. *Nurse Education Today* **5**: 41–46.

ARMSTRONG, F., WALDRON, R. (1991) A complementary strategy. *Nursing Times* **87**(11): 34–35.

BAILLIE, L. (1993) A review of pain assessment tools. *Nursing Standard* **7**(23): 25–29.

BEAUCHAMP, T.L., CHILDRESS, J.F. (1994) *Principles of Biomedical Ethics* (4th edition). p. 199. Oxford. Oxford University Press.

BENDELOW, G. (1993) Pain perceptions, gender and emotion. *Sociology of Health and Illness* **15**(3): 273–294.

BENDELOW, G., WILLIAMS, S. (1995) Pain and the mind–body dualism: a sociological approach. *Body and Society* **1**(2): 83–103.

BEYER, J.E., BYERS, M.L. (1985) Knowledge of pediatric pain: the state of the art. *Children's Health Care* **13**(4): 422–424.

BISHOP, G. (1959) The relationship between nerve fibre size and sensory modality: Phylogenetic implications of the afferent innervation of the cortex. *Journal of Nervous and Mental Disorders* **128**: 89–114.

BISHOP, G. (1946) Neural mechanisms of cutaneous sense. *Physiology Review* **26**: 77–102.

BONICA, J.L. (1990) *The Management of Pain* (2nd edition). Philadelphia. Lea and Febiger.

BONICA, J.L. (1979) The need of a taxonomy. *Pain* **6**: 247–252.

BROOME, M.E., LILLIS, P.P. (1989) A descriptive analysis of pediatric pain management. *Applied Nursing Research* **2(2)**: 74–81.

BROOME, M.E., SLACK, J.F. (1990) Influences on nurses management of pain in children. *American Journal of Maternal Child Nursing* **15(3)**: 158–162.

BUCKINGHAM, S. (1993) Pain scales for toddlers. *Nursing Standard Supplement* **7(25)**: 12–13.

CARRIGAN, J.T. (1994) The psychsocial needs of patients who have attempted suicide by overdose. *Journal of Advanced Nursing* **20(4)**: 635–642.

CARROLL, D., BOWSHER, D. (1993) *Pain Management and Nursing Care.* Oxford. Butterworth–Heinemann.

CHARLESWORTH, W.R. (1982) An ethological approach to research on facial expressions. In Izard, C.E. (ed.) *Measuring Emotions in Infants and Children.* pp. 317–334. Cambridge. Cambridge University Press.

COANCH, P., HOCKENBERY, M., HERMAN, S. (1995) Self hypnosis as antiemetic therapy in children receiving chemotherapy. *Oncology Nursing Forum* **12(4)**: 41–46.

CRAIG, K.D. (1992) Pleasure and pain: A scientist/professional looks at organized psychology. *Canadian Psychology* **33(1)**: 45–60.

DARWIN (1794) cited in Dallenbach, K. (1939) Pain: history and present status. *Journal of Psychiatry* **52**: 331–347.

DAVENPORT, D. (1993) Structured support at a time of crisis: treatment of paracetamol overdose. *Professional Nurse* **8(9)**: 558–562.

DAVIES, J., DAVIS, J. (1992) Where naming cuts confusion. *Nursing Times* **88(37)**: 43–45.

DEPARTMENT OF HEALTH (1971) *Misuse of Drugs Act.* London. Her Majesty's Stationery Office.

DEPARTMENT OF HEALTH (1987) *Promoting Better Health.* London. Her Majesty's Stationery Office.

DEPARTMENT OF HEALTH (1989a) *The Report of the Advisors Group on Nurse Prescribing.* London. Her Majesty's Stationery Office.

DEPARTMENT OF HEALTH (1989b) *The Children Act.* London. Her Majesty's Stationery Office.

DEPARTMENT OF HEALTH (1991) *The Patient's Charter.* London. Her Majesty's Stationery Office.

DEPARTMENT OF HEALTH AND SOCIAL SECURITY (1987) *Neighbourhood Nursing – A Focus for Care. Report of the Community Nursing Review.* London. Her Majesty's Stationery Office.

DESCARTES, R. (1664/1972) *Treatise on Man* (M Foster Trans). Cambridge.

Harvard University Press.

DEVINE, T. (1990) Pain management in paediatric oncology. *Paediatric Nursing* **2(7)**: 11–13.

DOUTHIT, J.L. (1990) Psychosocial assessment and management of pediatric pain. *Journal of Emergency Nursing* **16(3)**: 168–170.

ELAND, J. (1985) The role of the nurse in children's pain. In Copp, L.A. (ed.) *Perspectives on Pain.* pp. 29–45. London. Churchill Livingstone.

ELAND, J., ANDERSON, J. (1977) The experience of pain in children. In Jacox, A.K. (ed.) *Pain: A Source Book for Nurses and Other Health Professionals.* pp. 453–473. Boston Little Brown and Co.

ELLIOTT, P.A. (1995) The development of advanced nursing practice. *British Journal of Nursing* **4(11)**: 633–636.

ELLIS, J.A. (1988) Using pain scales to prevent under medication. *American Journal of Maternal and Child Nursing* **13**: 180–182.

FORDHAM, M., DUNN, V. (1994) *Alongside the Person in Pain. Holistic Care and Nursing Practice.* London. Baillière Tindall.

GEE, K. (1995) Competency through being the enemy within? *British Journal of Nursing* **4(11)**: 637–640.

GILLIES, M.L. (1993) Post-operative pain in children: a review of the literature. *Journal of Clinical Nursing* **2**: 5–10.

GILLIES, M.L., PARRY–JONES, W.L., SMITH, L.N. (1995) The pain we overlook: postoperative pain in children under five years. *Child Health* **3(1)**: 31–33.

HAWLEY, D. (1984) Postoperative pain in children: misconceptions, descriptions and interventions *Pediatric Nursing* **10**: 20–23.

HELMAN, C. (1990) *Culture Health and Illness* (2nd edition). London. Wright.

JANAL, M.N., COLT, E.W.D., CLARK, W.C., GLUSMAN, M. (1984) Pain sensitivity, mood and plasma endocrine levels in man following long distance running: effects of naloxone. *Pain* **19**: 13–25.

JESSEL–KENYON, J., CHENG NI BLOTT, B., HOPWOOD, V. (1992) Studies with acupuncture using a SQUID bio-magnetometer: a preliminary report. *Complementary Medical Research* **6(3)**: 142–151.

KANITSAKI, O. (1993) Acute health care and Australia's ethnic people. *Contemporary Nurse* **2**: 122–127.

KENWORTHY, N., SNOWLEY, G., GILLING, C. (eds) (1992) *Common Foundation Studies in Nursing.* Edinburgh. Churchill Livingstone.

KNAPP–SPOONER, C., KARLIK, B.A., PONTIERI–LEWIS, V., YARCHESKI, A. (1995) Efficacy of patient-controlled analgesia in women cholecystectomy patients. *International Journal of Nursing Studies* **32(5)**: 434.

LATHAM, J. (1991) *Pain Control* (2nd edition). London. Mosby.

LIPTON, J.A., MARBACH, J.J. (1984) Ethnicity and the pain experience *Social Science and Medicine* **19(12)**: 1279–1298.

LIVINGSTONE, W. (1943) *The Mechanism of Pain.* New York. Macmillan.

LLOYD–THOMAS, A.R. (1990) Pain management in paediatric patients. *British Journal of Anaesthesia* **64**: 85–104.

MACKEY, R.B. (1995) Discover the healing power of therapeutic touch. *American Journal of Nursing* **95(4)**: 27–32.

MALLIK, M. (1994) An impossible ideal? The role of the child advocate *Child Health* **2(3)**: 105–109.

MARSHALL, H. (1894) *Pain, Pleasure and Aesthetics.* London. Macmillian.

MATHER, L., MACKIE, J. (1983) The incidence of post-operative pain in children. *Pain* **15**: 271–283.

MASON, D.J. (1981) Investigation of the influence of selected factors on nurses' inferences of patient suffering. *International Journal of Nursing Studies* **18(4)**: 251–259.

MAY, L. (1992) Reducing pain and anxiety in children. *Nursing Standard* **6(44)**: 25–28.

McBRIDE, M. (1977) Can you tell me where it hurts? *Pediatric Nursing* **3(4)**: 7–8.

McCONNAN, L. (1992) Measuring a child's pain. *The Canadian Nurse* **88(6)**: 20–22.

McCAFFERY, M. (1972) *Nursing Management of the Patient in Pain.* Philadelphia. Lippincott.

McCAFFERY, M. (1977) Pain relief for the child. *Pediatric Nursing* **3(4)**: 11–16.

McCAFFERY, M. (1983) *Nursing the Patient in Pain.* London. Harper and Row.

McCAFFERY, M., BEEBE, A. (1989) *Pain Clinical Manual for Nursing Practice.* St Louis. The CV Mosby Company.

McCAFFERY, M., BEEBE, A. (1994) *Pain Clinical Manual for Nursing Practice,* UK edition. London. The CV Mosby Company.

McCREADY, M., MacDAVITT, K., O'SULLIVAN, K. (1991) Children and pain. Easing the hurt. *Orthopaedic Nursing* **10(6)**: 33–42.

McGEE, P., CASTLEDINE, G., BROWN, R. (1996) Survey of specialist and advanced nursing practice in England. *British Journal of Nursing* **5(11)**: 682–686.

McGRATH, P.A. (1989) Evaluating a child's pain. *Journal of Pain and Symptom Management* **4(4)**: 198–214.

McSHARRY, M. (1995) The evolving role of the clinical nurse specialist. *British Journal of Nursing* **4(11)**: 641–646.

MEINHART, N.T., McCAFFERY, M.

(1983) *Pain: A Nursing Approach to Assessment and Analysis.* p. 195. East Norwalk CT. Appleton and Lange.

MELZACK, R. (1978) Pain mechanisms recent research. *Acupuncture Electrotherapy Research Journal* **3**: 109–112.

MELZACK, R. (1981) Current concepts of pain. In Saunders, C., Summers, D.H., Teller, N. (eds) *Hospice: The Living Idea.* London. Edward Arnold.

MELZACK, R., WALL, P. (1965) Pain mechanisms: a new theory. *Science* **150**: 971–979.

MELZACK, R., WALL, P. (1973) Psychophysiology of pain. *International Anaesthesiology Clinics* **8**: 3–34.

MELZACK, R., WALL, P. (1982) *The Challenge of Pain (Volume 1).* London. Penguin.

MELZACK, R., WALL, P. (1988) *The Challenge of Pain (Volume 2).* London. Penguin.

MERSKEY, H. (1970) On the development of pain. *Headache* **10**: 116–123.

NORDENBOS, W. (1959) *Pain.* Amsterdam. Elsevier.

PARSONS, E.P. (1992) Cultural aspects of pain. *Surgical Nurse* **5(2)**: 14–16.

PRICE, S. (1990) Pain: its experience, assessment and management in children. *Nursing Times* **86(9)**: 42–45

PUNTILLO, K.A. (1988) The phenomenon of pain and critical care nursing. *Heart and Lung* **17(3)**: 262–272.

ROGERS, J. (1995) Remedy of detox. *Nursing Times* **91(38)**: 44–46.

ROYAL COLLEGE OF NURSING (1992) *The Named Nurse: Implications for Practice. Paper 14 Issues in Nursing.* London. Royal College of Nursing.

ROYAL COLLEGE OF NURSING (1995) *Advocacy and the Nurse. Paper 22 – Issues in Nursing.* London. Royal College of Nursing.

SOCIAL SECURITY SERVICES COMMITTEE (1987) *Report on Primary Health Care.* London. Her Majesty's Stationery Office.

STEVENS, B. (1990) Development and testing of a pediatric pain management sheet. *Pediatric Nursing* **16(6)**: 543–548.

STEVENS, B., JOHNSTON, C. (1992) Assessment and management of pain in infants. *The Canadian Nurse* **88**: 31–34.

STEVENS, B., JOHNSTON, C.C. (1993) Pain in the infant: theoretical and conceptual issues. *Maternal Child Nursing Journal* **21(1)**: 3–14.

STEVENS, B., HUNSBERGER, M., BROWNE, G. (1987) Pain in children. Theoretical, research and practice dilemmas. *Journal of Pediatric Nursing* **2(3)**: 154–166.

STEVENSEN, C.J. (1994) The psychophysiological effects of aromatherapy massage following cardiac surgery. *Complementary Therapies in Medicine* **2**: 27–35

STEWART, A.C., THOMAS, S.E. (1995) Hypnotherapy as a treatment for atopic dermatitis in adults and children. *British Journal of Dermatology* **132(5)**: 778–783.

THOMPSON, I.E., MELIA, K.M., BOYD, K.M. (1988) *Nursing Ethics* (2nd edition). Edinburgh. Churchill Livingstone.

TREVELYAN, J., BOOTH, B. (1994) *Complementary Medicine for Nurses, Midwives and Health Visitors*, p. 62.

London. Macmillan.

UKCC (1996) *Guidelines for Professional Practice.* p. 33. London. UKCC.

UKCC (1994) *The Future of Professional Practice: The Council's Standards For Education and Practice Following Registration.* London. UKCC.

UKCC (1992a) *Code of Professional Conduct* (3rd edition). London. UKCC.

UKCC (1992b) *The Scope of Professional Practice.* London. UKCC.

WACHTER-SHIKORA, N.L. (1981) Pain theories and their relevance to the pediatric population. *Comprehensive Pediatric Nursing* **5**: 321–326.

WAKEFIELD, A.B. (1995) Pain: an account of nurses' talk. *Journal of Advanced Nursing* **21(5)**: 905–910.

WALKER, A.C., TAN, L., GEORGE, S. (1995) Impact of culture on pain management: an Australian nursing perspective. *Holistic Nurse Practitioner* **9(2)**: 48–57.

WALL, P.D., MELZACK, R. (1989) *Textbook of Pain.* Edinburgh. Churchill Livingstone.

WALSH, M., FORD, P. (1989) It can't hurt that much! *Nursing Times* **85(42)**: 35–38.

WELLS, N. (1984) Responses to acute pain and the nursing implications. *Journal of Advanced Nursing* **9**: 51–58.

ZBOROWSKI, M. (1952) Cultural components in response to pain. *Journal of Social Issues* **8**: 16–30.

ZOLA, I. (1966) Culture and symptoms: an analysis of patients' presenting complaints. *American Sociological Review* **31**: 615–630.

2.4 Skin Integrity

K. Lewis and L. Roberts

KEY ISSUES

■ SUBJECT KNOWLEDGE
- structure and function of the skin
- ageing and the skin
- wound healing processes
- importance of appearance
- cultural influences related to skin care and adornment

■ PRACTICE KNOWLEDGE
- assessment of the skin
- assessment and management of a person with a wound
- evaluation of the effectiveness of wound management
- management of acute and chronic wounds

■ PROFESSIONAL KNOWLEDGE
- nurse's role in promoting skin health
- nurse's role in developing and maintaining quality systems of care
- continuing education in relation to skin integrity
- role of the nurse specialist
- skin integrity and the scope of professional practice

■ REFLECTIVE KNOWLEDGE
- developing research-based expertise
- involvement in nurse-led initiatives
- reflective diary
- developing decision-making skills

▶ INTRODUCTION

The skin or integument is a major organ of the body, providing a barrier between the internal and external environments. It is also an organ that is highly visible to others, and therefore any damage, alteration or deformity in its structure can cause not only physical, but also psychological, social and environmental problems. Skin integrity is concerned with the maintenance of this barrier in its optimum condition.

The aim of this chapter is to provide the requisite knowledge and decision-making skills to enable the nurse, within the limitations of his or her role, to nurse patients with skin problems. It also intends to help the nurse to reflect on current practice relating to skin care and maintaining their own skin health.

▶ OVERVIEW

▶ Subject Knowledge

The biological section covers basic anatomy and physiology of the skin. The level addressed is related to the knowledge you need in order to understand and apply the information that appears in this chapter. A more in-depth knowledge can be gained by reading specific anatomy and physiology books. The process of skin healing will be explored.

The importance of appearance and its effect on self-image is highlighted in the psychosocial section. Cultural influences are included and you are encouraged to reflect on how your own self-image is at times affected by your appearance.

▶ *Practice Knowledge*

Assessment of the skin is discussed. The knowledge, skills and understanding required to assess, plan, implement and evaluate the care of patients with wounds are addressed in broad terms. This is followed by a more in-depth discussion of the management of three common types of wound.

▶ *Professional Knowledge*

The contribution of nurses to the development of quality systems of care relating to skin integrity is explored. The need for and opportunities available to nurses in the development of their knowledge and expertise in relation to different aspects of skin care are examined. The roles of different specialist nurses who may be called upon to give expert help to patients with different problems relating to skin integrity are outlined.

▶ *Reflective Knowledge*

In this section you are encouraged to learn from your practice experience by keeping a journal of the types of skin conditions and wounds you see in practice.

Consolidation of your learning from the chapter and from practice experience is achieved through completing decision-making exercises based on four case studies.

On pp. 277–279 there are four case studies, each one relating to one of the branch programmes. You may find it helpful to read one of them before you start the chapter and use it as a focus for your reflections while reading.

SUBJECT KNOWLEDGE
Biological

The skin is one of the largest organs in the body. An adult's skin covers an area of about 2 m^2 and weighs approximately 3 kg. Every square centimetre of skin contains approximately 125 sweat glands, 25 sebaceous glands, 250 nerve endings, 50 sensors to pain, pressure, heat and cold, approximately 1 m of blood vessels, and millions of cells. Skin is made up of three main structures (Figure 2.4.1):

- ▶ the epidermis or outer layer;
- ▶ the dermis or base layer;
- ▶ the skin appendages such as hairs, nails and glands.

These structures are also termed the integumentary system.

▶ EPIDERMIS

The epidermis is the outer or cuticle layer of the skin, and consists of several layers of cells. It contains no blood vessels or nerve endings and its main function is to protect the underlying dermis. It has four or five different layers of cells depending on its location. From the deepest to the most superficial these are:

- ▶ stratum basale (or germinating layer);
- ▶ stratum spinosum;
- ▶ stratum granulosum;
- ▶ stratum lucidum (not present on hairy skin);
- ▶ stratum corneum (or cornified layer).

Figure 2.4.1: Skin section. (Adapted from Cull, 1989.)

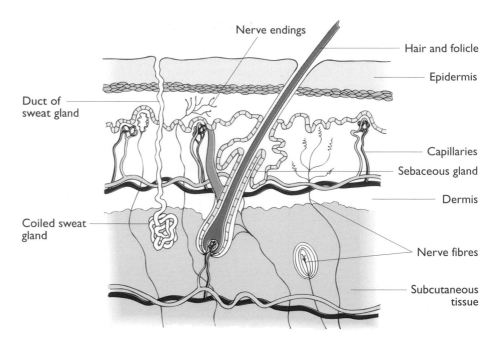

The cells in the stratum basale undergo mitosis and reproduce themselves. This enables the skin to repair itself when injured, and ensures an effective barrier against infection. As new cells are produced they migrate to the surface of the skin. During this movement the cells' normal cytoplasm is replaced by keratin, a waterproof substance, which gives the external layer of skin, the stratum corneum, its tough protective quality.

The majority of the epidermis is made up of keratinocytes, the cells that produce the outer surface of the skin. Scattered among these cells are two other types of cells known as melanocytes and Langerhans' cells.

Melanocytes are responsible for producing melanin, which produces the skin's pigmentation or colouring. White- and black-skinned people have the same number of melanocytes per unit of surface area, but in black-skinned people the melanocytes are more active and produce pigment at a faster rate. Melanin protects other cells of the skin against the damaging effects of strong sunlight. Exposure of the skin to the sun stimulates the melanocytes to produce more melanin. This reaction causes the characteristic darkening of the skin (suntanning). Black-skinned people are therefore better protected against the sun's ultraviolet rays.

Overexposure to sunlight can cause sunburn and skin cancers such as malignant melanomas and non-melanotic skin cancers (NMSC), primarily basal cell and squamous cell cancers. The number of people developing skin cancers in England has been rising rapidly in recent years (Table 2.4.1). Half of the people who develop malignant melanoma die as a result (Department of Health, 1993a, p. 24).

Langerhans' cells are thought to be important in the body's immune responses. They absorb small particles of foreign material such as nickel in jewellery and are responsible for setting up the allergic reaction common in contact allergic eczema (dermatitis). The resultant rash usually clears up within one week following removal of the irritant once it has been identified. The key to managing this condition in the long term lies in identifying and avoiding contact with the allergen.

	Malignant melanoma	NMSC
1980	1827	18 965
1981	1952	20 035
1982	1990	19 742
1983	2080	20 981
1984	2083	20 892
1985	2494	21 994
1986	2635	25 265
1987	2936	24 604

Table 2.4.1 Skin cancer incidence in England 1980–1987 (Department of Health, 1993a, p. 24).

DERMIS

The dermis is the deepest layer of the skin. It is composed mainly of connective tissue and contains fewer cells than the epidermis, the main ones being fibroblasts, which produce collagen, a protein that attaches the skin layers to the rest of the body with tiny elastic fibres. These fibres give the skin its suppleness and ability to stretch. The upper part of the dermis contains rows of projections known as dermal papillae, which bind the two layers of skin together at the dermal–epidermal junction. The dermis contains a good blood supply and is responsible for nourishing and maintaining the epidermis, which does not have its own blood supply. The dermis also contains sensory receptors to heat, cold, touch and pain.

GLANDS

Three types of glands are present in the skin:

- sebaceous or oil glands secrete an oily substance known as sebum, which lubricates and protects hair and skin;
- sudoriferous or sweat glands assist in the regulation of body temperature through evaporation;
- ceruminous glands produce cerumen or wax, which is found within the outer ear where it protects the ear by preventing the entry of foreign bodies.

Information on hair and nails can be found in Chapter 3.1 on hygiene care.

FUNCTIONS OF THE SKIN

The skin has five main functions.

Regulation of Temperature

The production of sweat by the sudoriferous glands during hot weather helps reduce the body temperature through a process of evaporation. Changes in blood flow also occur. During hot weather peripheral blood vessels dilate, enabling heat loss by radiation. Conversely, in cold weather peripheral blood vessels constrict in order to maintain vital organs at an optimum temperature for functioning (see Chapter 2.2 on homeostasis).

Protection

The skin provides a physical barrier against harm, protecting the underlying tissues from abrasion and bacterial invasion. The melanin prevents damage from the sun's ultraviolet rays and the waterproof quality of the skin stops excessive loss of body fluid.

Excretion

Sweat contains water, salts, urea, ammonia and several other compounds. During sweating small amounts of these substances are excreted.

Stimuli Reception

The skin contains many different types of receptors. The most common are receptors to temperature, pain and touch. These provide information about the external environment.

▶ Synthesis of Vitamin D

The skin aids in the synthesis of vitamin D. The precursor to vitamin D, 7-dehydrocholesterol, is present in the skin and is converted to chole-calciferol in the presence of ultraviolet light. After further conversion in the liver and then the kidneys, 1,25-dihydroxycalciferol is produced. This aids in the absorption of calcium from the dietary intake.

▶ AGEING AND THE SKIN

During an individual's life span, changes occur in the physical properties of the skin. In order to maintain a healthy skin different requirements must be met at different stages of an individual's life. For instance during infancy the skin is delicate and until the child is continent the skin requires protection from the damaging effects of urine and faeces. Similarly, during adolescence skin changes result in increased perspiration and oil production, sometimes leading to the development of acne.

During pregnancy there is an increase in activity of the sebaceous glands and melanocytes, resulting in increased oil production and patches of darker pigmentation on the skin – commonly linea nigra, which is a pigmented line down the abdomen, and chloasma, which are darker areas on the face often referred to as the 'mask of pregnancy'. Although the skin has the ability to stretch, during pregnancy the increase in size of the abdomen can be so great that the collagen fibres rupture, leaving visible scars. These are known as striae gravidarum or 'stretch marks'.

In old age, the production of cells slows down and they become smaller and thinner. The collagen and elastic fibres lose their shape and elasticity, and the amount of fat stored in the subcutaneous tissues lessens, resulting in skin wrinkles. There is a decrease in the number and an increase in the size of active melanocytes, producing concentrated areas of pigment commonly known as liver spots. There is also a reduction in the amount of intracellular fluid resulting in dry skin, which can lead to itching or 'senile pruritus', and increased skin fragility. The use of moisturisers or emollients can help to prevent excessive flakiness of skin.

For many people the desire to preserve a youthful complexion brings with it the necessity of a continued battle against the ageing process. Although creams and lotions may result in a superficial improvement in skin texture, prevention is obviously better, and protection of the skin against sun damage from an early age is of great benefit. Collagen injections, drugs such as tretinoin and surgical interventions such as a 'face lift' are effective but non-permanent ways of improving the skin's appearance as the ageing process will continue (Tortora and Anagnostakos, 1990)

▶ SKIN HEALING

Should the skin become cut or damaged, creating a wound, the process of healing has four distinct phases:

▶ coagulation;
▶ inflammation;

Trevelyan (1996) highlights the different skin care requirements of different groups of individuals, for example, infants, older people and different ethnic minority groups.

- *Reflect back on clients you have nursed who fall into the above groups and compare individual skin care requirements, accounting for any differences.*

DECISION MAKING

Liza Gordon is an 18-year-old student who enjoys holidays abroad with her friends. She has been admitted to the day care ward for a biopsy of a 'suspicious' mole, which turned out to be benign. Liza is very concerned about her appearance and is anxious to protect her skin against sun damage and the long-term effects of ageing.

- *What skin care advice would you give to Liza before discharge?*
- *Read chapter 5 of Health Promotion. Foundations for Practice (Naidoo and Wills, 1994) in which the authors discuss the five approaches to health promotion (i.e. medical, behavioural change, educational, empowerment and social change). Which approach do you consider would be most effective in helping Liza to maintain skin health in the long term?*

> ▶ regeneration;
> ▶ maturation.

Skin heals by primary or secondary intention.

▶ *Primary Intention*

This type of healing occurs when the edges of the wound are opposed, as in a surgical incision. Healing tends to be rapid due to the close proximity of the wound edges (Figure 2.4.2), and involves:

> ▶ coagulation – within eight hours following surgery the cut surfaces become inflamed, a blood clot fills the incision track, and phagocytes and fibroblasts migrate into the area;
> ▶ inflammation – phagocytes begin to break down the clot and cell debris and collagen fibres are produced by the fibroblasts and begin to bind the two surfaces together;
> ▶ regeneration – after 3–4 days epithelial cells spread across the incision track, the section of clot above the new cells becomes a scab, the clot in the incision track is absorbed, and myofibroblasts draw the edges of the wound together by a process of contraction;
> ▶ maturation – epithelial cells continue to be laid down until the full thickness of skin is restored.

▶ *Secondary Intention*

This type of healing occurs where there is a significant loss of tissue or where the skin edges are not opposed, as in an ulcer. Healing tends to be slower, but the exact time will depend on the extent of the damage (Figure 2.4.3). It involves:

> ▶ coagulation – the surface of the wound becomes acutely inflamed and phagocytes start to break down the necrotic tissue;
> ▶ inflammation – granulation tissue develops at the base of the wound and starts to grow up towards the wound surface;
> ▶ regeneration – phagocytosis causes the necrotic tissue to separate, exposing a new layer of epidermal cells, and there is contraction to reduce the size of the wound (as wound contraction is a normal process, it is important not to pack the wound with dressings unless specifically indicated, for example for a wound sinus, as it interferes with this process);

Figure 2.4.2: Wound healing by primary intention. The wound edges are in close proximity (often brought together by sutures). Healing occurs rapidly along the length of the wound.

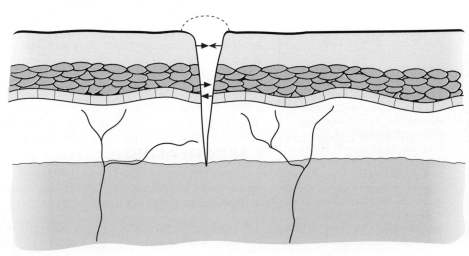

Figure 2.4.3: Wound healing by secondary intention. The wound edges are distanced due to crater formation. Healing is slower and begins at the bottom of the crater.

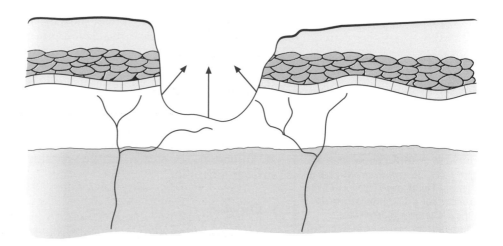

 ▶ maturation – when granulation tissue fills the wound cavity and reaches the level of the dermis epithelial cells migrate across the wound towards the centre, forming a single layer of cells. Epithelialization continues until full-thickness skin is restored.

▶ THE OPTIMUM ENVIRONMENT FOR WOUND HEALING

A variety of factors need to be present to create the optimum environment for wound healing to take place. These include:

 ▶ a good blood supply;
 ▶ optimum temperature;
 ▶ moisture;
 ▶ oxygen;
 ▶ freedom from contaminants and necrotic tissue.

▶ *Blood Supply*

Healing requires an integral blood supply to provide oxygen and nutrients to the developing cells. Reconstitution of the blood supply is termed angiogenesis and occurs during the regeneration phase of healing. Care must be taken not to disturb this process by inappropriately using dressings, for example dry dressings such as gauze can stick to wound beds, resulting in trauma when they are removed.

▶ *Temperature*

The optimum temperature for human cell growth is 37°C. Wounds kept at a constant temperature of 37°C will heal faster than those exposed to thermal shock (i.e. extreme changes in temperature). To keep wounds at a constant temperature unnecessary wound cleansing and dressing changes should be avoided.

▶ *Moisture*

The exudate produced by a wound contains nutrients, enzymes and growth factors that can aid the healing process. Lytic enzymes found in the exudate autolyse (break down) any necrotic tissue present, and growth factors increase the development rate of cells and result in less scarring.

A moist wound environment facilitates wound healing, reduces the amount of tissue inflammation, produces less scarring and results in less pain for the patient. If the wound is allowed to dry out, a scab or eschar forms. This impedes cell migration and consequently slows down the healing process. Excessive exudate may indicate that the wound is remaining in the inflammatory stage, which may suggest the presence of infection. It needs to be contained to prevent damage to the surrounding skin.

Oxygen

All cells require oxygen in order to develop and mature. Therefore, an integral blood supply is essential to ensure that cells receive an adequate oxygen supply in order to remain viable. The external administration of oxygen to the wound site, for example via an oxygen mask and tubing, will not benefit tissue perfusion, but will dry the wound site and delay wound healing.

Freedom from Contaminants and Necrotic Tissue

The presence of foreign bodies and dead or devitalized tissue delay wound healing and provide a focus for infection, which will in turn also delay wound healing.

RESEARCH BASED EVIDENCE

There is some debate on whether occlusive or semi-occlusive dressings are more effective for moist wound healing. Pandit and Feldman (1994) carried out a study comparing the efficacy of oxygen-permeable dressings with oxygen-impermeable dressings. The findings suggested that treatment with oxygen-impermeable dressings is more effective in the early stages of healing, but that once granulation has started to take place, oxygen-permeable dressings perform considerably better. It should be noted that this study was carried out on animal specimens. (See also Annotated Further Reading – Proven and Phillips, 1991; Kerstein, 1995.)

Psychosocial

THE IMPORTANCE OF APPEARANCE

Physical appearance is important to most people. As the skin is visible to others, its condition often influences how an individual feels about him or herself. People who feel attractive often feel positive about themselves.

Images in the media of suntanned, high profile individuals such as fashion models may help to encourage the idea that a suntan is both healthy and desirable. Accordingly, suntanned skin can promote a sense of psychological wellbeing. Therefore, despite current health education concerning the dangerous effects of ultraviolet light, sunbathing – either in natural or artificial sunlight – remains a popular pastime. The Department of Health (1993b, p. 67) recognizes the need to 'secure an alteration in people's attitude to a tanned appearance' in order to reduce the incidence of skin cancer. It is necessary to address the conflict between the improvement to psychological health and its detrimental effect on an individual's physical health. Gross (1992, p. 532) examines Festinger's theory of cognitive dissonance. Cognitive dissonance is a state of 'psychological discomfort and tension' caused by a person knowing that an action may cause harm, but at the same time participating in that action. Gross puts forward a way of choosing between two activities that are equally attractive that involves highlighting the undesirable features of each activity in order to help with the decision-making process. Although this may help in deciding whether or not to sunbathe it must be acknowledged that an individual may still decide that the psychological benefits of sunbathing are more important and therefore continue the activity.

You may wish to extend your personal reflection here into a debate with your fellow students on the choices to be made.

- **Is an individual's psychological or physical health more important?**
- **If it is necessary to make one dimension of health a priority which would take priority for you at a personal level? Justify your decision.**

Although the nurse should aim towards holistic care there are times in a person's life when choices have to be made. The nurse has an important role in helping the individual decide whether the psychological or the physical dimension of health should take priority.

Just as a healthy skin can help to promote a positive self-image, a skin disorder can have a detrimental effect. For thousands of years skin disorders have often been regarded as unclean: lepers, for instance, have often been treated as social outcasts. It may be argued that certain more common skin disorders continue to evoke a less than compassionate reaction nowadays, particularly those that are visible such as eczema. The impact of a skin disorder on a person's self-image can depend very much on the individual's ability to cope with it. If the disorder affects the person's ability to carry out and meet their self-care needs or if it causes stress to the individual or the family, it can seriously undermine their self-regard. The disorder can come to be viewed in a way that is out of all proportion to the problem itself and overshadow the individual's entire life.

> Think back to a time when you developed something as innocuous as a pimple on your face before an important social function.
> * *How did it make you feel?*
> * *How did it affect your self-image?*
> * *Did anyone else even notice it?*

▶ SELF-IMAGE

It is important to understand that the nurse's approach can have a significant effect on how the client responds to a skin disorder. Any signs of disgust, alarm or even fear may encourage the client to view their condition as offensive to others. Furthermore, the nurse needs to be aware of any signals that may be conveyed to the client. With thought the nurse can project and encourage a more positive self-image. If the skin disorder is not infectious and does not require the use of gloves when handling, the client's self-image can be enhanced if the nurse touches the affected area with unprotected hands. In addition, the client will benefit from being able to discuss any feelings about the condition with both relatives and the nurse. Moreover, a simple explanation of the aetiology (cause), and prognosis (probable course) of the condition may help the client to accept it. Some conditions of the skin, for example burns, ulcerations and extensive surgery, can cause great distress to both the client and the nurse. In order to help the client accept the condition, the nurse will first need to come to terms with it him or herself.

> * *Are there times when a nurse should be able to say that he or she is unable to cope with the nursing care of a particular patient or should nurses be able to nurse any patient with any condition?*
> * *If forced to care, how do you think this could affect the therapeutic relationship between the nurse and patient?*

▶ EXPOSURE THERAPY

There are two distinct ways of helping a client come to terms with any bodily disfigurement – gradual exposure and confrontation (see the section on desensitization in Chapter 4.1 where the terms 'graded exposure' and 'flooding' are used),

▶ *Gradual Exposure*

This is a process by which a client is gradually exposed to a disfigurement over an extended period of time in order to give him or her time to accept it. In the case of a patient who has undergone a mastectomy, for instance, the patient can first of all be shown the dressing so that she can get used to the size of the wound. The dressing can then be removed and the patient given time to come to terms with the appearance of the wound. This gradual exposure continues at a rate with which the patient can cope. It has been argued, however, that the gradual exposure of a disfigurement subconsciously compounds the view that it is offensive to others.

▶ *Confrontational*

The confrontational approach proposes that the patient should be encouraged to come to terms with the disfigurement quickly and that such an approach is in the long term less traumatic. The confrontational approach aims to encourage a frank and open technique with exposure taking place as quickly as the patient can tolerate (Marks, 1987). It can be argued, however, that patients need more time to adapt to physical change. Moreover, nursing and medical staff may be unable to provide the degree of support necessary if the patient has to adjust rapidly to a new body image.

▶ CULTURE AND APPEARANCE

Different cultures have very different approaches to and ideas about physical appearance. What is considered to be attractive in one culture may be regarded as physically unattractive in another. While a sun-tanned appearance may be desirable in western culture, some eastern cultures, notably Japan, may favour an altogether paler complexion. The traditional 'geisha' look was originally achieved using face whitening powder from dried nightingale droppings.

> Think of people you know who come from different cultures or alternatively collect together pictures of people from different cultures.
>
> • *Which do you consider to be the more attractive and why?*

Some cultures use skin decoration to produce the opposite effect. The Tuareg paint their skin with turmeric to make themselves less desirable and therefore less vulnerable to evil spirits. In Ethiopia, the Surma women insert clay discs into their lower lip to cause it to protrude. This is thought to have been first done to make the women less desirable to slave traders.

Beauty is a matter of subjective judgement (i.e. 'beauty is in the eye of the beholder'). To some extent, the skin plays an important part in the perception of an individual's attractiveness, and for hundreds of years has been decorated in many ways to enhance or diminish its appeal.

▶ SKIN ADORNMENT

▶ *Cosmetics*

These are used to accentuate attractive facial features and disguise imperfections. In many cultures they have religious significance, for example in Hindu society three stripes painted across the forehead signifies a holy devotee of the Lord Shiva (Jacobson, 1992)

▶ *Decorative Tattoos*

These have developed from ancient origins and are often related to religious ceremonies and marriage rites. Tattoos involve staining the skin using coloured pigments and should be considered permanent. They often result in stereotyping the wearer and several articles highlight the problems wearers come up against (Armstrong, 1991; Anonymous, 1992; Litt,

---

DECISION MAKING

During a trip to the seaside, Mandy, a student nurse aged 18, had a large tattoo put onto her right upper forearm. The tattoo is of a large red heart with the name of her current boyfriend etched through the centre. She did not tell anyone of her intention to do this. The tattooed area is very sore and Mandy is a little concerned about how she will cope on night duty that evening.

- *Decide on the possible short- and long-term implications of Mandy's actions.*

- *The next morning Mandy is very tearful and regretful and as you come on duty she takes you on one side and asks you what she can do about the tattoo. What advice would you give her?*
- *How do you think patients may react to Mandy given that they may have particular views of what is acceptable in the visual appearance of nurses?*

1994). During the 1990s the number of people with tattoos has risen sharply as they became a fashion accessory for both males and females. Most noticeable was the increase in the number of adolescents having tattoos (Armstrong and McConnell, 1994). As a result there was a corresponding increase in the number of people requesting tattoo removal as the novelty factor wore off.

Tribal Markings

These are a form of tattooing where patterns are cut directly into the skin. They often hold religious significance or show membership of a particular tribe or group. They are deemed to be an essential feature of some cultures and are considered attractive in both males and females.

Piercing

The 1990s saw a huge increase in the popularity of body piercing. Ears, nose, navel, eyebrows and nipples were all being subjected to the piercing trend and became fashion statements, particularly with teenagers and young adults (Armstrong, 1996).

PRACTICE KNOWLEDGE

Problems affecting skin integrity are wide ranging, varying for example from nappy rash to disfiguring wounds. Although core areas of knowledge and skills such as the prevention of cross-infection and asepsis are applicable in many instances, the management of specific skin conditions and disorders may demand more specific expertise. The role of the nurse will differ according to the type and extent of the skin problem. For example, when caring for an adult with a chronic skin condition such as atopic eczema, the focus of the nurse's role will primarily be that of a health promoter, empowering the individual to manage and live with his or her condition.

The wide range of conditions and possible therapeutic interventions prohibit detailed discussion of every example. Instead, the following discussion will focus on a general assessment of skin and then on one of the common problems of skin integrity, namely wounds. The many common skin conditions cannot be dealt with in this chapter as they are numerous and demand a specialist knowledge base in dermatology nursing.

ASSESSMENT OF THE SKIN

Assessment of the skin not only gives an indication of the condition of the skin itself, but can also help in identifying the client's physical health, emotional state and lifestyle. As assessment is undertaken in circumstances other than those purely related to problems of skin integrity, it will be discussed as a separate entity. Assessment requires

RESEARCH BASED EVIDENCE

Seymour (1995) cites a number of studies that suggest latex allergy is a growing problem for health care workers. For example, an American and a French study found, respectively, that 17.6% and 10.7% of nurses were sensitive to latex. If nurses or patients have an allergy to latex – either to the chemical additives used during their manufacture or to the proteins in natural rubber – hypoallergenic gloves and latex-free gloves are available.

close observation of the skin and includes visual inspection, palpation and noting skin odour. In addition, it is important to ask the client questions about his or her skin. Good illumination is necessary, and if there is any discharge from skin lesions, the nurse should wear disposable latex gloves. Above all, it is important that the nurse employs a sensitive approach and respects the dignity and privacy of the client.

Assessment of the skin should include observation of each of the following aspects of the skin:

> ▶ colour;
> ▶ temperature;
> ▶ moisture;
> ▶ texture;
> ▶ thickness;
> ▶ turgor;
> ▶ the presence of blemishes and lesions.

▶ Colour and Areas of Discoloration

Skin colour varies between individuals, most obviously between people of different races. There are also differences in skin colour in different parts of the body of each individual. For example, the nipples and areolae are darker than the rest of the skin, particularly in women during pregnancy. Similarly, areas that are exposed to sunlight, such as the face and the arms, tend to be darker due to increased melanin concentration. These differences aside, and with the exception of older people in whom pigmentation can increase unevenly, skin colour is usually uniform within an individual.

An assessment of skin colour should first of all involve looking at areas that are not generally exposed to sunlight, such as the palm of the hand. It should be noted, however, that for the first few days of life the hands and feet of newborn babies are a bluish colour, termed acrocyanosis, due to inadequate peripheral vasculature. Assessment thereafter should involve looking for specific changes in skin colour, for instance:

> ▶ cyanosis (a bluish colour);
> ▶ pallor (a decrease of colour);
> ▶ jaundice (a yellow–orange colour);
> ▶ erythema (redness).

These changes in colour are most obvious in certain parts of the body. For example cyanosis and pallor are particularly evident at the nail beds and buccal (mouth) mucosa. It is especially important to look at these areas in dark-skinned clients, as changes in general skin colour are less evident. Asian children may have Mongolian blue spots, which are very common and are normal. In addition, the nurse should note any bruising. Although bruising can be normal, extensive or fingertip-type bruising can be a sign of abuse and should be investigated further.

▶ Temperature

Skin temperature is best assessed by feeling the client's skin with the back of your hand. The temperature of the skin increases or decreases with an increase or decrease of blood circulating through the dermis. Although it is normal for hands and feet to be colder than the rest of the body when exposed to a cold environment because of reduced peripheral blood flow, localized areas of increased or decreased temperature may indicate a problem. For example, if the skin surrounding a wound is hot, inflamed, red and painful, a wound infection may be present. Similarly, if a limb is cold and pale, there may be circulatory impairment. Therefore, when clients have had vascular surgery or a plaster cast or bandages applied to a limb, it is important to assess for skin changes that may indicate impaired blood flow.

▶ Moisture

Moisture refers to the wetness and oiliness of skin. It is related to the level of hydration and general condition of the skin. Normally the skin is smooth and dry except in the folds of the skin where it is moist. An increase in skin temperature arising from a hot environment or exercise is accompanied by perspiration and is a normal phenomenon. However, when a client has a fever resulting from for example an infection, the skin may initially feel dry and hot, but becomes damp from perspiration as the fever breaks. In older people dry skin, which is often accompanied by itchiness, may be a problem.

▶ Texture

Usually the skin is smooth, soft and flexible, although in older people it sometimes becomes wrinkled and leathery. Skin thickness varies in different parts of the body: for example, skin is thickest on the palms of the hands and soles of the feet. Skin texture can be assessed by stroking and palpating the skin with the fingertips, which enables the nurse to gauge smoothness, thickness, suppleness and softness. Localized areas of changes to skin texture may indicate previous trauma or lesions. Should such changes be apparent, the nurse should ask the client about them. Rough dry skin may result from exposure to cold weather or overwashing.

▶ Turgor

Turgor refers to the elasticity of the skin, which is normally elastic and taut. It can be assessed by gentle pinching, lifting and letting go of an area of skin, usually on the back of the hand. Normally, the skin should quickly return to its former position. If it does not, it may indicate that the client is dehydrated. However, some loss of skin elasticity is normal in older individuals. Excessive accumulation of fluid in the tissue – termed oedema – gives the skin a taut shiny appearance. It results from either direct trauma to the skin or an underlying condition. The presence of oedema increases susceptibility to further skin damage and delays wound healing.

▶ Blemishes and Lesions

Many skin blemishes and lesions are normal, for example birthmarks, moles, freckles, and minor cuts, abrasions and blisters. Equally, nappy rash and heat rash are common among babies and children and mild acne is not uncommon in adults. Other blemishes and lesions, however, may require further investigation and the client may need to be referred to a doctor. For example changes in an existing mole may indicate the development of a malignant melanoma.

Rashes may be caused by infection, for example a postviral rash, chickenpox, meningitis and shingles, or an allergic response, for example to particular chemicals, food products or medication. Other lesions may

---

RESEARCH BASED EVIDENCE

According to McHenry et al. (1995), the prevalence of atopic eczema (or dermatitis) has increased substantially over the past 30 years. It affects 5–15% of children and 2–10% of adults. The condition appears to develop from a complex interplay between genetic, immunological and environmental factors. The two most commonly cited environmental factors are house dust mites and certain foods, particularly milk, dairy products and eggs.

Where individuals have existing skin conditions or diseases that cannot be completely cured, effective assessment and management will focus on minimizing the effects of the skin problem and maximizing health potential and quality of life. The effect of such chronic conditions can have a profound effect on the individual and his or her family (Table 2.4.2).

Scratching affects concentration and may cause bleeding
Disrupted sleep results in tiredness and irritability
Social and intimate relationships affected
Embarrassment
Poor self-image
Reduced self-esteem
Lack of confidence
Reduced socialization
Reduced participation in certain social activities (e.g. swimming)
Teasing and taunting by others
Self-disgust
Restrictions on career and occupational opportunities
Anger, frustration and despair resulting from lack of control of eczema
Increased washing of clothing and bedding
Time-consuming management
Restricted choice of some products (to avoid exacerbating eczema)
Increased expenditure on treatments and some products (to improve management of eczema)

Table 2.4.2 Effects of atopic eczema on the individual and his or her family.

DECISION MAKING

Carole, aged 28, is admitted to the mother and baby unit of a psychiatric hospital with her three-week-old daughter Jasmine. Carole is suffering from postnatal depression and has for the past week been neglecting herself and has shown little interest in caring for Jasmine.

- *What aspects of skin assessment would you focus on when determining Carole's and Jasmine's skin health?*
- *In what ways could the assessment of a patient's skin lead you to suspect underlying health problems?*

arise from skin infestations such as scabies, as a result of accidental or intentional trauma to the skin, or as a result of skin disease such as psoriasis or eczema. When abnormal blemishes, including scars or lesions are detected, their colour, size, location and specific characteristics, and, where appropriate, distribution and grouping, should be noted. Clients should be asked about such blemishes in particular to determine their cause.

▌ CLASSIFICATION OF WOUNDS

Wounds can be classified in a variety of different ways. They can be classified according to:

- ▌ cause (e.g. stab-wound);
- ▌ status of skin integrity (e.g. open or closed wound);
- ▌ cleanliness of wound (e.g. presence or absence of infection or foreign bodies);
- ▌ the characteristics of the wound bed of open wounds;
- ▌ severity of skin damage (e.g. full-thickness burn).

However, Westaby (1985) suggests that there are really only two types of wound:

- ▌ wounds characterized by skin loss;
- ▌ wounds where there is no skin loss.

In practice, wound classification systems are often incomplete and overlap. For example a surgically closed infected wound and an open chronic sloughy bacterially-contaminated wound. A simple wound classification system is given in Figure 2.4.4

Acute wounds result from surgery or accidents. However, in some instances acute wounds progress to chronic wounds as a result of complications. Acute surgical wounds tend to be surgically closed and clean, while accidental wounds may be either clean or infected and can also be open or closed. Chronic wounds result from underlying diseases and tend to be open, for example pressure sores and leg ulcers. Chronic wounds are more likely to be colonized or infected.

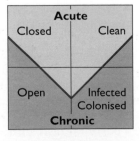

Figure 2.4.4: Wound classification table.

Open wounds can be further classified according to the observable characteristics of the wound bed as:

▶ granulating (red);
▶ epithelializing (pink) ;
▶ sloughy (yellow);
▶ necrotic (black).

▶ SEVERITY OF SKIN DAMAGE

It is not always easy to determine the extent of skin damage in terms of whether there is superficial, partial or full-thickness skin damage, but it is sometimes useful to do so. For example, burns and pressure sores are often graded and described in these terms (Table 2.4.3).

Despite the limitations of wound classification, it is nonetheless useful as it helps to identify both the potential complications of a given wound and the implications for wound care in each case and this can guide decision making when planning wound care. Algorithms or flow charts based on the classification of wounds aid in identifying priorities in wound care, and have been devised to guide nursing decisions and actions in wound management.

Grade	Features
I	Discoloration, persistent erythema of intact skin
II	Partial-thickness skin loss involving the epidermis and/or dermis. Abrasion, blister or shallow crater
III	Full-thickness skin loss involving damage or necrosis of subcutaneous tissue; a deep crater without undermining of adjacent tissue
IV	Full-thickness tissue loss with extensive destruction, tissue necrosis or damage to muscle, bone or supporting structures

Table 2.4.3 Classification of pressure sores. (Reproduced with permission from Benbow, 1994.)

▶ WOUND MANAGEMENT

The management of wounds will be discussed in general terms, followed by a more in-depth discussion of three specific types of wounds, namely accidental wounds, closed surgical wounds and chronic wounds.

▶ *Assessment of a Person with a Wound*

When undertaking an assessment of a person with a wound, it is necessary to consider the person as a whole and not just to focus attention on the wound itself. Morison (1992, p. 22) states that assessment can be thought of on four levels, namely assessment of:

'▶ general patient factors that could delay wound healing;
▶ immediate causes of the wound and any underlying pathophysiology;
▶ local conditions at the wound site;
▶ potential consequences of the wound for the individual.'

Localized pain

Localized erythema

Localized rise in skin temperature

Local oedema

Excess exudate

Pus

Offensive odour

Pyrexia

Table 2.4.4 Signs of clinical wound infection.

Morison's approach (1992) allows the nurse to:

◗ determine whether any health promotion activity is necessary to prevent a recurrence of the wound (e.g. advice on how to prevent sunburn);
◗ consider any factors that may retard wound healing and take measures to overcome these (e.g. inadequate nutrition);
◗ plan and provide holistic care that meets the needs of a person with a wound rather than just treating a wound per se.

The immediate and longer term care of a patient with a wound requires an assessment and understanding of the psychological effects and the functional, social and economic consequences of a wound for the patient if holistic care is to be provided. It is likely that besides nurses several other members of the multidisciplinary team will be involved in the care of a patient with a wound. Good communication between team members to facilitate the sharing of information is essential for achieving agreed goals.

◗ Assessment of the Wound Site

When assessing the wound site itself, the following should be noted:

◗ the location of the wound;
◗ the size of the wound;
◗ the characteristics of the wound bed (in open wounds) and wound margin;
◗ the degree of exudate;
◗ the presence of infection (Table 2.4.4);
◗ odour from the wound;
◗ pain;
◗ the condition of the surrounding skin;
◗ signs of other specific complications such as a haematoma;
◗ where appropriate, the presence of foreign bodies, the type of skin closure and the presence of drains and details of drainage.

Open wounds can be traced onto plastic film to obtain a visual record of the wound size. These films can be annotated to show areas of the wound bed with different characteristics. Maximum wound dimensions can be taken from the tracing. Wound depth can be measured using sterile probes. Serial photographs can also be taken to show wound changes over time, which will give some indication of the effectiveness or otherwise of treatment regimens.

If patients have existing wounds or have received wound care in the past, it is important during assessment to establish whether the patient has had any allergies to wound care products. Details of existing wound care should be recorded. Patch testing for allergies to any proposed wound care products is useful, particularly if large areas require dressing, for example an extensive venous leg ulcer.

Wound assessment charts can be useful tools when undertaking and recording the findings of wound assessments. Figure 2.4.5 shows an example of an open wound assessment chart developed by Morison (1992).

OPEN WOUND ASSESSMENT CHART

Type of wound (e.g. pressure sore, fungating carcinoma, etc.) ....
Location ....
How long has wound been open? ....
General patient factors which may delay healing (e.g. malnourished, diabetic, chronic infection) ....
Allergies to wound care products ....
Previous treatments tried (comment on success/problems) ....
Special aids in current use (e.g. pressure-relieving bed, cushion) ....
....
....

TRACE THE WOUND WEEKLY, ANNOTATING TRACING WITH NATURE OF WOUND BED, ORIENTATION OF WOUND, POSITION/EXTENT OF SINUSES, AND UNDERMINING OF SURROUNDING SKIN
All other parameters should be assessed at every dressing change.

Wound factors/Date									

I.   NATURE OF WOUND BED
  a.   healthy granulation
  b.   epithelialization
  c.   slough
  d.   black/brown necrotic tissue
  e. other (specify)									

2.   EXUDATE
  a.   colour
  b.   type
  c. approximate amount									

3. ODOUR Offensive/some/none									

4.   PAIN (SITE)
  a.   at wound site
  b. elsewhere (specify)									

5. PAIN (FREQUENCY) Continuous/intermittent/ only at dressing changes/none									
6. PAIN (SEVERITY) Patient's score (0–10)									

7.   WOUND MARGIN
  a.   colour
  b. oedematous									

8.   ERYTHEMA OF SURROUNDING SKIN
  a.   present
  b. maximum distance from wound (mm)									

9. GENERAL CONDITION OF SURROUNDING SKIN (e.g. dry eczema)									

10. INFECTION
  a.   suspected
  b.   wound swab sent
  c. confined (specify organism)									

WOUND ASSESSED BY:

Figure 2.4.5: Open wound assessment chart. (From Morison, M. (1992)
A Colour Guide to the Nursing Management of Wounds. p. 25. London. Wolfe Publishing Ltd.)

Facilitating Wound Healing

The general aim of wound management is to provide optimum conditions for facilitating natural wound healing as quickly and comfortably as possible with minimum scarring. This includes identifying and addressing factors that may affect wound healing. These can be divided into three broad categories as follows:

- local factors relating to the wound environment (e.g. presence of necrotic tissue, oedema);
- general client factors (e.g. nutritional status, compliance with treatment);
- treatment – nursing and medical factors (e.g. radiotherapy, dressing choice).

Successful wound healing is dependent on the body's ability to heal and wound care can only help to facilitate this process. Some wounds will not heal, for example inoperable fungating carcinoma, and here the aim of wound management is to contribute to an optimum quality of life for the client by containing wound odour and discharge, protecting the wound and controlling any pain.

The aims of local wound management are to provide an optimum environment to facilitate natural wound healing processes, to remove causes of delayed healing and to protect the wound from further damage (see Subject Knowledge).

If a wound is necrotic, one of the first priorities is to remove the necrotic tissue. This can be achieved by mechanical means, chemical means or by providing the right local conditions for autolysis to take place.

Wound sites also need to be free of clinical infection. If a clinical wound infection is suspected (see Table 2.4.4) a wound swab should be taken before wound cleaning and sent for microscopy, culture and sensitivity. An appropriate systemic antibiotic may be prescribed. The use of topical antibiotics is rarely indicated because of the risk of contact sensitivity and bacterial resistance (Podmore, 1994). Chronic wounds in particular may be colonized by microorganisms that do not cause clinical infections and do not appear to affect wound healing.

Consideration should be given to whether the wound needs to be cleansed or redressed as unnecessary intervention delays wound healing. Wounds should be cleaned if there is superficial slough, pus, excessive exudate or visible debris such as grit or residue from previous dressings.

Generally if wounds require cleansing they should be cleaned with warm sterile sodium chloride 0.9% solution. Unlike antiseptics, sodium chloride 0.9% solution does not have a toxic effect on skin tissue. Although antiseptics may be used in specific circumstances, such as heavily contaminated wounds, the benefits need to be weighed against the possible tissue damage they may cause (see Annotated Further Reading – Murphy, 1995). Preference should be given to irrigating wounds under moderate pressure rather than using cotton wool or gauze, which shed fibres into the wound, thereby delaying wound healing and providing a focus for infection. In addition, such mechanical cleansing can damage newly formed tissue.

The choice of dressing, if required, depends on a variety of factors. These include:

- the local conditions of the wound site and surrounding skin;
- other requirements arising from the individual patient's needs, wishes and lifestyle;

▶ cost-effectiveness and product availability.

Although it is not possible to determine the ideal characteristics of a wound dressing to suit all wounds, there are some features that the 'ideal' dressing should possess (Table 2.4.5).

In many instances, a single dressing will not suffice, for example, a primary dressing may meet the requirements of the wound–dressing interface, but may not possess the absorptive qualities needed to contain exudate, so a secondary absorbent dressing will need to be applied. Secondary dressings, including bandages, have the following functions:

▶ to protect and support the wound and surrounding skin;
▶ to maintain the position of primary dressings;
▶ to absorb moisture;
▶ to control bleeding or oedema (as a result of pressure exerted by secondary dressings).

In selecting a dressing the nurse needs to understand the properties, actions, indications and contraindications for the use of each dressing being considered and match this information to the specific requirements of the patient and the wound. The use of an algorithm and a dressing formulary will help nurses in decision making in this area of wound management (see Annotated Further Reading – Rodgers, 1991).

When undertaking wound care, it is essential that the nurse understands and adheres to the principles of asepsis to promote the prevention of cross-infection (see Chapter 1.3). If the client has several wounds that require redressing, the cleanest wounds should be dressed first.

There are occasions where wounds can be cleaned and dressed using a clean technique rather than an aseptic technique. Heavily contaminated minor wounds resulting from accidents do not need to be treated aseptically until the gross contaminants have been removed. Moffatt and

---

DECISION MAKING

Mr Heron, a 60-year-old farmer, has a venous leg ulcer, which is shallow, clean, granulating and 5 cm x 5 cm. There is a moderate amount of exudate. He has no known allergies to specific dressing products. In the role of the community nurse:

- *Select an appropriate dressing for the wound.*
- *Justify your choice in terms of promotion of wound healing, patient comfort and cost-effectiveness.*
- *Did you give consideration as to whether or not your choice of dressing would be available?*
- *Do you think you had enough information on which to base your decision? If not, what other information would you require before making a decision?*

References that will aid you in your decision making are Ertl (1993b) and Inman (1994).

Maintains a moist wound environment

Provides thermal insulation

Provides a barrier to microorganisms

Protects from trauma

Is non-toxic and non-allergenic

Is absorptive and removes excess exudate

Is sterile

Will not shed fibres into the wound

Is non-adherent and easily removed

Is flexible and conforming

Is comfortable

Controls odour

Is acceptable to the patient

Is easy to use

Requires infrequent dressing change

Is cost-effective

Has a reasonable shelf life and storage requirement

Is available

Table 2.4.5 Features of an ideal dressing.

Oldroyd (1994) suggest that chronic leg ulcers treated in the community may be cleaned by immersing the leg in a bowl of clean water to remove heavy exudate and debris from previous dressings. In a hospital setting, however, it is advisable that an aseptic technique is used because of the greater risk of cross-infection (see Annotated Further Reading – Mallett and Bailey, 1996).

▶ EVALUATION OF THE EFFECTIVENESS OF WOUND MANAGEMENT

The evaluation of wound management may take place at two levels:

- ▶ first, an organization may wish to keep a record of specific wounds and evaluate the effectiveness of the measures taken to deal with and minimize the incidence of these wounds;
- ▶ at the level of individual wounds, an evaluation should be made each time the dressings are changed by observing and measuring to see if the wound is healing as expected.

Evaluating individual wounds is important for two reasons. First, as wound healing progresses and the characteristics of the wound change, different dressings may be required. Second, if there is no change or the wound has deteriorated, it is necessary to reflect on the factors that may be responsible for delayed healing. The dressing choice may need to be changed or other treatment options considered. However, unless the wound has changed significantly, sufficient time must be given to allow the dressing to become effective before changing to another product. All members of the multidisciplinary team may need to be involved in the discussion and reappraisal of care. It is also important to evaluate the patient's progress as a whole and to ascertain their views on the progress they are making, so that areas of concern can be addressed.

▶ ACCIDENTAL WOUNDS

An accidental wound is defined here as an acute wound that has occurred as a result of an accident or a specific non-medical incident. They are sometimes referred to as traumatic wounds. Accidental wounds involving the skin can range from minor cuts and abrasions to major wounds such as the loss of a limb or crush injuries. Also included are burns, scalds, bites and stings.

Although the focus of this discussion is on the management of patients with accidental wounds in the accident and emergency department, the principles of first aid care are applicable in all situations. In all cases, it is necessary to assess the patient, and if possible to obtain a history of the wound. This includes the cause, circumstances, time of accident and any other information relevant to the management of the patient. Psychological care of the patient – and any accompanying relatives or friends – is extremely important, as the suddenness of the situation can cause considerable distress and anxiety. It is also important to identify and address any pain the patient is experiencing.

The management of major accidental wounds is decided and directed by the casualty officer. Rapid accurate assessment of the client's condition and underlying pathology is essential. Priority must be given to the re-establishment and maintenance of the airway, breathing and

---

RESEARCH BASED EVIDENCE

Bux and Malhi (1996) carried out an audit into the use of dressings in practice. The correct choice of dressing was made for only 48% of the 50 wounds observed. The correct choice and use of dressings was observed for only 20% of the wounds. The importance of training and information related to wound care was highlighted and the development of wound care guidelines and a hospital wound product formulary were encouraged.

DECISION MAKING

The mother of a 10-year-old child with a mild learning disability expresses concern to you that the wound on her child's leg is taking a long time to heal and looks lumpy. Although the wound has been infected, it is now clean, granulation tissue has formed and epithelialization is taking place at the wound margins.

- *How would you address the mother's concerns and convey to both the mother and child that the wound is healing well?*

circulation, and the control of bleeding before dealing with the wound itself. A head-to-toe examination must then be conducted to ensure that there are no other injuries that need to take priority over the management of the wound. The detailed management of the wound, as Wijetunge (1992) identifies should only commence once the patient's condition is stable.

In the case of minor wounds, such as slight cuts and abrasions, an initial assessment of the patient is still necessary, but attention can quickly be focused onto wound care to minimize the risk of infection. Other measures may, however, be necessary; for example, depending upon the circumstances, it may be appropriate to take the opportunity to offer health education or the patient many require a tetanus injection.

The cause of the wound will give an indication of the likely damage and complications, and will help to guide wound management decisions. For example, puncture wounds caused by stabbing have only a small entry site, but cut a deep track and may damage internal tissue and organs. As such a wound goes deep into the body, the risk of infection is high. Abrasions, on the other hand, can result in large tender areas where the superficial layers of skin have been removed. They often contain foreign particles such as grit, which can cause infection and tattooing if not effectively removed. If a large foreign body is embedded in the patient, it must be removed in theatre as there is a risk of major haemorrhage when it is removed (see Annotated Further Reading – David, 1986).

Accurate documentation is essential. In cases of criminal or civil prosecution or claims for industrial injury compensation the patient's records may be used as evidence. Where a patient is a victim of a non-accidental injury that warrants police investigation such as a stabbing or a road traffic accident, particular care must be taken with the patient's property, including clothing, as it may be required for further examination and used as evidence. Where child abuse is suspected, for example if a child appears to have cigarette burns on its buttocks, it is essential to follow the local hospital policy regarding the management and reporting of such cases, so that further action can be taken as appropriate. The nurse must use considerable tact when dealing with such situations.

> **DECISION MAKING**
>
> A ten-year-old boy is taken to the accident and emergency department after sustaining injuries when he was knocked off his bicycle outside his school. On arrival, the boy is unconscious and has a deep laceration on his forehead and several abrasions. His parents have been informed and are on their way.
> - *Identify management priorities.*
> - *Outline the care required for the laceration giving a rationale for your decision.*

▶ SURGICAL WOUNDS

Surgical wounds may be open or closed depending upon the reasons for surgery. In this section the role of the nurse in the promotion of wound healing by primary intention is discussed. The role of the nurse is to:

- ▶ prevent infection;
- ▶ monitor the wound to detect the onset of any complications;
- ▶ prevent trauma to the wound site;
- ▶ promote nutritional and fluid intake.

To prevent infection the nurse must prevent the chain of infection from completing all the links (Watson and Royle, 1987). The nurse will need to consider his or her own health: a nurse with a cold or sore throat will be a reservoir for infective organisms and should not be involved in wound care. Gloves may be worn when carrying out wound care to reduce contamination of the nurse's hands (Wilson, 1995). The use of aseptic technique during wound care is important (Briggs *et al.*, 1996).

To prevent the entry of infective organisms, wounds should be left undisturbed for 48 hours after surgery to allow the wound to seal itself

effects – some drugs such as glucocorticosteroids may alter the texture of the skin, while others such as sedatives may reduce the patient's level of alertness resulting in the associated problems of reduced movement and decreased awareness of risk;

▶ reduced 'consciousness' can lead to a patient being unable to identify the need to move, and can prevent him or her from doing so;.

▶ loss of 'sensation' can result in a patient being unaware of the position he or she is in and the need to change it;

▶ faecal and urinary 'incontinence' can cause contamination of wound sites, excess moisture in the wound area and problems with adherence with certain dressings, particularly in relation to pressure sores on the buttocks, sacrum or hips;

▶ 'external environment' covers a large area relating to resources – the general environment in which the patient is being nursed (e.g. own home, hospital single room or multi-occupancy room, nursing or residential care) can affect the type of dressing or treatment available or possible, as can the amount of assistance the patient can expect from nursing staff, other carers and relatives or significant others;

▶ it is important to identify the 'probable cause of the sore' developing as this may influence the care required – if shearing force is suspected attention may be focused on handling and positioning patients to prevent further damage, but if direct pressure has caused the problem the main objective is to remove the pressure;

▶ the patient's 'diagnosis' can sometimes affect the wound healing – conditions such as diabetes mellitus, vascular disease, malignancy and anaemia can alter the cellular environment and therefore interfere with the healing process;

▶ the 'aim of care' is not always apparent – for patients in the terminal stages of illness, it may not be possible to heal the pressure sore in the time the patient has left to live in which case the aims of care may be to prevent the wound from deteriorating and to increase patient comfort rather than to heal the sore;

▶ 'patient understanding' of his or her condition and treatments and the patient's ability to comply with regimens may also affect the overall choice of treatment;

▶ a current assessment score using a risk calculator such as that produced by Norton in the early 1960s or Waterlow in 1985, help to identify future risks and allow the implementation of preventive treatment to prevent further development of sores (see Annotated Further Reading – Wardman, 1991).

The outer ring of the assessment wheel consists of the factors you should consider when dealing with the wound itself. These factors have been covered earlier in the Practice Knowledge section under General Assessment of Wounds.

In addition to the points above, it is important to assess and manage the psychological impact of living with a chronic wound on the patient.

Any plan of care relating to pressure sore management needs to contain a core of information as follows:

▶ an up-to-date assessment of the wound;
▶ current at-risk assessment score and review dates;
▶ cleansing solution to be used;
▶ primary dressing requirements;
▶ secondary dressing requirements – padding, bandaging;
▶ method of carrying out dressing;

RESEARCH BASED EVIDENCE

The impact of pressure sores on a patient's quality of life is an area that is largely unexplored by research. Charles (1995) addressed the issue of quality of life in relation to the other major type of chronic wound, leg ulcers. She carried out a small scale project involving four patients who had suffered from leg ulcers for between five and 35 years. The subjects identified three main areas of concern: the physical impact of pain, sleeplessness, impaired mobility, no one listens and no one explains; the psychological impact of hopelessness, helplessness and lack of control; and the social impact of altered working life and diminished human interaction. Many of these concerns can be applied to patients with pressure sores.

> ▶ frequency of dressing changes;
> ▶ referrals made and advice received;
> ▶ associated factors – use of pressure relieving aids and mattresses, mobility programme and turning regimen;
> ▶ patient and relative involvement;
> ▶ patient and relative educational needs.

Pressure sores should not be seen as a nursing problem, but rather as a challenge to the full multidisciplinary team, in which each member has a role to play. The flow chart showing multidisciplinary involvement (Figure 2.4.7) is not exhaustive, but serves to highlight the level of integration that may be required. Care should be implemented in accordance with the written patient care plan. It is advised that a limited number of nurses are involved in implementing the wound care. Continuity and consistency are important if the pressure sore is to be given the best chance of healing. Different nurses may use slightly different techniques, therefore dressings may be applied in a different manner and this may affect the rate and amount of wound healing; for instance, one nurse may pack a wound tighter than another or one nurse may irrigate a wound while another nurse keeps the wound dry. Continuity of care also helps in terms of evaluation as the nurse becomes familiar with the wound and is better able to detect changes in its size, shape and general condition.

If a pressure sore does not heal, surgical intervention may be an option. This could entail surgical debridement or skin grafting. Surgical debridement is usually carried out under a general or spinal anaesthetic. It involves surgically excising all necrotic and infected tissue and any fibrosed tissue surrounding the wound. The wound bed is left clean and bleeding so that granulation can take place (David, 1986). There are many different types of skin graft, for example full- or partial-thickness, pedicle and flap grafts. The main objective of grafting is to provide an open wound with a covering layer of healthy skin. This skin can be of varying

---

RESEARCH BASED EVIDENCE

Boyce et al. (1995) carried out a pilot study into the treatment of chronic wounds with cultured skin substitutes. Sheets of cultured allogenic keratinocytes were used on the chronic wounds and found to offer an effective alternative method of accelerating wound closure.

Figure 2.4.7: Multidisciplinary involvement in the management of pressure sores.

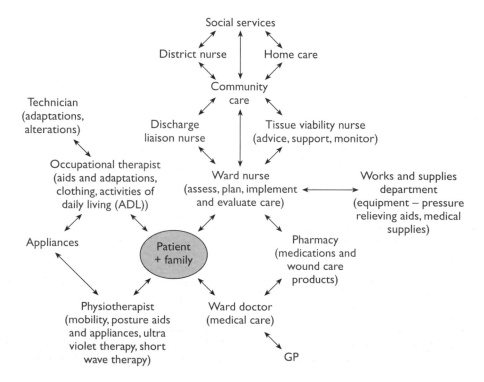

thickness, ranging from the very thin epidermal layer through to the grafting of full-thickness skin and muscle, and in some cases underlying bone. There have been many technological advances in the areas of grafting and replacing skin. As well as autografting (taking skin from one site to a second site on the same person), it is now possible to carry out homografting (between two human subjects) and xenografting (between different species – often using porcine (pig) tissue on human subjects). More recent advances have included growing tissue in laboratories from deoxyribonucleic acid (DNA) samples and producing synthetic skin substances.

PROFESSIONAL KNOWLEDGE

This section focuses on professional issues that are relevant to the quality of care provision relating to skin integrity. Examples are given to illustrate how nurses can influence the development of quality systems of care at an organizational level. The responsibility of the nurse to provide safe effective care – either by developing his or her professional competence or by acknowledging his or her limitations and seeking appropriate expert help – is explored.

▶ THE NURSE'S ROLE IN PROMOTING SKIN HEALTH

The nurse has an important role to play in promoting health. Rule 18(A) of Statutory Instrument 1989 makes specific reference to this aspect of the nurse's role. There is considerable potential for nurses in all care settings to promote skin health. Health promotion activities can range from teaching parents the necessary skin care for their newborn babies to empowering individuals to manage their chronic skin conditions such as psoriasis and eczema.

How nurses fulfil a role in promoting skin health in part depends on individual situations and circumstances. The knowledge base provided in this chapter, along with a more in-depth understanding of health promotion (see Naidoo and Wills, 1994), will enable the nurse to select the appropriate health promotion activity to assist specific individuals to achieve and maintain optimum skin health. To be effective it is essential that such activities are planned to achieve identified health goals. It is also important that the nurse recognizes individual limitations, and where necessary ensures that patients receive specific expert help. In addition, where longer term interventions are needed and input from other health care professionals or agencies is required – as is often the case with chronic skin problems – consideration must be given to how continuity can be ensured.

The nurse also has a responsibility to maintain his or her own skin health. This is not only important with respect to the nurse's health, but also to that of the patients in his or her care, particularly with respect to the prevention of cross-infection.

▶ THE NURSE'S ROLE IN DEVELOPING AND MAINTAINING QUALITY SYSTEMS OF CARE

There is considerable scope for nurses, along with other health care professionals, to be involved in the development and maintenance of quality systems of care relating to skin integrity. Examples include involvement in the development of standards of care, clinical guidelines and protocols, procedures, policies, managed care programmes and auditing clinical practice.

The development of clinical guidelines and protocols help to maintain standards and the continuity of care by providing an agreed framework for decision making for the treatment and management of specific aspects of care. Two examples relating to skin integrity are protocols for the prevention of pressure sores and wound management. Rodgers (1991) discusses the development of a wound care protocol with a central formulary that includes wound care products that meet agreed criteria. This approach provides nurses with guidance to the most appropriate treatment and wound care products available for a given type of wound. In addition, access to product information allows the nurse to make an informed decision about the wound care product selected for use. Rationalization of wound care products also enables bulk purchasing, which reduces costs. Rodgers (1991) highlights the need to review wound care protocols constantly as new products and information become available. This also enables nurses using wound care protocols to remain updated on wound management.

A relatively recent development in the UK health care system in which nurses are able to make an important contribution is the development and implementation of managed care programmes (Benton, 1995). Nurses also have a significant role in developing, undertaking and participating in the audit of clinical practice. As an example relating to skin integrity, a hospital may keep records of the incidence of pressure sores and may wish to investigate what measures were taken to prevent the development of pressure sores and what care was given when pressure sores developed. Auditing may be undertaken to see if the agreed standard for the assessment and prevention of pressure sores was being met through the correct implementation of a pressure sore prevention protocol. Equally, the management of existing pressure sores may be audited to see if the actual management reflects the agreed wound care protocol, and whether specific aspects of care follow established procedures.

▶ CONTINUING EDUCATION IN RELATION TO SKIN INTEGRITY

Several post registration courses are available that relate to the topic of skin integrity. Some of these courses, such as courses in burns and plastic surgery and dermatology, cover specific aspects of skin and wound management and are recommended for nurses working within these specialized areas of nursing. Other courses are suitable for nurses who intend to practice as nurse specialists and wish to gain expert knowledge in specific areas related to skin integrity. These include breast care, stoma care, infection control and continence courses. Courses that are wound specific are starting to emerge. These include a course on leg ulcer management, which is suitable for any nurse who may have to deal with patients with leg ulcers during their working day. Other courses that have some relevance to dealing with patients who have skin disorders include those that teach counselling and advocacy skills. Although not directly concerned with skin integrity these courses can provide the nurse with skills that are invaluable when supporting patients with skin disorders or deformities.

▶ THE ROLE OF THE NURSE SPECIALIST

Skin integrity is a huge topic that requires a diversity of knowledge and skills. Although nurses should work to increase their competence in both these areas they should also be able to recognize situations where experienced specialist help is beneficial. There are several nurse specialists who can become involved in skin and wound care, for example, infection control nurses, breast or stoma care nurses and tissue viability nurses. Most hold post registration qualifications. They provide help, support and education to both professionals and patients in their specialist area of practice. Other nurse specialists may be involved on an *ad hoc* basis depending on the requirements of the staff and patients, for example, continence advisers, nutrition and dietetics nurses, pain control nurses, discharge liaison nurses and any other specialist that may be relevant to a particular underlying disease process, for example a diabetic nurse or a MacMillan nurse in cancer care.

▶ LINK NURSE

In recent years, the number of nurse specialists has increased. However, it is common to have only one or two nurses available locally in each speciality. These nurse specialists may have to cover a large number of areas and so their input into direct patient care is limited. The use of specialist link nurses in wards and departments is becoming increasingly popular. The link nurse is usually a registered nurse who has an interest in a particular area of care, for example tissue viability. These nurses increase their knowledge in their chosen area by working with the appropriate nurse specialist and attending study days. In promoting the link nurse role the ward develops a team of nurses who have specialist knowledge in their chosen field. These nurses can then provide support and advice for the ward staff, and the nurse specialist is only required when a problem falls outside the scope of the link nurse. Furthermore, keeping wards up to date is easier as the specialist nurse is able to pass any new information on to the link nurses. The link nurses can then disseminate the information to their own areas of responsibility. The link nurse role not only improves communication and nursing care, but, also enables nurses to develop expertise in their chosen area of practice.

▶ SKIN INTEGRITY, THE NURSE AND THE SCOPE OF PROFESSIONAL PRACTICE

The UKCC (1992) *Scope of Professional Practice* sets out guidelines for extended nursing practice. Paragraph 3 states that 'Pre registration education prepares nurses, midwives and health visitors for safe practice at the point of registration... Post registration education equips practitioners with additional and more specialist skills necessary to meet the special needs of patients and clients'.

With ever growing technological development, nurses are being expected to take on additional roles. With this comes the need for a higher level of skill and knowledge. As nurses are responsible and accountable for their own practice, the following framework raises several professional issues that the individual nurse will need to address before taking on an extended role:

▶ Is this within my role as a nurse?
▶ Will the nursing profession support me if I carry out this extended role?
▶ Will my employer support me if I carry out this extended role?
▶ Is the practice research based?
▶ Do I have the knowledge, expertise and time to carry out this extended role?
▶ What are the risks and benefits to the patient or client?
▶ Am I willing to take responsibility for carrying out this extended role or would it be better carried out by another health professional?

The nurse should only consider taking on an extended role when he or she is satisfied that these issues have been appropriately addressed. There are many opportunities within the sphere of skin integrity for the nurse to undertake an extended role. Several of these are discussed below, although this list is not exhaustive.

▶ Nurse Suturing

A post registration course on suturing is concerned with providing suturing training for selected registered nurses working in the area of accident and emergency. There are several benefits of including suturing as part of the role of the accident and emergency nurse:

▶ cost-effectiveness to the organization in terms of time and resources;
▶ continuity of care and reduced waiting times for the patients;
▶ widened scope of professional practice and the opportunity to provide a comprehensive service to patients for the nurse (see Annotated Further Reading – Royal College of Nursing, 1996).

▶ Nurse Prescribing

In 1995, 60 nurses at eight pilot sites in England were involved in a trial on nurse prescribing. A 'community nurse' survey highlighted the fact that many nurses outside the pilot sites were engaged in 'prescribing behaviours', for example influencing the choice of prescribed drugs (Anderson, 1995). Of the 1108 nurses who completed the questionnaire, 94% thought that nurse prescribing should be extended. Within the area of skin integrity nurse prescribing could allow nurses to prescribe wound dressings, wound cleansing products and topical medications, providing better continuity and cost-effectiveness of care. It is hoped that by the year 2005 nurse prescribing will be commonplace.

▶ Nurse-led Clinics

The recent changes in the scope of professional practice (UKCC, 1992) has allowed nurses to make better use of their skills and knowledge. A recent innovation has been the development of nurse-led clinics. In the late 1980s a nurse-run minor injuries centre was established in

---

DECISION MAKING

You are a newly qualified staff nurse working in a busy accident and emergency department. A young woman is admitted who has fallen off her bicycle sustaining a laceration to her left forearm. Having assessed the wound, the doctor asks you to insert five black silk sutures. He says that he is aware that you have not yet undergone your suturing training, but as you have observed this procedure many times he is happy to take responsibility for your actions.

- *Decide whether or not you would be happy to carry out the doctor's request and give a rationale for your decision. You may find it helpful to use the framework given earlier in this section for deciding whether or not to accept the responsibility for carrying out extended practice.*

Manchester (Simon, 1992). Patients are only referred for medical intervention if the nurses feel their own expertise is insufficient. The majority of the nurses' work involves treating cuts, soft tissue injuries and dog bites. Suturing is carried out when appropriate and tetanus vaccinations given as required. Several other clinics of this type have since developed. The Riverside Community Leg Ulcer Project initially established six community clinics to provide care for patients with leg ulcers (Moffatt and Oldroyd, 1994). These are nurse-led, as is the wound healing clinic supported by the Tissue Repair Research Unit at Guys and St Thomas's Hospitals in London (Miller, 1994).

In any care setting nurses will meet patients or clients with a variety of problems and needs relating to skin care. This chapter provides the knowledge and decision-making skills that nurses will need (within the limitations of their roles) to make informed decisions about and provide appropriate effective care for patients or clients and their families in order to achieve and maintain optimum skin health. The importance of a holistic problem-solving approach to care is stressed, as is the need for effective communication between health care professionals. The roles of a number of specialist nurses to whom the nurse can turn for help, support and advice, are discussed.

As the scope of professional nursing practice extends, there will be greater opportunities for nurses who are caring for patients with a variety of skin-related problems and needs to become involved in the nurse-led care initiatives. It is therefore imperative that nurses develop specific research-based expertise so that they are able to assume responsibility and accountability for their future roles. Keeping a reflective diary will help you reflect on current nursing practice and to consider the knowledge base underpinning nursing decisions and the appropriateness and effectiveness of the nursing care of clients or patients with skin problems. Developing an enquiring approach to care will also help you question your own decision making and nursing practice.

▶ REFLECTIVE DIARY

Keep a diary of the nursing care of patients with problems and needs relating to skin integrity. Make sure you maintain confidentiality by omitting information that would make patients identifiable. For each case, address the following questions:

- ▶ What was the nature of the skin problem?
- ▶ How was it assessed?
- ▶ What specific care was proposed?
- ▶ What was the rationale for the proposed care?
- ▶ What specific skills were needed to implement the proposed care?
- ▶ What other health care professionals were involved in the patient's care?
- ▶ Was the care appropriate and effective? How was this determined?
- ▶ Were there any other care options that may have been more effective?

▶ CASE STUDIES

The following case studies will help you bring together the knowledge and decision-making skills required to address the needs of specific individuals with a variety of different skin problems.

▶ CASE STUDY: ADULT

Miss Green is 75 years old and lives alone in a one-bedroom ground floor flat. One morning, after the arrival of the district nurse, Miss Green slips on the kitchen mat and falls, sustaining a deep laceration to her head. The hot tea she is carrying splashes onto her arm causing a large but superficial burn.

■ **Decide what first aid treatment the district nurse should administer for the two skin injuries.**

■ **On arrival at the accident and emergency department the doctor examines Miss Green and finds that during the fall she has sustained a fractured neck of femur. Miss Green subsequently requires a hip replacement. Decide what care Miss Green will require in respect of her hip wound for the first ten postoperative days.**

▶ CASE STUDY: CHILD

Margaret and David MacDonnell take their five-year-old son Robert on holiday to a well-known seaside resort. As it is an overcast day Margaret has not applied any sun protection to Robert. Robert spends the whole day in just a pair of trunks playing on the beach. That evening Robert complains that his skin hurts and when David examines Robert he finds that his back is badly sunburnt.

■ **Decide what immediate measures should be taken to treat the effects of Robert's sunburn?**

■ **Given the opportunity, how would you help Mr and Mrs MacDonnell ensure effective sun protection for Robert in the future?**

▶ CASE STUDY: MENTAL HEALTH

Josie is 28 years old and single. She is attending a day unit for the adult mentally ill for treatment of anxiety-depression. During the post lunch rest period Josie shouts for you to come to the female toilet where she says she requires your help. When you arrive you find that Josie has inflicted several superficial lacerations to her wrists and forearms using the broken handle of a teaspoon from her lunch tray.

■ **What immediate first aid measures are needed?**

■ **Decide what measures the nurse will need to take to ensure that Josie receives appropriate wound care until her lacerations heal.**

■ **Decide what actions the nurse should take to ensure appropriate reporting and recording of the incident and to minimize the risk of Josie repeating the behaviour.**

▶ CASE STUDY: LEARNING DISABILITIES

Joseph is 40 years of age, has Down's syndrome and lives in residential care. He has developed the habit of picking the skin on the back of his hand, which has resulted in a small but deep wound. Although the wound has been covered with a plaster, Joseph continues to pick at the wound site and the nurse thinks that the present dressing is inadequate.

- **Decide what factors should be taken into account when choosing an appropriate dressing for Joseph?**

- **What nursing knowledge and skills would the nurse require to facilitate wound healing in Joseph's case?**

▶ ACKNOWLEDGEMENT

We would like to thank Mrs D.E. Cotrel-Gibbons, Nurse Teacher, for her advice and work on the surgical wounds section.

▶ ANNOTATED FURTHER READING

DEALEY, C. (1994) *The Care of Wounds*. Chapter 2. Oxford. Blackwell Science.
    This chapter outlines numerous types of wound dressings and wound cleansing products and gives information on their action.
DAVID, J.A. (1986) *Wound Management. A Comprehensive Guide to Dressing and Healing*. Chapter 4. London. Martin Dunitz.
    This is a useful chapter on wound care in accident and emergency departments.
KERSTEIN, M.D. (1995) Moist wound healing: the clinical perspective. *Ostomy Wound Management* **41(7a Suppl.)**: 37–50.
    This is a well referenced article discussing the use of moist wound healing techniques and comparing moisture-retentive dressings.
MACKIE R.M. (1992) *Healthy Skin. The Facts*. Oxford. Oxford University Press.
    A useful family guide to skin care that addresses common skin problems associated with different stages of life.
McHENRY, P.M., WILLIAMS, H.C., BINGHAM, E.A. (1995) Management of atopic eczema. *British Medical Journal*. **310**: 843–847.
    This article offers a comprehensive framework for good practice in the management of atopic eczema based on the consensus of opinion of the participants of a joint workshop of the British Association of Dermatologists and the Research Unit of the Royal College of Physicians of London.
MALLETT, J., BAILEY, C. (eds) (1996) *The Royal Marsden NHS Trust Manual of Clinical Nursing Procedures* (4th edition). Chapter 4. Oxford. Blackwell Science Publications.
    This is an informative chapter on aseptic technique.
MURPHY, A. (1995) Cleansing solutions. *Nursing Times*. **91**: 78, 80.
    This article provides a concise guide to wound cleansing agents.
PROVEN, A., PHILLIPS, T.J. (1991) An overview of moist wound dressings: the undercover story. *Dermatology Nursing*. **3**: 393–396.
    A useful article that discusses the merits of the major types of moist wound dressings.
RODGERS, S. (1991) Using proper protocol. *Nursing Times* **87**: 76, 78, 80.
    This article discusses the development – and consequent benefits – of a wound care protocol and central formulary.
ROYAL COLLEGE OF NURSING (1996) Suturing. *Nursing Standard*. **10(51)**: 49–56.
    This article, part of the Royal College of Nursing's continuing education series, describes the skills and techniques involved in suturing. In addition the article sets questions and activities for the reader to attempt.

ROYAL COLLEGE OF NURSING/SMITH AND NEPHEW (1991) *Wound Management Education System*. Smith and Nephew Medical Ltd, PO Box 81, Hessel Road, Hull HU3 2BN.

This is a five-module training package covering: 1. skin anatomy and physiology; 2. wound healing dynamics; 3. factors influencing wound healing; 4. practical wound management; and 5. risk assessment and early intervention: pressure sores. Each pack consists of slides and an accompanying booklet.

WARDMAN C (1991) Norton v Waterlow. *Nursing Times* **87**: 74, 76, 78.

This study carried out in a nursing home setting compares the effectiveness of two risk assessment tools, Norton and Waterlow.

▶ REFERENCES

ANDERSON, P. (1995) Your role in nurse prescribing. *Community Nurse* 1995; 1:20, 22.

ANONYMOUS (1992) Tattoos on women: a unique conversation piece or a career risk. *Reflections* **18(3)**: 35.

ARMSTRONG, M.L. (1991) Career-orientated women with tattoos. *Image – the Journal of Nursing Scholarship* **23**: 215–220.

ARMSTRONG, M.L. (1996) You Pierced What? *Paediatric Nursing* **22**: 236–238.

ARMSTRONG, M.L., McCONNELL, C. (1994) Tattooing in adolescents: more common than you think – the phenomenon and risks. *Journal of School Nursing* **10**: 26–33.

BENBOW, M. (1994) Improving wound management. *Community Outlook* **January**: 21, 22, 24.

BENTON, D. (1995) The role of managed care in overcoming fragmentation. *Nursing Times* **91**: 25–28.

BOYCE, S.T., GLATTER, R., KITZMILLER, W.J. (1995) Treatment of chronic wounds with cultured skin substitutes: a pilot study. *Wounds – A Compendium of Clinical Research and Practice* **7**: 24–29.

BRIGGS, M., WILSON, S., FULLER, A. (1996) The principles of aseptic technique in wound care. *Professional Nurse* **11**: 805, 806, 808, 810.

BUX, M., MALHI, J.S. (1996) Assessing the use of dressings in practice. *Journal of Wound Care* **5**: 305–308.

CASSIDY, J. (1995) Sun spots. *Nursing Times* **91**: 16.

CULL, P. (ed.) (1989) *The Sourcebook of Medical illustration*. Lancs. Parthenon Publishing Group.

CHAPMAN, E.J., CHAPMAN, R. (1986) Treatment of Pressure Sores: The State of the Art. In Tierney, A.J. (ed.) *Clinical Nursing Practice*. p. 105–124. Edinburgh. Churchill Livingstone.

CHARLES, H. (1995) The impact of leg ulcers on patients' quality of life. *Professional Nurse* **10**: 571, 572, 574.

DAVID, J.A. (1986) *Wound Management. A Comprehensive Guide to Dressing and Healing*. London. Martin Dunitz.

DEALEY, C. (1994) *The Care of Wounds*. Oxford. Blackwell Science.

DEPARTMENT OF HEALTH (1993a) *The Health of the Nation. Key Area Handbook: Cancers*. London. Department of Health.

DEPARTMENT OF HEALTH (1993b) *The Health of the Nation. One year on. . . A Report on the Progress of the Health of the Nation*. London. Department of Health.

ERTL, P. (1993a) Planning a route to treatment. A framework for leg ulcer assessment. *Professional Nurse* **8**: 675–679.

ERTL, P. (1993b) The multiple benefits of accurate assessment. Effective management of leg ulcers. *Professional Nurse* **9**: 139–144.

GROSS, R.D. (1992) *Psychology. The Science of Mind and Behaviour* (2nd edition). p. 532. London. Hodder and Stoughton.

INMAN, A. (1994) Leg ulcers in the community. *Primary Health Care* **4**:18, 21, 23.

JACOBSON, D. (1992) *India: Land of Dreams and Fantasy*. New York. Todtri Publications.

LITT, I.F. (1994) Self graffiti? Self image? Self destruction? Tattoos and adolescents. *Journal of Adolescent Health*. **15(3)**: 198.

MARKS, I.M. (1987) *Fears, Phobias and Rituals*. Oxford. Oxford University Press.

McHENRY, P.M., WILLIAMS, H.C., BINGHAM, E.A. (1995) Management of atopic eczema. *British Medical Journal* **310**: 843–847.

MILLER, M. (1994) Setting up a nurse-led clinic in wound healing. *Nursing Standard* **9(6 Tissue Viability)**: 54, 56.

MOFFATT, C.J., OLDROYD, M.I. (1994) A pioneering service to the community. The Riverside Community Leg Ulcer Project. *Professional Nurse* **9**: 486, 488, 490, 492, 494, 497.

MORISON, M. (1992) *A Colour Guide to The Nursing Management of Wounds*. pp. 37–39. London. Wolfe Publishing Ltd.

NAIDOO, J., WILLS, J. (1994) *Health Promotion. Foundations for Practice*. London. Baillière Tindall.

PANDIT, A.S., FELDMAN, D.S. (1994) Effect of oxygen treatment and dressing oxygen permeability on wound healing. *Wound Repair Regeneration* **2**: 130–137.

PODMORE, J. (1994) Leg ulcer: weighing up the evidence. *Nursing Standard* **8**: 25, 27.

RODGERS, S. (1991) Using proper protocol. *Nursing Times* **87**:76, 78, 80.

RUSSELL, G., BOULES, A. (1992) Developing a community based leg ulcer clinic. *British Journal of Nursing* **7**:337–340.

SEYMOUR, J. (1995) Gloves. Alternatives to latex. *Nursing Times* **91**: 46, 48.

SIMON, P. (1992) No doctor in the house. *Nursing Times* **88**:16.

STATUTORY INSTRUMENT (1989) No. 1456. Nurses, Midwives and Health Visitors (Registered Fever Nurses Amendment Rules and Training Amendment Rules) Approval Order 1989. Found in EEC Directive: 77/453/EEC. Annex to UKCC Circular PS&D/89/04 (C).

TORTORA, G.J., ANAGNOSTAKOS, N.P. (1990) *Principles of Anatomy and Physiology* (6th edition). London. Harper and Row.

TREVELYAN, J. (1996) Skin care for special groups. *Nursing Times* **92**: 48, 50.

UKCC (1992) *The Scope of Professional Practice*. London. UKCC.

WATSON, J.E., ROYLE, J.A. (1987) *Watson's Medical-Surgical Nursing and Related Physiology* (3rd edition). London. Baillière Tindall.

WESTABY, S. (ed.) (1985) *Wound Care*. London. William Heinemann Medical Books Ltd.

WIJETUNGE, D. (1992) An A & E approach. *Nursing Times* **88**: 70, 72, 73, 76.

WILSON, J. (1995) *Infection Control in Clinical Practice*. London. Baillière Tindall.

2.5 | *Aggression*

M.F. Taylor

▸ INTRODUCTION

This chapter addresses the topic of aggression and how nurses may respond to this danger. It does this by explaining aggression from its theoretical and practical aspects. An important feature of the chapter is the application to nursing care of the concepts discussed.

▸ OVERVIEW

▸ *Subject Knowledge*

This part of the chapter explores what is understood by the term aggression and the situations in which it occurs. Aggression is considered in terms of its biological and psychosocial explanations.

▸ *Practice Knowledge*

This section explores the nursing management of aggression. Models of aggression management are considered and applied to the nursing situation. Both aggression management and methods to reduce the aggressive action are key elements of this section.

▸ *Professional Knowledge*

In this part there is a discussion of the professional issues that stem from aggression. This section ranges across the whole spectrum of nursing practice from the nursing management of aggression to legal, preventive and safety issues.

▶ *Reflective Knowledge*

The Reflective Knowledge provides exercises for you to complete and to increase awareness of your own responses to aggression. In addition, this section contains four case studies that explore issues of aggression management in each of the four branches of nursing.

On pp. 306–308 there are four case studies, each one relating to one of the branch programmes. You may find it helpful to read one of them before you start the chapter and use it as a focus for your reflections while reading.

SUBJECT KNOWLEDGE

▶ DEFINITIONS OF AGGRESSION AND VIOLENCE

Many authors make distinctions between violence and aggression (Farrell and Gray, 1992; Breakwell, 1995). They contend that violence refers to actual physically destructive acts carried out by one person upon another. This behaviour is intended to produce physical harm. Violent acts are therefore characterized by the use of physical force. They may be directed outwardly towards others or inwardly at the individual (self mutilation). Aggression, on the other hand, refers to a range of behaviours including verbal, emotional or physical actions, that are intended to produce harm upon another. Aggressive acts range on a continuum from verbal or emotional acts to serious physical harm and, in contrast to violent acts, physical harm is not essential. It is also important to stress that the perception of what is an aggressive act may vary. For example, what is deemed a verbal assault by one person, may be identified by another as 'assertion' or a 'defensive' act.

As you will see, the distinction between violence and aggression is not clearcut, and blurring of the two concepts is common. Kaplan *et al.* (1994), for example, use the terms aggression and violence almost synonymously in describing violent fantasies that may become converted into aggressive behaviours. An important element of aggressive acts is that they are intended by the perpetrator to produce harm. This rules out harmful actions that occur accidentally such as in a road traffic accident where someone may be injured, but usually this is not intended by the driver. In the health care context, Bibby (1995) defines health related aggressive actions as those occurring when a health care worker feels threatened or abused or is assaulted by a member of the public during the course of their duties.

▶ CONTEXT AND AGGRESSIVE BEHAVIOUR

The context in which aggressive behaviour occurs is another factor that must be considered. Aggressive acts carried out by competitors in certain sports, such as football or boxing, may be accepted by society in general, whereas the use of these same acts elsewhere would constitute a violent or aggressive act. In health care, an operation produces harm to the patient, but this harm is intended by the surgeon to produce a longer term beneficial effect and so does not meet the criteria of an aggressive act. The social context in which aggression occurs is therefore important.

> Acts of aggression range from harsh words to physical assault. Think of a time when you became angry. Spend a few minutes focusing on:
>
> - *What you thought about.*
> - *How you felt.*
> - *What you wanted to do.*
> - *Having considered these questions is there a major difference between the experience of aggressive thoughts and feelings and the expression of these same feelings?*

▶ PREVALENCE: WHAT IS THE RISK?

As nurses treat the general public they will be exposed to some members of this public who commit aggressive acts. Two topics need to be considered here.

▶ one, comprises the incidence of aggression in society at large;
▶ the second, the incidence of aggression in the health care sector.

It may be argued that an increase in society's level of aggression will be reflected in an increase of aggression in the health caring agencies.

▶ *Social Incidence of Aggression*

The Central Statistics Office (1995) estimated the number of reported violent offences against the person in England and Wales in 1981 was 100 200. In 1991 this had increased to 190 000, and in 1993 was 205 100. These figures need to be understood in relation to a more general increase in crime levels, however. In 1989 total crimes reported were 3 870 700, but by 1994 had risen to 5 521 100. Additionally, these figures should be interpreted within their sociocultural context. For example, increasing social deprivation leading to crime might be one possible explanation, while an increase in social stressors such as long working hours might be an alternative explanation. Nevertheless, irrespective of causes, crimes against the person appear to be increasing.

As well as general increases in crime other contextual observations should be made. For example, fear of crime is far higher for females than for males. In the age range 16–29 years 13% of males express a fear of mugging compared to 33% of females. These figures are important when considering the relative proportions of females and males in the nursing profession.

▶ *Health Related Aggression Incidents*

Many people experience aggression or the fear of aggression in their workplace. The Home Office Research and Statistics Department (1988) found that 25% of crime victims identified their work as the site of the aggression incident, and 14% of respondents said they had been verbally abused at work at least once in the previous year. Work can also be dangerous, not just by being at work, but also in travelling to and from work. For nurses this risk can be especially pertinent as shift work means travel often occurs at times when the protection of busy streets is missing or lonely car parks have to be used (Orr, 1984; Campbell *et al.*, 1989).

Health care itself can be a hazard in that the problems in society will be reflected, and sometimes more sharply focused in health care settings. Some health workplaces are especially vulnerable to aggressive acts. Accident and emergency departments have to deal with alcohol related aggression regularly (Farrel and Gray, 1992; Phil *et al.*, 1993). Psychiatric nursing facilities are also susceptible to the experience of aggression (Fottrell *et al.*, 1978; Vincent and White, 1994; Whittington and Wykes, 1989). Kidd and Stark (1995) noted particular danger in mental health settings, general practice establishments, accident and emergency departments and in facilities caring for the elderly mentally ill. In these situations aggression is exacerbated by high stress levels in which the individual's coping responses may be exceeded. (Chapter 4.1 outlines the range and effect of stressors in the health care environment that may induce coping failure.) Nurses working in these facilities therefore have an increased risk of experiencing acts of aggression.

RESEARCH BASED EVIDENCE

Ryan and Poster (1993) conducted a postal survey for the Nursing Times *comprising the return of 554 questionnaires from readers. Of the respondents 75% were female and the majority were in their 20s and 30s, with 54% working in adult nursing and 32% working in mental health settings. More than 50% of respondents reported 1–9 assaults of some kind in their career: 22% reported being attacked over 15 times; 12% experienced between 10 and 15 assaults; 27% reported 4–9 assaults; 30% experienced 1–3 assaults; and only 8% reported no assaults.*

Hodgkinson et al. (1984) found that the number of assaults on staff was rising at a psychiatric hospital despite a continuous decrease in the number of patients (see also Fottrell et al., 1978).

Although some areas of health care are more susceptible, aggressive acts can occur in all areas of health care. Thoughts of immunity from aggressive acts are a fantasy (Rogers and Salvage, 1988) that may incur severe penalties if resulting complacency has led to a lack of preparation to manage such incidents.

Biological ❯ **THEORIES OF AGGRESSION**

The next step then is to consider the mechanisms, both bodily and psychosocially, by which aggression occurs.

❯ *Biological Theories*

Biological theories focus upon the somatic phenomena underpinning aggression. These physical effects invariably arise and are directed towards the individual's psychosocial environment. Therefore although in this part of the chapter the biological aspects of aggression are considered, the link to the psychosocial environment remains important. Three biological theories of aggression will be explored:

❯ neurological structure and neurotransmitter regulation;
❯ hormonal constitution;
❯ genetic constitution.

❯ *Neurological Structures and Neurotransmitters*

❯ Neurological structures

Stoudemire (1990) and Owens and Ashcroft(1985) discuss the different brain structures that have been identified in the aggression response in animals. These include the preoptic and lateral hypothalamus and the limbic brain regions, including the septum and amygdala. Although these are associated with aggression in different animal species such as rodents, problems occur when attempting to extrapolate this theory to humans because aggression has not been associated with specific human brain structures (Owens and Ashcroft, 1985; Kaplan *et al.*, 1994).

❯ Neurotransmitters

Two neurotransmitters, noradrenaline and serotonin, have been the prime focus of studies into aggression. Briefly, serotonin is thought to inhibit aggressive responses while noradrenaline increases them. To support this contention, low serum concentrations of serotonin have been found in aggressive individuals (Hollin, 1992). A two-way process therefore emerges in which a high serum concentration of noradrenaline increases aggression, while a high serum concentration of serotonin counteracts aggressive impulses. Similarly if the serotonin serum concentration falls, noradrenaline becomes more able to exert aggressive impulses.

Although an attractive theory, a simple chemical cause of aggression has not in fact been found (Moyer, 1979; Owens and Ashcroft, 1985; Hollin, 1992). Chemical influences do not cause aggression on their own, although they may contribute to it.

One way in which an individual's internal chemistry can be changed is by the use of chemical substances such as alcohol and other 'leisure' drugs. Raistrick (1994) debates whether it is the drugs that cause individuals to act aggressively or the individuals themselves. Some drugs such as alcohol are associated with violence (Phil *et al.*, 1993). These authors argue that violence with alcohol results from an inhibition of control. Again it may be the underlying personality's desire for aggression rather than the alcohol that incites aggressive behaviour.

Other drugs, such as opiates decrease aggressive behaviour, yet their use is also associated with violence. Here their association is indirect, such as in fights between drug dealers.

Figure 2.5.1 outlines the main ideas by which neurological structure and function produce aggressive behaviour.

> If a patient or client exhibited more aggression than others would this mean he possessed abnormally aggressive brain structures or chemicals?

RESEARCH BASED EVIDENCE

In a study by Shachter and Singer (1962) subjects were told they were being given vitamin injections, when in actual fact they were given adrenaline (a substance related to noradrenaline) or a harmless placebo. These subjects were then placed into either 'happy' or 'angry' situations. The major effect of the adrenaline was to enhance the subject's response to the situation they were in. Adrenaline did not produce the emotion itself.

This study provides an important insight into chemical research and aggression-producing substances. In human subjects it appears that almost irrespective of the various chemicals circulating in the blood that could facilitate an aggressive response, humans first interpret their situation before making a response. The site of this interpretation appears to reside in the cerebral cortex, which is the site of cognition or thinking activity. Within this cognitive dimension, action is geared to the social environment in which the individual's internal chemical environment serves a secondary function.

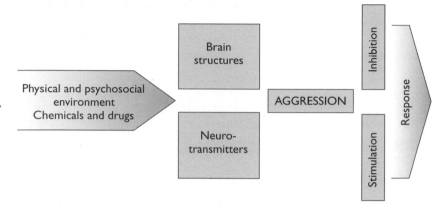

Figure 2.5.1: Neurological structure, function and the occurrence of aggression. This shows how environmental factors provide input to the brain structures and how the neurotransmitter state of the individual can give rise to aggression or aggression inhibition.

▶ *Hormones*

Most research into hormones and the aggressive response has concerned the sex hormones. These are thought to act at two levels:

▶ first, by predisposing the individual to become biologically developed in terms of muscular and other body systems to enable aggression to be used in the pursuit of sexual or other drives;

▶ second, by the direct incitement to act aggressively under the influence of sexual hormones.

Owens and Ashcroft (1985) noted how the male sex hormone, androgen, influenced aggressive responses. They discussed how castrated rats became less aggressive – probably due to their removed androgen supply – and how monkeys with high serum androgen concentrations were associated with higher levels of aggressive responses. The problem is that it is difficult to replicate these same findings in human subjects. Although it can be shown that males are more involved in violent and sexual crimes, and that male delinquency is associated with the onset of puberty (Hollin, 1992), attributing such behaviour to high serum testosterone levels has not been proven in human subjects. It can be argued that the social and economic environments are more important determinants of aggressive behaviour as men with high levels of testosterone may never commit violent or sexual offences.

One other area of hormonal influence on aggressive behaviour is the role of hormones in the menstrual cycle (Prentky, 1985). This was prompted by women attributing violent or aggressive actions to the premenstrual stage of their menstrual cycle. Again problems establishing a definite causal linkage are the major issue and as yet this has not been established.

One of the major problems with research in this area is that it is usually individuals who have come to the attention of medical or other authorities who become the subjects of study. Healthy individuals who do not have similar problems are not usually studied in sufficient number to provide evidence of causality.

▶ *Genetic Factors*

Owens and Ashcroft (1985) identified three major genetic influences on aggressive behaviour:

▶ one concerned how certain abnormal chromosome patterns influence aggressive behaviour;

RESEARCH BASED EVIDENCE

Prentky (1985) carried out research into falls in the serum concentration level of progesterone, a substance considered to possess tranquillizing properties. Tension and irritability appeared to increase during the time in the menstrual cycle when progesterone fell to its lowest serum concentration values, resulting in aggression in a small proportion of women. However, Prentky failed to establish a specific link between falls in progesterone serum concentration level and aggression.

> the second, considered personality to be genetically determined;
> the third identified specific sex chromosomal abnormalities associated with aggression – some patterns increasing and others decreasing aggressive behaviour.

Eysenck and Gudjonsson (1989) argued for a genetic influence in offending as monozygotic (identical) twins were found to be more likely to offend than dizygotic (fraternal) twins. This similarity may also be explained by similarities of upbringing rather than genetic factors, although Bouchard *et al.* (1990) found that twins raised apart demonstrated similar behaviour.

Jeffrey (1979) also attributed aggressive behaviour to genetic makeup. He considered that an extra Y chromosome in male prisoners was associated with aggressive behaviour. Additionally, he considered there was also a greater proportion of such individuals in secure mental hospitals. The findings of this research have been questioned, however, as other studies have found that such individuals commit crimes against property rather than against people (Casey *et al.*, 1973; Price, 1978). Consequently, a similar problem emerges to that of the other biological explanations of aggression. It is difficult to separate factors like genetic makeup from the other complex variables that make up human individuals.

> Imagine you experienced an aggressive incident and the perpetrator suggested afterwards that it was mainly a physical response on his part over which he had little control.
>
> • **What would your response be to this individual?**

Psychosocial ▶ PSYCHOSOCIAL THEORIES

Three major psychosocial theories of aggression will be considered (Howells and Hollin, 1989; Lloyd and Mayes, 1990; Feldman, 1992; Hilgard *et al.*, 1993):

> psychoanalytic theory;
> frustration–aggression hypothesis;
> social learning theory.

The Psychoanalytic Theory of Aggression

Freud's model of the person comprised a bipolar model (Frankl, 1990):

> at one pole is an eros drive – the instinct for life;
> at the other pole is a thanatos drive – the death or destructive instinct.

It is the death instinct when turned outwards that results in aggressive impulses, and when turned inwards creates self-destructive impulses (Bocok 1986; Aronson 1995). Freud saw society controlling the release of this death energy by socializing controls. When such control is not achieved then aggression occurs. From this perspective aggression is an instinctual response that enables the individual to survive. According to Frankl (1990, p. 46) the aggressive drive 'is a compensatory response of the life-seeking instinct to the dangers of loss or negation of libidinous flow, an attempt to regain it by attacking the depriving object and breaking through its inhibitions'.

Aggression arises when a threat has occurred to the life seeking drive (eros) of an individual. As a response the individual releases the opposing (thanatos) drive to attack the causes of the threat. Aggression is therefore a reaction to frustrations of the eros drive.

Psychoanalytic literature identifies the origins of aggression from infancy (Freud, 1920; Fenichel, 1982; Klein, 1988; Frankl, 1990). During

Imagine the situation where you have made plans to pursue a particular project. You have been planning this project for many months. Suddenly, your employer insists you have to work. This will mean you will miss your project.

- *Where does your experience of aggression arise from?*
- *Is it deep within you or is it related to your employer and therefore outside yourself?*

DECISION MAKING

Lee, aged 22 years, has been admitted to the orthopaedic ward following his involvement in a fight at a night club earlier in the evening. He has sustained a possible fracture in his hand, which will require manipulation later the next day and has been admitted for this procedure. The ward has been particularly busy lately, and on the night shift Lee has been particularly demanding. He still smells of alcohol, and he is asking for one thing and then another. As he senses the attitude of the nursing staff he becomes even more demanding and hostile.

- *Name three theories of aggression that may explain Lee's currently aggressive and demanding behaviour.*
- *Which theory of aggression do you consider best explains Lee's current responses on the orthopaedic ward?*

feeding infants suffer frustrations, which manifest as aggressive actions directed towards their mother and environment. Human infants are not capable of understanding all that is happening about them even if it is for their own good. So, when their immediate desires are not met, they become frustrated and express this as aggression. Therefore aggression in the adult is viewed as regression to an early period of experience.

Frustration–Aggression Hypothesis

This theory was first proposed by Dollard *et al.* (1939) and proposes that aggression is not tied to instinctual drives, but to the social environment. The common precipitant of aggression arises from frustration to some ongoing activity. When an individual is blocked or frustrated from reaching a desired goal then aggression is deemed likely to occur. A distinction needs to be made from psychoanalytic theory where the frustration in the child arises from within – from the child's thanatos impulses. Conversely, in the frustration–aggression theory, the actual occurrence of aggression is linked to the emergence of anger and negative feelings in response to situations individuals find themselves in. The trigger for aggression therefore arises outside the individual (Berkowitz, 1969, 1990). It follows then that aggressive impulses can be controlled if all experiences are kept frustration free.

Figure 2.5.2 depicts the location of aggressive impulses: the level of shading in the different boxes illustrates the openness of the individual to their social world. Theories that rely on purely innate states possess little contact with the social environment, while drive theories and social learning theories propose greater social influence.

Social Learning Theory

Malim and Birch (1989) identify two major sources of aggression:

- one arises from the provocation of other people;
- the other arises by exposure to aggressive models of responding.

For example, if an individual believes him or herself to be under attack from others then it is likely to result in attack as a response. (Attack is the best form of defence.) In this case, emotional arousal results from aversive experiences. One option that is learned in this situation is to respond aggressively as a form of survival. When the individual observes aggressive behaviour from other people, they deduce that there are incentives for them to act aggressively.

Individuals learn to respond violently to a range of cues. These include factors in the social environment such as overcrowding, heat, noise and drugs that reduce inhibition such as alcohol. The watching of violence on television (Eron *et al.*, 1972; Gerbner and Gross, 1976) has also been suggested as an aggression-inducing factor.

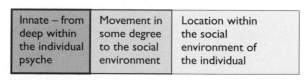

Figure 2.5.2: Location of aggressive impulses.

Biological theories and psychosocial theories of aggression have been discussed. Although no one particular theory appears to offer a complete explanation for aggression, they all provide insight into the aggressive process. The theories of aggression must therefore be viewed eclectically. That is that they originate in the individual's biological, psychological and social environment. This knowledge then forms the platform upon which nursing insight may be gained in terms of the later construction of nursing interventions.

PRACTICE KNOWLEDGE

This section starts with the nursing assessment, the purpose of which is to:

◗ predict risk;
◗ plan for de-escalation of the risk;
◗ aim to prevent aggression.

◗ PREDICTION OF RISK OF AGGRESSION

Pollock *et al.* (1989), Hinde (1993) and Farrington (1994) identified factors implicated in aggressive behaviour and these have been combined into Tables 2.5.1 and 2.5.2. Table 2.5.1 focuses on the individual. It is important not to pre-judge individuals who may have experienced previous problems with aggression. It is, however, also important to be prepared for any contingencies. Table 2.5.2 focuses on the individual's interaction with the environment. These factors may predispose individuals to take on an aggressive role. An awareness of such predisposing factors is therefore necessary in the nursing assessment of aggression risk.

DECISION MAKING

You are working in an accident and emergency unit situated in a busy inner city area.

• *What factors may predispose the unit staff to experience aggressive incidents?*

Prediction category	Examples
Personality factors	• Low threshold of frustration or impulsivity • Increased liability to become aroused · • An antisocial personality such as someone who is habitually aggressive or undercontrolled · • Substance abusers
Previous history of aggression or violence	• An institutional record where violence has been a factor may mean an increased risk of violence
Biological factors	• A genetic constitution that tends towards a lack of control • Disinhibitory factors such as caused by brain damage, and some organic mental illnesses
Mental disorder	• Psychotic individuals who experience a build up of tension before a violent outburst • Some depressed individuals may attempt to kill others for altruistic reasons – to relieve their supposed suffering
Fear, pain or frustration	• Frustration, fear or pain may lead to aggressive responses

Table 2.5.1 Prediction of aggression: the individual.

Prediction category	Examples
Peer influences and group pressures	• Peer and group pressures to act aggressively may be exerted on individuals • Certain geographical areas may possess more aggressive cues than others • School influences can occur with some schools possessing relatively more offenders in their pupils compared with other schools • Generally, the culture that individuals may have been exposed to that do not denigrate aggression may predispose certain individuals to an aggressive response pattern
Economic, social and environmental influences	• Economic and social deprivation tend to be associated with offending and sometime aggressive responses • There may be an association between situational influences and aggressive behaviour – such as the availability of weapons • Additional social factors include extrafamilial roles, peer group and media influences • Uncomfortable or stressful social or physical conditions can predispose to aggression
The presence of a victim	• As a subject upon whom aggression is expressed is necessary, so victims are essential in the expression of aggression – the assertion is made here that aggression is not likely to occur without the presence of someone on whom to carry out the aggressive act • As nurses it is essential that taking on the identity of a victim or potential victim is kept to a minimum

Table 2.5.2 Prediction of aggression: the social environment.

▶ IDENTIFYING CUES THAT WARN AGGRESSION IS IMMINENT

Individuals usually give warning that an act of aggression is about to occur. Littlechild (1996) and Breakwell (1992) listed verbal and non-verbal cues that often precede aggressive or violent acts and may herald an aggressive action (Table 2.5.3). Usually, an aggressive individual will exhibit some of these verbal and non-verbal cues before the aggressive act. Wright (1989) observed that often the precursor to aggression is a build-up of anger. Denial and avoidance of potential aggression are likely to increase the danger, therefore an awareness of the escalation of aggression by the nurse is essential. Once the danger signals have been picked up by the nurse, action needs to be taken. De-escalation is the term used to refer to the process of reducing the threat posed by a potential aggressor. The next section will consider how de-escalation can be achieved.

▶ WHAT TO DO ABOUT ANGER AND IMPENDING AGGRESSIVE ACTIONS

Before actions can be taken to de-escalate a potentially aggressive incident it is essential that nurses are aware of their own feelings. Fear in this situation is to be expected, and can be used to provide the impetus necessary to take the actions required. Three actions are essential (Table 2.5.4).

Body language	Movements become jerky
	Pacing
	An aggressive posture in relation to others
	Threatening gestures
	Physical closeness
	A stiff posture
	Objects may be broken
	Clenching of fists
	Drumming of fingers
	Tight facial musculature
	Heightened respiratory rate
	Pointing
Eyes	Fixed eye contact
	Looking away
	Long periods of silence
Voice	Raised voice
	Verbal threats
	Shouting
	Pressure of speech
	Obtaining the help of others

Table 2.5.3 The non-verbal cues that may precede aggression. Adapted from Breakwell (1992) and Littlechild (1996).

Actions	Rationale
Listen to what the aggressive individual is saying	This will provide the information necessary to identify and deal with the source of the individual's anger
Focus on the source of the individual's anger	This will help to prevent the conversion of the focus of aggression to a more physical process
Try not to mirror aggressive body posture	Adopting an aggressive body posture in response to that of the potential aggressor is likely to be interpreted as the nurse's own preparation for aggression (Braithwaite, 1992).

Table 2.5.4 Actions to deal with the potential aggressor.

▶ WASP (Wait – Assess – Slowly – Proceed) and RAP/Review (Recognition – Awareness – Planning – Review)

Waring and Wilson (1990) in providing assistance for aggressive individuals give the following advice in the form of the acronym WASP, which stands for:

- ▶ wait;
- ▶ assess;
- ▶ slowly;
- ▶ proceed.

Wait means to stop and see what is taking place. It is important to not simply react. Meeting an aggressive verbal response with an equally aggressive verbal response is likely to result in each person increasing the stakes with more emotional input. It is important here to stop and consider what is happening. Assess means to focus on the important issue that is the trigger for this particular incident. What is it that this person is responding to with this aggressive style of expression? Slowly indicates that an attitude of calmness is necessary. As you slow down, so the other person is likely to as well, and so you will both be helped. Proceed means to use assertive or other skills to bring about a de-escalation of the problem. Focus on the issues that are disturbing this person. Although this advice was primarily intended for the perpetrators of violent acts it is good advice for nurses who may need to deal with violence.

This WASP model is similar to the RAP/review model proposed by Littlechild (1996), which stands for:

▶ recognition;
▶ awareness;
▶ planning;
▶ review.

Recognition of anger and impending aggression is essential if measures are to be taken to de-escalate this risk. Awareness on the part of nurses is also essential if they are to take effective action. Planning to deal with both anger and aggression ensures the safety and wellbeing of all concerned. Review means that all aggressive incidents are subject to later analysis from the clinical practitioners and the larger agency structures. While planning should take place before an aggressive incident, the review stage should take place afterwards and so assist in dealing with any future incidents. This latter process of review by the agency managers may be taken some time from the initial incident and may include a review of similar incidents.

▶ The First Two Rules for Managing a Potential Aggressor

It is often useful to use rules to help planning to deal with aggressive situations (Smith, 1986; Burrow, 1994). At this stage then we can generate a rule for managing with a potential aggressor.

> ▶ **Rule 1:** Summon provisional help while you deal with the individual's anger first – before it escalates into aggressive actions

Cembrowicz and Ritter (1994) provide the following advice for dealing with the angry person:

▶ pay close attention to him or her;
▶ stand just outside his or her personal space – out of arm's reach;
▶ stand on his or her non-dominant side (locate the non-dominant side by observing the hand on which the wrist watch is worn or what side the hair is parted);
▶ use a quiet, calm, but determined manner;
▶ use calm body language – avoid mirroring the angry individual's body expression;
▶ avoid staring eye contact;
▶ avoid pointing or touching or entering his or her personal space.

At this point another rule can be made.

> ▶ **Rule 2:** If the individual remains verbally, or emotionally aggressive, and you consider violence is likely, then help is needed at this time

If no help is available, then ascertain avenues of escape. Do not let the individual come between you and your escape route.

▶ *The Assault Cycle*

If the point has been reached where the potential for aggressive acts has been reached then an assault cycle is entered. Smith (1977), Rowett and Breakwell (1992) and Leadbetter and Paterson (1995) describe how this is structured. Using the five-stage assault cycle (Figure 2.5.3) helps to understand how aggression occurs and how intervention may be planned.

Figure 2.5.3: The assault cycle.

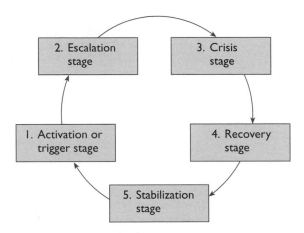

▶ 1. Activation or trigger stage

The individual becomes aroused by some event or interpersonal situation. In this stage the nurse needs to identify and reduce aggression triggers. This means that clients need to be listened to and understood. Client anxieties need to be dealt with and nurses must communicate effectively to direct clients to alternative courses of action. Communication becomes less effective if the client proceeds to the crisis phase. Leadbetter and Paterson (1995) emphasize 'personalizing the self'. By 'personalizing the self', these authors mean making reference to the individual in terms of their needs and feelings, and not referring to them as the occupant of a social or other role. This means talking to the client as an individual.

▶ 2. Escalation stage

Stress and frustration increase. The client feels helpless and the probability of conversion to physical expression increases. Calming measures need to be kept active. Communication needs to be maintained in a non-threatening stance. A return to the previous stage is possible, and this should be the aim of intervention.

▶ 3. Crisis stage

Physical, emotional, and psychological impulses are expressed. The client is in the fight or flight phase of the stress response. Blood supply is diverted to skeletal muscles, cardiac and respiratory systems.

If escalation to the crisis stage occurs communication is more difficult. If physical aggression occurs then help from other staff members is essential. Bystanders need to be removed, as do any objects that could be used as weapons. Verbal communication still needs to be maintained. At this stage it becomes essential to observe the third rule for managing a potential aggressor.

The Third and Fourth Rules for Managing a Potential Aggressor

Rule 3: It is essential that all nurses are aware of how to summon help

This rule includes a sound knowledge of all agency policies in relation to client aggression. Such knowledge is required before an aggressive incident. Check aggression management policies immediately when entering new clinical areas and keep revising your knowledge of these procedures.

Being prepared is essential for all nurses at this stage. Remember that aggression can occur in any area. Adequate preparation before an encounter helps effective management of aggressive incidents.

During the crisis stage all avenues available to communicate with the client should be used. A raised voice may be necessary to make a point. It may be necessary to bargain in some measure. However, it is also important not to give in completely to clients as this could reinforce future use of aggression to further their own ends. If control becomes lost then escape, physical restraint or self-defence become essential. Bibby (1995) and Leadbetter and Paterson (1995) discuss responses to physical violence as comprising:

- fight;
- flight;
- compromise.

Farrell and Gray (1992) emphasize the need for an effective self-presentation, that is, appearing non-threatened and non-intimidated, which may preclude the need for self-preservation. However, if self-preservation is needed then another rule can be made.

Rule 4: Never attempt to physically restrain a client without assistance from others

Use all means necessary to call for help. This may include the use of a panic button, the telephone, shouting or sending other people. Ideally, such preparations are made before the crisis phase is reached. Leadbetter and Paterson (1995) call this part of the crisis stage the destructive phase, and they indicate the necessity for the skills of risk assessment, breakaway techniques and staff coordination. This chapter will not discuss breakaway and restraint techniques, which lie in the province of specialist teaching units. However, effective practice of physical restraint skills is a necessary part of nursing care, both for the protection of nurses and for the safety of clients.

The Fourth and Fifth Stages of the Assault Cycle

4. Recovery stage

Agitation decreases, anxiety lessens, and communication becomes possible. At this stage the acute crisis has ended and the need for physical control of the client has ended. However, caution still needs to be maintained as the individual may feel upset at how he or she has been treated and can still revert to the crisis stage.

It is necessary that staff maintain control of the situation and contain the risk. This may require the use of sedation or seclusion, in which case local policies for observation will need implementing. Staff members who have been called to help will also need to maintain their presence.

Calm, but firm communication is needed. Generally, people who have witnessed part of the proceedings may be apprehensive and so a calm manner is needed to progress to the next stage.

5. Stabilization stage

The client is able to regain control of outward behaviour. Often a post-crisis depression occurs in which the individual's professional performance is guarded and uncertain, so resulting in less efficiency in their place of work. At this stage he or she is most likely to be receptive to clinical interventions and may feel remorse, guilt or shame for the behaviour. It is important to maintain communication with the client and to investigate with them the reasons for the crisis that has occurred. A quiet area where the nurse and client can talk undisturbed is necessary. The client needs to know that he or she is still accepted and the emphasis needs to be on how the client can be helped to avoid future repetition of the aggression. The role of nursing staff is not to judge nor punish such clients, but to assist them to live more effective and less problematic lives. It is not only the client who needs attention at this time, but all the staff who have been involved in the incident. Here another rule – the fifth rule for managing a potential aggressor – may be applied.

The Fifth Rule for Managing a Potential Aggressor

Rule 5: Staff who have been involved in an act of physical aggression from a client will need debriefing

The aim of staff debriefing is to fulfil three functions:

- to enable a review of the whole incident and plan future client care appropriately;
- to enable a review of the procedures carried out and to advise whether modification is necessary in the light of information obtained from the incident;
- to enable staff to ventilate their feelings and review their own coping resources.

It is also important at this stage to consider the effects of the incident upon other clients who may have been present. A policy of open communication is essential and clients should be allowed to express their concerns and anxieties about the incident they have witnessed. They need to be reassured that the needs of the client in crisis were uppermost despite any physical restraint carried out. Such reassurance will enable other clients to come to terms with the event they have witnessed. It is essential that clients are aware that nurses act in the interests of the client in crisis.

DECISION MAKING

You are working on an acute psychiatric admission ward. A male client, aged 23 years, has recently been admitted under section 4 of the *Mental Health Act* (DHSS, 1983). His behaviour has become increasingly bizarre, and he tried to set fire to a bus on which he was a passenger. He is restless and keeps asking to leave the ward. Gradually, his stance becomes more threatening, and he approaches staff very close and stares directly at them. He has been prescribed chlorpromazine syrup, 100 mg orally four times a day, which can be repeated as required. You are the nurse in charge and have three staff members, two female, and one male.

- *What phase of the assault cycle is this client in?*
- *What calming measure would you use?*
- *How would you respond to his demands to leave the ward?*

PROFESSIONAL KNOWLEDGE

The nursing interventions so far have provided understanding of a strategy for dealing with aggression. This section will consider the wider issues involved in the professional nursing management of aggression. The following headings will be explored in the light of nursing care:

- safety of others;
- nursing management following an aggressive incident;
- legal issues;
- resourcing to maintain a safe environment;
- the ramifications of inappropriate nursing behaviour in response to aggressive situations;

- client abuse and aggressive staff;
- planning for non-aggressive units;
- community care.

▶ SAFETY OF OTHERS

The need to manage aggression to minimize harm has already been mentioned. As a professional dealing with aggression the nurse has responsibility not only to the person experiencing aggression, but to all others in the area in which aggression occurs. This includes:

- the individual experiencing aggression, who needs to be kept as safe as possible; staff should not carry out acts of retribution;
- any victim of the attack or assault, who needs to be cared for and their future safety ensured, and this may involve medical care, and counselling;
- the nurse involved and other nursing colleagues, who need to be assured of their safety; plans need to be made and communicated in the event of further aggression;
- other clients in the immediate vicinity, who should be firmly asked to leave during the early stages of any aggressive incident, but if this has not been possible they may need checking for physical or psychological injury;
- other bystanders, for example visitors to the unit, who should preferably have been asked to leave in the early stages, but if they have been present they need to be talked to, their impressions confirmed, and provided with any needed reassurance. This means taking active steps to talk to visitors, to allow them to express their opinion, and to assure them that control has been achieved, and that the aggressive individual and others involved will be helped to deal with the incident.
- other professional staff, who may need help before they leave the area;
- if property has been damaged it needs to be inspected and repaired to ensure future safety.

▶ NURSING MANAGEMENT FOLLOWING AN AGGRESSIVE INCIDENT

The nursing management following an aggressive incident falls into two main areas: the first immediately following the incident, and the second concerning the time up to a few days later.

▶ *Immediately Following the Incident*

During this time it is important to allow a gradual return to the usual level of activity in the unit. This return to routine allows a sense of control and stability to emerge. During this time it is important to document the names of all present. This allows for future debriefing and it may also be necessary to contact them should legal proceedings follow. As soon as calm has been restored to the unit, agency policy documents relating to the incident should be completed and debriefing undertaken.

◗ *Up to a Few Days Following the Incident – Debriefing*

Debriefing allows individuals to deal effectively with the aggressive incident and not suffer long-term psychological damage as a result. It is of special importance in enabling staff to learn from the incident and avoid self-blame or guilt. It is also helpful in the prevention of post-traumatic stress disorder (PTSD). Any staff who need to, should be allowed to talk at this stage before the debriefing described below, and reassured that there will be later support and an opportunity for them to talk.

Cembrowicz and Ritter (1994) state that the aim of debriefing is to assure the individual that:

◗ their feelings and thoughts are normal;
◗ their feelings are important;
◗ their feelings are recognized.

This is supported by Robb (1995) who adds that 'critical incident' debriefing should be undertaken 48–72 hours after the incident and suggests that all involved should be asked:

◗ what happened?
◗ how he or she felt at the time of the incident?
◗ how he or she feels now?

Asking 'what happened?' allows the individual give his or her account and helps to gain some perspective of his or her role in the incident. It is important to allow this to proceed at the pace the individual requires to explain it in full. This helps to prevent suppression of important elements of what happened and, in turn, prevent later problems.

Asking 'how did you feel?' provides an opportunity to contact and deal with negative emotions. The feelings generated by an aggressive incident are likely to be highly negative and unpleasant. This means the individual has two options available – to either discuss and bring into the open negative emotions or to deny them. Bringing negative emotions into a discursive format may be unpleasant at the time, but once talked about and shared with others, these emotions begin to lose their power to adversely affect the individual. Alternatively, if negative emotions are suppressed or denied they may exert a later unconscious influence over the individual who can go on to develop long-term emotional problems. Emotional disinhibition, in which the control of emotional expression is lost, is another important sequel to aggression. This also needs to be explored with a view to facilitating an effective emotional contact with the incident so that effective emotional expression followed by appropriate levels of emotional control is achieved.

Asking 'how do you feel now?' helps to bring feelings into the present. This gives an indication of how the incident is being dealt with. If denial is suspected or other emotional reactions are present, more specialized help may be required. It is important that emotional responses to aggressive incidents are accepted as a normal and expected reaction. Nurses do not need to demonstrate a hard exterior and be completely emotionless and in control. Nurses are human, and therefore subject to feelings of fear, anger, guilt and shame – all of which are common and expected reactions to aggression. To talk about such emotions in an attentive and caring manner is perhaps the most important element in caring for carers after aggressive incidents.

▶ *Debriefing Sessions*

Debriefing can take many forms and can range from individual meetings with the team leader or another skilled helper to the use of larger group meetings. Cembrowicz and Ritter (1994) suggest the use of three team meetings, noting that even if only one team member is involved he or she still needs team support, as follows:

▶ a first informal meeting over tea or coffee and soon after the event at which a skilled leader facilitates the group to discuss informally about what has happened and the feelings of staff who were present or involved;

▶ a second meeting of at least two hours 1–2 days after the event, which takes place in a more formal setting and allows members to re-live the event and their responses to it and to talk about how the event has influenced their home or social life, and at which educational material may also be provided;

▶ a third meeting to address unresolved issues from the second meeting and to conclude the debriefing.

If someone has been either physically or psychologically damaged then psychological support from skilled professionals may need to be arranged. Such support will require the assistance of counsellors skilled in the treatment of PTSD. The symptoms of PTSD include the following (World Health Organization,1992):

▶ flashbacks;
▶ emotional numbing;
▶ hypervigilance;
▶ avoidance;
▶ confusion, anxiety and depression.

It is most important to prevent this disorder and so effective debriefing is therefore essential.

▶ *Clinical Supervision*

An adjunct to the debriefing session is the use of supervision meetings. Clinical supervision is concerned with assisting nurses to practice and improve helping skills with the aid of a long-term relationship with another clinical practitioner. Clinical supervision offers the opportunity to bring the experience of aggression into a long-term support meeting where all aspects of the incident and its experience can be dealt with.

▶ *Reviewing the Incident*

Earlier in the chapter the use of RAP/review model suggested by Littlechild (1996) was considered. Integral to this model is the process of review. When all accounts of participants have been made and strategies for help obtained, then further actions can be taken to learn from the incident and assist in minimizing the risk of aggression in the future. It is important that it does not degenerate into attributing blame as this often leads to those who feel 'wronged' to seek retribution. The purpose of review is to take positive learning from the incident to reduce the likelihood of similar situations developing or to review how such incidents might be more effectively managed.

Littlechild (1996) suggests that strategies for managing aggression should exist at three levels – with practitioners, with managers and at agency level. This structure should subsequently form the basis of the review:

▶ at the practitioner level opportunities are present for individuals to learn from their experience and they may need to adopt different or modified personal strategies;

▶ at the manager level learning points can be identified and questions concerning issues such as the availability and skill of help provided and the speed of response should be asked;

▶ at the agency level issues of policy amendment or change may need to be addressed and the effectiveness and availability of post-incident support can be identified.

▶ LEGAL ISSUES

During the review it may be concluded that the general safety of the clinical environment should be examined. It is the duty of the employer to ensure a safe workplace as far as possible. Specific legislations that set out these conditions are the:

▶ *Health and Safety at Work Act* (DHSS, 1974);
▶ *Management of Health and Safety at Work Regulations* (Health and Safety Commission, 1992).

These place a responsibility for safety and employee training upon the employing authority if five or more staff are employed. Employers therefore have a duty to ensure that their staff are equipped with training and, in terms of their workplace, to ensure a safe environment. It follows then that employee training in techniques such as restraint and breakaway, under these acts, is the responsibility of the employer.

As the employers have the responsibility to provide a safe environment and adequate staff training, so a responsibility also rests with the nursing staff to provide a professional level of intervention. Here the nurses' need to carry out defensive measures against a possible assailant is contrasted against any possible harm that may occur to an assailant. Nurses possess a 'duty of care' to assist clients. When clients are aggressive, it may be argued that nurses are not under such duty if they feel threatened. The answer to this problem is that where aggression is likely, such as in psychiatric wards or casualty departments, employers have a duty to provide written instructions and training for managing aggressive clients with which nurses must be acquainted and follow (Aiken and Tarbuck, 1995).

If a nurse is attacked the law allows for 'such force as is reasonable in the circumstances in the prevention of crime . . .' according to section 3(1) of the *Criminal Law Act* (Home Office, 1967). The issue here is that any actions by the nurse need to be reasonable to prevent further attack or assault. However, any response by the nurse needs to be taken within the context of the nurses' *Code of Professional Conduct* (UKCC, 1984), which in Rule 1 states that nurses 'act always in such a way as to promote and safeguard the well-being and interests of patients and clients'. This means that nurses who need to carry out restraint or self-defence must ensure that their actions do not go beyond the point at which unnecessary harm is done to the client. The *Code of Practice of Mental Health Act* (DHSS, 1993) offers guidance in dealing with mentally ill people. Aiken and Tarbuck (1995) discuss how this code enables restraint to be carried out in a safe manner (without the infliction of pain) and the use of seclusion. The *Code of Practice of Mental Health Act* (1993) also offers advice for psychiatric staff in terms of ensuring effective communication, personal space, acting therapeutically, monitoring client mix and staff skills, and facilitating client complaints procedures.

Before leaving the topic of legal issues it is necessary to emphasize that accurate record keeping is an essential component in the management of aggressive incidents. Personal biographic and contact data need to be obtained from all those involved. Full statements, including events before, during, and following the aggressive incident need to be recorded, as well as the times of and the actions carried out. Different health care agencies possess their own documentary systems for recording these data. It is essential that all documentary procedures are carefully followed to avoid later legal problems.

▶ RESOURCING TO MAINTAIN A SAFE ENVIRONMENT

The *Health and Safety at Work Act* (DHSS, 1974) aims to ensure a safe working environment. The issue for nursing practice is that plans are made not only to maximize safety during an aggressive incident, but also to minimize the incidence of aggressive events. All acts of aggression take place in particular environments so elements in the environment need to be screened to assess their contribution to the development or escalation of anger in clients. For example, if aggressive outbursts are more common at particular times such as at meal times, then actions can be taken to reduce this risk. The RAP/review model (Littlechild, 1996) suggests that clinical practitioners as well as management are essential participants for planning and dealing with aggression. Safety for staff and clients must be a priority if health care work is to continue safely.

▶ THE RAMIFICATIONS OF INAPPROPRIATE NURSING BEHAVIOUR IN RESPONSE TO AGGRESSIVE SITUATIONS

A case (Holland, 1992) is mentioned (Professional Conduct Committee Case no. A5) in which an enrolled nurse pulled a patient to the floor and dragged him several feet. This action could be described as either an over-response, or an attack by the nurse upon the patient. The nurse was dismissed from his employment, but was allowed to remain on the professional register by the Professional Conduct Committee. The nurse was deemed to have been unwise and overconfident in his abilities to manage difficult patients. The issue here is that a line may be drawn between actions that are necessary and those that are unnecessary in terms of controlling aggressive clients. Sometimes discrimination between sufficient and excess control is difficult to ascertain. Overzealous physical control can occur with the implications of client assault. As a guide to what level of control is necessary in any given situation imagine that all the nurse's actions are being filmed for public showing and consider whether any of the actions would cause a public outcry in terms of their degree of physical attack or force. Often cases have arisen where cruelty, defined as unnecessary harm, has occurred to clients and public enquiries have been mounted to ascertain fault. Such actions can reduce the public's confidence in the nursing profession.

▶ CLIENT ABUSE AND AGGRESSIVE STAFF

Client abuse falls into two categories:

- ▶ the first is where physical restraint escalates beyond the point of need and becomes converted into client attack;
- ▶ the second is where no preliminary contact is made and clients are attacked without provocation.

In both situations the UKCC *Code of Professional Conduct* (UKCC, 1984) is explicit that client care is the priority. Physical assault that takes place outside the legal framework constitutes an infringement of human rights and becomes a potential criminal issue. Nursing staff are often in positions of power relative to clients, and such power needs to be handled within a philosophy of care to clients. Being alert to abuses of this power is a necessary aspect of professional nursing. Staff who abuse clients must be reported to their employers, and criminal proceedings may follow. If this course of action is to be undertaken then it is essential that records are kept and are accurate. 'Hearsay' evidence is open to debate, and human memory can fail. Full recording of any incidents of abuse need to be made stating the date, times, those present, the staff member/s involved, and the actions taken at the time. Medical staff may be needed to examine clients to confirm any injuries sustained.

▶ PLANNING FOR NON-AGGRESSIVE UNITS

Prevention of aggressive incidents is, of course, the preferred action. Gould (1994) describes several practical ways in which violence was reduced on a psychiatric continuing care ward. Among his recommendations are:

- ▶ allowing patients privacy;
- ▶ providing good and comfortable facilities to indicate to patients that they are valued;
- ▶ treating patients as partners in care;
- ▶ listening and responding to patient requests;
- ▶ consistency in the nursing and care team;
- ▶ providing clear leadership.

Undoubtedly, if these recommendations are not implemented clients will be more likely to feel the need to respond aggressively to make themselves heard. Contrast this list with the precipitants to aggression identified by Burrow (1994):

- ▶ overcrowding;
- ▶ inappropriate temperature;
- ▶ restricted movement;
- ▶ lack of available information;
- ▶ inhospitable decor;
- ▶ lack of facilities to occupy patients;
- ▶ perception that patients are less of a priority than staff members.

▶ COMMUNITY CARE

Although the issues raised so far relate in some ways to the situation of community care, one important difference exists – that is that nurses working in community care often work on their own in clients' homes. Such work may also involve travelling alone at night, which carries its own attendant risks. Planning should always take account of the safety of the practitioner. Before making visits other agency staff should be made aware of intended destinations, and expected return times, and if staff become overdue then an action plan should be carried out. Staff should also make use of mobile telephones or radios, if available, to update their base of their whereabouts.

If aggressive words or actions occur, then community care nurses need to make rapid exits. Pre-planning in case of the need for a quick exit will assist the community nurse. If concern is raised about a possibly violent client then visits should be made by more than one member of staff or the individual should be asked to visit the health centre or clinic.

REFLECTIVE KNOWLEDGE

This chapter emphasizes the need to be aware of potential outbursts of aggression in nursing practice. This requires a deeper level of analysis than presented by the surface events. The theories of aggression offer different explanations, but no one theory is entirely comprehensive.

The predisposing factors in aggression have been identified and these provide clues or warnings that can be used to prepare staff for aggressive clients. Dealing with anger in clients is especially important if the assault cycle is to be curtailed before an assault occurs. You also need to develop an awareness of your own responses to aggression. The WASP (wait – assess – slowly – proceed) procedure has been used as a basis for analysing your responses to a situation and the exercises are to help you develop strategies to cope effectively in aggressive situations.

The professional implications for nurses who deal with aggressive clients have also been discussed, and the importance of safety and accurate record keeping emphasized.

It is from this base that professional decision making can develop. To consolidate your learning you should now attempt the exercises that follow.

▶ PERSONAL ATTITUDES TOWARDS PHYSICAL OR VERBAL AGGRESSION

The following six exercises are designed to help you become aware of your own reactions to aggression and to explore alternative responses.

▶ EXERCISE I

Littlechild (1996) developed a checklist to help people monitor their liability to fear and uncertainty when entering different situations. In the following exercise Littlechild's checklist has been applied to nursing. Fill in Table 2.5.5 by ticking the appropriate box to assess your levels of confidence and fear levels when entering a variety of situations. The list in Table 2.5.5 is not definitive and more situations specific to your circumstances can be added in the vacant rows.

All responses that do not fall in the fully confident column need to be given attention. Examples of actions that can be taken include:

- Provide for contact with others (i.e. If alone at night);

- Increase security measures – personal attack alarms, defensive training;

- Check out employer training, advice, and policy in the event of aggression;

- Reassess the justification for threat assessment;

- Check that others are aware of your location.

Sometimes aggression can be read into situations in which it is not justified. For example, a client may joke that he is a 'karate expert' and could 'take anyone out'. This may not actually be a threat; however, if a threat is perceived, then it is best to check out with the individual concerned. For example, with this client it would be possible to ask him to clarify what he means, such as by asking why he feels the need to make the statement.

Type of situation	Fully confident	Feel threatened	Very threatened	Would avoid the situation
When with male or female patients				
Accident and emergency department				
Acute psychiatric unit				
Surgical ward				
Medical ward				
The staff car park at night				
Adolescent unit				
Elderly confused ward				
Elderly day hospital				
Client's home				
Walking alone at night				
Late night social events				
Driving alone in the car at night				
At home alone at night				

Table 2.5.5 Table to assess levels of confidence and fear levels when entering a variety of situations.

▶ PERSONAL COPING STRATEGIES WITH AGGRESSION – BECOMING ASSERTIVE

Clients can become angry, and the nurse's ability to respond non-aggressively to anger is important. Giving way to angry or aggressive clients will probably encourage them to use such tactics more often. Farrell and Gray (1992) make the observation that assertion is an effective way of dealing with aggression. Assertion, according to Farrell and Gray is the acknowledgement of self and others' worth, which is accomplished by stating the individual's rights and views.

Aggression is characterized by a stiff threatening posture, loudness, and accusatory and rapid speech. This is meant to produce a response of passivity in the recipient so that compliance occurs. Such passivity is transmitted by quietness, looking away and an apologetic manner and verbal response. Assertion is characterized by relaxation, appropriate eye contact and confidence in posture and speech. The use of the personal pronoun 'I' is a good guide to assertion. Statements like 'I believe that . . .', 'I'd like us to consider . . .', 'Tell me your views on . . .', indicate assertion.

▶ EXERCISE 2

■ Make a list of the situations in which you feel you can be assertive. For example at home, with friends, at college in small groups, in the clinical situation.

■ Now make a list of situations where you do not feel assertive. For example, in large groups in college, in certain clinical situations, when someone is being angry, in the presence of authority figures.

■ What are the differences between the two lists of situations? Probably you will find that you can be assertive in situations where you do not feel under threat. In fact this process of modifying your response to events means that your ability to be assertive depends upon how you interpret the situation you are in.

▶ EXERCISE 3

This exercise enables you to challenge your interpretations of situations where you feel threatened. You can either complete it by yourself or work with a friend.

■ Think of a situation where you feel threatened and unable to be assertive.

■ Question why you feel this way and make a list of your reasons.

■ Now go through the reasons and challenge them. Do they stand up to being challenged? Your reasons for apparent fear may not be justified. We often act more upon the basis of habit than reason!

▶ EXERCISE 4

Experiment with assertive responses in situations that you find difficulty with. Two examples you might use are: you have bought a new CD player which is faulty and have returned to the shop that you bought it from who want to send it away for repair, but as the CD player is brand new, you want a replacement; on clinical placement, the ward manager is persistently late in completing the duty rota and you rarely know what shifts you will be working more than one week in advance so you want the ward manager to complete the duty rota at least two weeks in advance.

■ If you are working with a friend then ask your friend to adopt the role of the other person and act the scenario through. If you are working on your own you can do a similar exercise using thought rehearsal. This is similar to working with a friend except that you think the scenario through adopting both roles. Try to include different responses and determine the consequences.

■ Remember that changing habitually submissive patterns of responding can take some time, so carry out small changes, and gradually increase your assertiveness strategy. If things do not work at first keep trying!

▶ EXERCISE 5

This exercise asks you to make a record of the aggression you have witnessed with a view to using such personal accounts to develop your coping strategy in future experiences of aggression. Make a table with the headings shown in Table 2.5.6, which has been completed to show how such a table can be used. The purpose of providing this form of analysis is to identify what can be learned for the future and to ask yourself:

■ Would I deal with the same situation in the same way now?

■ What changes would I now make?

■ What alternative responses could I have made.

Then construct a table identifying your own situations. If you cannot recall other specific situations, compile some imaginary situations that you might meet in your future clinical nursing.

Incident of aggression experience: brief description of incident	What happened from about ten minutes before the incident	How the incident unfolded	What I said and what I did	How I felt afterwards and how others felt afterwards
A patient on an acute psychiatric ward shouts abuse after I advised him it was meal time	The patient was playing darts, and kept losing. He was becoming more angry each time. The patient he was playing darts with suggested he should learn how to play.	The nurse giving out the meal asked me to tell the patient that the supper had arrived. He was throwing darts at the dart board on his own when I approached and told him about supper. Then he responded with his verbal abuse. I stood there and 'took it' and left the area. He eventually came for his supper.	I told the patient supper was ready. When the verbal abuse was given out I stood there and then left.	I felt humiliated and angry. I avoided the patient until his discharge some days later.

Table 2.5.6 A record of witnessed aggression.

▶ DEVELOPING ANALYTICAL SKILLS

▶ EXERCISE 6

This exercise is intended to increase your analytical skills with regard to aggressive incidents. From your own experience or from peers or from other professional nurses think of an aggressive incident that occurred during practice. Find out as much detail as you can. Then answer the following questions:

- Were there predisposing factors in the client's history?

- What triggers can be identified that led to the incident?

- How was the increasing escalation dealt with by those present?

- What happened during the assault cycle and how far did it progress?

- Could an earlier intervention have been made?

- What things can be changed to avoid such an incident in the future?

- What can be learned from this incident about the future management of aggressive incidents and client management?

▶ CASE STUDY: ADULT

Staff nurse Bill Grey is working the Friday night in the casualty department. This is the fourth consecutive Friday night he has worked. 'More drunks again' he thinks as he drives to work. The night starts early and by 9 p.m. several young patients have come into the department who have been drinking. One of them called Colin is 18 years old and keeps demanding to be seen for what appears to be a relatively superficial abrasion to his arm. He has been in the department with his friends on previous occasions when alcohol played a significant role in the minor injuries they have suffered. When in the department they are usually noisy and demanding. Bill calls him into the cubicle to be seen. 'Let the lads come in as well' is Colin's response. 'Only you' shouts Bill. The young men then proceed to keep mimicking Bill. Bill eventually persuades Colin to go into the cubicle, and he starts cleaning the graze on Colin's forearm. 'Ouch' Colin yells, 'You did that on purpose'. He then shoves Bill against a trolley. Bill is then very angry, grabs hold of Colin, drags him out of the casualty building and deposits him outside. An hour later Colin, accompanied by the police and his parents, arrives in the casualty department.

- Need the aggression have occurred?

- How could Bill have dealt with the group that accompanied Colin?

- How could Bill's treatment of Colin have been changed to prevent Colin's reaction?

- If Bill approached you before this incident, what advice would you have given him to enable him to cope more effectively?

▶ CASE STUDY: CHILD

Dean is aged nine years. He is described as being 'highly strung' and is prone to tantrums when he is unable to do as he wishes. Dean's parents separated three years ago. For about two years before splitting up they used to have regular, sometimes violent, arguments. This worsened during the last six months of their marriage when Dean's father became unemployed. Dean's mother confides to you during a visit to the well woman's clinic that she feels unable to control Dean. He shouts at her when he does not get his own way and on several occasions he has physically attacked her. The school has complained to her that he bullies other children. Recently he has joined a group of older children and failed to attend school on several occasions. He has subsequently been found at the local amusement arcade. Dean's mother has noticed that Dean sometimes develops a rash around his mouth. She has noticed tubes of empty wood adhesive in Dean's room, but cannot find anything that he has been sticking together.

■ **What violent behaviour is Dean displaying?**

■ **Referring to the theories identified in this chapter, explain what has led Dean to behave in this way.**

■ **Why does Dean continue to behave in this way when both his mother and the school wish him to stop?**

■ **How might Dean's mother help to reduce the violent behaviour?**

▶ CASE STUDY: LEARNING DISABILITIES

Louise is 38 years of age and has a severe learning disability. For most of her life she has lived in an institution. However, due to changes in the provision of health care, she was transferred into a local authority group home three months ago. The care home is several miles away from the old hospital. This has made visiting by her elderly parents difficult and they are now only able to visit once a fortnight instead of twice weekly. Louise has difficulty in communicating. The staff that had looked after her while she was in hospital had developed a system of communication with her, but were not transferred to the group home. The group home staff comprise mainly of care assistants. They find it difficult to communicate with Louise and tend to avoid contact with her. Louise is reported to be deteriorating in behaviour since her transfer and occasionally strikes out at staff.

■ **With reference to knowledge you have gained from this chapter, offer explanations as to why Louise's behaviour has changed to become aggressive.**

■ How should carers approach Louise to minimize aggressive outbursts?

■ How could this situation have been better managed to prevent distress and aggression?

▶ CASE STUDY: MENTAL HEALTH

Joe, aged 22 years, has a long history of admissions to the mental health unit. His mother left the family home when he was three years of age and he lived with his father until he was ten, when he was placed into local authority care following his father's conviction for armed robbery. During the period he lived in the local authority home he become implicated in several petty thefts. He was also noted to have a low frustration threshold and became involved in numerous fights. Later he began to experiment with drugs. This led to his first contact with the mental health services.

Joe has a girlfriend with whom he lives. He tells the staff that he believes that she is playing around with other men. Joe's girlfriend on the other hand is fed up with Joe's tantrums and accusations. She speaks to the ward manager and informs him that it is her intention to terminate the relationship while Joe is in hospital as she is frightened about what his reaction will be if she waits until he is discharged. The ward manager however, does not pass this message on to the other members of the team. You are on duty in the mental health unit and Joe's girlfriend is visiting him in the day area where there are other clients and visitors. Suddenly you hear the sound of furniture being broken and screaming from the day area. You arrive on the scene to find Joe's girlfriend lying on the floor with blood coming from her mouth. Joe is standing alongside her calling her a slut and kicking her.

■ What should your immediate action be?

■ Referring to Tables 2.5.1 and 2.5.2 earlier in this chapter, how might this response have been predicted?

■ What actions can be taken, and with whom, following the incident?

■ What advice would you offer the staff to enable them to manage similar situations more effectively?

▶ ANNOTATED FURTHER READING

▶ *Theories of Aggression*

BREAKWELL, G. (1995) General and specific clues and dangerousness checklist. In KIDD, B., STARK, C (eds) (1995) *Management of Violence and Aggression in Health Care*. London. Gaskell.
For a concise account of the current theories concerning aggression this chapter by Breakwell in Kidd and Stark (1995) is an excellent resource of recent developments. This chapter also contains an account of the assault cycle.

HILGARD, E.R., ATKINSON, R.C., ATKINSON, R.L. (1993) *Introduction to Psychology*. New York. Harcourt Brace.
This book contains an accessible section on aggression theories.
STORR, A. (1992) *Human Aggression*. Harmondsworth. Penguin Books.
For a wider view of aggression in terms of social, individual and interpersonal factors, this book by Anthony Storr makes interesting and useful reading.

▌ *Management of Aggression*

FARRELL, G.A., GRAY, C. (1992) *Aggression: A Nurse's Guide to Therapeutic Management*. London. Scutari Press.
A useful book for nurses in that it offers an adaptation of aggression management strategies specifically to the nursing situation.
KIDD, B., STARK, C. (1995) *Management of Violence and Aggression in Health Care*. London. Gaskell.
This book offers useful chapters on the practical management of aggression.
SHEPHERD, J. (ed.) (1994) *Violence in Health Care: A Practical Guide to Coping with Violence and Caring for Victims*. Oxford. Oxford University Press.
For a comprehensive set of papers by leading workers in the field, this book offers the reader a wide range of interventions in different health care situations.

▌ *Personal Safety*

BIBBY, P. (1995) *Personal Safety for Health Care Workers*. Aldershot: Arena.
The book on personal safety for health care workers by Pauline Bibby from the Suzy Lamplugh Trust offers a more personally orientated approach and gives advice for personal safety. Very useful chapters include assertiveness and practical steps to safety, as well as travelling guidelines. This book also contains a chapter devoted to trainers in the management of violence.

▌ REFERENCES

AIKEN, F., TARBUCK, P. (1995) Practical, ethical and legal aspects of caring for the assaultive client. In Kidd, B., Stark, C. (eds) *Management of Violence and Aggression in Health Care*. London. Gaskell.

ARONSON, E. (1995) *The Social Animal*. New York. W.H. Freeman & Company.

BERKOWITZ, L. (1969) Frustration–aggression hypothesis: Examination and reformulation. *Psychological Bulletin* 106: 59–73.

BERKOWITZ, L. (1990) On the formation and regulation of anger and aggression: A cognitive–neoassociationist analysis. *American Psychologist* 45: 494–503.

BIBBY, P. (1995) *Personal Safety for Health Care Workers*. Aldershot. Arena.

BOCOCK, R. (1986) *Freud and Modern Society*. Wokingham. Reinhold (UK) Co Ltd.

BOUCHARD, T.J., LYKKEN, D.T, McGUE, M., SEGAL, N.L., TELLEGEN, A. (1990) Sources of human psychological differences: The Minnesota study of twins reared apart. *Science* 350: 223–228.

BRAITHWAITE, R. (1992) *Violence: Understanding , Intervention and Prevention*. Oxford. Radcliffe Professional Series.

BREAKWELL, G. (1995) General and specific clues and dangerousness checklist. In Kidd, B., Stark, C. (eds) *Management of Violence and Aggression in Health Care*. London. Gaskell.

BURROW, S. (1994) Nurse-aid management of psychiatric emergencies: 3. *British Journal of Nursing* 3(3): 121–125.

CAMPBELL, B., STUART, J., SUTHERLAND, E. (1989) A high occupation risk? *Nursing Times* 85(13): 37–39.

CASEY, M.D., BLANK, C.E., McLEAN, T.M., KOHN, P., STREET, D.R.K., McDOUGALL, S.M., GOODER, J., PLATTS, J. (1973) Male patients with chromosome abnormality in the state hospitals. *Journal of Mental Deficiency Research* 16: 215–256.

CEMBROWICZ, S., RITTER, S. (1994) Attacks on doctors and nurses. In Shepherd, J. (ed.) *Violence in Health Care: A Practical Guide to Coping with Violence and Caring for Victims*. Oxford. Oxford University Press.

CENTRAL STATISTICS OFFICE (1995) *Social Trends*. London. Her Majesty's Stationery Office.

DEPARTMENT OF HEALTH AND SOCIAL SECURITY (1974) *Health and Safety at Work Act*. London. Her Majesty's Stationery Office.

DEPARTMENT OF HEALTH AND SOCIAL SECURITY (1983) *Mental Health Act*. London. Her Majesty's Stationery Office.

DEPARTMENT OF HEALTH AND SOCIAL SECURITY (1993) *Code of Practice. Mental Health Act (1983)*. London. Her Majesty's Stationery Office.

DOERING, C.H., BRODIE, H.K.H., KRAEMER, H.C., BECKER, H.B. (1974) Plasma testosterone levels and psychologic measures in men over a 2-month period.

DOLLARD, J., HAMBURG, D.A., DOOB, L., MILLER, N., MOWER, O.H., SEARS, R.R. (1939) *Frustration and Aggression*. New Haven, CT. Yale University Press.

ERON, L.D., HUESMANN, L.R., LEFKOWITZ, M.M., WALDER, L.O. (1972) Does television violence cause aggression? *American Psychologist* 27: 253–262.

EYSNECK, H.J., GUDJONSSON, G.H. (1989) *The Causes and Cures of Criminality*. New York. Plenum.

FARRELL, G.A., GRAY, C. (1992) *Aggression: A Nurse's Guide to Therapeutic Management.* London. Scutari Press.

FARRINGTON, D.P. (1994) The causes and prevention of offending, with special reference to violence. In Shepherd, J. (ed.) (1994). *Violence in Health Care: A Practical Guide to Coping with Violence and Caring for Victims.* Oxford. Oxford University Press.

FELDMAN, R.S. (1992) *Elements of Psychology.* London. McGraw-Hill Inc.

FENICHEL, O. (1982) *The Psychoanalytic Theory of Neurosis.* London. Routledge & Kegan Paul.

FOTTRELL, E., BEWLEY, T., SQUIZZONI, M. (1978) A study of aggressive and violent behaviour among a group of psychiatric in-patients. *Medicine Science and Law* **18(1)**: 66–69.

FRANKL, G. (1990) *The Unknown Self.* London. Open Gate Press.

FREUD, S. (1920) Beyond the pleasure principle. In Strachey, J. (ed.) (1921) *The Standard Edition of the Complete Works of Sigmund Freud.* London. Hogarth Press.

GERBNER, G., GROSS, L (1976) The scary world of TV's heavy viewer. *Psychology Today* **9**: 41–45.

GOULD, J. (1994) The impact of change on violent patients. *Nursing Standard* **8(19)**: 38–40.

HEALTH AND SAFETY COMMISSION (1992) *Management of Health and Safety at Work Regulations.* London. Her Majesty's Stationery Office.

HILGARD, E.R., ATKINSON, R.C., ATKINSON, R.L. (1993) *Introduction to Psychology.* New York. Harcourt Brace.

HINDE, R.A. (1993) Aggression at different levels of social complexity. In Taylor, P.J. (ed.) *Violence in Society.* London. Royal College of Physicians.

HODGKINSON, P., HILLIS, T., RUSSELL, D. (1984) Aggression management: Assaults on staff in a psychiatric hospital. *Nursing Times* **80(16)**: 44–46.

HOLLAND, S. (1992) *Managing Care Pack 17.* London. Distance Learning Centre.

HOLLIN, C.R. (1992) *Criminal Behaviour.* London. The Farmer Press.

HOME OFFICE (1967) *Criminal Law Act.* London. Her Majesty's Stationery Office.

HOME OFFICE RESEARCH AND STATISTICS DEPARTMENT (1988) *British Crime Survey.* London. Her Majesty's Stationery Office.

HOWELLS, K., HOLLIN, C.R., (1989) *Clinical Approaches to Violence.* Chichester. John Wiley & Sons.

JEFFREY, C.R. (1979) *Biology and Crime.* London. Sage Publications.

KAPLAN, H.I., SADOCK, B.J., GREBB, J.A. (1994) *Kaplan and Sadock's Synopsis of Psychiatry, Behavioural Sciences, Clinical Psychiatry,* 7th edition. Baltimore. Williams & Williams.

KIDD, B., STARK, C.R. (1995) *Management of Violence and Aggression in Health Care.* London. Gaskell.

KLEIN, M. (1988) *Envy and Gratitude.* London. Virago Press.

LEADBETTER, D., PATERSON, B. (1995) De-escalating aggressive behaviour. In Kidd, B., Stark, C. (eds) *Management of Violence and Aggression in Health Care.* London. Gaskell.

LITTLECHILD, B. (1996) The risk of violence and aggression to social work and social care staff. In Kemshall, H., Pritchard, J. (eds) *Good Practice in Risk Assessment and Risk Management.* London. Jessica Kingsley.

LLOYD, P., MAYES, A. (1990) *Introduction to Psychology.* London. Fontana.

MALIM, T., BIRCH, A. (1989) *Social Psychology.* Bristol. Introductory Psychology Series.

MOYER, K. (1979) Biology and the individual offender: what is the potential for biological control? In Jeffrey, C. (ed.) *Biology and Crime.* London. Sage Publications.

ORR, J. (1984) Violence against women. *Nursing Times* **80(17)**: 34–36.

OWENS, R.G., ASHCROFT, J.B. (1985) *Violence: A Guide For The Caring Professions.* London. Croom Helm.

PHIL, R.O., PETERSON, J.B., LAU, M.A. (1993) A biosocial model of the alcohol–aggression relationship. *Journal of Studies on Alcohol, Supplement* **11**: 128–139.

POLLOCK, N., McBAIN, I., WEBSTER, C.D. (1989) Clinical decision making and the assessment of dangerousness. In Howells, K., Hollin, C.R. (eds) *Clinical Approaches to Violence.* Chichester. John Wiley & Sons.

PRENTKY, R. (1985) The neurochemistry and neuroendocrinology of sexual aggression. In Farrington, D.P., Gunn, J. (eds) *Aggression and Dangerousness.* Chichester. John Wiley & Sons.

PRICE, W. H. (1978) Sex chromosome abnormalities in special hospital patients. In Owens, R.G., Ashcroft, J.B. (eds) (1985) *Violence: A guide for the Caring Professions.* London. Croom Helm.

RAISTRICK, D. (1994) Alcohol, other drugs, and violence. In Shepherd, J. (ed.) *Violence in Health Care: A Practical Guide to Coping with Violence and Caring for Victims.* Oxford. Oxford University Press.

ROBB, E. (1995) Post-incident care and support for assaulted staff. In Kidd, B., Stark, C. (eds) *Management of Violence and Aggression in Health Care.* London. Gaskell.

ROGERS, R., SALVAGE, J. (1988) *Nurses at Risk: A Guide to Health and Safety at Work.* London. Heinemann.

ROWETT, C., BREAKWELL, G.M. (1992) *Managing Violence at Work.* Slough. NFER Nelson.

RYAN, J., POSTER, E. (1993) Workplace violence. *Nursing Times* **89(48)**: 38–41.

SCHACHTER, S., SINGER, J.E. (1962) Cognitive, Social and physiological determinants of emotional states. *Psychological Review* **69**: 379–399.

SMITH, P. (1977) *Management of Assaultive Behaviour (Training Manual).* Sacramento. California Department of Developmental Services.

SMITH, R.E. (1986) Handling aggression. *The Professional Nurse* **January**: 91–94.

STOUDEMIRE, A. (1990) *Human Behaviour: An Introduction for Medical Students.* London. J. B. Lippincott Company.

UKCC (1984) *Code of Professional Conduct.* London. UKCC.

VINCENT, M., WHITE, K. (1994) Patient violence toward a nurse: predictable and preventable? *Journal of Psychosocial Nursing* **32(2)**: 30–32.

WARING, T., WILSON, J. (1990) *Be Safe.* Bolton. M.O.V.E.

WHITTINGTON, R., WYKES, T. (1989) Invisible injury. *Nursing Times* **85**: 30–32.

WORLD HEALTH ORGANIZATION (1992) *The ICD–10 Classification of Mental and Behavioural Disorders.* Geneva. World Health Organization.

WRIGHT, B. (1989) Threatening behaviour. *Nursing Times* **85**: 26–27.

Supportive practice

3.1 Hygiene

M. Mallik

KEY ISSUES

■ SUBJECT KNOWLEDGE

▶ structure and functions of the skin, the mouth, the eyes, hair and nails as they relate to hygiene care
▶ history of hygiene care practices in society
▶ the impact of individual, cultural and spiritual beliefs on individual hygiene practices

■ PRACTICE KNOWLEDGE

▶ assessment of an individual's hygiene needs in relation to care of the body, mouth, hair and eyes
▶ the relative value of assessment tools in relation to oral care
▶ differing modes of delivery of hygiene care for all body parts

■ PROFESSIONAL KNOWLEDGE

▶ the impact of the historical place of hygiene care on the image of the nurse today
▶ ritualization of hygiene care and its impact on present day skill mix debates
▶ the resourcing of hygiene care in the community

■ REFLECTIVE KNOWLEDGE

▶ personal feelings regarding the facilitation of hygiene care
▶ consolidation of learning from the chapter through case study work

▶ INTRODUCTION

Maintaining hygiene according to one's personal and cultural norms is a basic human need. Helping individuals maintain their own hygiene is recognized as a fundamental role for the nurse. In partnership with the client and carer, the nurse is the primary decision maker in this area of health care practice. However, the role of the nurse in the delivery of care will alter depending upon the particular context in which hygiene care is delivered and the specific needs of the individual.

Children and teenagers need varying levels of support and teaching to help them meet their hygiene needs. Health educator to the child and the family may be an important role to fulfil for this client group in whatever context. Children and adults with deficits in learning ability may need extra encouragement, time and teaching in order to meet their needs. The person with a mental illness who has become demotivated about maintaining personal appearances and hygiene may need the nurse to act as advisor and counsellor. The nurse needs to be highly sensitive to the client's personal wishes while still encouraging normal hygiene behaviour. Adults whose health status is compromised by acute or chronic illness will need specific support within a continuum from total self care to being totally dependent upon the nurse for hygiene care. The dignity and privacy of all clients, especially the elderly, will need to be facilitated and protected by the nurse whatever the context of hygiene care delivery.

The context of care will have important implications on decision making about hygiene because of the environmental conditions in which the education, support and care may be delivered. The nurse will need to adapt to the resources available. There may be a need to become active politically to obtain better resources or facilitate these resources through other professionals.

The content of this chapter will outline both the scientific and practice-based knowledge needed by the nurse to promote and deliver hygiene care. The aim of this chapter is to explore fully this domain of nursing and to outline clearly the knowledge base needed for decision making for all aspects of hygiene care.

▶ OVERVIEW

General and specialist knowledge is needed in decision making on the delivery of hygiene care. Specialist knowledge is related to hygiene care for specific body parts. For this reason the Subject Knowledge and Practice Knowledge subdivisions of the chapter are further divided into the relevant specialist sections involved in the administration of hygiene care. These sections include:

- ▶ body hygiene care;
- ▶ oral hygiene care;
- ▶ eye hygiene care;
- ▶ hair and nails hygiene care;
- ▶ perineal hygiene care.

▶ *Subject Knowledge*

In the Biological part of Subject Knowledge, knowledge from the physical sciences is explored in relation to the skin, mouth, eyes, hair, nails and perineum. In each section the focus is on the applied knowledge needed to make decisions about hygiene care. The psychosocial knowledge base integrates these specific body parts in order to outline issues in hygiene care related to development and individuality. The historical and social dimensions of hygiene care and cultural and spiritual norms are explored.

▶ *Practice Knowledge*

This part follows a similar format as the Subject Knowledge section, but concentrates on the knowledge needed in the assessment and delivery of hygiene care to and with patients and clients.

▶ *Professional Knowledge*

The professional, political and social dimensions of hygiene care are addressed. Hygiene care as a ritual within nursing is discussed more fully with a particular focus on the role of the nurse as the key decision maker in this area of health care practice.

▶ *Reflective Knowledge*

There is a particular focus in this part on the reflective experiences of students in the delivery of care that is intimate and private. Case studies are used to help consolidate knowledge gained from practice and the chapter content.

On pp. 340–342 there are four case studies, each one relating to one of the branch programmes. You may find it helpful to read one of them before you start the chapter and use it as a focus for your reflections while reading.

SUBJECT KNOWLEDGE
Biological

▶ THE SKIN

The structure and functions of the skin are more fully outlined in Chapter 2.4 on skin integrity. Reference will be made here to some of the specific structures that are pertinent to skin and body hygiene. A key function of the skin is protection. Its unique structures protect the body from:

▶ undue entry or loss of water;
▶ pressure and friction;
▶ microorganisms;
▶ chemicals (weak acids and alkalis);
▶ most gases;
▶ physical trauma (alpha rays, beta rays to a limited extent, and ultra-violet radiation) (Hinchliff, 1996).

The two layers of the skin, the epidermis and dermis, function as a single layer. However, the outer layer, the epidermis, has five layers of cell types, each of which has its own unique function. The innermost cell layer of the epidermis (the stratum basale) is important in skin regeneration as the cells are constantly dividing and reproducing, the life cycle of skin cells being approximately 35 days (see Chapter 2.4). These new cells move through the epidermal layers to the surface of the skin. For the purposes of hygiene care, the stratum corneum, the outermost horny cell layer is therefore of primary interest. The cells or squames of the stratum corneum are all dead and are constantly being shed from the surface of the body. According to Hinchliff (1996) up to one million of these cells are shed every 40 minutes through the process of desquamation or exfoliation.

Keratin helps the epidermis form a tough protective barrier. The process of keratinization, which begins in the basal layer, means that the horny cells of the stratum corneum are filled with this protein. Keratin is most evident in areas of the skin exposed to stress, for example the palms of the hands and soles of the feet. Both psoriasis (a skin condition characterized by rapid and excessive production of keratin cells) and dandruff (hyperplasia of the scalp) result in the exfoliation of flakes of keratin (Hinchliff, 1996).

Certain bacteria are normally present on the skin's outer surface, for example *Staphylococcus epidermidis* and *Corynebacterium* (Gould, 1991). They are classified as normal flora (commensals) and are protective in function because they inhibit the multiplication of disease-causing organisms. These normal commensals, which inhabit the deeper layers of the stratum corneum, are not usually shed with exfoliation. Commensals use healthy skin scales as a source of food and also rely on the skin having a slightly acid pH in order to maintain their protective function in preventing disease (Hinchliff, 1996).

The dermis layer of the skin contains collagen and elastic fibres, nerve fibres, blood vessels, sweat glands, sebaceous glands and hair follicles. The latter three are particularly significant in relation to hygiene care.

▶ *Sweat Glands*

Eccrine and apocrine glands are two types of sweat glands, are distributed throughout the skin, and assist in temperature control. They produce sweat when the skin temperature rises above 35°C. Approximately 500 ml of sweat is produced each day in temperate climates. Secretion of sweat also occurs in response to stress and anxiety as well as to certain spicy foods. Both the production of sweat and its evaporation from the skin

---

DECISION MAKING

Given that commensals are a normal feature of human skin investigate the following:

- *How might the use of soaps affect the activity of normal skin flora?*
- *How will babies born with no resident skin commensals gain these normal bacteria?*
- *What will be the effect of lack of hygiene care on these skin commensals?*
- *What effect might alcoholic skin preparations used both in cosmetic preparations and surgical lotions have on the normal skin flora?*

(See Annotated Further Reading – Bolander, 1994; Hinchliff *et al.*, 1996.)

assist in heat loss from the body, and the rate of evaporation is particularly important in the patient with pyrexia (raised body temperature) (see Chapter 2.2).

Sweat left on the skin, especially if from the apocrine glands of the axilla and genital areas, is responsible for body odour through the process of bacterial decomposition (Hinchliff, 1996). There are racial differences in the structure of apocrine glands, which are more developed in African races than Asian races (Bolander, 1994). The apocrine glands are dormant during childhood, but begin to actively secrete sweat during puberty and continue to do so throughout adult life. The widespread use of deodorants in developed countries is based on the principle that these solutions will kill the bacteria and mask any odour produced. Anti-perspirant sprays block the openings of the ducts to the sweat glands with metal salts such as aluminium (Hinchliff, 1996).

▶ Sebaceous glands

Sebaceous glands secrete sebum into the hair follicles. This sebum is an oily odourless fluid containing cholesterol, triglycerides, waxes and paraffins that lubricates the skin and keeps it supple and pliant. Sebum also has a role in waterproofing the skin. Sebaceous glands are found in highest numbers over the scalp and face, the middle of the back and the genitalia, and in the auditory canal.

Babies and young children have relatively fewer and less active sebaceous glands and are therefore more prone to skin redness and excoriation in damp conditions, while the loss of sebaceous glands in old age also makes the skin of the elderly more vulnerable to damp conditions, redness and to breakdown. During the menarche (puberty), however, the secretion from sebaceous glands increases in response to an increase in adrenocortical hormones. The increasing output of sebum during the teenage years combined with hereditary factors can contribute to the development of acne vulgaris (common acne) (Wong, 1995).

▶ Hair

The hair follicle is situated in the dermis and is surrounded by its own nerve and blood supply (Figure 3.1.1). Sebaceous glands and sweat gland ducts open directly into the hair follicle causing the scalp to become moist and oily, particularly in a hot environment (Bolander, 1994). The cycle of hair growth comprises a period of growth for up to two years followed by a rest period and then atrophy. About 70–100 scalp hairs are normally lost each day (Hinchliff, 1996).

Certain factors affect the rate of normal hair growth and loss. These include:

- ▶ nutrition;
- ▶ hormones (puberty and the menopause);
- ▶ hereditary factors (baldness);
- ▶ age (decreased number of hairs with old age).

Most of the body is covered by hair, but it varies in type. Lanugo is the fine silky hair found on the fetus *in utero* and on premature babies and is lost from the body soon after birth. Vellus is colourless hair found on the female face. Terminal hair is found on the adult head and pubis and is the subject of hygiene care in relation to maintaining healthy hair covered later in this chapter.

Abnormal hair loss can occur in times of stress, trauma, and poor

---

DECISION MAKING

Sarah Woodford a 14-year-old schoolgirl has developed acne, which makes her very self-conscious about her appearance in front of her peer group, many of whom pass on their tips for cleaning her skin. Following repeated unsuccessful attempts to control the condition, Sarah finally goes to see the practice nurse at her local health centre.

- *How would the practice nurse explain to Sarah the cause of her condition?*
- *What methods are available from which the practice nurse could choose a treatment for Sarah's individual needs?*
- *What other advice could be given to Sarah about her general health and hygiene at this time?*

(See Annotated Further Reading – Wong, 1995)

Figure 3.1.1: Diagram of a hair. (Redrawn from Hinchliff *et al.*, 1996.)

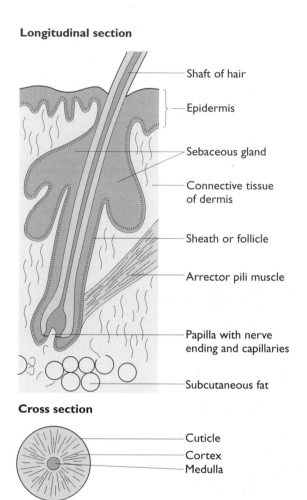

Longitudinal section

Shaft of hair

Epidermis

Sebaceous gland

Connective tissue of dermis

Sheath or follicle

Arrector pili muscle

Papilla with nerve ending and capillaries

Subcutaneous fat

Cross section

Cuticle

Cortex

Medulla

nutrition and as a result of drug therapies, especially cytotoxic drugs used in cancer cell treatment. Alopecia is the term given to hair loss of unknown cause.

▶ *Nails*

Nails are keratinized plates resting on the highly vascular and sensitive nail bed (Hinchliff, 1996). The external appearance of the nail bed is often used to indicate general health status as the shape, colour and condition of finger nails are easily observed. Toe nails cause more problems for individuals than finger nails. Debilitated adults may have difficulties in maintaining adequate care and hygiene for their feet which will lead to their toe nails becoming thick, brittle and prone to fungal infections (Table 3.1.1). Children may have problems with ingrowing toe nails because of difficulties in maintaining good fitting shoes, especially in times of rapid growth such as during adolescence. It may be necessary to resize children's feet every three months to maintain the correct shoe size.

▶ THE PERINEUM

The perineum is the area located between the thighs and extends from the anus (posterior) through to the top of the pubic bone (anterior).

Specific risks	Biting and improper care
	Exposure to chemicals
	Frequent and prolonged immersion in water
	Ill-fitting shoes
	Ingrowing nails
	Bacterial and fungal infection of the feet.
General health risks	Poor nutrition
	Peripheral vascular disease
	Diabetes mellitus

Table 3.1.1 Health risks to nails. (Adapted from Bolander, 1994)

Anatomical structures in this area are concerned with the expression of sexuality, reproduction and elimination (see Chapter 3.3 on continence and Chapter 4.3 on sexuality).

In the female, the external genitalia (vulva) consists of the mons pubis, clitoris, urethral and vaginal orifices, the labia majora and minora. The normal moist environment around the vaginal orifice is maintained by secretions from Bartholin's glands, which are mucus-secreting glands in the lateral wall of the vagina. The slightly acid secretion varies in amount during the ovulation cycle, has a slight odour and helps to inhibit bacterial growth.

In the male, the perineal area includes the penis, the scrotum and the anus. The end of the penis (glans penis) through which the urethra opens in the centre is covered with a skin flap or foreskin in the uncircumcized male. Because the skin of both the penis and scrotum is thin and hairless it is more easily irritated and injured than skin elsewhere.

The perineal areas of both men and women are prone to infections because they contain openings into the body and are also warm and moist environments. In both sexes, the urethral orifices lead to sterile bladders, but are in close proximity to the anus, which opens into the 'unclean' rectum. The main aim for hygiene care in this area is to prevent or eliminate infection. Prevention of odour is closely linked to the prevention of infection and is a cultural preoccupation in developed countries.

▶ THE MOUTH AND TEETH

The mouth has many physical and psychosocial functions that are important in supporting the health and wellbeing of an individual (Table 3.1.2). The nurse has an important role to play in helping patients and clients sustain their oral health through advice, support and delivery of oral hygiene.

The mouth or oral cavity forms the first part of the gastrointestinal tract (Figure 3.1.2). It is lined by mucous membrane, which along with the three pairs of salivary glands – the parotid, sublingual and submandibular – secretes mucus and saliva to aid the mastication and digestion of food. The tongue is a large muscular organ involved in taste,

Ingestion and digestion of food
Taste
Speech
Psychosexual – expression of intimacy
Social interaction – nonverbal expressions

Table 3.1.2 Functions of the mouth.

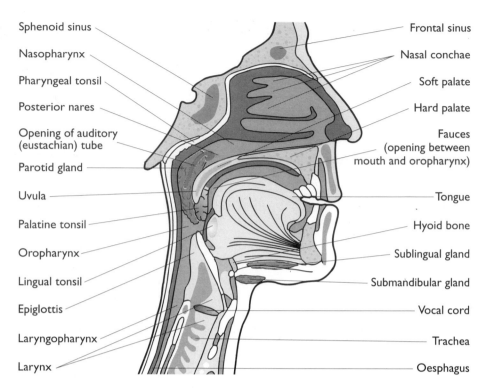

Figure 3.1.2: The oral cavity. (Redrawn from Hinchliff *et al.*, 1996.)

Sphenoid sinus
Nasopharynx
Pharyngeal tonsil
Posterior nares
Opening of auditory (eustachian) tube
Parotid gland
Uvula
Palatine tonsil
Oropharynx
Lingual tonsil
Epiglottis
Laryngopharynx
Larynx

Frontal sinus
Nasal conchae
Soft palate
Hard palate
Fauces (opening between mouth and oropharynx)
Tongue
Hyoid bone
Sublingual gland
Submandibular gland
Vocal cord
Trachea
Oesphagus

speech and swallowing. There are numerous papillae and taste buds on the upper surface of the tongue. The teeth masticate food, help to shape the mouth and are involved in the formation of speech sounds. The deciduous teeth begin to erupt between five and eight months of age. In childhood there are normally 20 deciduous teeth. From the age of six, most of these deciduous teeth are gradually lost and replaced by 32 permanent teeth, 16 in the lower and 16 in the upper jaw. This knowledge can be important to the nurse caring for a child going for surgery under a general anaesthetic as loose teeth may fall out and be inhaled during induction of anaesthesia.

The structure of the adult tooth contains three parts, the exposed section labelled as the crown, the root which is held in place in the jaw bone by cementum, and the pulp cavity, which contains the blood vessels and nerves (Figure 3.1.3).

▶ *Dental Hygiene*

The two major types of oral problems in the normally healthy individual are dental caries (cavities) and periodontal disease. The prevention of both these problems is necessary to prevent abnormal tooth loss thoughout the life span. Particularly vulnerable times for tooth loss are during childhood and teenage years, pregnancy and the third age (over 50 years old).

Health promotion strategies addressed to all ages must take into account the interaction between the oral environment of the individual and dental plaque. As soon as food and drink are ingested the acidity in the mouth increases. The pH is lowered considerably by foods containing sugar and until the acidity is buffered there is a risk of demineralization of the teeth with subsequent decay. The mouth contains many varieties of bacteria, which do not cause problems if suspended in saliva. However, once these organisms attach themselves to the teeth, gums or tongue surfaces via a mucopolysaccharide glue they become insoluble in water

Figure 3.1.3: Structure of a tooth. (Redrawn from Hinchliff *et al.*, 1996.)

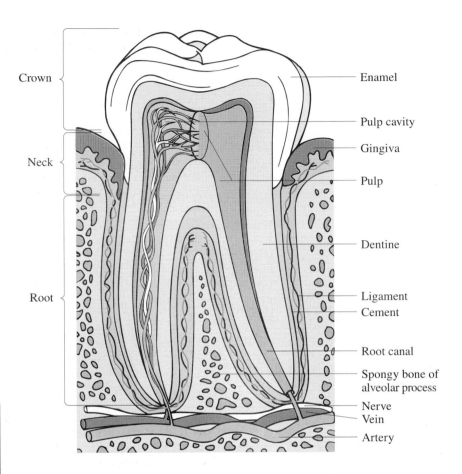

Crown — Enamel

— Pulp cavity

Neck — Gingiva

— Pulp

— Dentine

Root — Ligament

— Cement

— Root canal

— Spongy bone of alveolar process

— Nerve

— Vein

— Artery

and problems begin. The bacterial deposits cannot be rinsed away and dental plaque forms. Plaque takes 24 hours to develop. It causes dental caries and periodontal disease, which may eventually lead to systemic disease (Clarke, 1993).

Saliva plays an essential role in maintaining a healthy mouth. Thin watery saliva flushes away debris from around the gums and teeth and buffers any acids in the mouth. Thick sticky saliva will aid the formation of plaque and therefore increases the risk of periodontal disease and dental caries (Griffiths and Boyle, 1993).

Dental caries involve the calcified structure of the tooth. Bacterial enzymes combined with the dental plaque produce organic acids, which decalcify the tooth enamel (hard protective covering). Cavities or caries begin to develop once the bacteria have access to the central matrix of the tooth.

Periodontal disease is a chronic process that leads to the destruction of the structures supporting the teeth, that is the gingivae (gums). If allowed to progress, the underlying bone is destroyed causing periodontitis, the gums recede and the teeth become loose and fall out. Gingivitis, which is characterized by bleeding gums and halitosis, occurs during the early stages of periodontal disease.

Halitosis, also labelled as 'oral malodour' or 'foetor oris', is common in healthy people, especially after sleep. It is due to the metabolic activity of bacteria present in oral plaque. People who stop cleaning their mouths will soon develop halitosis. Many foods and drinks can cause transient malodour, especially garlic, onions, curries, smoking, drugs and alcohol. Any form of oral sepsis such as gingivitis or periodontitis will produce a degree of halitosis. Rarer causes include diabetic ketoacidosis and severe renal or hepatic problems (Scully *et al.*, 1994).

▶ THE EYES

The eye is a delicate organ with its own built-in mechanisms for protection and hygiene. The conjunctiva covers the exposed surface of the eye and the inner surface of the eyelids and helps to prevent drying of the eye. The eye produces tear fluid, which is washed across the eyes by the regular blinking action of the eyelashes. Tear fluid contains salt, protein, oil from sebaceous glands and a bactericidal enzyme called lysozyme, which helps protect the eye against infection. Tears are produced by the lacrimal and accessory glands, which respond to reflexes and the autonomic nervous system. Tears need a drainage system if the eye is not to become 'watery' (epiphora). Drainage is normally via canaliculi at the inner end of the lid margin into the lacrimal sac and duct and finally into the nasal cavity. Any condition that interferes with these three protective mechanisms may cause problems:

> **RESEARCH BASED EVIDENCE**
>
> *Cochrane (1993) reviewed studies that examined the rate and type of viral and bacterial contamination of contact lenses. There have been outbreaks of epidemic keratoconjunctivitis resulting from contamination by the adenovirus. After reviewing studies that focused on different methods of decontamination of lenses, it was concluded that provided the lenses were cleaned daily with a surfactant cleaner and that lens cases were regularly cleaned and replaced, the risks of developing microbial infections are very low.*

- ▶ people who wear contact lenses, particularly in a dry centrally heated building for long periods, may be at risk of excessive drying of the cornea and subsequent inflammation (Hinchliff, 1996);
- ▶ the person who has had a stroke or is unconscious for any reason may be vulnerable to eye infections without adequate eye hygiene;
- ▶ many elderly people suffer from 'watery eye' and may require surgery to prevent secondary infections (Hinchliff, 1996);
- ▶ neonates and young children are prone to get what is known as 'sticky eyes' and the condition may be due to blockage or malformation of the lacrimal ducts and require surgery;
- ▶ *Chlamydia* infection passed from the mother to the baby during childbirth can cause serious eye infection in the neonate;
- ▶ bacterial conjunctivitis can be a common problem in children's nurseries and schools, especially as children are prone to rub their eyes with dirty hands (Wong, 1995).

Psychosocial ## ▶ INDIVIDUAL ASPECTS OF HYGIENE CARE

Beliefs and attitudes to personal hygiene are developed during childhood and are strongly influenced by social and cultural norms. Nurses may be aware of the scientific principles on which they base their beliefs about hygiene care, but need to be sensitive to the family and cultural influences on their clients.

Historically, hygiene practices have been influenced by:

- ▶ social norms;
- ▶ religious rituals;
- ▶ the environment (accessibility of water for bathing)
- ▶ evolution of hygiene aids (e.g. showers, soaps, razors, electric toothbrushes, hair dryers) (Bolander, 1994).

Hygiene maintenance is a normal daily occupation and promotes a feeling of security and stability alongside wellbeing and self-esteem (Roper *et al.*, 1996). An important stage in the development of independence in hygiene self care in childhood occurs during the toddler and

- *Review your own personal hygiene routines and practices over one week.*
- *What or who have the most influence on your practices?*
- *What standards of hygiene practices would you find intolerable for yourself? (Recall situations when you did not have access to hygiene facilities for whatever reason.)*
- *Reflect on how your particular personal standards might influence your approach to patients and clients who may have very different beliefs about hygiene care.*

pre-school phase (i.e. at 1–6 years of age). During this time children develop physically, learn to gain self-control and mastery over body functions, and become increasingly aware of their own dependence and independence (Wong, 1995). The social and cultural beliefs of the family are of great importance in this pre-school period in influencing attitudes and practices in hygiene care and health promotion is usually directed through the parents and carers of the child. Peer influences become increasingly important through the school years and hygiene habits for both sexes may be influenced more by advertising, peer support and the wish to conform to group and sexual norms. Health promotion strategies by health care professionals during this phase of development need to consider these predominant social influences. During the late teenage years, values and attitudes become internalized and each individual justifies for themselves their choices in hygiene care.

▶ CULTURAL AND SPIRITUAL ASPECTS OF HYGIENE

Historically, bathing was an important social activity and public baths were a feature of ancient Greek, Egyptian and Roman society (Encarta, 1995). The ancient Roman facilities included exercise rooms, hot, warm and cold baths, steam rooms and dressing rooms and are now being mimicked by the modern gym facilities with their saunas and jacuzzis, which are becoming an increasingly common feature of hotels and health clubs. Sociologists have argued that this recent trend is linked with treating 'the body' as a consumer commodity that must be maintained and groomed to achieve maximum market value (Lupton, 1994). Body maintenance in the interest of good health is linked with the desire to appear sexually attractive for both sexes, but more especially for women (Bordo, 1990). However cultural habits in hygiene care still demonstrate links with past beliefs, which are often expressed culturally (Helman, 1978).

The early Christian church considered physical cleanliness as less important than spiritual purity and after the decline of moral standards in the Roman Empire discouraged public bathing. Bathing, even in private, came to be regarded as unhealthy and was considered an indulgence. In the middle ages, the use of water to clean the body was rare and the only areas that needed to be cleansed were those visible to others. Even then, the 'dry wash', which involved rubbing one's face and hands with a cloth, was considered healthy right up to the seventeenth century (Vigarello, 1988). The use of hot water was considered unhealthy as people believed that the pores of the skin would open and allow infection to penetrate the body, therefore being covered up meant that the body was protected from disease. Lay beliefs about how we become susceptible to colds can echo these earlier beliefs (i.e. 'not allowing one's head to get wet', 'not going outside after washing one's hair', 'getting one's feet wet', 'getting caught in the rain' (Helman, 1978).

The relationship between bathing, body hygiene and becoming healthy changed with the industrial revolution when the body could then be compared with a machine; the use of cold water was seen as invigorating and helping to firm up the body and also became associated with moral austerity. With the scientific discovery of microbes, washing became important to rid the body of disease, touching of certain body parts considered 'dirty' became prohibited and more frequent washing was encouraged (Vigarello, 1988). At this time, buildings did not include bathing facilities and it was not until the level of dirt and disease increased after the industrial revolution that there became an increased demand for good bathing facilities to reduce cross-infections such as cholera. By the late nineteenth century, private homes of the upper classes began to have separate rooms set aside for bathing, and municipal baths were built for the general public to use (Encarta, 1995). In developed countries today most private homes have their own bathroom facilities, which are often multiple as *en suite* bathrooms have become the norm in new housing at the end of the twentieth century. There is now a more marked preoccupation with cleanliness and showers have become more commonplace, even in temperate climates. Cleansing products and deodorants are heavily marketed as body odour can be regarded as the ultimate 'social sin'. However, the preoccupation with 'smelling good' is being counterbalanced by a movement that accepts natural odours as normal and antipathy to the use of 'chemicals' on the skin (Bolander, 1994).

Bathing has also been an integral part of the ritual cleansing of religious practices over many centuries. Baptism in Christianity and the mikvah in Orthodox Judaism are derived from bathing rituals, while bathing is an important part of Muslim and Hindu religious ceremonies. Muslims perform ablutions before prayer and are very particular that all bodily excretions are removed.

Culturally certain hygiene habits may appear distasteful and noisy to nurses in developed countries. Internal cleansing rituals such as sniffing water up into the nose and blowing it out into a basin may provoke disgust, but this can be a normal practice among Muslims and Hindus, while colonic irrigations are a favoured method of internal cleansing of the gut among those who practice yoga.

The 'short back and sides' image of hair hygiene in developed countries is not relevant to a Sikh, to whom the hair (Kes) is sacred and should not be cut, but should instead be kept covered by a turban. Rastafarians do not like to wash their long hair.

Certain items of clothing are also sacred in certain cultures and should not be removed during hygiene care. These can include neck threads (marriage thread for Hindu women), bangles and comb (Kara and Kasngha – Sikhs), nose jewels (wedding symbols for Bangladeshi women), and a stone or medallion around the neck (protection for Muslims) (Sampson, 1982). There are many other cultural and religious habits among different cultural and religious groups that have an important impact on the delivery of appropriate and sensitive hygiene care. It is important to be sensitive to any requests that may seem strange, but are in fact normal to the individual concerned.

PRACTICE KNOWLEDGE

Knowledge for the assessment of needs and implementation of care will be the main focus within this section. Although in most instances hygiene care is delivered to meet the total needs of the patient, in order to incorporate the specific knowledge underpinning practice, the material in this section will be presented under four headings as follows:

▶ body hygiene care, including reference to foot and nail care and perineal hygiene;

▶ oral and dental hygiene;
▶ hair care;
▶ eye care.

▶ BODY HYGIENE CARE

Decision making around the delivery of hygiene care to a patient or client is dependent upon many factors, which include the patient's ability to self care, the facilities available, including family members or informal carers, and the nurse's expertise and time. According to Wilson (1986), accurate assessment of the individual patient's needs and level of participation should be encouraged wherever possible. Although there is still a need for the timing to be negotiated to fit organizational needs, the ritualization of bed bathing to the morning shift whether in hospital, hostel or community should become a thing of the past.

With children, infants and babies, bath times and routines in any health care facility should mimic as closely as possible the child's normal routine with the parents or significant carer being involved directly in providing care. Although the child may view hygiene rituals as unpleasant, they can be fun. There should be facilities both in time and the design of the environment that will maintain and encourage playtime for the infant and young child during the delivery of hygiene care. Children also need privacy, but there should be a balance between allowing them privacy and understanding how much help they require in order to be safe and achieve the goals of good hygiene. A baby needs a warm environment and less exposure to prevent chilling. Teenagers will expect that facilities will allow them to maintain their privacy, while older adults may expect the nurse to respect their usual routines for bathing and not demand bathing as a daily ritual if their normal habit is to bath less frequently (Jones, 1995).

The ability to care for one's own hygiene needs is important to all individuals and is a prime motivating factor in focusing the nurse on teaching self care to children or adults with learning difficulties. Goals set should be commensurate with the individual's ability and may need to be frequently revised in order to allow feelings of achievement if progress is slow. The motivation to maintain personal hygiene as part of a personal self-image can be lost when a person is depressed or disturbed mentally. The nursing role is then focused on encouraging self care through specific behaviour modification techniques or other counselling approaches that aim to improve the individual's feeling of self-esteem. Equally, the individual may be confused or have a loss of short-term memory and need constant direction in order to be encouraged to maintain his or her independence in hygiene care.

Overall goals for hygiene care will vary depending upon the particular circumstances and needs of the individual patient. These include some or all of the following:

▶ providing comfort and relaxation for the patient;
▶ ensuring cleanliness through the removal of secretions, micro-organisms and surface dirt;
▶ improving self-image by removing odours and enhancing physical appearance;
▶ improving skin and muscle condition by stimulating the circulation and massage (Bolander, 1994).

RESEARCH BASED EVIDENCE

In a study that examined the behaviour of 33 clients with cognitive impairment during bathtime, Kovach and Meyer-Arnold (1996) found that 73% of these adults displayed agitated behaviour during personal hygiene care. The clients used strategies that included attaining control, sharing control, resigning control and regaining inner control. Their coping mechanisms were needed because of the conflicting agendas between them and their carers.

If patients or clients need help from the nurse in meeting their hygiene needs, the following elements should be considered when making an assessment (Wilson, 1986):

▶ psychosocial needs: the need for privacy, aesthetic values of the patient, personal habits of the patient, cultural background of the patient;
▶ physical needs: level of dependence or independence, temporary or long-term dependence, therapeutic value of hygiene care;
▶ facilities and time available: choice of method to deliver care, time of day (patient choice where possible), aids required.

The activity of washing removes sweat, sebum, dried skin scales, dust and microorganisms from the skin's surface. If not removed, microorganisms multiply and lead to body odour and infection. When ill, increased anxiety can lead to increased sweating and therefore the need to wash more frequently (Spiller, 1992). In surgical patients, prevention of wound infection and cross-infection is a paramount consideration in the decision making about how often and by what method to deliver hygiene care. Patients who are incontinent may need more frequent and sensitive attention to their hygiene needs.

Decision making around hygiene care is concerned with skilful adaption of practice when the facilities within the context of care and the actual needs of the patient are incongruent.

Aesthetically care should be given according to the norms of good taste and culturally specific values. The method selected should be effective in terms of the patient's and the nurse's time and energy. It should promote and maintain the patient's independence, enhance the nurse–patient relationship and provide an opportunity for two-way information processes such as health promotion activities. Body hygiene care may also be therapeutic if part of a treatment regimen which includes the need for exercise of joints and muscle relaxation while the individual is submersed in warm water. Perineal hygiene care post childbirth also promotes wound healing in the mother who has perineal sutures.

▶ Facilitating Body Care

There are many different ways of delivering body hygiene care (Table 3.1.3). Although some or all of these methods are used on a daily basis by nurses in multiple contexts, textbooks generally concentrate on the techniques of bed bathing the highly dependent patient. There has been a major shift in conventions around decision making in this area of total body hygiene as the emphasis is placed on patient independence in maintaining his or her own hygiene care.

Conventional methods of bed bathing are physically tiring for the patient and the nurse. To overcome some of the disadvantages of bed bathing, towel bathing has been used in the USA for some time and

---

DECISION MAKING

You are allocated on a morning shift to work with a primary nurse who has responsibility for the care of six elderly women with varying degrees of mental and physical disabilities. Your partner is keen that all hygiene care should be delivered by the end of the morning.

• *Decide on what information you need to collect in order for you to make decisions on how to prioritize the care you give.*
• *Reflect on and discuss how you would cope with the wishes of your primary nurse to complete the care by lunchtime.*

(In completing this exercise, cross reference to any work you have done on assertiveness and dealing with potential conflicts of opinion.)

RESEARCH BASED EVIDENCE

In an early study in the USA, Barsevick and Llewellyn (1982) studied the effects of a towel bath and a bed bath on anxiety. They found that both techniques of bathing helped to reduce patient anxiety, but those patients receiving the towel bath had significantly lower anxiety scores.

After a visit to the USA, Wright (1990) introduced the towel bath to a unit in a UK hospital and surveyed 25 patients in a surgical ward: 92% preferred the towel bath.

Bath (tub or bath)
Shower
Complete bed bath
Towel bath
Partial bed bath or 'top and tailing' in infants and small children
Therapeutic baths

Table 3.1.3 Methods for body hygiene.

Reflect on your own personal choices when purchasing products such as soaps and lotions for your personal hygiene.
- *At a personal level, reflect on those factors that influence how you choose these products.*
- *At a professional level, reflect on how much knowledge you may need about the content of these products in order to give relevant advice to patients or clients about buying them.*

RESEARCH BASED EVIDENCE

Rhode and Barger (1990) completed a major review of the history of perineal care in postpartum women (following childbirth): they describe practice that used to be common in the past and compare the results of research into the various methods of care from 1951 through to 1989. In order to expand your knowledge in this specialist area of practice, review the contents of this article and compare it with what advice is given to newly delivered mothers in your local mother and child unit at present.

has been introduced into the UK on a limited basis (Wright, 1990). A seven-foot towel is soaked in a solution that contains a cleansing agent at a temperature of 110°F for which no rinsing is required. The patient is wrapped in the towel and massaged clean.

Although bathing is usually associated with the use of soap and water, various bath and shower gels containing an emollient have become increasingly popular as an alternative. Soap lowers skin surface tension by removing sebum (oily substance) from the skin, which facilitates cleaning. Care should be taken as some soaps remove too much sebum, and in the elderly with frail skin this may cause excessive drying of the skin. Special hypoallergenic soaps are available for people who experience allergic reactions. For babies and young children integral 'baby baths', which include bath cleanser and shampoo, for example Infacare, are readily available. People have individual preferences for the fragrance of the soap, the type of deodorant and other lotions and powders used following skin hygiene.

Special Areas for Care: the Perineal Area

In children care of the genitalia or perineum is important. For babies and young children who are not yet toilet trained, this area needs extra hygiene care and the application of water repellent creams to prevent skin damage. Children should generally be encouraged to self care, but in the older child there is a tendency to avoid cleaning this area (Wong, 1995). For boys over three years of age who are not circumcised, the foreskin should be retracted and the exposed surface cleaned (except in circumstances where cultural beliefs will not allow this). However, care must be taken to retract the foreskin very gently as it may be tight (phimosis) and overstretching can create scarring, leading to sexual and micturition (passing urine) difficulties in the future.

In adults of both sexes who cannot maintain their own hygiene, extra sensitivity is needed in dealing with perineal care because of cultural and spiritual taboos in exposing this area of the body. Perineal care in women following childbirth is managed differently, especially if there is a surgical wound in the area (Rhode and Barger, 1990).

Special Areas for Care: Nails and Feet

Although nails can be subjected to much abuse, especially finger nails, most people can maintain nail hygiene according to their own particular standards and values. In children, hygiene care to keep nails clean is particularly important after outdoor play, toileting and before meals as the eggs from intestinal parasites or helminths (roundworms, hookworms, pinworms, threadworms or *Toxocara* from dogs or cats) can be ingested and the child then becomes infected. Besides good hand and nail hygiene, children should be discouraged from biting their nails and from scratching the bare anal area (Wong, 1995).

Foot care and good nail care is also important in the elderly, and especially in any person who has diabetes mellitus as poor peripheral circulation makes this group of people vulnerable to skin breakdown with subsequent delayed healing. Specialist foot nail care is required through the expert skills of the chiropodist and the nurse's role is primarily in recognizing the need to refer clients and in providing preliminary care and advice. Primary health care nurses and specialist diabetic nurses, however, will be expected to give additional health education and care to the diabetic client (Childs, 1994; George, 1995).

▶ Therapeutic Baths

The temperature of the water in a bath can be used for therapeutic reasons as well as hygiene. Baths at skin temperature (37°C) are relaxing, those hotter or colder can be stimulating. Hot baths can help to relieve pain and discomfort and may control convulsions and induce sleep. Cold baths can be helpful in reducing fever and inflammation. All the body can be submerged or only a body part such as the perineum in a sitz bath or a foot bath. If any substance is added to the bath to have an effect on a disease, the bath can be termed as 'medicated'. Alkaline baths have been used extensively in the treatment of rheumatic conditions. Steam baths use medicated vapours to help lung conditions. Mineral baths are usually public baths that use the natural warm mineral springs of a certain region to aid in the recovery of numerous conditions. These are the fashionable spas of the nineteenth century and are still used today to promote general health (Encarta, 1995). Alternative therapies, which include aromatherapy oils added to the bath water and therapeutic massage given during a bed bath, may be used as an adjunct to hygiene care to promote healing and a general feeling of wellbeing (Price and Price, 1995; Tiran, 1996).

▶ Bathing Aids

For the disabled patient or client, particularly if confined to a wheelchair, bathing is potentially a very important time. Warm water will help to relax stiff muscles, there is the opportunity to increase the range of muscle movement, and there is also a change of position and atmosphere, which promotes a general feeling of wellbeing. To be able to get in and out of the bath in comfort and to be able to remain in the bath is a much appreciated luxury and one that can be difficult in institutional care where time and staffing is in short supply. Special facilities for the disabled include the Parker bath (Figure 3.1.4), with its unique design features, which allow the client to slide into the bath. It can be moved into several positions to aid both the client and the nurse. There are many different aids for bathing for the disabled on the market (see Chapter 3.4 on mobility) that can be used in the home in an ordinary bath (Milne, 1988).

▶ Principles of Care

Whatever procedure is selected to deliver body hygiene, the principles of safety, prevention of cross-infection and privacy should be followed. Safety extends to promoting good back care and posture for the nurse or carer by encouraging the use of appropriate bathing aids. Parents of babies and infants, in preparation for bathing their baby, should be aware of the dangers in lifting baby baths when full of warm water and also when disposing of the water after bathing. Children should never be left alone in the bath as there is always a danger of drowning regardless of the water level.

The process of providing care should be methodical, logical and safe, taking into consideration the specific limits of the patient, whether temporary, for example post surgery, or permanent, for example due to physical disability. If teaching or encouraging a child or adult with a learning disability or the frail elderly, goals should be set for what the patient can realistically do without causing undue discomfort and exposure during the bathing process. Being sensitive and not taking over is very important as most people are intrinsically motivated to participate

Figure 3.1.4: A Parker bath.

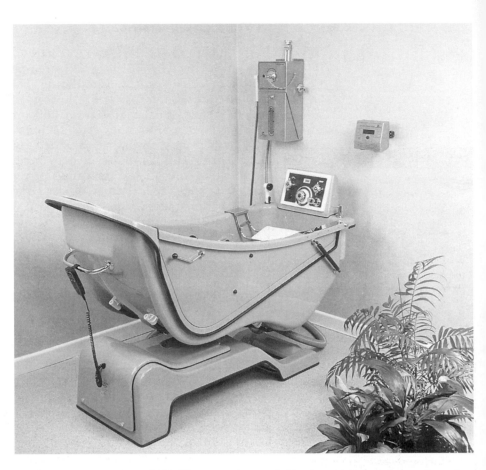

in their own care and dislike any loss of dignity and freedom of action (Wilson, 1986).

Giving hygiene care also allows the nurse to undertake other activities that are necessary for the overall decision making about care for the clients (Table 3.1.4). This particular aspect is often overlooked in skill mix debates when it is argued that hygiene care does not need the skills of a registered nurse. The opportunity to make relevant observations, to initiate and sustain the nurse–patient relationship, to explore the patient's

Type of activity	Details
Observations	Observe for signs and symptoms of physical problems Note any nonverbal expressions of anxiety and fear
Interpersonal communication	Encourage disclosure by patient (intimate procedure) Time for trusting and building relationships Opportunity to offer empathy and support
Health promotion	Information giving about the immediate condition and its treatment Advice and support for self care strategies on discharge or in the long term
Social interaction	Recognition of the influence of family, life and work on the patient or client Growth and development of the nurse as a person and a practitioner

Table 3.1.4 Nursing activities that can be incorporated into the delivery of hygiene care. (Adapted from Wilson, 1986)

concerns and to promote a healthy lifestyle is a fundamental part of the delivery of body hygiene care.

ORAL AND DENTAL HYGIENE

Assessment

The nurse's role in the maintenance of oral hygiene involves the use of general observation skills and specific assessment tools. Although it has been recognized that much of the responsibility for the delivery of oral care in an institutional setting has devolved to the junior or untrained nurse, the initial and ongoing assessment is the responsibility of the registered practitioner. Specific assessment tools should aid this process. However, to date, these tools are not yet in common use and reliability is dependent upon the same nurse carrying out the assessment in order to reduce the subjective nature of the decision making about oral care. It is important to encourage the use of an objective assessment tool that is valid, reliable and practical to use on a day to day basis.

The content of the various oral assessment tools include:

- direct observation of areas of the oral cavity;
- assessment of the functions of the mouth;
- risk factors that have the potential to create oral problems.

All tools include scoring systems that indicate the severity of the patient's oral condition. Jenkins (1989) developed a practical tool that acts as an 'at risk' calculator. Table 3.1.5 demonstrates the common features of the various assessment tools presented in the literature.

As it is important to use an objective measure, especially where care is being delegated to many (including junior) staff, the registered nurse may need to assess which of the tools will provide the most valid and reliable information for the particular client group in his or her care.

In the assessment of different client groups it is important to remember

Feature	Details
Observation of areas within mouth	Lips: colour, moisture, texture Tongue: colour, moisture, texture Gingiva: colour, moisture, haemorrhage, ulceration, oedema Teeth: shine, debris Palate: moisture, colour, ulceration
Functions within the mouth	Saliva: thin, watery, hypersalivation, scanty, absent, thick, ropey Voice: normal, deep, raspy, difficult or painful speech Swallow: normal, difficult, pain on swallowing fluids or solids, diminished or no gag reflex
Predisposing stressors	Mouth breathing Oxygen therapy Mechanical ventilation Restricted oral intake Chemotherapy or radiotherapy Drugs and concurrent diseases.
Subjective data from patients	Taste changes Pain profile

Table 3.1.5 Common features of different oral assessment tools.

that specific predisposing factors may put them at considerable risk of developing oral problems. Children with Down's syndrome and other disabling conditions tend to have thick ropey sticky saliva that fails to 'wash' food debris away and adheres to the tooth surface. This process encourages the early formation of plaque (Lloyd, 1992). For the older client, the ageing process leads to a decreased salivary flow. If the client is wearing dentures, these should be checked for fit to prevent trauma to the palate and gums (Barnet, 1991). If the individual client has diminished neuromuscular control he or she may have difficulty in maintaining oral care through lack of hand to mouth coordination. Teenagers wearing orthodontic appliances (braces) and those with an oral deformity such as a cleft lip or palate who have removable or fixed appliances will need special advice on how to maintain their oral hygiene, but may need encouragement from the nurse to sustain these practices (Griffiths and Boyle, 1993). For the elderly mentally infirm, it may be the client's behaviour that needs to be targeted during rehabilitation so that the individual's coping strategies can be improved. This assessment will involve other members of the health care team in order to measure the client's progress against pre-set short- and long-term goals. The Simon Nursing Assessment for the elderly mentally infirm includes an assessment section for oral hygiene (O'Donnovan, 1992). There are many risk factors to optimum oral health in the mentally ill. These arise from the condition itself (see Annotated Further Reading – Griffiths and Boyle, 1993) or the drug treatment to control the symptoms of the illness (Table 3.1.6).

Many other conditions, treatments and drugs can put the individual client at particular risk of developing oral problems. Some of these treatments are included in the risk assessment tools referred to earlier (see Table 3.1.5). Many drugs cause xerostomia (dry mouth) and damage the normal defence and healing processes of the oral cavity and are detailed in Table 3.1.6.

DECISION MAKING

A 13-year-old boy with a severe learning disability is subject to seizures for which he is taking anticonvulsants. He has some difficulty in cleaning his teeth due to physical disabilities.

- *Using an oral assessment tool (selected as a result of the previous Decision Making Exercise) decide on the level of risk of this boy.*
- *Discuss and make a decision on your strategy for health promotion in order to maintain this boy's oral hygiene.*

Drug group	Mechanism of action
Antihistamines	
Antispasmodics	
Anticholinergics	
Antidepressants	
Antipsychotics	Reduce salivary production
Tranquillizers	
Anticonvulsants	
Narcotic analgesics	
Antibiotics	Alter the balance of commensal organisms so that candidal organisms can invade the mouth
Cytotoxics and chemotherapeutics	Reduce the autoimmune response and therefore allow easy growth of invading organisms
Corticosteroids	Reduce the healing properties of tissues
Diuretics	Potential dehydration resulting in a reduction in salivary flow

Table 3.1.6 Drug groups that cause xerostomia (Gooch, 1985; Torrance, 1990; Thurgood, 1994).

If an individual complains of halitosis there is a need to establish the cause and assess its severity. A subjective assessment of the degree of severity of the halitosis by the individual concerned has been shown to correlate well with measurements of the amount of sulphide in the mouth. A portable sulphide monitor is used and gas chromatography can provide an accurate assessment of the wider range of compounds that can be responsible for halitosis. Usually such a full assessment is carried out by a dentist or periodontologist. Treatment is aimed at reducing any oral flora and is best achieved by brushing the teeth and cleaning between the teeth.

Overall there are many assessment tools now being researched, even if they are not yet being used in practice. Many of these tools do not include the subjective views of the client, which are important in increasing the validity of the assessment and in encouraging compliance with subsequent oral hygiene practices (Hoade–Reddick, 1991).

▌ *Facilitating Oral Care*

In the delivery of oral care to clients or patients the nurse has many decisions to make concerning the most appropriate tools and solutions to use in caring for the dependent patient. Likewise in the health promotion role, the advice and education given to the independent client needs to be specific to the individual client needs. It is therefore necessary to have knowledge of and experience in using the various tools and solutions available.

▌ *Methods for Dental and Oral Care*

The single most effective method of promoting dental health is to encourage a reduction in the consumption of refined sugars in the diet (see Chapter 3.2 on nutrition). Oral hygiene itself aims to reduce dental caries and maintain a healthy mouth. Various tools and solutions are used to achieve these aims. For the individual, having clean 'white' teeth and fresh breath may be even more important social goals and the timing of care may vary according to the family and cultural norms.

The toothbrush is the most effective method for removing plaque. Ideally the design should include a small head with soft multitufted nylon bristles (Alderman, 1988). Recent developments in toothbrush design have produced the circular head brush. Used as a battery-operated device, the oscillating movement of the brush head is efficient in removing debris without causing undue harm to the gums (Thurgood, 1994). Manually, a good simple technique is to brush in small circles dividing the mouth up into sections and systematically brushing each section. Brushing gums is just as important as the area between the teeth and gums can trap plaque, which will lead to gingivitis. Single-tufted brushes with a pointed tip are useful for patients with trismus (limited mouth opening). The use of dental floss or tape is recommended to clean between the teeth. All the above tools are relatively easy to use when the client can understand how and can control their use. Problems arise when the client is dependent on the nurse for oral care.

Although toothbrushing is the method of choice, in the past, nurses have failed to use them with clients, particularly because they feared causing trauma and perceived them as unsuitable for an edentulous mouth (Harris, 1980; Roth and Creason, 1986). The choice of toothbrush and method for using it are of prime importance for different client groups.

Young children need to have their teeth brushed for them and the nurse involved in giving advice to parents and carers should be able to provide the correct information. As flossing between teeth can potentially cause gum damage, it is important to avoid flossing for a child under ten years of age and to get expert advice if the older child needs this doing for them (Lloyd, 1992). For the disabled child or adult, electric or specially adapted standard toothbrushes are necessary. In school-aged children, recent studies have shown that chewing gum (even sucrose gum) for 20 minutes has a positive effect on salivary flow and will return the pH of the mouth to neutral, even after a meal high in carbohydrates (Lloyd, 1992). However, chewing gum is not recommended for the pre-school child.

Toothpaste is the most common substance used to clean teeth and since the introduction of fluoride into toothpaste there has been a large reduction in dental decay, especially in children (Rugg–Gunn and Murray, 1990). The fluoridation of water has been widespread, although the ethical debates related to personal choice have prevented its implementation in some areas. Although special fluoride supplements (rinses, gels, tablets and drops) have been available for children, there is concern that with the increasing amounts of fluoride in toothpaste, there may be a danger of the child developing fluorosis. Ensuring that children do not swallow toothpaste and rinse their mouths carefully is important in order to prevent fluorosis. Fluoride supplements should only be used on the advice of a dentist.

Other solutions in common use are listed in Table 3.1.7. Overall chlorhexidine is the most effective antiplaque agent. There is still a need to research more fully the effectiveness of some of the solutions that are still in common use in institutional health care settings. Commercially available solutions may contain alcohol, which has no benefit.

Other tools used for giving oral care to the dependent patient include foam sponges, swab on forceps and the swab on the finger technique. Foam sponges have the advantage of causing little oral trauma, but are ineffective at removing debris from the surface or in between teeth (Howarth, 1977). The swab on a forcep technique can be difficult to manipulate and may be more prone to causing trauma (Harris, 1980). The swab on the gloved finger if used with a gentle sweeping action can be effective in removing debris without causing undue trauma (Griffiths and Boyle, 1993). However, in any dependent person with facial muscle weakness that affects the mouth it is important that food and debris are not missed as the action of the swabbing may cause food to be compressed into one part of the mouth (Shepherd *et al.*, 1987).

▶ *Denture Care*

Dentures, both full and partial, are the most common oral appliance, especially among the elderly population and need regular rinsing and cleaning, particularly after eating. Dentures should be removed at night to prevent the development of oral candidiasis (thrush). As with teeth, the most effective method for removing plaque is through brushing and rinsing. Proprietary denture cleaners are available as solutions, brush-on cleaners or pastes, but all have some disadvantages such as staining, bleaching and corrosion of metal. Regular brushing with unperfumed soap and water is considered one of the best methods of cleaning dentures (Griffiths and Boyle, 1993). A common problem may be loose-fitting dentures, especially if the wearer is ill and poor nutrition leads to physical deterioration. A temporary method to overcome this problem is to insert a soft lining until a new set of dentures can be made. In residential

---

RESEARCH BASED EVIDENCE

Roth and Creason (1986) in a comprehensive review of selected nursing, medical and dental literature suggest that convenience and lack of the potential for trauma influence the nurse in her choice of tools for mouth care. Toothpaste and toothbrushes were not used because they were not easily available.

A recent review by Moore (1995) found that there has been little change in oral care practices over the past 30 years and that there has been neither enough research into oral care nor application of the research findings available in the assessment and decision making about oral care for specific client groups.

Solution	Action	Limitations
Chlorhexidine gluconate (solution, gel, spray)	Effective antiplaque Well tolerated by most client groups	Reversible staining of teeth
Hexetidine and cetylpyridinium, (mouthwash, gargle)	Antiplaque	Not as effective as chlorhexidine
Hydrogen peroxide and sodium perborate (diluted as mouthwash at 3%)	Mucosolvent that breaks down thick and viscous saliva	Unpleasant taste Short-term use only Incorrect dilution leads to chemical burns Risk of borate absorption
Sodium bicarbonate (powder diluted in water)	Mucosolvent Cleansing	Unpleasant taste Further research needed to ascertain how useful in practice
Thymol (mouthwash)	Antibacterial at high concentrations Refreshing taste	Little to no antibacterial action at low concentrations
Sodium chloride (mouthwash, gargle)	Effective cleansing agent Well tolerated	None indicated
Lemon and glycerine (impregnated swabs on a stick)	Lemon is a salivary stimulant Glycerine for lubrication, but astringent	Overuse can lead to salivary gland exhaustion and increased xerostomia Low pH increases the risk of dental caries
Phenol (mouthwash, gargle, spray)	Cleansing	Epiglottic and laryngeal oedema Contraindicated in children Needs further research to test effects on plaque
Povidone–iodine 1% (mouthwash/gargle)	Cleansing	Mucosal irritation Hypersensitive reactions No antiplaque activity
Benzydamine hydrochloride (mouthwash, spray)	Relief of oral ulceration	Numbness or stinging

Table 3.1.7 Solutions in common use for oral hygiene: actions and limitations. (Adapted from Griffiths and Boyle, 1993.)

or nursing home care many of the elderly residents have dentures, but loss of dentures can now be prevented by labelling dentures using a commercially available naming kit (i.e. Indenture).

▶ HAIR CARE

Hair styling and grooming feature very highly in maintaining physical and psychological health and a positive body image. Most people can and wish to maintain their own hair according to their own choice. In institutions where the individual is unable to care for themselves it is often therapeutic for both the client and his or her family if a member of the family or a friend provides this aspect of hygiene care. Self care may be a significant goal to achieve for those with physical and mental disability.

Reflect on your own experiences of cleaning dentures for a particular client group.

- *How did you feel about completing this task?*
- *What effect do you think your feelings would have in your decision making for providing optimum oral hygiene for a group of elderly patients who are receiving institutionalized care because of dementia?*

(For reference, see Boyle, 1992.)

Hair care among different ethnic groups can be part of deeply embedded beliefs that are cultural as well as religious (see Psychosocial part of Subject Knowledge) and these need to be respected. Hair care for black children or adults, if dependent, may need specific combs and techniques (Joyner, 1988). Hair loss from the head from whatever cause can be a significant source of worry, especially if it occurs for no known cause in children and adolescents (Clore and Corey, 1991)

All of the above variations in hair care need to be taken into account in assessing and facilitating hygiene care. Resources, which include time, should be available to provide optimum hair care in any health care institution. Daily combing and brushing can usually be maintained through self care, family support and nursing care. However, standards of care for shampooing can vary, and in the acute care setting may inevitably be given lower priority when resources are stretched. Many institutions for both acute and long-term care have back-up hairdressing services available, but often at a financial cost to clients.

▶ *Hair infestation*

Head lice are endemic and although they are not responsible for the spread of any disease, they are responsible for considerable social distress. They are cosmopolitan in that they can infest anybody and do not discriminate between class or cleanliness (Chunge *et al.*, 1991). Infestation with head lice can be quite debilitating if left untreated. However, this rarely happens today. The term 'feeling lousy' originates from feeling weak and 'nitwit' refers to poor performance at work due to untreated infestation (Sinclair, 1994).

Head lice eggs hatch after 7–10 days and the eggshell that remains is called the 'nit'. New hatchings are about 1 mm long and females do not mate until fully grown (i.e. six days old) and about 3 mm in length. Spread is through contact, and can be very quick as the two heads need only have direct contact for approximately one minute to allow the lice (usually fully grown lice) to move across from one hair to the other. Lice usually prefer short clean hair to long greasy hair (Sinclair, 1994).

School nurses, practice nurses and health visitors are key health care workers in dealing with head lice in children (Black, 1991). Both education and public health acts make it mandatory for health professionals to monitor and diagnose the presence of head lice in schoolchildren, but it is then the responsibility of the parents to cleanse the head. Free prescriptions for head lice preparations are available for children under 16 years of age. Most health districts now use a rotational policy for the main chemical treaments for head lice as there is evidence that resistance has developed. Table 3.1.8 shows the main lotions in use. All treatments

Compound	Lotion	Limitations
Organochlorines	Lindane	Resistance is becoming widespread Not often used
Anticholinesterases	Malathion Carbaryl	Inactivated by heat, some hair products and chlorine from swimming pools Shampoos weaker than the lotions
Pyrethroids	Permethrin Phenothrin	Generally wide margin of safety Mild itching or burning Shampoos have been used successfully

Table 3.1.8 Lotion groups for treatment of head lice.

for head lice are chemical in origin and can cause undue irritation of the skin.

A nonchemical approach to the treatment of head lice has been developed by Ibarra (1988, 1995). It involves removing the lice from the head before they are large enough to spread or reproduce. The method involves shampooing and conditioning the hair twice a week followed by combing with a fine-toothed plastic comb when the hair is wet. It was found through measuring the lice (1 mm long is newly hatched) that it was possible to clear the hair of lice within a fortnight by completing this treatment twice weekly.

▶ EYE CARE

In general, eye hygiene is part of the process of maintaining personal hygiene and practices from washing the area around the eyes with a clean face flannel through to using commercial products for cleansing lids and lashes (e.g. Lid-Care by CIBA Vision) and the removal of eye cosmetics is a matter for individual choice. The normal defence mechanisms of blinking and washing tears over the eye are sufficient to maintain healthy eyes. However, in health care particular groups of people can be at risk and need special eye hygiene care. These include:

- ▶ the newborn;
- ▶ the unconscious person;
- ▶ following eye injury or surgery.

Although pupillary and corneal reflexes are present in the newborn infant, the tear glands do not begin to function properly until the infant is 2–4 weeks old. Particular risks for the newborn include ophthalmia neonatorum, an infectious conjunctivitis that needs specific treatment with antibiotic drops (guttae) or ointment (ung.). The eyes are usually cleansed with sterile water before the insertion of drops or ointment. Conjunctivitis is common in infants and older children and the many different causes need specific treatments and eye hygiene measures (Wong, 1995).

In the unconscious person, the corneal reflex is lost and the eyes may tend to remain open and become dry. Drying of the eyes can lead to corneal ulceration and susequent loss of sight. Regular cleaning of the lids and lashes, the installation of an eye lubricant, and keeping the eyes closed are necessary to prevent damage to the eyes.

Following eye surgery or eye injury specific hygiene practices are usually instigated by the specialist ophthalmic nurse, but a key role is in health promotion in order to prepare the patient for continuing self care following discharge. As the eye is such a sensitive organ, self care is often difficult to achieve, especially by the elderly and those who have difficulty in remembering instructions or in manipulating the dropper or the ointment tube. It may be more important to educate relatives and friends to deliver the care (Latham *et al.*, 1992; Higgins and Ambrose, 1995).

PROFESSIONAL KNOWLEDGE

The imagery and politics of hygiene care are important areas for discussion with a particular focus on the continuing role of nurses in decision making and controlling this area of their professional practice.

The words 'basic nursing care' have been adopted by nurses as synonymous with meeting the hygiene needs of patients. Dictionary meanings for the word 'basic' are given as 'forming the base or essence' or 'fundamental' (*Oxford English Dictionary*, 1989). The dictionary also acknowledges a meaning for 'basic', which implies having relatively little value. Professionalization of nursing seems to have permitted the word 'basic' to become synonymous with the notion of being 'simple' or 'easy', thus implying a hierarchy of skills with 'technical' nursing skills where less body care is involved having greater importance and status (Lawlor, 1991). Acceptance of the 'simple and easy' meaning allows this fundamental aspect of the professional nurse's role to be delegated to the most junior member of the nursing team or the unqualified nurse (Badger *et al.*, 1989). Hygiene care, however, remains a core activity for the development of knowledge and decision making within the domain of nursing practice.

▶ THE RITUALIZATION OF HYGIENE CARE

The nursing profession has in the past been preoccupied with learning techniques for the delivery of hygiene care, in particular the bed bath. In the context of nursing within an institution there was a habit of giving hygiene care at a fixed time of the day (e.g. during the morning shift only) (Walsh and Ford, 1989). These factors have led to the ritualization of hygiene care, particularly in an institutional context. Clients are often given little choice in how their individual preferences are met (Jones, 1995) and nurses themselves accept hygiene care as a routine chore that requires little decision making.

Adams (1984) traces the obsessional concern of nurses for soap and water to aspects of institutional life bequeathed by the Poor Law. An immediate bath on admission was an institutional rule, part of an initiation cermony. There were often 'bath teams', with each member of the team carrying out a specific task, for example one undresses, one baths and one dries. The general public regard 'frequency of bathing' as one of the main criteria for assessing standards of care for the elderly in community institutions. Being kept clean and looking clean is associated with being respectable. It may be that little has changed in long-term care for the elderly, as for this particular client group 'cleanliness is next to godliness'.

▶ HYGIENE CARE AND THE IMAGE OF THE NURSE

According to Foucault (1975) when an individual becomes ill and enters an institution for care the boundaries of what might be considered normal in society are breached. This contention has particular implications for the breaking of the rules of privacy associated with the delivery of hygiene care. The body of the individual becomes 'objectified' in a way that allows health care professionals to observe and treat the individual without seemingly having to consider the emotions that body exposure may arouse both in the patient and in the nurse (Lawlor, 1991; Seed, 1995).

Nursing is also considered as 'dirty work' because it deals with the 'body' and body products. It is viewed as acceptable that people of low

---

RESEARCH BASED EVIDENCE

In a small study of nurses' and patients' opinions about bathing, Webster et al. (1988) found that 91% of nurses thought that bathing was very important in patient care. The patients in the study would have preferred to stick to their home routines, but felt that the nurses should make the decisions about bathing routines while they were in hospital.

status should do this work and it has been argued historically that women are best suited to this type of care giving. Paradoxically the women (nurses) who administered body care were expected to be both morally and physically pure (Wolf, 1986).

Sexual stereotypes of female nurses are perpetuated by the media and by film and TV dramas (Kalisch and Kalisch, 1982; Salvage, 1985). These stereotypes can be selected by male patients and instigated as part of the banter with female nurses, especially when having to subject themselves to the intimacy of hygiene care. Wearing a uniform may be important not just for cross-infection protection, but also because it is symbolic in that it gives the nurse permission to administer intimate care (Seed, 1995). In units where a uniform is not now worn, special garments such as plastic aprons may still be worn during the process of facilitating hygiene care.

There are equally powerful boundaries that the male nurse needs to cross in caring for female patients. The male nurse's role in giving hygiene care is more atypical of the accepted status quo in society in that nursing is seen in the context of 'motherhood', with a predominantly female profession giving intimate care. Therefore the need to seek permission may be more prominent when a male nurse seeks to give hygiene care to a female, especially if of a similar age. Seed (1995) found that male students were confronted with the feeling that they were doing something immoral in delivering intimate care to women.

RESEARCH BASED EVIDENCE

Lawlor (1991) describes her research into body care by nurses. She shows from her interview data that nurses learn through experience to touch and handle other people's bodies in a way that is deemed nonsexual and minimizes embarrassment. Elements used to do this included defining the situation as a professional encounter, displaying a 'matter of fact' manner, careful use of language, avoiding overexposure of a body part, the use of humour to minimize embarrassment, and the expectation that the patient and the nurse will behave 'properly'.

▶ THE POLITICS OF HYGIENE CARE

Government policy for the past 30 years has focused on the premise that where at all possible the chronically sick, disabled and frail elderly should be cared for in their own homes. Although the burden for initial assessment of overall needs has been transferred to the social worker (Department of Health, 1989), professional nurses are still involved in the detailed assessment of hygiene care needs. Added to this workload are the current increases in day case surgery, early discharge from hospital policies and home treatment, even for acute illnesses. A large part of the overall workload of the professional nurse working in the community is the prioritization of patient need within a framework of diminishing resources.

Generally, the actual routine delivery of hygiene care in the community, like institutions, is primarily undertaken by care assistants and is beholden to strict budgetary limits (Badger *et al.*, 1989). This leaves the biggest burden of care with relatives and friends or informal carers (Green, 1988; Atkinson, 1992). For informal carers there are major difficulties that need to be overcome. According to Atkinson (1992) these include:

- ▶ the physical cost of hygiene care – it can be heavy, time consuming and dangerous;
- ▶ resouces (e.g. hoists and shower units) can be slow to arrive and suffer from 'cut-backs';
- ▶ community nurse visits once a fortnight and then only if no relatives are available;
- ▶ little instruction is given to carers about how best to manage – 'relatives have to rely on hints from neighbours';
- ▶ restricted entry into day centres, especially if in the middle of a 'career of disablement';
- ▶ carers are reluctant to ask for help outside the home even if experiencing considerable physical problems with giving care.

Attitudes to the importance of hygiene care are a factor in the allocation of resources. Porter and James (1991) found that bathing received low priority compared to other client needs and was not considered as essential as dressing, toileting and feeding. Priorities set by community nurses were to visit the most vulnerable who include:

▶ older clients on their own;
▶ those who have no lay support;
▶ those who have been on their 'books' for a long time.

The average frequency of bathing in the home was either weekly or fortnightly, and the deciding criterion was often whether the patient was continent (Badger *et al.*, 1989).

Patients and families in the community were concerned with the quality of service, the main areas of concern being:

▶ time allocated for care was very short (e.g. 'a mad rush', 'not dried properly');
▶ lack of information and advice;
▶ lack of cultural awareness (e.g. importance of rinsing for an Asian client);
▶ frequency of the service was generally not often enough.

Equally there is also a need to monitor who assesses and makes decisions about the delivery of hygiene care within health care institutions. Skill mix debates, which at present focus on obtaining the best value for money, may in the future shift the balance of care delivery from a primary nursing model back to a system where the limited numbers of registered nurses in an area preclude adequate professional assessment and facilitation of hygiene care (National Association of Hospitals and Trusts, 1996). The shift of the nursing workload towards more 'technical' care may undermine the central role of the registered nurse in this key aspect of health care.

The material presented in this chapter demonstrates the potentially large quantity of knowledge needed by the nurse in order to make decisions about hygiene care and work collaboratively with the multidisciplinary team. It may be necessary to clarify and audit more carefully the critical and supportive activities undertaken by the nurse, similar to the classification system undertaken by nursing in the USA (Titler *et al.*, 1991). The classification system used in the USA presents a list of 'critical activities' and 'supportive activities' for interventions which are closely related to hygiene care and include among others: bathing, bedrest care, hair care, oral health maintenance, oral health promotion and oral health restoration. In order to support a case for retaining and strengthening the role of the registered nurse in this fundamental domain of nursing practice, such a classification system should be developed in the UK.

DECISION MAKING

Obtain a copy of the study by Badger *et al.* (1989) and review the findings and recommendations made at the end of the study.

- *Compare the findings with your own experiences when allocated to a community placement.*
- *Check for any more up-to-date studies that may have produced different findings to those of Badger* et al. *(1989). Discuss the implications of these differences with members of the primary health care team*

When making decisions about hygiene care within a system where resources are limited what should be the priority for the community nurse who has to make these decisions. Consider your answer by examining which of the following should take priority.

- *Patient-defined needs.*
- *The nurse's perceptions of what the patient needs.*
- *The resources available.*

The delivery of high standards of hygiene care requires the nurse to have detailed knowledge and skills and to be able to take appropriate and sensitive decisions in facilitating hygiene care for each individual client. Research-based evidence is needed to set standards and the nurse should be actively engaged in reviewing and applying such evidence in daily practice. This chapter should provide a starting point in the development of your knowledge, which needs to be constantly updated.

It is important to reflect, integrate and consolidate the knowledge gained from this chapter with the knowledge gained from your practice experience. This can be achieved through reflection on your own personal experiences and those of your peer goup of students and through the case study work, which you can complete on your own or may form the basis for a group seminar.

▶ EXPERIENTIAL EXERCISES IN PRIVATE OR PRACTICUM

Learning about all aspects of hygiene care for all client groups is a fundamental part of any nursing course. Much of your practice experience is gained directly with patients or clients in partnership with an assigned clinical supervisor or mentor. Expert nurses forget how embarrassed a student may feel when they first have to deliver intimate hygiene care to a client and take for granted their own knowledge and skills in the delivery of hygiene care. Reflective notes made in a personal learning diary will be useful so that you can discuss your feelings later if you wish (Jones, 1995). Problems faced by students in the delivery of hygiene care are often not discussed (Orr, 1987).

You may, however, get the opportunity to practice and reflect on your own personal feelings and reactions in the relatively safe environment of a 'practicum' or 'learning laboratory'. Experiential exercises in assessing 'the normal' in your fellow students and in providing hygiene advice and care to your fellow students under different circumstances will help you gain confidence in your own ability before being exposed to patients and clients.

These exercises are not so much concerned with the technique of delivery of hygiene care (although this can be included), but with issues surrounding the 'taken for granted' aspects of hygiene care delivery, especially in an institutional care setting. These exercises can form the basis for feedback within a group discussion session or for reflective notes in your journal or learning diary.

▶ *Examples of Experiential Exercises*

1. Complete an oral assessment and give or facilitate oral care to your student partner who can 'role play' circumstances such as being confined to bed in the supine position, being paralysed, being blind, being non-cooperative and aggressive, being confused and unable to follow your instructions.
2. Reflect on your own needs while giving yourself a 'strip wash' at home. Consciously note the temperature of the water, how often you change it, how much soap and rinsing you like, what movements you use in washing, how much pressure you apply in drying your skin, and how you deal with cleansing your face, eyes and ears. Discuss your findings with your peers. Appraise how you may need

---

RESEARCH BASED EVIDENCE

Through participant observation and interviews Seed (1995) explored the experiences of a cohort of student nurses as they coped with intimate body care during the various phases of their training. Early in the course, students found giving intimate care stressful, particularly when it involved a member of the *opposite sex. With increasing experience, both male and female students developed means of coping. Although it signalled their occupation, the students found that wearing a uniform was seen as self-protective and legitimized them in crossing social boundaries in the delivery of intimate care.*

to adapt personal habits to fit the needs of different client groups.

3. Experience the feeling of being helpless, dependent and embarrassed because someone else has to wash you through exercises in washing one another in the safe environment of a learning laboratory. Explore feelings around being washed by a member of the opposite sex.

▶ CASE STUDIES

The following case studies will help you consolidate knowledge gained through studying this chapter and completing any relevant reading outside the chapter content.

▶ CASE STUDY: LEARNING DISABILITIES

David Hargreaves, aged 25 years, has recently been discharged from a longstay hospital to the care of his ageing parents. He has been in institutional care for most of his life because of a severe learning disability. He is also physically disabled and requires much support and encouragement in maintaining his own hygiene care. He can wash his face and clean his teeth regularly, but it needs two people to give him full body hygiene care. His parents are finding it increasingly difficult to provide this care because of their age and lack of strength. They had been waiting some years for a grant to make suitable alterations to their home that would allow them to have a purpose-designed shower unit built.

■ **What other information would you need in order to make decisions regarding responsibility for support and care for this family?**

■ **How would you prioritize their needs?**

■ **Who do you think has the ultimate responsibility for decisions about resourcing the needs of this family?**

▶ CASE STUDY: MENTAL HEALTH (AND CHILD)

Li is a second generation member of a Vietnamese family who have settled in England. She has married a fellow Vietnamese and has recently given birth to her second child, a daughter.

Her son is two years old. Li has become depressed after the birth of her son and is beginning to show the same symptoms again. Her husband has become anxious as she is neglecting herself and the children. He has sought help from the health visitor (whom the family know) at the local health centre. Because her condition has deteriorated and it is difficult for her husband to cope with the newborn baby and his son, Li is admitted along with her two children to a special family unit that cares for women with postnatal depression.

■ **How might the needs of this family be assessed by the multidisciplinary team of the family unit?**

■ **In relation to self care, what strategies might be employed to encourage Li to care for her own hygiene needs initially?**

■ **How much self care might you expect Li's son to be able to perform for his stage of development.**

■ **Are there any special cultural practices among Vietnamese people that the multidisciplinary team need to be sensitive to in relation to the hygiene practices of Li and her two children?**

■ **On what basis might the multidisciplinary team make a decision that Li can return home with her two children?**

▶ CASE STUDY: ADULT

John is a 75-year-old retired lecturer. He is married and has two sons who are also teachers. Three years ago he had a stroke, which has left him with weakness of the left arm and leg. He has been feeling weak and unwell for the past three months. He has lost his appetite and a considerable amount of weight. After a visit to his general practitioner he is admitted to an acute medical unit for investigation of his weight loss.

■ **What factors should be considered in assessing John's specific hygiene needs?**

■ **When facilitating John's hygiene care, what other observations can be made by the nurse that will help with the overall assessment of John's problems?**

■ **Because of weight loss, John's dentures are ill-fitting. Decide on the specific advice and care John may need in relation to his oral hygiene.**

▶ CASE STUDY: CHILD

Simon is three years old and has recently complained to his dad about pain on passing urine. He has not spoken at all about this to his mum and appeared acutely embarrassed when dad mentioned this problem. It is clear that Simon's mum will need to take him to see the family doctor since his dad will be unable to due to work commitments. Simon is diagnosed as having balinitis (infection under the foreskin). He is prescribed systemic antibiotics and his mother is advised to cleanse the area and apply an antiseptic cream. Simon is cared for by a childminder and his mum and dad.

■ **Initially what strategies could the mother be advised to use in order to introduce Simon to the idea of being seen and examined by the doctor? How would this advice relate to your role in dealing with children who need help with intimate hygiene care delivery in hospital?**

■ **Consider the impact that this special hygiene care and treatment might have on Simon's privacy and dignity. How could he be helped to cope with the childminder administering this care?**

■ **Simon becomes very interested in this 'new' aspect of hygiene and begins to retract his foreskin when using the toilet. How could his family manage this new habit?**

▶ ANNOTATED FURTHER READING

BOLANDER, V. (1994) *Sorenson and Luckmann's Basic Nursing – A Psychophysiologic Approach* (3rd edition). Chapter 38. Philadelphia. W.B. Saunders Co.
This current chapter does not cover the actual techniques for delivering hygiene care. There are many textbooks on the market that will describe 'how to do it'. Sorenson and Luckmann's text is one that comprehensively covers all aspects of 'basic' nursing care and is a very useful resource text, especially Chapter 38.

GRIFFITHS, J., BOYLE, S. (1993) *Colour Guide to Holistic Oral Care: A Practical Approach*. Aylesbury. Mosby Year Book.
Overall this is a very good book for much more in-depth information on all aspects of oral and dental hygiene. Chapters focus on different client groups and their special needs and will be particularly useful when you move into your specialist branch of nursing.
Chapter 12 is a particularly good chapter for students caring for patients or clients with mental health problems. It covers the oral health problems that can occur in people with many different types of specific mental health disorder and refers to relevant research in this field.

HINCHLIFF, S., MONTAGUE, S., WATSON, R. (1996) *Physiology for Nursing Practice* (2nd edition). Chapter 6.1. London. Baillière Tindall.
This well-produced second edition of a popular physiology book is a very good reference book for filling in the gaps on the biological basis of hygiene care and providing relevant material for most of the other chapters in this book.

LAWLOR, J. (1991) *Behind the Screens: Somology and the Problems of the Body*. Edinburgh. Churchill Livingstone.
Lawlor conducted her research in the Australian nursing context, but her book is a very accessible, reflective and analytical account on all the rituals and practices that surround the personal and cultural management of the delivery of hygiene care in institutional settings.

LUPTON, D. (1994) *Medicine as Culture – Illness, Disease and the Body in Western Societies*. London. Sage Pub.
For those interested in the sociology of health, disease and medicine this is an interesting book that provides many references for further reading for studying the sociology of health care in more depth. It includes chapters on power relations between medicine and nursing and also the feminist perspective on health care issues.

SAMPSON, A.C. (1982) *The Neglected Ethic: Cultural and Religious Factors in the Care of Patients*. London. McGraw–Hill.
Although there is now an increasing number of texts on the ethnic and cultural

aspects of health care, Sampson's earlier text is the only one to date that provides concrete practical information that can be applied in the practice setting.

WONG, D. L. (1995) *Whaley and Wong's Nursing Care of Infants and Children* (5th edition). Chapter 20. St Louis. Mosby.

For students who wish to specialize in children's nursing, this book is a very comprehensive resource book for all aspects of infant, child and teenage care.

▶ REFERENCES

ADAMS, J. (1984) Soap opera. *Nursing Mirror* **159(22)**: 22, 31–32.

ALDERMAN, C. (1988) Oral hygiene. *Nursing Standard* **40(2)**: 24.

ATKINSON, F.I. (1992) Experience of informal carers providing nursing support for disabled dependents. *Journal of Advanced Nursing* **17**, 835–840.

BADGER, F., CAMERON, E., EVERS, H. (1989) The nursing auxiliary service and the care of elderly patients. *Journal of Advanced Nursing* **14**: 471–477.

BARNET, J. (1991) A reassessment of oral healthcare. *Professional Nurse* **6(12)**: 703–704, 706–708.

BARSEVICK, A., LLEWELLYN, J. (1982) A comparison of the anxiety-reducing potential of two techniques of bathing. *Nursing Research* **31(1)**: 22–27.

BECK, S. (1979) Impact of a systematic oral care protocol on stomatitis after chemotherapy. *Cancer Nursing* **2(3)**: 3, 185–189.

BLACK, K. (1991) Campaigning against head lice in schools. *Midwife, Health Visitor and Community Nurse* **27(1)**: 14.

BOLANDER, V. (1994) *Sorenson and Luckmann's Basic Nursing – A Psychophysiologic Approach* (3rd edition). Philadelphia. W.B. Saunders Co.

BORDO, S. (1990) Reading the slender body. In Jacobus, M., Keller, E.F., Shuttleworth, S. (eds) *Body Politics: Women and the Discourses of Science*. New York. Routledge.

BOYLE, S. (1992) Assessing mouth care. *Nursing Times* **88(15)**: 44–46.

CHILDS, M.B. (1994) Footcare for the diabetic patient: an overview. *Journal of Vascular Nursing* **12(3)**: 65–67.

CHUNGE, R., SCOTT, F., UNDERWOOD, J., ZAVARELLA, K. (1991) A review of the epidemiology, public health importance, treatment and control of head lice. *Canadian Journal of Public Health* **82(3)**: 196–200.

CLARKE, G. (1993) Mouth care and the hospitalized patient. *British Journal of Nursing* **2(4)**: 225–227.

CLORE, E.R., COREY, A. (1991) Hair loss in children and adolescents. *Journal of Pediatric Health Care* **5(5)**: 245–250.

COCHRANE, C. (1993) Contact lenses and bacterial infections. *Nursing Standard* **7(20)**: 32–34.

DEPARTMENT OF HEALTH (1989) *Working for People – Community Care Act*. London. Her Majesty's Stationery Office.

EILERS, J., BERGER, A.M., PETERSON, M.C. (1988) Development, testing and application of the oral assessment guide. *Oncology Nursing Forum* **15(3)**: 325–330.

ENCARTA (1995) CD Rom. Seattle. Microsoft Corporation, Funk and Wagnalls Corporation.

FARRELL, M., WRAY, F. (1993) Eye care for ventilated patients. *Intensive and Critical Care Nursing* **9(2)**: 2, 137–141.

FOUCAULT, M. (1975) *The Birth of the Clinic: an Archeology of Medical Perception*. New York. Vintage Books.

GEORGE, M. (1995) A feat for nursing? *Nursing Standard* **9(31)**: 22.

GOOCH, J. (1985) Mouth care. *Professional Nurse* **1(3)**: 77–78.

GOULD, D. (1991) Skin bacteria: what is normal? *Nursing Standard* **5(52)**: 216–228.

GREEN, H. (1988) *Informal Carers. General Household Survey 1985*. Series GH5, No.15, Supplement A. London. Her Majesty's Stationery Office.

GRIFFITHS, J., BOYLE, S. (1993) *Colour Guide to Holisitic Oral Care: A Practical Approach*. Aylesbury. Mosby Year Book.

HARRIS, M.D. (1980) Tools for mouthcare. *Nursing Times* **76(8)**: 340–342.

HELMAN, C. (1978) 'Feed a cold, starve a fever' – folk models of infection in an English suburban community and their relation to medical treatment. *Culture, Medicine and Psychiatry* **2**: 107–137.

HENDRICKS, S.J.H., FREEMAN, R., SHEIHMAN, A. (1990) Why inner city mothers take their children for routine medical and dental examinations. *Community Dental Health* **7**: 33–41.

HIGGINS, L., AMBROSE, P. (1995) The effect of adjunct questions on older adult's recall of information from a patient education booklet. *Patient Education and Counselling* **25(1)**: 67–74.

HINCHLIFF, S. (1996) Innate defences. In Hinchliff, S., Montague, S., Watson, R. *Physiology for Nursing Practice* (2nd edition). London. Baillière Tindall.

HOADE–REDDICK, G. (1991) A study to determine oral health needs of institutionalised elderly patients by non-dental health care workers. *Community Dental Oral Epidemiology* **19**: 233–236.

HOLMES, S., MOUNTAIN, E. (1993) Assessment of oral status: evaluation of three oral assessment guides. *Journal of Clinical Nursing* **2**: 35–40.

HOWATH, H. (1977) Mouthcare procedures for the very ill. *Nursing Times* **73(10)**: 354–355.

IBARRA, J. (1988) How to detect head lice: the changing emphasis in health education. *Health at School* **3**: 109–112.

IBARRA, J. (1995) A non-drug approach to treating head lice. *Community Nurse (Nurse Prescriber)* **1(25)**: 25, 27.

JENKINS, D.A. (1989) Oral care in the ICU: an important nursing role. *Nursing Standard* **4(7)**: 24–28.

JONES, A. (1995) Reflective process in action: the uncovering of the ritual of washing in clinical nursing practice. *Journal of Clinical Nursing* **4(5)**: 283–288.

JOYNER, M. (1988) Hair care in the black patient. *Journal of Pediatric Health Care* **2(6)**: 281–287.

KALISCH, P.A., KALISCH, B.J. (1989) *The Changing Image of the Nurse*. Menlo Park. Addison–Wesley Press.

KOVACH, C.R., MEYER–ARNOLD, E.A. (1996) Coping with conflicting agendas: the bathing experience of cognitively impaired older adults. *Scholarly Inquiry for Nursing Practice* **10(1)**: 23–42.

LATHAM, B., HIGGINS, L., AMBROSE, P. (1992) Cataract patients' post-op eye care: development and evaluation of a teaching programme. *Australian Journal of Advanced Nursing* **10(1)**: 4–9.

LAWLOR, J. (1991) *Behind the Screens:*

Somology and the Problems of the Body. Edinburgh. Churchill Livingstone.

LEVINE, R.S. (1989) *The Scientific Basis of Dental Health Education* (3rd edition). London. Health Education Authority.

LLOYD, S. (1992) Brushing up on children's mouth care. *Professional Care of Mother and Child* **21(2)**: 16–17

LUPTON, D. (1994) *Medicine as Culture – Illness, Disease and the Body in Western Societies.* London. Sage Pub.

MILNE, J. (1988) Bathing aids for handicapped children. *British Journal of Occupational Therapy* **51(6)**: 207–209.

MOORE, J. (1995) Assessment of nurse-administered oral hygiene. *Nursing Times* **91(9)**: 40–41.

NATIONAL ASSOCIATION OF HEALTH AUTHORITIES AND TRUSTS (1996) *The Future Healthcare WORKFORCE.* Birmingham. N.A.H.A.T.

O'DONNOVAN, S. (1992) Simon's nursing assessment. *Nursing Times* **88(2)**: 30–33.

ORR, J. (1987) Arn't misbehaving? *Nursing Times* **83(9)**: 25.

OXFORD ENGLISH DICTIONARY (1989) 2nd edition. Oxford. Clarendon Press.

PASSOS, J., BRAND, L. (1966) Effects of agents used for oral hygiene. *Nursing Research* **15(3)**: 196–202.

PORTER, J., JAMES, F. (1991) To bath or not to bath? A joint initiative to resolve the problem of increasing demand for bath assessment. Part I. *British Journal of Occupational Therapy* **54(3)**: 92–94. Part II. *British Journal of Occupational Therapy* **54(4)**: 135–138.

PRICE, S., PRICE, L. (1995) *Aromatherapy for Health Professionals.* Edinburgh. Churchill Livingstone.

RHODE, M.A., BARGER, M.K. (1990) Perineal care—then and now. *Journal of Nurse Midwifery* **35(4)**: 220–230.

ROPER, N., LOGAN, W., TIERNEY, A. (1996)*The Elements of Nursing* (4th edition). Edinburgh. Churchill Livingstone.

ROTH, P.T., CREASON, N.S. (1986) Nurse administered oral hygiene: is there a scientific basis? *Journal of Advanced Nursing* **11(3)**: 323–331.

RUGG-GUNN, A.J., MURRAY, J.J. (1990) Current issues in the use of fluorides in dentistry. *Dental Update* **17(4)**: 154–158.

SALVAGE, J. (1985) *The Politics of Nursing.* London. Heinemann.

SAMPSON, A.C. (1982) *The Neglected Ethic: Cultural and Religious Factors in the Care of Patients.* London. McGraw–Hill.

SCULLY, C., PORTER, S., GREENMAN, J. (1994) What to do about halitosis. *British Medical Journal* **308**: 217–218.

SEED, A. (1995) Crossing the boundaries – experiences of neophyte nurses. *Journal of Advanced Nursing* **21**: 1136–1143.

SHEPHERD, G., PAGE, C., SAMMON, P. (1987) The mouthtrap. *Nursing Times* **83(19)**: 25–27.

SINCLAIR, A. (1994) Head lice and scabies. *Professional Care of Mother and Child* **4(8)**: 241–242.

SPILLER, J. (1992) For whose sake – patient or nurse? Ritual practices in patient washing. *Professional Nurse* **7(7)**: 431–432, 434.

THURGOOD, G. (1994) Nurse maintenance of oral hygiene. *British Journal of Nursing* **3(7)**: 332–334, 351–353

TIRAN, D. (1996) *Aromatherapy in Midwifery Practice.* London. Baillière Tindall.

TITLER, M., PETTIT, D., BULCHER, G. et al. (1991) Classification of nursing interventions for care of the integument. *Nursing Diagnosis* **2(2)**: 45–56.

TORRANCE, C. (1990) Oral hygiene. *Surgical Nurse* **13(4)**: 16–20.

TRENTOR-ROTH, P., CREASON, N. (1986) Nurse-administered oral hygiene – is there a scientific basis? *Journal of Advanced Nursing* **11(3)**: 323–331.

VIGARELLO, G. (1988) *Concepts of Cleanliness: Changing Attitudes in France since the Middle Ages* (translated by J.Birrell). Cambridge. Cambridge University Press.

WALSH, M., FORD, P. (1989) *Nursing Rituals, Research and Rational Actions.* London. Heinemann.

WEBSTER, R., THOMPSON, D., BOWMAN, G., SUTTON, T. (1988) Patients' and nurses' opinions about bathing. *Nursing Times Occasional Paper* **84(7)**: 54–57.

WILSON, M. (1986) Personal cleanliness. *Nursing (London): The Journal of Clinical Practice, Education and Management* **3(2)**: 80–82.

WOLF, Z. R. (1986) Nursing work: the sacred and profane. *Holistic Nursing Practice* **1(1)**: 29–35.

WONG, D.L. (1995) *Whaley and Wong's Nursing Care of Infants and Children* (5th edition). St Louis. Mosby.

WRIGHT, L. (1990) Bathing by towel. *Nursing Times* **86(4)**: 36–39.

3.2 Nutrition

T. Hoyle

▶ INTRODUCTION

Most major improvements in health have had little to do with the high-technology and expensive treatments of individuals that are associated with modern medicine. The biggest advances have been made as a result of improvements in housing, sanitation and general improvements in living standards. One of the most important of these is in the supply of plentiful, good quality food.

In affluent countries, the fear of starvation has been replaced by the worry of obesity and heart disease caused by overeating or eating the 'wrong' foods. It is important then that nurses are able to give well-informed, impartial advice to clients. This is not the simple matter it may at first appear because of the vast amount of often conflicting information that both clients and nurses may encounter. Nurses must also be cautious because there is a belief, often promoted by politicians and the media, that diseases do not just happen, but that they are caused by something that the individual has done or failed to do. This is the process of 'victim blaming', a popular strategy employed by governments who need to reduce expenditure on health (Naidoo and Wills, 1994). It would be quite easy therefore to engender guilt and make clients feel that it is their fault that they have developed an illness.

▶ OVERVIEW

▶ Subject Knowledge

In this section, the functions of food as a source of energy, growth and repair are explored. The physiological processes that allow the body to

Identify some of the information you have encountered about food, diet or nutrition in the past week. Sources of such information may include television, radio, newspapers, posters, magazines and books, as well as friends.

• *How do you think this information has affected your attitudes and behaviour?*

utilize nutritional components of food are detailed, and throughout this section you are asked to compare the physiological evidence against common contemporary dietary myths. Social and psychological factors and their influences on diet are then discussed. In particular, while reading this chapter, you should consider how social changes and pressures within different sections of society have influenced diet.

▶ Practice Knowledge

In this section, the main focus is on the nursing assessment of clients' nutritional status. Nutritional needs vary according to a client's age, gender and lifestyle. In addition, women who are pregnant or breast-feeding have particular nutritional needs to ensure their own health and that of their babies. Strategies for the planning and implementation for nursing care follow, and alternative methods of feeding for use when clients are unable to eat normally are discussed.

▶ Professional Knowledge

This section outlines legislative issues and focuses on the Code of Professional Conduct (UKCC, 1992) in respect to food and diet. Finally in this section, three common dietary disorders – diabetes mellitus, anorexia nervosa and obesity – are discussed. This forms the rationale for the nursing strategies used when working with clients suffering from one of these conditions.

▶ Reflective Knowledge

The final part asks you to reflect on the chapter.

On pp. 370–371 there are four case studies, each one relating to one of the branch programmes. You may find it helpful to read one of them before you start the chapter and use it as a focus for your reflections while reading.

SUBJECT KNOWLEDGE

▶ HISTORICAL AND SOCIAL PERSPECTIVES

Many people refer back to a golden age when everything was organic, and feel that many of our problems would be solved if only we could achieve a 'natural' diet. The difficulty is in identifying such an elusive concept. How far back in history should we go to find the diet we were 'designed' to consume?

In hunter gatherer societies, it appears that the men did the hunting and the women collected roots, nuts, seeds and berries (Blaxter, 1993). The diet, therefore, would have contained very few simple sugars and would have been high in fibre, low in protein and low in fat. Animal fat would have been very scarce as wild game is generally exceptionally lean. The mixture of many different foods reduced the risk of deficiency diseases and although the nomadic lifestyle is impractical for most of us, we can still learn some lessons from it about the balance of foods in our diet.

Most people do not now hunt to survive and food is purchased from growers and farmers. Therefore, the type of diet people have is largely determined by the amount of money they spend on it. During the nineteenth century it was considered that the working classes had a generally small stature and low intelligence because they were genetically inferior. Work by Boyd Orr (1936) showed that the differences between public school and council school boys were due to protein deficiency, and more recently a return to similar class differences has been noted (Reading *et al.*, 1993). At the time that Boyd Orr published his findings, it was recommended that people should increase their intake of dairy foods. This was good advice at the time, but it has caused confusion because it is now advised that the intake of cheese, eggs and whole milk should be reduced.

For many years now the percentage of our income that we spend on food has been declining, leaving a larger proportion for non-essential items. This is the result of remarkable advances in agriculture, which have enabled us to grow more and more food from the same area of land. Intensive agriculture has its critics, especially in the areas of animal husbandry and the use of pesticides and chemical fertilizers. However, there is no doubt that it has made a significant contribution to the availability of sufficient cheap food and therefore the material wealth of all of us. It has in fact been so successful that we produce far more food than we can consume.

Biological ▶ **ENERGY-PRODUCING FOODS**

All of the activities we undertake involve the expenditure of energy. Even when we are asleep or unconscious the muscles of our heart and respiration need energy. Heat energy is needed to maintain body temperature and cells are constantly being replaced as they wear out and die. All of the energy for these processes is derived from food in the form of carbohydrates, fats or proteins.

The amount of food we need is controlled by our energy expenditure. This is called the energy balance. If we take in less energy than we are using we are said to be in negative energy balance and will lose weight. On the other hand taking in excess energy, regardless of the type of food eaten, is a positive balance and will result in weight gain. Many people maintain the same weight for many years, which indicates very accurate control of energy balance, although how this regulating mechanism works is uncertain.

The amount of food we actually eat is determined to a large extent by appetite. The main control of appetite is physiological, involving two centres within the hypothalamus – the feeding (hunger) centre and the satiety (full) centre – which work in opposition to each other. The satiety centre is mainly stimulated by the blood glucose concentration and functions to suppress the hunger centre. As the blood glucose concentration decreases, however, the power of the satiety centre is lowered and the hunger centre becomes active, giving rise to the feeling of hunger and desire to eat. This explains why something sweet at the end of a meal (consequently containing a large amount of simple sugars, which are rapidly absorbed to raise the blood sugar level) leaves an individual feeling satisfied and in need of no further food.

Other physiological influences on appetite are body fat deposits and distension of the gut. Psychosocial factors are also important as will be discussed later in this chapter.

How the body uses carbohydrates, proteins and fats is discussed below.

▌ *Carbohydrates*

Carbohydrates should account for more than half the energy intake in the diet. They have the general formula $(CH_2O)_n$ and are manufactured by plants from carbon dioxide, water and energy from sunlight through the process of photosynthesis. By this means the energy of the sun is trapped and made available to animals when they eat the plants.

The most simple carbohydrates, such as glucose, fructose and galactose, contain six carbon molecules and are called monosaccharides. These three monosaccharides all have the formula $C_6H_{12}O_6$ but the positions of the carbon atoms in relation to the oxygen atoms differ. These monosaccharides can combine to form pairs of molecules called disaccharides. This is achieved by the removal of a water molecule and is known as the condensation reaction (Figure 3.2.1). Depending on the combination of monosaccharides, different disaccharides are produced. For example:

▌ the disaccharide we are most familiar with is sucrose, which is table sugar, and this is simply one glucose molecule joined to one fructose molecule;

▌ two molecules of glucose form maltose, which is also a disaccharide;

▌ one molecule of glucose and one molecule of galactose form lactose.

Because of their relatively uncomplicated molecular structure, mono-

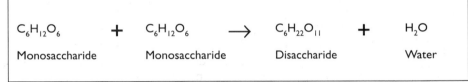

$$C_6H_{12}O_6 \quad + \quad C_6H_{12}O_6 \quad \longrightarrow \quad C_6H_{22}O_{11} \quad + \quad H_2O$$

Monosaccharide   Monosaccharide   Disaccharide   Water

Figure 3.2.1: The condensation reaction.

saccharides and disaccharides are quickly absorbed and utilized. They are also referred to as simple sugars. Many glucose molecules joined together form a polysaccharide called starch, which plants use as an energy store, for example the starch in potatoes and cereals. Foods containing these will therefore be high in complex carbohydrate.

Plants also use another form of carbohydrate called cellulose to form their structure. Humans are unable to digest this structural carbohydrate, but ruminants such as cows and sheep are able to break it down and use it for energy.

▌ Common misconceptions

Many people believe that some forms of simple carbohydrates are more natural and therefore healthier than others and these myths are often exploited by the food industry who try to convince us that their products are more healthy than those of their competitors. It is worth remembering that, from a nutritional viewpoint there is no difference between glucose, fructose and sucrose, and certainly no advantage to cane sugar over beet sugar. Pure carbohydrate from whatever source releases 4.1 kcal/g when metabolized, although foods containing a high proportion of water and cellulose will have a lower energy density.

▌ Digestion, transport and storage of carbohydrates

All complex carbohydrates must be broken down by the digestive system into monosaccharides before they can be absorbed. The process begins with the action of salivary amylase, which converts cooked starch into the disaccharide, maltose. Other starches are split into disaccharides by pancreatic amylase. The final step is for a series of enzymes in the small intestine

---

DECISION MAKING

Peter is extremely keen on football and regularly plays for the school football team. At half time his mother ensures that he drinks an expensive soft drink that had been advertised as an energy supply for footballers.

• *What advice would you give to Peter's mother, who is giving her child expensive glucose drinks because she thinks they are more healthy than sugary drinks?*

to break the disaccharides into monosaccharides. There is a specific enzyme for each disaccharide, but the names are easy to remember:

- maltose is split by maltase;
- sucrose is split by sucrase;
- lactose is split by lactase.

Splitting disaccharides also involves putting the water back, a process called hydrolysis ('hydro' means water, and 'lysis' means breaking down). This is the opposite process to that of the condensation reaction, which removes water to join the two monosaccharide molecules.

Once broken down to monosaccharides in the digestive system, carbohydrates are absorbed in the small intestine and transported via the portal vein to the liver. This raises the concentration of plasma glucose and stimulates the secretion of insulin by the beta cells of the pancreas. This in turn increases the rate which the large glucose molecules are able to pass through the cell walls into the cells where they will be broken down to provide energy.

Excessive plasma glucose can be converted into an insoluble carbohydrate, glycogen, which is similar to starch in plants, through the process of glycogenesis. Glycogen is stored mainly in the liver and muscles, where it is readily converted back to glucose (glycogenolysis) when the plasma glucose concentration falls. When the glycogen stores are full, any remaining glucose may be converted into fat and stored until it is needed, although studies show that this process is not really significant in humans (Hellerstein *et al.*, 1991). As the glucose in the blood is used up, insulin secretion decreases and glucagon secretion from the alpha cells of the pancreas increases. Glucagon converts glycogen back into glucose to restore the blood glucose concentration and mobilize the stored fat.

> Utilization of carbohydrates: respiration

Carbohydrates are made in the chloroplasts of plant cells through the action of photosynthesis as follows:

$$6H_2O + 6CO_2 + Energy \rightarrow C_6H_{12}O_6 + 6O_2.$$

When the equation is moving in this direction, energy from the sun is used to form carbohydrate. However, in the mitochondria of animal cells this action is reversed, in the process of respiration, as follows:

$$C_6H_{12}O_6 + 6O_2 \rightarrow 6H_2O + 6CO_2 + Energy.$$

The energy produced in respiration takes two forms: heat energy and chemical energy. The heat energy maintains body temperature. This explains why we get hot when we exercise as more metabolism of food in the muscles generates more heat. The chemical energy is used to join phosphate to another molecule to store energy for future use. The commonest example of this action is phosphate (P) joining adenosine diphosphate (ADP) to form adenosine triphosphate (ATP). When energy is required the phosphate bond is broken to revert back to ADP and P, so releasing the stored energy.

The process of obtaining energy from glucose occurs in three stages.

- The first stage, glycolysis (Figure 3.2.2a), takes place in the cytoplasm of the cell. Here the six-carbon glucose molecule is split into two three-carbon pyruvate molecules. Glycolysis releases eight ATP molecules.
- If there is no oxygen present (i.e. anaerobic conditions) pyruvate is converted to lactate, which will be reconverted to pyruvate when oxygen becomes available. This costs six ATP molecules. Therefore,

---

DECISION MAKING

The hormone glucagon is secreted by the alpha cells of the pancreas when the blood glucose concentration falls. This causes a reduction in glycogenesis and an increase in glycogenolysis, which leads to an increase in blood glucose concentration. Glucagon can be manufactured synthetically and administered by injection.

- *What are the indications for the use of synthetic glucagon?*
- *What is the usual dosage?*
- *What are the limitations of using synthetic glucagon?*

in the absence of adequate oxygen, the energy yield from glycolysis drops to two molecules of ATP. In the presence of oxygen, however, the pyruvate is transported into the mitochondria where it is converted to carbon dioxide and acetyl coenzyme A (acetyl CoA). The acetyl CoA enters the Krebs cycle (Figure 3.2.2b) where the hydrogen is removed and carbon dioxide is released (aerobic metabolism).

▶ In the third stage of the process, called the electron transport chain, the energy is once more used to combine phosphate with ADP to produce ATP. The hydrogen is then combined with oxygen to form water.

The three stages of this glucose metabolism will release sufficient energy from one molecule of glucose to produce 38 molecules of ATP.

The more mitochondria there are in a cell the more reactions can take place and the greater the amount of energy available. The mitochondria therefore increase in response to the energy demand made upon a cell. Consequently this increases the individual's basal metabolic rate. When less demand is made upon a cell the number of mitochondria and the energy capacity of the cell decrease. You may notice this effect if you decide to improve your fitness by training. You will notice that as you continue a programme of training the length of time you are able to engage in activity increases. You see yourself becoming fit. Cells are able to engage in more activity as the number of mitochondria increase in response to the demand made upon them during training.

Figure 3.2.2: (a) Glycolysis. (b) Krebs cycle. (Redrawn from Hinchliff *et al.*, 1996.)

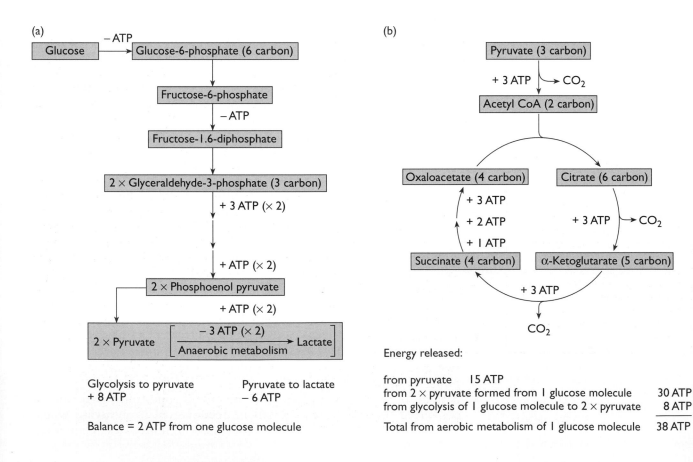

(a)

Glucose → Glucose-6-phosphate (6 carbon)   − ATP

Fructose-6-phosphate

Fructose-1.6-diphosphate   − ATP

2 × Glyceraldehyde-3-phosphate (3 carbon)

+ 3 ATP (× 2)

+ ATP (× 2)

2 × Phosphoenol pyruvate

+ ATP (× 2)

2 × Pyruvate   − 3 ATP (× 2) / Anaerobic metabolism → Lactate

Glycolysis to pyruvate +8 ATP   Pyruvate to lactate − 6 ATP

Balance = 2 ATP from one glucose molecule

(b)

Pyruvate (3 carbon)

+ 3 ATP → CO_2

Acetyl CoA (2 carbon)

Oxaloacetate (4 carbon)   Citrate (6 carbon)

+ 3 ATP
+ 2 ATP   + 3 ATP → CO_2
+ 1 ATP

Succinate (4 carbon)   α-Ketoglutarate (5 carbon)

+ 3 ATP

CO_2

Energy released:

from pyruvate   15 ATP

from 2 × pyruvate formed from 1 glucose molecule   30 ATP

from glycolysis of 1 glucose molecule to 2 × pyruvate   8 ATP

Total from aerobic metabolism of 1 glucose molecule   38 ATP

▶ *Fats*

Fats are solid and oils are liquid, and they are referred to collectively as lipids. They are insoluble in water and have the general formula $CH_3(CH_2)_nCOOH$, which looks complicated, but like carbohydrates, they contain only carbon, hydrogen and oxygen. Most of the lipids in the diet are in the form of triglycerides. These comprise three fatty acids, each attached to a glycerol molecule to form a structure like a letter 'E', with the glycerol being the vertical stroke (Figure 3.2.3).

Figure 3.2.3: Diagram of triglyceride.

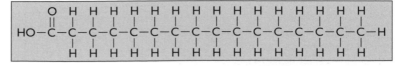

▶ Fatty acids

Fatty acids are a line of carbon atoms with hydrogen atoms attached (Figure 3.2.4). In Figure 3.2.4 all the adjacent carbon atoms have single valency bonds between them. This is therefore a saturated fatty acid. If one of the bonds is double, the fatty acid is a monounsaturated fatty acid, and if more than one of the bonds are double, the fatty acid is polyunsaturated.

Saturated fats are solid at room temperature whereas mono and polyunsaturates are liquid (oils). Generally animal fats are saturated whereas those from vegetables and fish are unsaturated, with the exception of palm oil and coconut oil, which are saturated. Saturated fat in the diet tends to raise the concentration of blood cholesterol, whereas monounsaturated fats such as olive oil tend to lower it. Because a high blood cholesterol concentration is linked to arterial disease, the current recommendation is to reduce the total amount of fat in the diet and to limit the intake of saturated fat so that it constitutes no more than 10% of the energy intake (Department of Health, 1992).

Examples of fatty foods include butter, margarine, lard, cooking oil and the fat on meat. Cholesterol is found in all animal products because it forms part of the cell membrane, but because it is manufactured in the liver, the amount in the diet has a modest effect on serum cholesterol concentration (Health Education Authority, 1996).

RESEARCH BASED EVIDENCE

Over recent years fats have gained a bad reputation as the cause of heart disease. The simple image of fat in the diet sticking to the walls of the arteries and blocking them is appealing, but research suggests that the explanation is not as clear cut as it may appear. The oxidation of fat in the body due to a lack of the antioxidant vitamins may be equally important (Stephens et al., 1996).

Figure 3.2.4: Diagram of a fatty acid (palmitic acid).

- *What have you read about saturated and unsaturated fats?*
- *What are The Health of the Nation (Department of Health, 1992) targets for total fat intake, and why does it recommend that we eat more poly-unsaturates and less saturated fat?*
- *Write a brief explanation for clients to help them identify saturated and unsaturated fats.*

▶ Common misconceptions

Fats are often thought of as being 'bad', but a certain amount is essential to our health and wellbeing. Fats are needed to make cell membranes, the steroid hormones, prostaglandins and bile, and to store energy. In fact they are a very efficient way of storing energy because they contain 9.3 kcal/g, which is more than double the energy content of carbohydrates and proteins. However, because fats pack many calories into a small volume it is easy to take too many calories in a high fat diet.

▶ Digestion, utilization, transport and storage of lipids

Lipids are insoluble and form large globules in water. They therefore need to be emulsified. This is achieved by the action of bile. Once emulsified the triglycerides are split by the enzyme lipase into fatty acids and monoglycerides. Short-chain fatty acids are absorbed into the blood directly at this point (Figure 3.2.5). Most fatty acids are long chain (i.e. have more than 12 carbon atoms) however, and these and the monoglycerides take a different pathway to the blood. By combining with bile salts, long-chain fatty acids and monoglycerides form micelles and in this form are then able to enter the epithelial cells of the villi. Once in the epithelial cells lipase acts on the monoglycerides to reduce them to glycerol and fatty acids. The fatty acids and glycerol are then combined to once again form triglycerides, which in turn combine with cholesterol and phospholipids

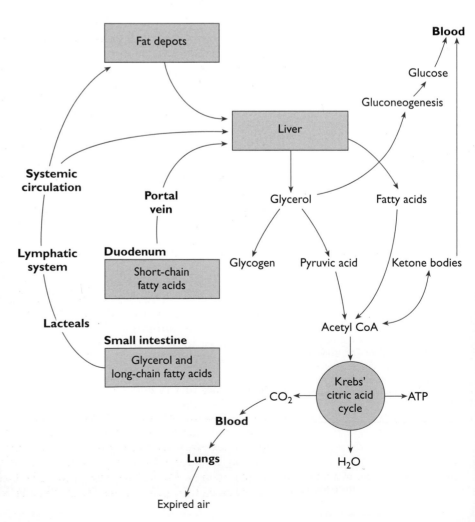

Figure 3.2.5: Diagram of fat metabolism. (Redrawn from Hinchliff *et al.*, 1996.)

to form chylomicrons. These are absorbed into the lymphatic vessels (lacteals) in the small intestine and transported through the lymphatic system to enter the blood at the subclavian vein.

As fats are insoluble, absorbed fats are either transported in the blood as chylomicrons or as free fatty acids attached to albumin. Another name for these transport molecules are lipoproteins (i.e. lipid + protein). Because fat is lighter than water, the higher the percentage of fat in a lipoprotein, the lower the density. The low density lipoproteins (LDLs) carry a high percentage of cholesterol and are therefore associated with a risk to health. High density lipoproteins (HDLs) on the other hand transport fat from the tissues to the liver to be excreted.

Lipids are either stored in adipose tissue as triglycerides or metabolized by the liver in a process called beta oxidation. The liver cells split pairs of carbon atoms from the fatty acid to form acetyl CoA, which can then enter the Krebs cycle. Excess acetyl CoA is converted into ketones and circulated to other tissues in the body where it is converted back to acetyl CoA and used for energy.

▶ Proteins

▶ Chemical structure

Proteins share many of the properties of fats and carbohydrates. They contain the same three chemicals – carbon, hydrogen and oxygen – but additionally, all proteins contain nitrogen. In a similar way to that of complex carbohydrates, which are made up of monosaccharides, complex proteins are made up of amino acids linked together by a peptide bond (Figure 3.2.6).

There is no general formula, but amino acids all have an amine group (NH_2) and an acidic carboxyl group (COOH) in common, with the remainder of the molecule varying depending upon which amino acid it is. Although there are only 20 amino acids, the number of possible combinations in which they can be joined to form proteins is almost infinite. One very important characteristic of proteins is that each one tends to fold itself into a specific shape, which will determine its function. For example, if the haemoglobin molecule does not assume its correct shape, sickle cell anaemia results. The action of enzymes, which are proteins, also relies on their shape, and if this is altered by heat or changes in pH they will be denatured and will not function.

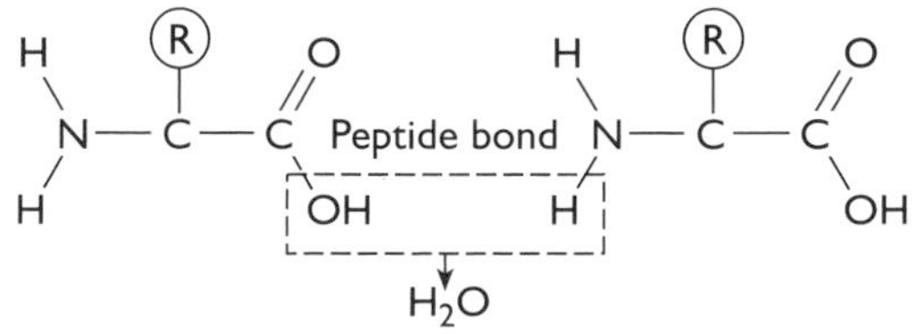

Figure 3.2.6: Peptide bonds linking amino acids to form protein chains.

▶ Sources

Many amino acids can be synthesized in the body, but those that cannot are called the essential amino acids and must be taken in the diet. Many plant proteins are deficient in one or more of the essential amino acids, but a mixture of plant proteins is capable of supplying all the amino acids needed. Meat, fish, eggs and milk have a high protein content. Plant sources rich in protein are mainly seeds, with beans, peas and nuts being

Babies

Birth weight is linked to maternal nutritional status and low birth weight is associated with perinatal mortality and the onset of heart disease in later life (Barker, 1995). The required energy intake of a baby is much higher than for an adult, even though the baby may not be very active. For babies up to six months of age the intake should be 110 kcal/kg of expected weight/day, which is more than double that of an adult. This equates to 150 ml/kg/day of breast or formula milk.

Details of recommendations on weaning can be found in the Department of Health Report *Weaning and the Weaning Diet.* (Department of Health, 1994). Some of the major recommendations are:

- weaning should begin at four months of age;
- semi-solids should be given by spoon and not mixed with milk;
- dietary recommendations on low fat do not apply to infants, but the amount should be reduced for children from two years of age until adult recommendations apply at five years of age;
- breastfed infants do not need vitamin supplements before six months of age;
- iron deficiency is the most common nutritional problem in early childhood, so care must be taken to ensure an adequate intake, particularly in vegetarian diets (soya milk inhibits iron uptake).

DECISION MAKING

In relation to the advantages and disadvantages, what information and advice would you give to a pregnant woman who wishes to bottle feed?

Schoolchildren

The nutritional status of schoolchildren affects their rate of growth and age of puberty (Reading *et al.*, 1993). Because of their rapid growth and high metabolic rate, a more energy-dense diet may be needed. Concern has been expressed at the reduced level of physical activity of children due to the dangers of allowing them out to play. This reduced activity and the increase in passive rather than active play (such as watching television) has implications for diet and the prevalence of obesity.

Teenagers

Teenagers are particularly susceptible to media images, which portray thinness as desirable, and this susceptibility is a factor in the development of anorexia nervosa, especially in young girls. Boys at this time may become involved in bodybuilding and eat a very high protein diet in the mistaken belief that it will build muscle mass. In fact a high protein diet tends to be associated with adverse effects on serum cholesterol concentration and may be unhealthy.

Adults

Reduced activity often accompanies increasing age, and energy intake must reflect this or the all too familiar 'middle-aged spread' will occur and may continue into old age. Postmenopausal women are prone to osteoporosis so an adequate intake of calcium should be encouraged.

Older people

Particular problems may arise if elderly people are living alone, are on a low income or have difficulty in moving around. Because of difficulties shopping, they may not buy fresh fruit and vegetables because tinned food is easier to store and this may lead to a lack of vitamin C. Elderly people also have a tendency to eat smaller amounts at more frequent intervals so large amounts of fibre may be too filling without providing the energy required. As always, the intake should be tailored to the level of physical activity and should provide an adequate supply of vitamins and minerals.

▶ *Conducting the Nursing Assessment*

As part of the nursing assessment of nutritional status, the information collected should include:

- ▶ an estimate of the basal metabolic rate (BMR);
- ▶ a calculation of the body mass index (BMI);
- ▶ an assessment of physical conditions affecting the client's ability to eat;
- ▶ a history;
- ▶ socioeconomic information;
- ▶ cultural and religious beliefs.

▶ An estimate of the BMR

The BMR of an individual varies according to surface area as this determines the rate of heat loss. Tall thin people lose heat faster than a short fat people because they have a larger surface area in relation to their volume. Babies have a very large surface area in relation to their volume and also have comparatively large heads with little hair so they can lose heat very quickly. The physical activity of an individual will affect their calorie requirements so a nursing assessment of nutritional status should take this into account.

▶ A calculation of the BMI

This is useful and easy to interpret as it is not necessary to have charts of normal weight and height. An individual with a BMI of:

- ▶ 20–24.9 is normal;
- ▶ 25–29.9 is overweight;
- ▶ 30 and over is obese;
- ▶ less than 20 is underweight.

Above 30 and below 20 the risk of disease increases in proportion to the deviation from the normal range.

BMI is calculated by measuring the height in metres (m) and the weight in kg. The formula is weight/height^2. For a 70 kg man who is 1.75 m tall, the calculation is $70/(1.75 \times 1.75) = 70/3.0625 = 22.8$. So the BMI for this man is 22.8, which is within the normal range of 20–25.

▶ Assessment of physical conditions affecting the client's ability to eat

Difficulties in eating may result from physical conditions such as arthritis, hemiplegia following a cerebrovascular accident (stroke), hand or arm injuries, dysphagia or a lack of motor skills, particularly in those with learning disabilities or in very young children. Ill-fitting dentures or no dentures at all will cause difficulty with chewing and may mean that certain foods are avoided or need special preparation.

- *Calculate your own BMI.*
- *When you are next on clinical placement use client records to calculate their BMIs.*

DECISION MAKING

Children with learning disabilities often have muscle spasms that cause them to arch their back and 'scissor' their legs and this can cause considerable problems when feeding them.
- *How would you position such a child when feeding him or her from a spoon?*
- *Check this with the local recommendations.*

DECISION MAKING

- *What specific information would you gather from the parents of a young child to enable you to plan the correct dietary regimen?*
- *Why would you collect this data?*

History

The history can include the following information:

- medical conditions, which may be related to diet;
- medication that may affect nutritional status (e.g. thiazide and loop diuretics can cause potassium deficiency, corticosteroids can cause sodium and water retention, and excessive vitamin and mineral supplements may lead to toxicity);
- a history of constipation or self medication with laxatives, which may indicate dietary fibre deficiency;
- information about current dietary habits, such as how many meals each day, at what times, and any snack foods, which may be helpful in planning meals;
- a history of high alcohol intake, which can cause vitamin deficiencies, particularly vitamin B_{12}, and lead to medical problems such as peripheral neuropathy and Wernicke–Korsakoff's syndrome;
- unexplained weight loss in the recent past, which may need investigation.

Socioeconomic information

Does the client live alone? If so he or she may feel that it is not worth cooking for one and may live on a monotonous diet of cold, easily prepared food, which may be deficient in vitamins, or may eat take-away foods, which tend to be high in fat and low in vitamins. Can the client afford an adequate diet and does he or she have access to shops with a good selection of fresh food? Has the client any refrigeration to store food safely? Does the client have adequate cooking facilities? It is also useful to find out if the client has or needs support from social services, meals on wheels, relatives or neighbours.

DECISION MAKING

- *On your next placement, check the care plans for evidence of nutritional assessment, make your own assessment and see how they compare.*
- *How does the meal system accommodate clients with specific dietary requirements such as vegan diets, halal meat or not eating during specific times of the day (such as in the Muslim Ramadan)?*
- *If the meal system is unable to accommodate the client's needs, what strategies could the nurse employ to meet the client's needs?*

Cultural and religious beliefs

Specific dietary requirements must be noted. Is the client vegetarian? If so is he or she vegan or does he or she eat fish and eggs or drink milk? Many ethnic groups have specific dietary requirements.

PLANNING

The nursing assessment will indicate what particular dietary requirements and conditions the client requires. In the institutional setting planning will ensure that the client is provided with a diet that meets these requirements and is able to eat it. Alternatively, if the client is in the community, it may be necessary to plan information-giving sessions to enable them to select and prepare appropriate foods within their financial means and own preferences.

Any temptation for the nurse to be prescriptive or tell the client what to eat must be avoided at all costs. It is all too easy to try to impose one's own ideas of a healthy diet onto the client. A little knowledge can transform the carer into a food evangelist, determined to shepherd everyone onto the path of high fibre, low fat or whatever dietary advice is fashionable. Planning should be a collaborative effort and very much client centred.

If, on the other hand, the client wishes to change his or her dietary

DECISION MAKING

- *What factors should be taken into account in order to avoid a prescriptive approach?*
- *What will be the benefits and drawbacks from the client's point of view?*

pattern, for example to lose weight or because of a fear of arterial disease, then a detailed planning procedure should be instituted. First, the client should be encouraged to identify the benefits and difficulties of the proposed course of action. It is very easy for the client to make a decision to lose weight without thinking of the fact that the change will affect their social life and will require a permanent change in lifestyle. Once the decision has been made the client should be involved in the planning. Giving the client a diet sheet and telling them to stick to it is neither helpful, client centred nor individualized. A useful strategy is for the client to record what food they consume and when in a diary. The nurse should then identify how difficult it would be for the client to omit or increase items in the diet. The aim should be to make the least possible changes consistent with achieving the outcome. It is essential that the client understands that a permanent change in eating habits is needed rather than a 'diet' that is to be tolerated only for the length of time it takes to achieve the goal. It is useful to plan with clients how they will deal with problems such as eating in restaurants or at a friend's house. This enables clients to be prepared rather than having to make a snap decision to refuse or accept a particular item.

▶ INTERVENTION

In the institutional setting, nursing intervention may involve ensuring that clients are provided with food, can reach it, can cut it up and transfer it to their mouths, and can chew, swallow and digest it. The nurse must ensure that the food is accessible and that the patients are sitting up and able to feed themselves. If chewing, swallowing or digestion are impaired or a patient is unconscious, artificial feeding may be necessary by either the enteral (e.g. nasogastric) or parenteral (e.g. intravenous) route.

In the community setting, the client may need help with shopping or cooking and the nurse may be involved in organizing the support services to provide this.

Mealtimes are a social event. In the institutional setting this is especially important as the day is usually structured around mealtimes, which become an important part of the daily routine. Mealtimes break the monotony, provide structure, are an opportunity to socialize and a topic of conversation (even if some of it is negative!). It is therefore important that the whole care team recognize this and do not regard meals as an interruption to *their* tasks. As far as possible the ward manager should ensure that meals are not interrupted by doctors rounds, drug rounds, dressings or other routine tasks.

▶ Feeding a Client

If clients require feeding they should be sat up in a position where they can see the food and the method of feeding should be as normal as possible. The nurse should sit in a relaxed manner to avoid any suggestion of hurry, be at the same eye level as the client and in a position to make eye contact. Every effort should be made to maintain the dignity of the client. Being unable to feed oneself is associated with early childhood and it is very easy to treat such clients as if they are children. The use of plastic bibs reinforces this image and they should be avoided. The use of normal napkins is much better. Whenever possible food should be cut up and given in the same way as the patients would eat it if they were able to feed themselves. The practice of cutting the food up all at

---

DECISION MAKING

- *What information and advice would you give to a 15-year-old girl who has decided to become vegetarian?*
- *How would you help her to maintain a healthy diet?*
- *Would you try to dissuade her?*

DECISION MAKING

- *What factors may make it difficult or impossible for someone to follow a healthy diet?*
- *What actions and advice could you give that may help?*

DECISION MAKING

Stress activates the sympathetic nervous system and releases adrenaline. This diverts blood from the digestive system and may cause anorexia and indigestion (see Chapter 4.1).
- *What measures have you seen in your clinical areas to reduce stress and make mealtimes relaxed and enjoyable?*
- *Can you think of any ways these measures could be improved?*

Ask a friend to feed you and give you a drink while you sit on your hands. You must not speak to your friend while this is being done. Swap positions so that you feed your friend in the same way and then discuss the following questions.

- *How did you feel while you were being fed?*
- *How easy was it for you to drink?*
- *What would it be like if you really were immobile and unable to speak?*
- *People who are immobile*

and unable to speak often have difficulty in chewing, swallowing and sitting straight. How do you think they feel?

- *What can you learn from this to improve your clinical practice?*

once and then feeding the client with a spoon should be avoided. Would you like to be fed like that? Although feeding patients is often left to the most junior members of staff, it requires considerable skill and sensitivity if it is to be done well.

▶ *Enteral and Parenteral Feeding*

If a client is unable to eat then it may be appropriate to feed him or her either via a tube into the digestive system (i.e. enteral feeding) or intravenously (i.e. parenteral feeding). There are three basic levels of problem that may occur:

- ▶ the client may not be well enough to take sufficient food;
- ▶ the client may be unable to swallow because of trauma, oropharyngeal surgery or an obstruction of the oesophagus such as a tumour;
- ▶ the client may not have a swallowing reflex, perhaps due to a head injury causing long-term unconsciousness.

▶ Enteral feeding

If the digestive system is functioning, enteral feeding is the simplest and safest method of feeding. If the client is unable to take sufficient food orally, more frequent but smaller meals may be appropriate or extra calories can be given as high energy drinks. Enteral feeding is not then required. If this is not successful, however, a nasogastric tube can be passed and used to supplement the oral intake (Barker, 1996).

If a client is unable to swallow, then total nasogastric feeding with such products as Ensure® or Osmolite® may be prescribed. These can be given by bolus injection using a funnel or syringe barrel by gravity infusion or by pump. Bolus injection is liable to cause diarrhoea or vomiting and is more appropriate if the feed is a supplement rather than the sole method of feeding. Gravity infusions are rather unreliable and need frequent checking to ensure that the rate is correct. Pumps are ideal if they are available as they save nursing time and cause fewer problems for the patient.

Long-term enteral feeding of an unconscious client is becoming more common as technology to maintain life develops. As an ordinary nasogastric tubes can cause erosion of the nasal passages or oesophagus and needs to be changed every week or so, it is better to use a fine-bore tube, which results in less trauma and is resistant to gastric acid. Consequently, these tubes can be left *in situ* for several months.

Enteral feeding has acquired a reputation for causing diarrhoea, but it is as well to remember there are other causes such as antibiotic therapy and infections. An osmotic diarrhoea may result, however, if the feed is given too quickly or is too concentrated (Barker, 1996).

▶ Parenteral feeding

If the digestive system is not functioning or if it is necessary to rest the gut, as for example in Crohn's disease, then the intravenous route can be used. To maintain sufficient calorific intake, concentrated glucose solutions used to be given. They tend to cause thrombophlebitis in small veins, however, so it was necessary to administer them via a central vein to ensure that they were diluted quickly by the rapid blood flow. Technology has since progressed and now fats are added to the feed. This increases their calorific value. As a consequence the glucose does not need to be so concentrated so peripheral veins can be used. Although the protocol varies, in most centres short-term parenteral feeding using such a solution will be via a peripheral vein. If the client is likely to need parenteral nutrition for more than one week, however, a central line will probably be inserted and used instead (Silk, 1994).

The general principle is to use the simplest method of ensuring adequate nutrition, progressing from small high-energy meals through the various methods of supplementation to total parenteral nutrition (TPN).

PROFESSIONAL KNOWLEDGE

The nurse should be aware of *The Food Safety Act* (1990) and the ensuing ramifications of labelling of food and food hygiene. These statutory instruments are enacted to ensure that food is safe and that any labelling is informative and not misleading. At the time of publication, legislative changes are being formulated to ensure parity across the European Union. For example, in the instance of vitamin supplements, the UK has no legislation other than that the supplements must be clearly labelled and conform to standards of purity. Conversely, in other European countries, vitamin supplements must not contain more than the recommended daily amount of any vitamin otherwise it is regarded as a medicine. This may give rise to some anomalies, for instance some natural foods such as sardines contain several times the recommended daily amount of vitamin B_{12} so should they be regarded as a medicine?

Information in *Hungry in Hospital*, a report published by the Community Health Council (1997) should remind nurses of their roles and responsibilities in relation to the nutrition of hospital patients. Within the *Code of Professional Conduct* (UKCC, 1992) there are a number of rules that should be kept in mind:

▶ '4. Acknowledge any limitations'... If you have not sufficient knowledge to give dietary advice it is best to refer the patient or client to a dietician;

▶ '5. Work in an open and co-operative manner with patients, clients and their families'... this approach is much more likely to be successful than being prescriptive;

▶ '6. Work in a collaborative and co-operative manner with health care professionals'... Having a good working relationship with hospital caterers, domestic staff and dietetic department will benefit the patient;

▶ '16. Be aware of the rules regarding endorsement of commercial products'... suggesting a particular slimming product may not be in the best interests of the patient/client.

▶ DISORDERS OF NUTRITION

In day to day practice, nurses are likely to be involved with three common dietary disorders. These are diabetes mellitus, anorexia nervosa and obesity.

Look at the evidence on one of the following topics: bovine spongiform encephalopathy; *Salmonella* contamination of food; *E. coli* contamination of meat; or, irradiation of food.

- *How is this reported in the newspapers, in professional journals and in government reports?*
- *How easy was it for you to find the information?*
- *How accurate was the information from each source?*
- *How might a nurse working in a school use this information when advising an anxious mother on the safety of food?*

(A useful source for UK government reports can be found on the Internet at address http//www.open.gov. uk)

◗ *Diabetes Mellitus*

This common condition is characterized by an inability to control plasma glucose concentration. In type I (insulin dependent diabetes mellitus or IDDM) the glucose spills over into the urine (glycosuria) and causes an osmotic diuresis, resulting in dehydration. In addition the body metabolizes excessive amounts of fat, resulting in a rise in plasma ketone concentration (ketosis), which may be sufficient to cause acidosis and coma. Type II (non-insulin dependent) diabetes mellitus usually results in hyperglycaemia, glycosuria and dehydration. It is important to realise that non-insulin dependent diabetes mellitus is not a mild form of the disease. If it is inadequately managed, complications are likely to occur that will lead to serious long-term health problems.

Although medication may be used, all clients with diabetes mellitus must follow a strict dietary regimen. Each client will have his or her individual diet based upon their basal metabolic requirements and level of physical activity. The principles of the diet are similar to those for any normal healthy diet, but the amount, type and frequency of carbohydrate is controlled to allow a constant blood glucose concentration to be maintained. The objectives of the diet are:

- ◗ to maintain or achieve desirable weight (i.e. BMI of 20–25);
- ◗ to maintain a low fat intake of 30–35% of calories, mainly as polyunsaturates;
- ◗ to take regular meals three times each day;
- ◗ to supplement the regular meals with snacks three times each day;
- ◗ to consume 50–55% of the diet as carbohydrates (mainly complex);
- ◗ to have a high dietary fibre content to slow the absorption of carbohydrate;
- ◗ to avoid excess simple sugars, which are absorbed quickly and increase the blood glucose excessively;
- ◗ to maintain normoglycaemia.

When planning the type of carbohydrates to include in the diet, the glycaemic index may be used. This is a measure of how blood glucose concentration is affected by eating a particular carbohydrate. Glucose itself has an index of 100 whereas the same amount of carbohydrate taken as pasta will be absorbed more slowly and cause a smaller increase in blood glucose concentration. This would consequently give a lower score on the glycaemic index. Combinations of high and low glycaemic index foods eaten together will cause a lower increase in blood glucose concentration than when the high index food is eaten alone.

One of the key factors in controlling diabetes mellitus is client education and the development of a partnership between the clients and those responsible for their care. Clients who do not understand their condition are less likely to comply with the diet and risk long-term complications, which may prove fatal. It is now recognized that it is possible to tailor the diet and drug therapy to suit the client's lifestyle rather than the other way round. It is the task of the nurse to encourage clients to follow the diet and drug regimens or to help them negotiate changes to aspects they find unacceptable.

DECISION MAKING

George Smith, aged 45 years, is a computer programmer. He has recently been diagnosed as having IDDM.

- *Decide on the extra knowledge you will need in order to support and advise George during this period when he has been newly diagnosed*
- *How could the Diabetic Nurse Specialist support George:*
    immediately following his diagnosis:
    following the stabilization of his diabetes?
- *Consider the development of clinical nurse specialists in nursing with reference to their impact on the role of the ward/unit nurse*

◗ *Anorexia Nervosa*

The name 'anorexia nervosa' suggests a loss of appetite and a lack of interest in food, but the reality is just the opposite. The sufferer experiences hunger and is concerned, indeed obsessed, with food, and this concern seems to replace any other interests. Anorexia nervosa primarily affects girls and young women aged 13–20 years, although it can also occur in males. One of the problems is in diagnosis: when does dieting to lose weight become anorexia nervosa? The generally accepted diagnostic criteria (Parkin, 1995) are:

- ▶ a body weight of 25% below normal for age, height and build;
- ▶ a morbid fear of being overweight;
- ▶ amenorrhoea.

Additionally, clients may perceive themselves as 'fat' despite being emaciated (Decker, 1989). Sufferers of anorexia nervosa are often described by their parents as being 'model' children, however, this may also mean that the child was non-assertive and complied with family norms and values. Minuchin *et al.* (1978) found that families of anorexics were frequently over involved in one another's lives. Individuals became lost in the family and unable to learn what their own needs were – they only knew those of their parents. Consequently the anorexia nervosa became a way of gaining control.

The desire to be thin is largely determined by culture. Surveys of women in developed countries have indicated that 75% want to be thinner than they are for cosmetic reasons rather than for health (Rolls *et al.*, 1991). The culture of thinness in developed countries is associated with affluence, whereas poorer societies value corpulence (Parkin, 1995). Is seems that as societies become richer, and sufficient food is available for all, being overweight becomes synonymous with sloth, self indulgence and greed. Thinness conversely, becomes associated with discipline and self control. This is reinforced by the media, particularly for women, who attempt to conform to this arbitrary ideal. It is therefore hardly surprising that there is an increasing incidence of eating disorders.

A client admitted with anorexia nervosa may have many physical problems, and although their care should include psychological support, the initial problem may be to ensure survival. In severe cases, enteral or parenteral feeding may be necessary.

Once out of immediate physical danger, the most common type of treatment will be based on behavioural therapy. At the start of the programme the client will be confined to bed and all privileges such as a radio, books or television are removed. Target weights are set and once they have been achieved rewards are given in the form of privileges. Without supportive therapy to address the underlying cause of the illness, however, in the long-term the programme is unlikely to be effective. Parkin (1995) argues that to help clients effectively the underlying psychological and social issues need to be addressed. A comprehensive plan of care should therefore include assertiveness training, psychotherapy, family therapy and incorporate measures to improve body acceptance and promote self esteem (Tennant, 1989; Meades, 1993; Halek *et al.*, 1995).

▶ Obesity

As Garrow (1981) points out, obesity is not a disease that people either do or do not have – it is a continuum with an arbitrary boundary between normal, being overweight and being obese. A commonly recognized definition is that 20% above normal weight is obese. Alternatively it may be graded by BMI:

- ▶ grade one is defined as a BMI of 25–29.9;
- ▶ grade two is defined as a BMI of 30–40.

- • *In what circumstances should patients be able to refuse food?*
- • *Does your decision alter according to the medical diagnosis?*
- • *How does this integrate with the responsibilities of the nurse stated in the Code of Profesional Conduct (UKCC, 1992)?*
- • *Should food ever be withheld from patients?*

(You may find it useful to refer to Jennett, 1996.)

RESEARCH BASED EVIDENCE

Dietary energy consumption of households in the UK has been declining since 1970, so we have the paradox of increasing weight in the face of decreasing energy intake. Physiologically, this must lead us to the conclusion that energy expenditure has decreased faster than energy intake. Prentice and Jebb (1995) suggest that low levels of physical activity are as important as energy intake in producing the increasing obesity being seen in the UK and the USA.

- *What are the social pressures that make thinness so desirable among women?*
- *Are there benefits to the individual in being thin or is it just fashionable?*
- *Reflect on how social pressures regarding bodyweight and image might affect your professional role in health promotion.*

Grade one obesity is not considered to constitute a serious health risk, but mortality and morbidity increase rapidly in grade two.

The prevalence of obesity increases with age and is steadily increasing in most developed countries. Approximately 30–40% of the population are overweight in surveys carried out in the UK and the USA. In some sections of the population in the UK the number of overweight people has doubled in less than a decade, so there is no doubting the extent of the problem (Prentice and Jebb, 1995).

Why obesity is increasing so rapidly is by no means clear, although a correlation with an increased dietary fat intake has been demonstrated. The intake of fat has increased by 50% over the past 50 years. One problem seems to be that fat does not increase the blood glucose concentration to give the feedback signals to the satiety centre to stop eating, whereas carbohydrate does (Lissner and Heitmann, 1995). In addition, if the intake of complex carbohydrates is increased there is an increase in carbohydrate oxidation to compensate. In fat metabolism there is no comparable mechanism. So is an increased fat intake in the diet of developed countries the cause of their obese populations?

It is clear that machinery at work and in the home has decreased the energy expenditure of most people and that this is not compensated for by increased physical activity in recreation. The individual doing light work (4 kcal/min) for seven or eight hours each day will use far more energy than someone doing half an hour of vigorous exercise (12 kcal/min) two or three times each week.

The question that must be asked is 'Does it matter if individuals are overweight?' Early work suggested that the excess mortality associated with obesity could be accounted for by other factors such as smoking, age, high blood pressure and cholesterol. It has since been shown, however, that obesity contributes to cardiovascular disease by increasing blood pressure and altering the blood lipid profile in a way that is detrimental (Bender and Brooks, 1987). Obesity is also associated with mature onset diabetes mellitus because it reduces sensitivity to insulin. Gallstones, some cancers and osteoarthritis are all more common in individuals who are obese (Garrow, 1981). Apart from the physical disorders, the stigmas attached to obesity and its association with laziness and gluttony may cause the obese individual to seek advice.

▶ Management of obesity

A walk around a bookshop will reveal a plethora of self-help books to overcome obesity ranging from a simple guide to the calorific value of foods to some very bizarre ideas with no scientific basis. The supermarkets contain a veritable Aladdin's cave of low fat, low sugar, low calorie, healthy option foods to be used 'as part of a calorie controlled diet'. The number of pills and potions reputed to cause weight loss without dieting is difficult to estimate, but at frequent intervals some entrepreneur comes up with something new and makes a great deal of money from the vulnerable and gullible individuals who are fooled by the pseudoscientific jargon and testimonials from satisfied customers.

The fact is that for every kilogram that someone is overweight, he or she has stored 7000 kcal of energy and the only way to get rid of it, short of surgery, is to metabolize it. This can be achieved by decreasing energy intake or increasing energy output by the requisite amount. The amount of energy used during exercise is actually very little, for example using an exercise bicycle at a pedal load sustainable for any length of time by an unfit individual will use approximately 5 kcal/min. In other words it would take about 24 hours of cycling to lose 1 kg of weight. This is clearly not a practical proposition, although exercise has other benefits. For example the individual who becomes fitter as a result of exercise is more likely to be active than the unfit person. Also exercise tolerance will increase, leading to an ability to exercise harder and for longer without discomfort. It is also helpful in maintaining lean body mass and metabolic rate, thus counteracting the tendency of the body to reduce the BMR when food intake is reduced. However, it really comes down to reducing energy intake by altering the diet, and whether this is a banana diet, grapefruit diet, high fibre diet or whatever, if it delivers too many calories it will fail. Success depends on finding a diet that contains less energy than the individual is metabolizing and that he or she is happy with.

For the nurse planning a reducing diet, permanent weight loss is likely to be achieved if the points outlined below are followed.

- Establish a realistic rate of weight loss. It may have taken years to gain the weight and it is unrealistic to expect to lose it in weeks. A target of 0.5–1 kg/week is reasonable, but the client may have seen advertisements saying lose 10 lb in one week so feel disappointed that you suggest so little. Point out that much of this loss would be water rather than fat and that even not eating anything would only result in the loss of 1.5–2 kg/week.
- Calorific intake should be reduced by 500–1000 kcal/day. A smaller reduction will mean that the weight loss will be very slow, a greater reduction may risk loss of lean body mass and vitamin and mineral deficiencies.
- Moderate exercise will help, but it should be something the individual enjoys doing otherwise they are unlikely to keep it up.
- Fats can be restricted quite drastically without essential fatty acid deficiency developing, and because of their high calorie content this can account for much of the reduction of calories in the diet.
- Some increase in fibre may help the client to feel satisfied after a meal.
- Several small meals will each increase the metabolic rate (postprandial thermogenesis) and reduce the chance of overeating, which can occur with one meal each day.
- A change in eating habits that results in slow weight loss is more likely to result in a permanent weight loss.

- Why does the BMR reduce when food intake or activity reduce?
- Why is exercise an important component of a weight loss programme?

(You may wish to refer back to the section on mitochondria and the Krebs cycle discussed earlier in this chapter in Subject Knowledge.)

RESEARCH BASED EVIDENCE

Perry (1997) conducted a small survey in one hospital in the south of England. Data collection included nursing documentation of nutrition related activities (141) and questionnaires to qualified nurses (110). She found that although there was evidence of knowledgeable and proactive practice, there were still widespread deficiencies in the knowledge, communication and co-ordination required to ensure consistent good practice

REFLECTIVE KNOWLEDGE

This chapter has introduced you to the various components of a balanced diet, the common sources from which these may be obtained, and the ways in which the various foods are digested and used within the body. Because of public interest in food and dieting, there is a need for nurses to be familiar with the research-based evidence to be able to give clear guidance to clients. In order to avoid causing undue anxiety it has been stressed that the general advice about a healthy diet is quite simple and that clients should not worry about the reports that appear in the press on an almost daily basis implying that a certain food will cause or prevent a particular disease. These reports are often gross oversimplifications of small scale research and do little other than provide a headline for the newspaper.

To consolidate your learning from this chapter, work through the following case studies.

▶ CASE STUDY: ADULT

Peter Dawson is a 58-year-old man who lives at home with his wife. He is very overweight, being 1.8 m tall and weighing 100 kg. He admits to drinking and smoking 'quite a bit' most evenings and says he has no time to exercise. He has recently been diagnosed as having non-insulin dependent diabetes mellitus, for which he has been prescribed a diabetic diet and a hypoglycaemic drug. Having been told that good control of his diabetes will reduce the probability of complications, he is keen to comply with the treatment.

■ **Calculate Peter's BMI. What grade of being overweight does this represent?**

■ **Apart from reduced insulin sensitivity, why might his diabetes mellitus be made worse by his obesity, smoking and drinking of alcohol?**

■ **What help and advice could Peter be given to improve his lifestyle?**

▶ CASE STUDY: MENTAL HEALTH

Sally, aged 17 years, lives at home with her mother, who is divorced. Sally started dieting two years ago, but continued to diet after reaching her target weight. She is now 20 kg under-weight, but says she still feels fat. Sally's mother has always believed that her place has been in the home looking after Sally and her younger brother, and is very worried because Sally looks so thin.

■ **Apart from lacking energy intake, what other factors may be missing in Sally's diet?**

■ **What sort of social pressures are there on young girls to account for the high incidence of eating disorders?**

■ **Consider how Sally's schoolfriends and her parents may have unwittingly contributed to her problems.**

▶ CASE STUDY: CHILD

Marcus and Yvonne are strict vegans. They have fed their son of four months, Jason, with soya milk and are now contemplating weaning to solids.

■ **What are the ramifications of Marcus' and Yvonne's dietary preferences on Jason's dietary needs?**

■ **Plan a diet that is both compatible with Marcus' and Yvonne's beliefs and Jason's nutritional needs?**

■ **How could the nurse later assess that the diet is meeting all Jason's nutritional requirements?**

▶ CASE STUDY: LEARNING DISABILITIES

Andrew is 38 years of age and suffers from a moderate learning disability. He attends a social centre on a daily basis, but otherwise lives with his parents. Andrew is 1.76 m tall and weighs 98 kg.

He enjoys his food and has a hearty appetite, eating a cooked breakfast every morning and a full dinner at night. This is supplemented by a cooked snack at the social centre every day and bars of chocolate. Andrew's parents feel that although Andrew is a little overweight he is otherwise happy. They have no time for special diets or 'rabbit food'.

■ **Calculate Andrew's BMI.**

■ **What are the long-term physiological consequences for Andrew should this situation continue?**

■ **How might the nurse help Andrew lose weight, but continue to eat the food he and his family enjoy?**

▶ ANNOTATED FURTHER READING AND RESOURCES

BOULTON HAWKER FILMS (1984) *Functional Chemistry in Living Cells.* Hadleigh, Ipswich, Suffolk. IP7 5BG.
This video is a useful introduction to basic chemistry and the chemical structure of food.

CREE, L., RISCHMILLER, S (1991) *Science in Nursing*, 2nd edition. Sydney. W.B. Saunders.
Chapter 10 is useful for a more in-depth look at energy and metabolism.

JAMIESON, E.M., MCCALL, J.M., BLYTHE, R., LOGAN, W.W. (1992) *Guidelines for Clinical Nursing Practices.* Edinburgh. Churchill Livingstone.
A useful 'how to do it' guide to practical nursing. Look at enteral and parenteral feeding sections.

SOLOMON, E.P., SCHMIDT, R.R., ADRAGNA, P.J. (1990) *Human Anatomy and Physiology.* Orlando. Harcourt Brace Jovanovitch.
Chapters 25 and 26 are very helpful in understanding the digestive system and metabolic processes.

BARKER, D.J. (1995) Fetal origins of coronary heart disease (Review). *British Medical Journal* **311**: 171–174.

▶ REFERENCES

BARKER, H.M. (1996) *Nutrition and Dietetics for Health Care* (9th edition). New York. Churchill Livingstone.

BENDER, A.E., BROOKS, L.J. (1987) *Body Weight Control.* Edinburgh. Churchill Livingstone.

BLAXTER, K. (1993) From hunting and gathering to agriculture. In Leathwood, P., Horisberger, M., James, W.P.T. *For a Better Nutrition in the 21st Century.* Nestle Nutrition Workshop Series Vol 27. New York. Raven Press.

CAMPBELL, B. (1984) *Wigan Pier Revisited: Policy and Politics in the 80s.* London. Virago.

COMMUNITY HEALTH COUNCIL (1997) *Hungry in Hospital.* London. Association of Community Health Councils for England and Wales.

DECKER, S.D. (1989) Eating disorders: anorexia nervosa and bulimia. In Shoen–Johnson, B. *Psychiatric–Mental Health Nursing* (2nd edition). Philadelphia. Lippincott.

DEPARTMENT OF HEALTH (1992) *Health of the Nation: A Strategy for Health in England.* London. Her Majesty's Stationery Office.

DEPARTMENT OF HEALTH (1994) *Nutritional Aspects of Cardiovascular Disease.* Report of the Cardiovascular Review Group of the Committee on Medical Aspects of Food Policy. London. Her Majesty's Stationery Office.

DEPARTMENT OF HEALTH (1994) *Weaning and the Weaning Diet.* Report on Health and Social Subjects No 45. London. Her Majesty's Stationery Office.

ENGLISH NATIONAL BOARD (1995) *Nutrition for Life.* London. English National Board.

GARROW, J.S. (1981) *Treat Obesity Seriously.* Edinburgh. Churchill Livingstone.

GARROW, J.S., JAMES, W.P.T. (eds) (1993) *Human Nutrition and Dietetics.* Edinburgh. Churchill Livingstone.

HALEK, C., CREMIN, D., CHANDRAN, U., PARNELL, J. (1995) Weights on the minds – anorexia nervosa, eating disorders, nursing development units. *Nursing Times* **91(48)**: 42–43.

HEALTH EDUCATION AUTHORITY (1996) *Nutritional Aspects of Cardiovascular Disease.* Nutrition Briefing Paper. London. Health Education Authority.

HELLERSTEIN, M.K., CHRISTIANSEN, M., KAEMPFER. S., KLETKE. C., WU, K., REID, J.S. (1991) Measurement of *de novo* hepatic lipogenesis in humans using stable isotopes. *Journal of Clinical Investigation* **87**: 1841–1852.

HINCHLIFF, S., MONTAGUE, S., WATSON, R. (1996) *Physiology for Nursing Practice* (2nd edition). London. Baillière Tindall.

JENNET, B. (1996) Managing patients in a persistent vegetative state since Airedale NHS Trust v Bland. In: McLean, S. (ed.) *Death, Dying and the Law.* Aldershot. Dartmouth Press.

LEADBETTER, J., BALL, M.J., MANN, J.I. (1991) Effect of increasing quantities of oatbran in hypercholesterolaemic people. *American Journal of Clinical Nutrition* **54**: 841–845.

LISSNER, L., HEITMANN, B.L. (1995) Dietary fat and obesity: evidence from epidemiology. *European Journal of Clinical Nutrition* **49**: 79–90.

McWHIRTER, J.P., PENNINGTON, C.R. (1994) Incidence and recognition of malnutrition in hospital. *British Medical Journal* **308**: 945–948.

MEADES, S. (1993) Suggested community psychiatric nursing interventions with clients suffering from anorexia nervosa and bulimia nervosa. *Journal of Advanced Nursing* **18(3)**: 364–370.

MINUCHIN, S., ROSEMAN, B., BAKER, L. (1978) *Psychosomatic Families: Anorexia Nervosa in Context.* Massachusetts, Harvard University Press.

NAIDOO, J., WILLS, J. (1994) *Health Promotion: Foundations for Practice.* London. Baillière Tindall.

ORR, J.B. (1936) *Food, Health and Income.* London. Macmillan.

PAGE, M. (1995) The role of diet in coronary heart disease. *Professional Nurse* **10(11)**: 691–696.

PARKIN, D. (1995) Interpretations and treatment of anorexia nervosa. *Mental Health Nursing* **15(1)**: 18–20.

PERRY, L. (1997) Nutrition: a hard nut to crack. An exploration of the knowledge, attitudes and activities of qualified nurses in relation to nutritional nursing care. *Journal of Clinical Nursing* **6(4)**: 315–324.

PRENTICE, A.M., JEBB, S.A. (1995) Obesity in Britain: gluttony or sloth? *British Medical Journal* **311**: 437–439.

READING, R., RAYBOULD, S., JARVIS, S. (1993) Deprivation, low birth weight and childrens height: a comparison between rural and urban areas. *British Medical Journal* **307**: 1458–1462.

ROLLS, B., FEDOROFF, I., GUTHRIE, J. (1991) Gender differences in eating behaviour and body weight regulation. *Health Psychology* **10(2)**: 133–142.

SILK, D.B.A. (ed.) (1994) *Organisation of Nutritional Support in Hospitals.* Report by the working party of the British Association for Parenteral and Enteral Nutrition, BAPEN, Maidenhead, Berks.

STEPHENS, N.G., PARSONS, A., SCHOFIELD, P.M., KELLY, F., CHEESEMAN, K., MITCHINSON, M.J., BROWN, M. (1996) Randomised controlled trial of vitamin E in patients with coronary disease: Cambridge Heart Antioxidant Study (CHAOS). *The Lancet* **347**: 781–785.

The Food Safety Act (C16) (1990) London. Her Majesty's Stationery Office.

UKCC (1992) *Code of Professional Conduct for the Nurse, Midwife and Health Visitor.* London. UKCC.

TENNANT, D. (1989) Tea for three – an anorectic girl was helped by treating her as part of her family system. *Nursing Times* **85(8)**: 72–73.

WHITEHEAD, M. (1988) The health divide. In Townsend, P., Davidson, N. (eds) *Inequalities in Health.* London. Penguin.

3.3 Continence

A. Kelley and S. Shepherd

KEY ISSUES

✳■ SUBJECT KNOWLEDGE
▷ definition of continence and incontinence
▷ biology of the urinary system
▷ the process of defecation
▷ different types of incontinence and their causes
▷ effects of the ageing process on continence
▷ psychological and environmental causes of incontinence
▷ behavioural problems caused by or causing incontinence
▷ the stigma of incontinence

■ PRACTICE KNOWLEDGE
▷ nursing assessment of urinary and faecal incontinence

▷ ways of promoting urinary and faecal continence
▷ aids and appliances used to manage incontinence

■ PROFESSIONAL KNOWLEDGE
▷ role of the continence advisor
▷ the link nurse scheme
▷ provision of a good quality and cost-effective service
▷ charter for continence

■ REFLECTIVE KNOWLEDGE
▷ empathy with the incontinent client
▷ exercises to enable holistic care for a person with continence problems
▷ consolidation of knowledge through case studies

▶ INTRODUCTION

'People have the right to be continent whenever that is achievable. When true continence is not achievable, people have the right to the highest standards of continence care and incontinence management, to enable social continence and maintenance of the individual's dignity'. (Philosophy of Association for Continence Advice – Association for Continence Advice, 1993)

Urinary incontinence is a distressing condition causing the patient and carer to feel shame and embarrassment. Faecal incontinence is seen as less socially acceptable and causes even more misery. Societies worldwide have rules and codes of behaviour that are only broken in exceptional circumstances, for example too young to know differently. Apparent disregard of these codes may lead society to feel disgust and hostility. Often incontinence can be seen as just such a violation (Mitteness, 1992), causing the sufferer to feel an outcast of society. A nurse caring for a client with continence problems not only has to be competent in dealing with their physical and psychological needs, but also has to cope with the misguided attitudes of others.

This chapter aims to introduce you to the concept of continence and the causes of incontinence, both urinary and faecal. It then focuses on the wide range of knowledge and skills needed to assess a client with continence problems and to plan the care needed to promote continence or in certain cases to manage incontinence efficiently and sympathetically.

The exercises used throughout the text are designed to help you develop a thorough understanding of how continence is maintained and how problems – physical, psychological and social – can cause incontinence in clients in all branches of nursing. They are also designed to explore the feelings and emotions evoked by these problems. The case studies are then used to combine and consolidate the knowledge you have gained to assess clients and plan care.

▶ OVERVIEW

▶ *Subject Knowledge*

The Biological part covers the applied physiology of the urological system and the lower bowels to explain how continence is maintained and how alterations in anatomy and physiology can give rise to incontinence. Changes in other physiological systems that may affect the continence of a client will also be discussed. In the Psychosocial part we show how continence is developed in children as they mature physiologically, and how society and its attitudes can affect elimination behaviour.

▶ *Practice Knowledge*

You will learn to develop skills needed to assess clients' problems, ways of promoting continence, how to manage incontinence and additional treatments that can be offered by referring clients to the continence advisor and the multidisciplinary team. These principles can be applied to clients of all ages in all branches of nursing, whether the client is being cared for in hospital or at home.

▶ *Professional Knowledge*

This part of the chapter examines the role of the continence advisor and the use of link schemes to disseminate knowledge needed to improve standards. The way the practitioner has to balance quality care and cost-effectiveness is also discussed briefly.

▶ *Reflective Knowledge*

The aim of the exercises is to aid your understanding of the knowledge required when caring for clients with elimination problems. All four branches of the nursing diploma are covered, but the principles reflected on lay down important foundations for all clients.

On pp. 412–414 there are four case studies, each one relating to one of the branch programmes. You may find it helpful to read one of them before you start the chapter and use it as a focus for your reflections while reading.

SUBJECT KNOWLEDGE

'Continence is a skill gained when a person learns to recognise the need to pass urine and/or bowel motion, has the ability to reach an acceptable place to void, is able to hold on until they reach there and is able to void/eliminate effectively on reaching that place' (Association for Continence Advice, 1993). The International Continence Society Committee on Standardisation of Terminology defines urinary incontinence as 'The involuntary loss of urine which is objectively demonstrable and a social or hygiene problem' (Anderson *et al.*, 1988).

It is thought that over three million people in the UK suffer from incontinence. A survey conducted by Thomas *et al.* in 1980 showed that approximately 5% of the population suffered from regular urinary incontinence (i.e. being incontinent more than twice a month) irrespective of age. Incontinence affected 1.65% of men and 8.5% of women between the ages of 15 and 65; among those over 65 years of age the percentage rises to 6.9% of men and 11.6% of women. However, these figures may not be accurate due to the reluctance of people to admit to these problems.

First we will look at the physiological mechanism used to achieve continence and then at how it may fail and cause urinary and faecal incontinence. Following that other types of physiological failures that may cause problems with elimination will be considered.

Biological ## ▶ ANATOMY AND PHYSIOLOGY OF THE LOWER URINARY TRACT

Urine is made in the kidneys and passes into the bladder where it is stored until it is convenient to void. To understand continence fully we need to look at the anatomy and physiology of the organs involved in storage and evacuation and how they relate to the lower bowel and the male and female reproductive organs (Figure 3.3.1).

The bladder is made of four layers of tissue:

▶ an inner layer of transitional epithelium;
▶ a connective tissue layer;
▶ smooth muscle;
▶ an outer coating covering the upper surface, the peritoneum (Figure 3.3.2).

The epithelial layer has the ability to stretch and also produces mucus to protect the tissues from the acidity of the urine. The smooth muscle is known as the detrusor muscle and is made up of layers of longitudinal and circular muscle to allow it to both expand and contract. Stretch receptors are found within these muscles and monitor the fullness of the bladder. Urine enters the bladder through the ureters and leaves through the urethra (see Figure 3.3.2). The triangular area between these openings is known as the trigone. The trigone contains many stretch receptors, which transmit sensory impulses as the bladder fills (Colborn, 1994). The urethra is a tube running from the bladder and is 3–5 cm long in the female and 18–22 cm long in the male. It has three layers:

▶ a mucosal lining;
▶ smooth muscle;
▶ a connective tissue lining.

The mucosal lining is thick and contains mucus-producing cells, and is folded to enhance the water-tight seal of the bladder.

At the bladder neck the smooth muscle passes from the bladder to the urethra, forming the internal closing mechanism. This is more distinct in men than women, being found just above the prostate gland (Figure 3.3.3). This closing mechanism's function is to prevent leaking during the filling phase of the bladder and retrograde ejaculation in males (Malone-Lee, 1989). The external sphincter is found in the urethra. In men it is a separate ring just below the prostate gland. It allows voluntary closure of the urethra and is thought to function in interrupting voiding (Cheater, 1992b).

The pelvic floor is a muscular sling supporting the abdominal organs. It is pierced by the rectum posteriorly and the vagina and urethra anteriorly. It is very important in continence, contracting to maintain urinary

Figure 3.3.1: Anatomy of the urethra. (Redrawn from Hinchliff and Montague, 1988.)

Female

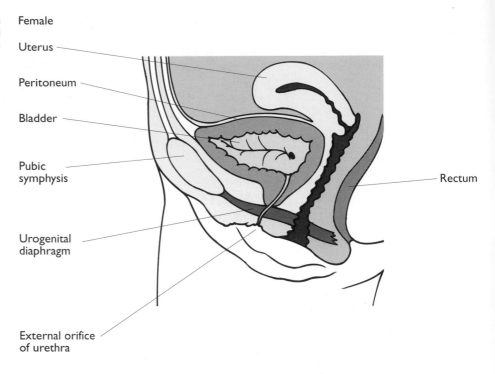

Uterus

Peritoneum

Bladder

Pubic symphysis

Urogenital diaphragm

External orifice of urethra

Rectum

Male

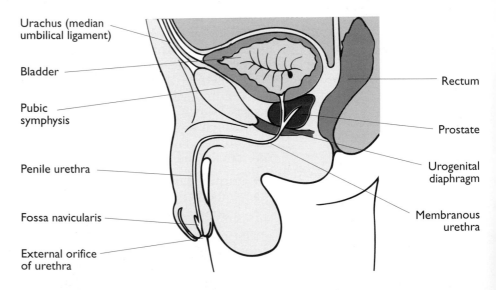

Urachus (median umbilical ligament)

Bladder

Pubic symphysis

Penile urethra

Fossa navicularis

External orifice of urethra

Rectum

Prostate

Urogenital diaphragm

Membranous urethra

and faecal continence, but relaxing to allow expulsion of urine and faeces (Lewis Wall, 1994). The bladder and the proximal urethra sit well supported above the pelvic floor, and this position is needed to maintain continence (see Figure 3.3.2). This will be discussed more fully when considering stress incontinence.

Figure 3.3.2: Cross section of urinary bladder (female). (Based on Cheater, 1992b.)

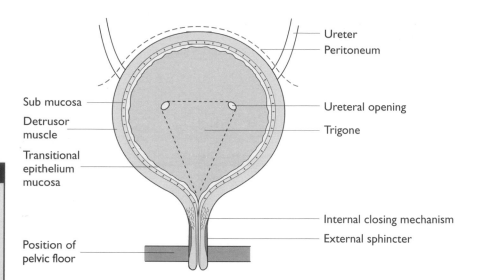

Sub mucosa

Detrusor muscle

Transitional epithelium mucosa

Position of pelvic floor

Ureter

Peritoneum

Ureteral opening

Trigone

Internal closing mechanism

External sphincter

The bladder is controlled by both the somatic and the autonomic nervous system, which allow it to store urine and then expel it at a suitable time. The sympathetic system innervates the detrusor muscle of the bladder, allowing the bladder to fill and the sphincters to remain closed, thus preventing leakage. The stretch receptors of the detrusor muscle will allow filling up to approximately 500 ml without registering changes of pressure. Once this volume is reached the parasympathetic nerves transmit impulses to the sacral area of the spinal cord (S2–S4) where the reflex arc is stimulated. If there is no voluntary control, a spinal reflex arc is completed, allowing impulses to pass back to the bladder through the parasympathetic motor nerves, causing the muscle to contract and the sphincter to open, and resulting in micturition (Figure 3.3.4).

Figure 3.3.3: The sphincters of the bladder.

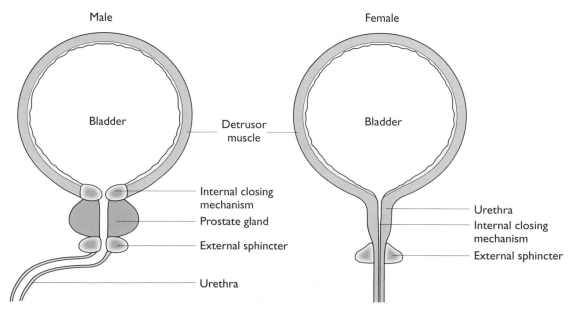

Male

Female

Bladder

Bladder

Detrusor muscle

Internal closing mechanism

Prostate gland

External sphincter

Urethra

Urethra

Internal closing mechanism

External sphincter

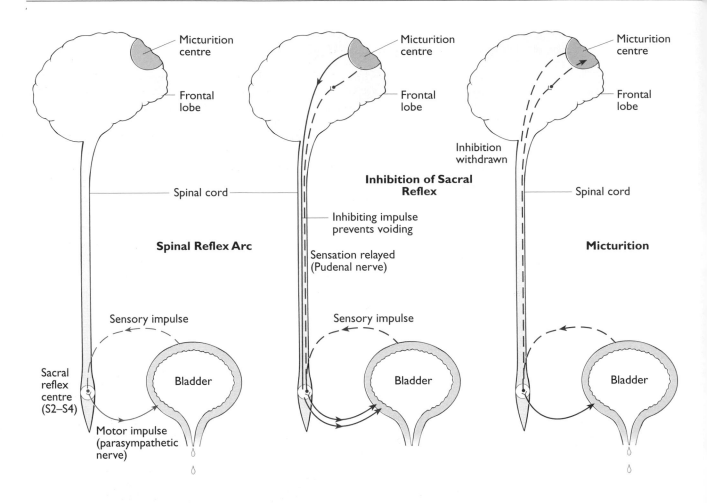

Figure 3.3.4: Involuntary and voluntary control of micturition.

The voluntary control works in an inhibitory manner: impulses are sent through the pudendal nerve to the cortical micturition centre in the frontal lobe of the brain informing it that the bladder is full. Impulses are passed back to the sacrum to prevent the sacral reflex action initiating micturition. This inhibition is lifted only when the individual is ready to pass urine (see Figure 3.3.4). The reflex arc action occurs in babies. The inhibitory process begins to develop in young children from the age of 18 months as the central nervous system matures.

▶ ALTERED PHYSIOLOGY OF THE LOWER URINARY TRACT

Four main types of incontinence result from an alteration of the normal physiology described above. These are:

▶ stress incontinence;
▶ detrusor instability;
▶ outflow obstruction;
▶ hypotonic bladder.

The conditions will be discussed separately so that you can understand the different symptoms of each type. This is important when you assess patients as some clients may have more than one condition causing their continence difficulties.

▶ *Stress Incontinence*

According to Cardozo *et al.* (1993) stress incontinence is 'the involuntary loss of urine when intravesical pressure exceeds the maximum urethral pressure in the absence of detrusor activity'.

Stress incontinence is most common in women and results when a rise in abdominal pressure caused by for example laughing, sneezing or lifting during the filling phase of the bladder exerts a pressure higher than that in the urethra causing leakage of urine. When held in the correct position by the pelvic floor the inner closing mechanism and the external sphincter of the bladder prevent leakage (Figure 3.3.5). True competence of the sphincter mechanism can be shown if a woman can perform a 'star jump' (a form of gym exercise) with a full bladder and experiences no leakage. If the pelvic floor is weak there is no compensatory pressure helping to counteract the pressure on the bladder and leakage may occur (see Figure 3.3.5); this is made worse if the urethral sphincter mechanism is also weak. Table 3.3.1 lists the common causes of stress incontinence.

Figure 3.3.5: Diagram showing the relationship between the bladder and the pelvic floor for continence and how a lax pelvic floor causes stress incontinence.

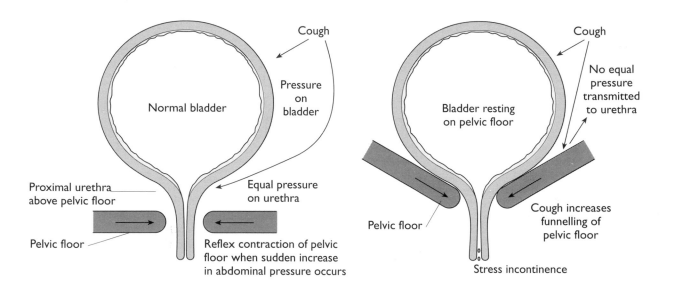

Mechanism	Cause
Weakness of pelvic floor muscles	Pregnancy Chronic constipation Obesity Prolonged lifting of heavy weights
Bladder or pelvic floor muscle damage	Childbirth Pelvic or prostatic surgery
Hormonal changes (lower levels of oestrogen)	Pregnancy Last part of menstrual cycle Menopause
External factors (exacerbate stress incontinence)	Chronic cough Urinary tract infections (UTIs) Lifting Poor fluid intake

Table 3.3.1 Common causes of stress incontinence.

◗ *Detrusor Instability*

Detrusor instability or unstable bladder is characterized by involuntary bladder contractions during its filling phase (Wells, 1996) and produces symptoms of urgency, frequency, urge incontinence, nocturia and nocturnal enuresis (Table 3.3.2). Simply the inhibition impulse from the cortical micturition centre of the cortex is not sufficient to prevent the sacral reflex action occurring, so the bladder starts to contract and voiding begins. This may be due to damage to the central nervous system, for example a cerebrovascular accident, tumours, spinal cord injuries or malfunction of the conduction of the nerve impulses (as seen in multiple sclerosis and parkinsonism). Local bladder factors may be responsible for causing spasm that overrides cortical inhibition, for example caffeine (Creighton and Stanton, 1990), urinary tract infections, concentrated urine or external factors such as prostatic enlargement or constipation. Detrusor instability may occur in the absence of any detectable pathology (Figure 3.3.6).

Urgency	The need to pass urine in a great hurry.
Sensory urgency	Urgency in the absence of unstable bladder contractions. The bladder is hypersensitive.
Frequency	Visiting the toilet to pass urine more often than is acceptable to the patient. This usually means more than seven times during the day and more than once at night.
Urge incontinence	While experiencing urgency the patient may not be able to get to the toilet in time and is therefore incontinent.
Reflex incontinence	Urine loss due to detrusor hyperreflexia (or involuntary urethral relaxation) when there is a neuropathic absence of sensation.
Hesitancy	Difficulty in initiating voiding.
Dribbling	Dribbling of urine after voiding, due to pooling of urine in the urethra between internal and external sphincter.
Nocturia	Waking at night to pass urine.
Nocturnal enuresis	Bedwetting while asleep.
Passive incontinence	Wetting at rest without any coincident activity or sensation.
Dysuria	Pain or burning while actually passing urine.
Haematuria	Blood in the urine.

Table 3.3.2 Definitions of terms.

◗ *Outflow Obstruction*

In some people the outlet of the bladder becomes blocked, for example in some elderly males with prostatic enlargement or clients with urethral stenosis or stricture following infections or instrumentation, though sometimes this narrowing can be congenital. When this occurs emptying is impeded and causes outflow obstruction (Figure 3.3.7) This condition causes a variety of symptoms including frequency, hesitancy, poor stream and urgency. In some cases the bladder is never completely emptied and a residual volume of urine builds up, causing overflow incontinence (Norton, 1986). This residual volume encourages urinary tract infections and recurrence of these is a further indication of this problem. The detrusor muscle of an obstructed bladder may become very powerful and hypertrophied in an attempt to overcome the high outflow resistance,

Figure 3.3.6: The unstable bladder: failure of inhibition of detrusor contraction. (Reproduced by kind permission of Coloplast Ltd.)

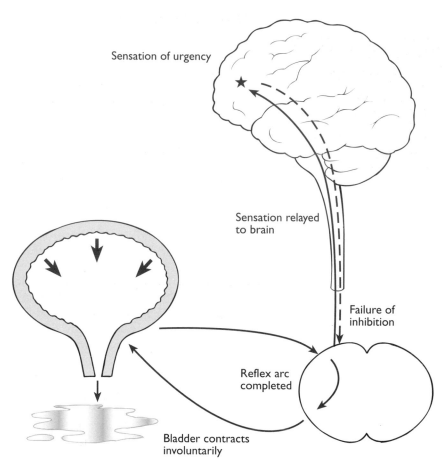

Sensation of urgency

Sensation relayed to brain

Failure of inhibition

Reflex arc completed

Bladder contracts involuntarily

Figure 3.3.7: Obstruction with overflow incontinence. (Reproduced by kind permission of Coloplast Ltd.)

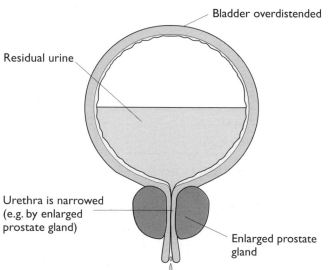

Bladder overdistended

Residual urine

Urethra is narrowed (e.g. by enlarged prostate gland)

Enlarged prostate gland

and in some instances this causes secondary detrusor instability and urge incontinence. If the obstruction is longstanding the bladder may eventually give up and become hypotonic.

▶ Hypotonic Bladder

A hypotonic bladder is one in which the detrusor muscle of the bladder does not produce a sufficiently powerful voiding contraction and may require manual expression to empty. Micturition becomes inefficient and a residual volume can build up (Figure 3.3.8). The bladder filling sensation may be absent or reduced and the large residual volume (i.e. more than 150 ml) may result in recurrent urinary tract infections and overflow incontinence (Roe and Williams, 1994). Cardozo *et al.* (1993) state that a residual volume of more than 100 ml should be considered significant. Symptoms are frequency, urgency, urge incontinence, hesitancy, poor stream, nocturia, nocturnal enuresis and straining. The working volume and working capacity are worked out as follows:

- ▶ volume of bladder – residual volume = working capacity;
- ▶ for example 600 ml – 0 ml = 600 ml normal working capacity;
- ▶ for example 600 ml – 450 ml = 150 ml working capacity with a hypotonic bladder.

The client's bladder will therefore have a low working capacity. The low working capacity may mimic that of detrusor instability, occasionally causing misdiagnosis.

Hypotonic bladder is found in people who have a damaged reflex arc, for example, due to lower spinal cord injury as found in spina bifida, peripheral neuropathy associated with diabetes mellitus (Diokno *et al.*, 1983), multiple sclerosis, spinal cord and pelvic injuries, tumours, dementia, strokes and parkinsonism.

Figure 3.3.8: The underactive detrusor. (Reproduced by kind permission of Coloplast Ltd.)

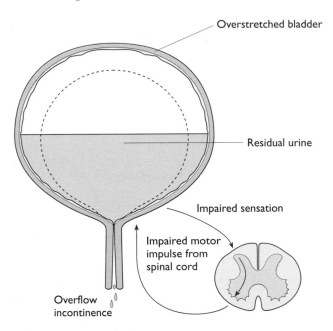

▶ ANATOMY AND PHYSIOLOGY OF THE LOWER BOWEL

Faecal incontinence is an even greater social stigma than urinary incontinence – it is poorly tolerated by carers and frequently leads to the breakdown of community care (Sandford, 1975). Less than 1% of clients with faecal incontinence live in the community, and 25–35% are found on longstay elderly wards (Barrett, 1992).

The large intestine consists of the caecum and colon and terminates with the rectum and anal canal. It receives 600 ml of chyme from the small intestine daily and reduces it to 150–200 ml of faeces by reabsorbing water from the chyme as it travels through the colon. Faeces are stored in the rectum and eliminated though the anal canal (Hinchliffe, 1988). The rectum has a mucosal lining (i.e. columnar epithelial), which produces mucus to lubricate the passage of stool. The anal canal has a squamous epithelial lining, which is dry and very sensitive and can distinguish between flatus and stool, allowing flatulence to escape to relieve gaseous distension, but retaining faeces. The muscle layer is smooth involuntary muscle and contains specialized stretch receptors, which monitor the fullness of the rectum. In the anal canal the smooth involuntary muscle thickens to form the internal sphincter, which is surrounded by a layer of voluntary muscle, the anal sphincter (Bendall, 1989) (Figure 3.3.9).

Figure 3.3.9: Section through lower rectum and anus. (Reproduced from Bendal, 1989, by kind permission of Wallace Ltd and Smith Industries Medical Systems.)

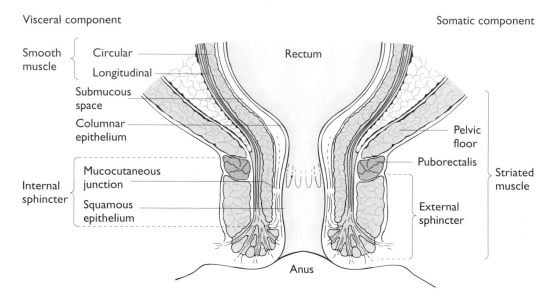

Faeces formed by the large bowel enter the rectum by a series of colonic movements known as the gastrocolic reflex, which is stimulated by physical activity and ingestion of food (Barrett, 1992). Once 150 ml or more of stool is in the rectum the individual gets a feeling of fullness and impending defecation and the internal anal sphincter relaxes and allows the stool to enter the anal canal. If defecation is not convenient, the external sphincter remains closed and the faeces return to the rectum (Alderman, 1988b). However, if it is appropriate, the external sphincter relaxes and defecation occurs. This is most efficiently achieved in a squatting position as pressure from the abdominal muscles will cause the external and internal anal sphincters to relax, the pelvic floor will drop down to form a funnel, and the bowel will empty easily (Chiarelli and Markwell, 1992).

The nervous control has yet to be fully elucidated (Barrett, 1992). It appears to be a reflex action involving the myenteric plexus and stimulated by a full rectum. The internal anal sphincter is controlled by the autonomic nervous system and the external sphincter is controlled by the somatic nervous system (pudendal nerve). Charlotte Alderman (1988b) suggests that there is a reflex arc in the spinal cord from which information is sent to the higher centres, which will regulate defecation by inhibition in a similar manner to bladder emptying (Figure 3.3.10)

If the defecation mechanism is working properly the individual should be able to pass 150–200 ml of formed but soft stool regularly. However, the interval of time between defecation varies between individuals, ranging from three times a day to once in three days (Chiarelli and Markwell, 1992).

Figure 3.3.10: Possible nervous control of the lower bowel.

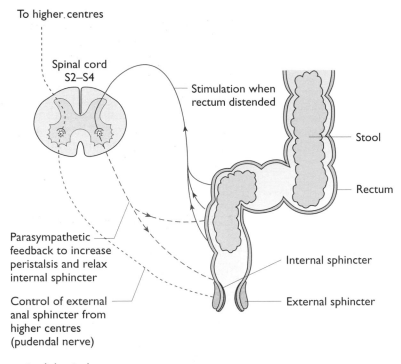

To higher centres

Spinal cord S2–S4

Stimulation when rectum distended

Stool

Rectum

Parasympathetic feedback to increase peristalsis and relax internal sphincter

Internal sphincter

Control of external anal sphincter from higher centres (pudendal nerve)

External sphincter

Figure 3.3.11: Faecal continence and incontinence and the anorectal angle. (Reproduced by kind permission of Coloplast Ltd.)

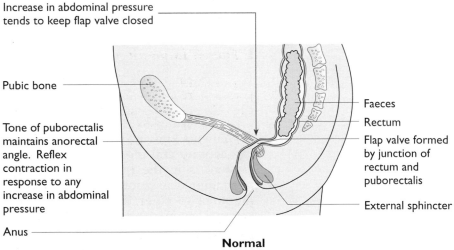

Increase in abdominal pressure tends to keep flap valve closed

Pubic bone

Tone of puborectalis maintains anorectal angle. Reflex contraction in response to any increase in abdominal pressure

Anus

Faeces

Rectum

Flap valve formed by junction of rectum and puborectalis

External sphincter

Normal

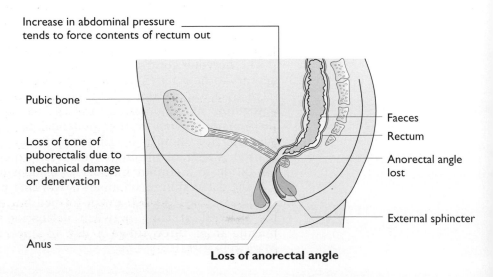

Increase in abdominal pressure tends to force contents of rectum out

Pubic bone

Loss of tone of puborectalis due to mechanical damage or denervation

Anus

Faeces

Rectum

Anorectal angle lost

External sphincter

Loss of anorectal angle

The pelvic floor is responsible for keeping the rectum in the correct position. The muscle of the pelvic floor, which anchors the rectum to the pubis (i.e. the puborectalis), is of great importance in maintaining faecal continence. The puborectalis maintains an angle of 60–105° between the rectum and the anal canal. This angle acts as a flap valve, which closes when abdominal pressures rise, for example due to sneezing or lifting, preventing leakage through the canal (Figure 3.3.11) The nerve supply of the pelvic floor is innervated by the same nerve as the external sphincter, the pudendal nerve. This nerve synapses with the autonomic system at sacral vertebrae 2–4.

▶ ALTERED PHYSIOLOGY OF THE LOWER BOWEL

Barrett (1992) classifies the causes of faecal incontinence under five headings as follows:

- ▶ faecal impaction;
- ▶ neurological – dementia; unconsciousness; behavioural; damage;
- ▶ anorectal incontinence;
- ▶ colorectal disease;
- ▶ immobility.

The first four physical causes from this list will now be discussed.

▶ *Faecal Impaction*

Faecal impaction can be the result of chronic constipation. If the constipation is rectal, it may exert pressure forcing the faecal matter through the anal sphincter. Colonic constipation, however, can also cause leakage of liquid stool (Colborn, 1994). This may be a seepage of liquid waste from above the obstruction or the result of bacterial breakdown of the hard faeces resulting in a slimy liquid with extra mucus (i.e. a foul smelling spurious diarrhoea). There are many causes of constipation and a complete list is given in Table 3.3.3. It most commonly occurs when there is insufficient material in the rectum to distend it and initiate the defecation reflex. This can be due to poor diet or fluid intake. Those at risk are the elderly, those on slimming diets or a gluten-free diet, and people who tend to eat only snack foods.

Slow peristaltic action increases the time the stool stays in the lower bowel and this will cause constipation. This may simply be due to lack of exercise. Some clients have a naturally slow motility rate, passing large stools and emptying their bowels less frequently than the rest of the population. In the elderly this can lead to terminal reservoir syndrome where the bowel is never emptied (Norton, 1986a).

Nerve damage affecting the rectum and anal canal can cause a loss of rectal sensation and propulsion of stool and sphincter malfunction (i.e. remaining closed and preventing evacuation), and all these effects may give rise to constipation. Faecal impaction is not always caused by hard stool, it may be caused by a large mass of soft or liquid stool. The presentation of this type of loading can be misleading as the patient may be passing stool daily, but does not empty the bowel. Such a patient will therefore be straining and have faecal incontinence due to the massive loading. 'Faecal impaction may therefore be better described as faecal loading of the rectum and/or colon with a large amount of stool of any consistency' (Barrett, 1992).

Mechanism	Causes
Insufficient material in the bowel	Lack of fibre in the diet Poor fluid intake
Abnormal neurological control	Spinal or nerve injury affecting autonomic nervous system Hirschsprung's disease (a condition where there is an absence of nerves in the wall of the bowel) Psychological factors, by an inhibitory effect on autonomic innervation
Obstruction	Tumours Diverticular disease Haemorrhoids Congenital abnormalities
Pregnancy	High progesterone levels causing decrease in motility of the gastrointestinal tract
Metabolic causes	Diabetes mellitus Hypothyroidism Dehydration
Drugs	Aluminium (antacids) Anticholinergics Diuretics Iron Analgesia opiates Verapamil
Laxative abuse	Over-use of laxatives can cause damage to the nerves in the colon, resulting in atonic bowel
Environmental	Anything preventing defecation e.g. lack of privacy; dirty toilets; insufficient toilets
Immobility	Lack of exercise means the bowel itself is less active The client may have difficulty reaching the toilet

Table 3.3.3 Causes of constipation.

▌ *Neurological Causes*

Norton (1986) says that any neurological disorders that prevent the individual from recognizing or inhibiting defecation, for example unconsciousness or dementia, can cause faecal incontinence. The demented person may suffer from unstable bowel, where the client experiences an urgent need to pass stool, resulting in faecal incontinence if they cannot reach the toilet in time. This is due to an inability of the higher centres to sufficiently inhibit the reflex arc (Alderman, 1988b). Damage in the spinal area of S2–S4, for example due to spina bifida or low spinal cord damage, can result in uncontrollable bowel evacuation as the patient has no rectal sensation or sphincter control.

▌ *Anorectal Incontinence*

Anorectal incontinence results from weakness of the pelvic floor, particularly the puborectalis muscle, and as a result the anorectal angle and therefore the flap valve are lost. Faecal incontinence may then occur when abdominal pressure increases, for example when sneezing or lifting (see Figure 3.3.11). This muscle weakness may result from damage to the nerves supplying the pelvic floor by chronic straining at stool, childbirth or forceps delivery. In the elderly, anorectal angle changes may be

DECISION MAKING

An important part of assessing for urinary incontinence is the state of a client's bowels. Relating this fact to the anatomy and physiology previously covered:

* *Decide why this may occur.*
* *Review the backgound information as well as the specific information you would need to collect before making any decisions about the care of an incontinent patient.*
* *At this stage identify any extra reading you would need to do to develop your knowledge further in this complex area of care*

exacerbated by nerve degeneration and muscle weakness (Barrett, 1992). Damage to the internal or external anal sphincters (or both) due to forceps delivery or perineal tears during childbirth are often responsible for faecal incontinence in younger women.

Colorectal Disease

A bad attack of diarrhoea may cause faecal incontinence, especially in those who are very ill, bedbound or have mobility problems.

▶ GENERAL ALTERED PHYSIOLOGY CAUSING CONTINENCE PROBLEMS

If we return to our original definition of continence, we can see that physiological changes in other systems of the body may affect the continence state of the client. For example when identifying the place for elimination the client needs to be orientated. We may get confused when in unfamiliar surroundings, as may some clients, who on entering a strange environment, for example hospital, become disorientated and unable to find the toilet (Stokes, 1987). Clients with dementia, confusion or disorientation, may become incontinent purely because they are unable to locate the toilet. Finding the correct receptacle may also be a problem: the demented patient may confuse washbasins with urinals (Norton, 1986). To locate a toilet a person needs to be able to follow a signed route, which can be difficult in dim corridors or if the person is blind or partially sighted. The sign also needs to be recognizable, so notices in small print or the modern stylized pictures may not be obvious to the disorientated. A sign only saying 'toilets' is also unsuitable, causing discomfort to people who fear sharing facilities with the opposite sex. People may have to ask for the toilet, which can be embarrassing for some, but very difficult for clients with communication problems due to physical illness (e.g. stroke) or mental illness (e.g. depression).

The ability to reach the toilet is essential and clients with problems like stiff joints or poor balance may find this difficult. In addition this effort may tire them, resulting in an incontinent episode before they reach the toilet. Obstacles en route such as stairs, narrow passages, sharp corners, loose mats and heavy doors can also hamper the journey to the toilet (Norton, 1986). Memory loss causes problems as the client may forget what their goal is after setting out to go to the toilet and wander around until it is too late (Stokes, 1987). On reaching the toilet itself the client needs dexterity to remove clothing, before eliminating; inappropriate clothing may slow the client so much that they may begin to void or defecate too soon and incontinence may occur (Fader and Norton, 1994). To complete the toileting sequence a

How accessible is our social environment for individuals who need to reach the toilet quickly and cannot get there as fast as others? Consider those with mobility or sight problems. Thinking of a pub or restaurant you have visited discuss the difficulties you think may arise.

* *How easy was it to identify the toilet?*
* *Was it easy to reach the toilet?*
* *What hazards were in the way en route to or in the toilet?*

Looking further afield look at the provision of the toilets in a town centre near you.

* *Does this provision meet the needs of the general public, people with continence problems and the disabled?*
* *Is there an even spread of toilet facilities throughout the town?*
* *What provisions are made in these toilets (e.g. hygiene facilities, disabled facilities, baby changing facilities, see Cunningham and Norton, 1993)?*
* *Check on their hours of opening – are they suitable? and note any difference between the opening times of the male and female toilets.*

person must be able to squat, or for men have the stability to stand, and this may cause problems for the disabled.

▶ *Ageing*

Any of the general physiological factors discussed above may be a problem for the elderly, but they are not inevitable (Brocklehurst, 1984). The ageing process may affect continence in many other ways and the following factors are some of the important ones.

- ▶ Loss of normal circadian rhythms – urine is produced continuously over 24 hours (Colborn, 1994) and this may lead to nocturnal enuresis.
- ▶ Hormonal change – the amount of oestrogen circulating in a woman's body decreases. As a result, the soft convoluted tissue of the vagina and urethra become less elastic with less pronounced folds, resulting in the loss of the watertight seal in the urethra.
- ▶ The elderly man has a tendency towards prostatic enlargement and therefore overflow incontinence.
- ▶ Loss in muscle tone of the pelvic floor leading to stress incontinence (due to decreased oestrogen levels in some cases).
- ▶ The muscle tone of the bladder may also become more lax and the sphincters do not relax as fully as before, so the bladder may not empty completely and a residual volume may build up (Norton, 1986).
- ▶ Deterioration of nerves – the sensation of bladder fullness becomes less acute, and the older person will feel the urge to urinate when the bladder is 90% full, and not 50%, as in the younger person. There is also a tendency towards an unstable bladder in the elderly due to neural changes (Roe and Williams, 1994).
- ▶ The immunological system becomes less efficient thus increasing the incidence of infections (Herbert, 1991) This coupled with a residual volume of urine in the bladder increases the likelihood of urinary tract infections. Roe and Williams (1994) list infections as one of the factors that can cause transient incontinence in the elderly.
- ▶ Polypharmacy – many drugs can encourage urinary incontinence, some cause urinary retention and some cause constipation.

> In your practice placements where there are elderly clients:
> - *Review the medicines that individual clients are receiving.*
> - *Explore the drugs' effects and side effects and review whether these could affect the continence of your client.*

Psychosocial ▶ DEVELOPMENT OF CONTROL

There are many physical and psychological skills needed to acquire continence and a child needs to reach 18 months to two years of age before being mature enough to be toilet trained. The child will need to have some control over both anal and urethral sphincter mechanisms, being able to hold urine for two hours and to hold on until reaching a potty. The urge sensation of passing urine or wanting to defecate should be recognized by the child and be associated with the feeling of wet or soiling. The gross motor skills of walking and sitting and the fine motor skills involved in dressing and undressing should be developed. The ability to be able to sit on the toilet for 5–10 minutes is important if toilet training is to be successful. The child must be able to convey the need to go to the toilet to a parent, so communication skills, verbal or nonverbal, are essential. At this stage of their development children will be uncomfortable when dirty or wet and will also have a desire to please their parents by being clean and dry. It is only at this stage that a child is ready for toilet training (Wong, 1993).

For toilet training to be successful parents need to encourage and help their children. Once the child is interested in using the toilet, it is important that a parent or carer can give time to help the child get used to the potty or toilet, allowing them time to practise. Praising the child when he or she successfully uses the potty is important, but praise and encouragement for cooperating is also necessary (Dobson, 1996). Toilet training may take some time and accidents may occur, especially if the child is engrossed in play. This will upset the child and the parent and reminding the child to use the toilet regularly will help.

Every child will become dry in their own time. Bowel control may be accomplished before bladder control as there is usually a more regular pattern and a stronger sensation in defecation. Night-time continence may take much longer than daytime continence and children may reach four or five years of age before this is achieved, and even then 15–20% of five year olds are still wet at night (Blackwell, 1989). Problems can arise during toilet training if the child is ill or experiences an emotional upset, for example divorce or a new baby sibling. This may prolong the training or even cause the dry child to start wetting again (regression). Usually with encouragement, care and time, the skill will be regained. Problems with wetting may continue into school age, for example nocturnal enuresis and diurnal enuresis.

The strict definition of enuresis is incontinence of urine, but it is usually used to describe bedwetting (i.e. nocturnal enuresis). Primary nocturnal enuresis differentiates those children who have never been dry at night from secondary enuresis, which arises after a period of complete control (Feneley, 1986). Nocturnal enuresis is twice as common in boys than girls, there are strong familial tendencies, and it is associated with stressful events in the third or fourth year of life (Dobson, 1996). In girls a urinary tract infection may lead to incontinence (Kalvin *et al.*, 1973).

Several theories have been suggested as causes of nocturnal enuresis. Genetic factors and delayed maturation of a child's nervous system are suggested by Eisberg (1995), while Simmonds (1977) stated that inadequate training and habit formation may be causes. Psychological or emotional disorders may also lead to delayed continence or other toileting problems including enuresis. Robbins (1985) reports that some children have an emotional or psychological block about elimination. Broomfield and Douglas (1985) say there is a link with lower social class and being disadvantaged.

Another area of nursing where acquiring continence is important, is in caring for those people who have a learning disability. Toileting is a complex operant and social learning process and this can be hindered by a reduced learning capacity and by institutionalization (Boulter, 1995).

▶ BEHAVIOURAL FACTORS

Incontinence in an individual cannot be explained by physical factors alone (Norton, 1986). The emotional and mental state of the individual, along with his or her attitude will also have a bearing on the problem. In children, regression may occur when a sibling is born, while in an adult the beginning of continence problems can sometimes be traced to emotional traumas, for example bereavement, rejection or moving to a new place (Stokes, 1987). Many people become incontinent on admission

---

RESEARCH BASED EVIDENCE

Bliss and Watson (1992) conducted a survey in two schools for children with severe learning difficulties, asking parents about toilet training their child. They found that although continence may be gained later than normal, eventually 88% were continent in the daytime. This shows that the nurse should have a positive approach to the client with learning disabilities becoming continent.

- *List the skills required by a healthy person for voiding or defecating from intially recognizing the need to actually passing urine in the toilet and returning to their original activity.*
- *From this list identify individuals who may have difficulty with any of these factors due to physical disease or disability, mental health problems or learning disabilities.*
- *When in practice placements observe how nurses use this knowledge in helping clients with their toileting needs. Ask those nurses you observe to explain the reasons for their particular actions.*

to residential care or soon after, and this may be related to the loss of independence and personal responsibility and a decreasing sense of self worth that often accompany their admission; thus by regressing to an infantile state such people may be able to avoid facing reality.

Incontinence may be an expression of anger, as one of the few weapons available to the individual against his or her carers, not only getting their own back, but also gaining attention. In some cases, incontinence can become rewarding since it gains attention and creates fuss, especially in understaffed institutions where a one to one relationship is only available during toileting or when an incontinent episode occurs.

Continence is an acquired habit, and the motivation to be continent can be diminished in the apathetic or confused elderly person, for example if a toilet is cold, unpleasant or a distance away the call to micturate or defecate may be ignored. Confused or demented people are very dependent upon familiar stimuli in order to maintain their activities. It is all too easy to upset these conditioned reflexes by offering confusing stimuli (Newman, 1962). Most people have a lifetime of conditioned reflexes to pass urine while seated with no clothing over the genital areas on a toilet in privacy and with the sensation of a full bladder. If an individual is taken to the toilet repeatedly when the bladder is not full the purpose of visiting the toilet will be destroyed. Also if a person is sat in a chair with a bare bottom on an underpad, he or she gets the message to go ahead and pass urine. This leads to paradoxical urination patterns. The individual does not pass urine in the toilet, but will do so when back in the chair. It must be understood that the individual is seldom trying to be awkward, but is merely responding to the confusing stimuli to which he or she is subjected.

DECISION MAKING

Most people have a lifetime of conditioned reflexes determining their toileting behaviour and it is all too easy to upset these reflexes by offering confusing stimuli.

- **List ways in which we can prevent the loss of the conditioned reflex of continence.**

Mr Jackson, a 45-year-old man, has spent the majority of his life in prison. He has recently been involved in a road traffic accident and sustained a head injury. He has made a good physical recovery, but now suffers from short-term memory loss and occasional confusion. On discharge from hospital he moves in with his sister. She reports to the community psychiatric nurse (CPN) that he has recently become incontinent and will only urinate in a wastepaper basket in his room.

- **Why do you think Mr Jackson does this?**
- **What could the CPN suggest in order to help Mr Jackson regain his continence?**

▌ STIGMA AND INCONTINENCE

Eliminating both urine and stool are very personal functions of the human body and one of the few things we do alone. We tend to be embarrassed about it, using euphemisms for passing urine and defecating. It was during the Victorian era that it was realised that poor sewage facilities and bad hygiene led to the spread of disease. The water closet was developed, giving a definite area for eliminating, and a system created to remove this waste from living areas. General standards of hygiene were improved and at the same time strict rules on self discipline and sexual conduct were expected.

Mrs Barton went to the doctor complaining she was unable to 'go round the corner'. After checking her mobility and her balance he could find nothing wrong with her. He asked her daughter for help, and she explained that this was the phrase her mother used for opening her bowels. List all the euphemisms you have heard for:

- *passing urine;*
- *passing stool.*

The expressions you have heard tend to be both personal and part of 'local culture'.

- **What are the implications for decision making in care if there is lack of understanding of these differing cultural expressions?**

The definition of incontinence is 'lacking restraint or unable to retain control; unable to control excreta' (*Concise Oxford English Dictionary*). A recent pilot study of a continence education programme showed that 42% of respondents considered that the word incontinence meant no control over bladder and bowels (H. Bayliss, 1996). These definitions mean that people labelled as incontinent of urine feel disgrace as if they are lax generally. The smell caused by wetting and soiling went against the Victorian ideal that 'cleanliness is next to godliness'. Therefore during the Victorian era to admit to incontinence was a great social stigma. The elderly patients we nurse today will have been raised by parents who were born in the Victorian times and who will have instilled in them their values. Many women relate incontinence of urine to having children and something to be borne without complaint. The frail elderly may become incontinent, which encourages the attitude that incontinence is an inevitable part of ageing. Thus there is a myth held by young and old alike that incontinence should not be mentioned and should be suffered in silence with no expectation of help or cure.

Passive acceptance coupled with extreme embarrassment means people often cope by adapting their lifestyle to hide their incontinence by not going out with friends or to social functions and giving up playing sport. Outings by bus or car can be an ordeal because of worrying about being able to get to a toilet when needed, and staying overnight with friends can be out of the question in case of wetting beds or furniture. This shame may go further than leading to social restriction and affect the individual's relationship with those closest to them. Some people find telling their spouses that they are incontinent is impossible. The guilt, shame, frustration and feelings of the hopelessness of a situation that does not seem to have a solution can then lead to depression. Therefore a problem that appears to be physical can cause severe social and psychological problems.

The sexuality of the individual is also affected by incontinence. There is a high correlation with impotence and it has been shown that stress incontinence is associated with sexual dysfunction among middle-aged women (Association for Continence Advice, 1995). The feeling of being unclean or smelly, and perhaps wearing incontinent aids will hamper a person's self image and may cause them to question their sexual attractiveness. Sex is regarded as a private and personal matter and like incontinence is also taboo. Discussing this dual problem needs to be conducted with delicacy. It is important to remember that clients who have to rely on pads or catheters may still wish to have a sex life, and if these are causing problems, help and counselling should be sought from a specialist.

RESEARCH BASED EVIDENCE

Veronica Haggar (1994, 1995) undertook a project in London's East End that examined ways that continence could be promoted among Bangladeshi women. Despite the importance of 'dryness' in their lifestyle, it showed that not only was there limited suitable information on the subject, but that many women would not seek medical help because their general practitioner was male. This study shows a need for special thought when helping ethnic minorities

---

Think of a secret that you have never divulged to anyone, not even your closest friend.

- *How would you feel if a situation arose where you had to tell someone?*
- *Keeping these thoughts in mind how would you feel if you were unable to control your bladder and or bowel?*
- *List the emotions that came to mind when you considered the two questions above, using these may help you to understand how the client you are assessing may be feeling.*
- *How would you feel if a person with a strong odour sat next to you on a bus?*
- *How would these feelings affect the advice and care you would need to give to a patient who is incontinent?*

PRACTICE
KNOWLEDGE

▶ ASSESSMENT OF URINARY INCONTINENCE

It has been shown at the beginning of this chapter that incontinence is a symptom and not a diagnosis and has multiple causes. Accurate assessment of the individual with incontinence is the key to a successful outcome (Winder, 1996). Ideally the assessment will be multidisciplinary, involving doctors, nurses, physiotherapists and occupational therapists in either the hospital or the community (Association for Continence Advice, 1993). However, a good nursing assessment provides a starting point. Although it does not need to be done by a nurse specialist, it should be carried out by someone with a sound basic knowledge of the subject (Colborn, 1994).

When assessing and caring for a client with elimination difficulties the nurse needs to understand how the client and his or her carer feels, and also be aware of her or his own feelings towards the situation. By pretending that there is nothing unusual happening and getting on with the job of clearing up, gives the impression that incontinence is not important enough to be discussed, and discourages clients mentioning their fears.

The environment where the assessment is made will also put the client at ease. The individual's own environment is preferable, but if this is not possible, a relaxed atmosphere somewhere private should be chosen. Make time for the assessment; if done in a rush the client will sense this and feel a nuisance. Using a mutually understood vocabulary will put the client and carer at ease. An assessment framework should include:

- ▶ the main complaint;
- ▶ urinary symptoms;
- ▶ medical history;
- ▶ bowel problems;
- ▶ mobility and dexterity;
- ▶ communication;
- ▶ environmental;
- ▶ diet and fluids;
- ▶ psychological;
- ▶ recreational;
- ▶ physical examination;
- ▶ residual volume;
- ▶ charting.

Each of these areas will be explored briefly.

▶ *Main Complaint*

It is important to gain the client's perspective in order to determine the severity of the problem to the client. Wetting a teaspoon a day into a panty liner may not seem much, but to certain individuals this loss of control can be devastating, both psychologically and socially. Therefore a discussion about when the problem started, whether this was associated with any particular event and how it affects lifestyle is a good starting point.

▶ *Urinary Symptoms*

Assess the bladder symptoms, and questioning should establish what type of urinary symptoms the client has. First an overall picture is needed, for example:

- how much and how often do you leak?
- when does it happen – on the way to the toilet? in bed? during intercourse?
- is the problem getting worse?
- do you have to wear a pad?
- have you ever seen anyone about your problem?

Then ask questions to establish more specific symptoms, for example:

- do you get any warning or do you have to rush to the toilet? (this will give an indication of urgency);
- stress incontinence may be determined by asking whether there is any leakage on exercise, laughing or lifting;
- getting the client to describe the stream of urine passed will enable the nurse to recognize whether there is a poor stream, hesitancy, dribbling, dysuria or haematuria;
- a description of the daily urinary pattern, the frequency of voiding and information about any night-time leakage are also needed;
- the client should be asked if he or she senses when the bladder is full and whether he or she needs to strain or apply pressure to empty the bladder.

Medical History

This should cover illnesses and surgery, especially for neurological, urological and gynaecological problems. A woman's menstrual history is taken, with details of the normal menstrual cycle and whether the problem is worse at a particular time during it. Similar information is obtained about the menopause in older women. The obstetric history (parity, weight of babies, type of delivery, if forceps were used) of a female client are noted to give an idea of the state of the pelvic floor. In men a history of prostatic problems is a vital part of assessment.

Bowel Problems

The client's normal bowel habit should be noted, covering the colour and consistency of the stool, how often the client defecates and the ease with which stool is passed.

Mobility and Dexterity

Any mobility difficulties making walking to or sitting on the toilet a problem, and poor dexterity making it difficult to open doors or to remove clothing must be explored.

Communication

Sight, hearing problems and any memory loss or confusion should be noted. In this and the previous assessment area, the nurse is looking for any problems the client has in answering the need to pass urine.

Environmental

The nurse needs to ask about the location of the toilet – up or downstairs? in or outdoors? the distance from the client's living area? The toilet itself may be the problem: is it the correct height? is it clean? how many people use the toilet? is it private? are there any problems that might deter the client from using it? Washing facilities should also be noted – can the client wash his or her hands after toileting, and if the client does have incontinence are there facilities to cope with the laundry? If the nurse is able to assess the client in his or her own home a clearer picture of the client's environmental circumstances can be obtained; embarrassment may cloud an assessment made purely in hospital or clinic.

▶ *Diet and Fluids*

Note the amount and type of fluid your client drinks to see whether he or she is drinking a sufficient amount and whether unsuitable fluids are being drunk, for example caffeine or fizzy drinks. A dietary history may reveal reasons for constipation (see Chapter 3.2 on nutrition).

▶ *Psychological*

The client's attitude to the problem is important and if the client is reliant on a carer it is worth finding out the carer's feelings about the incontinence problem. Note anything in the client's mental state that could encourage incontinence, whether the client is confused and if so how severe the confusion is, whether the client has memory loss? and whether the client is depressed or anxious?

▶ *Recreational*

The attitude of clients to their incontinence and to what extent it has affected their lives should be explored. Has it stopped them going out socially? Has it caused problems at work? Has it affected their family relationships? Has it caused sexual difficulties? This part of the assessment will begin to give a true picture of the patient's problem and must be included in the planning of treatment and care.

If information has to be obtained from a carer because the client is confused or unable to give a comprehensive history then factors like the behaviour of the client when he or she needs the toilet and whether the client can identify a suitable place to urinate should be recorded.

▶ *Physical Examination*

A nursing assessment should include a basic examination of the client, but the nurse must remember that the patient may find a physical examination embarrassing. The perineal area should be examined for signs of infection, prolapse, vaginitis and urethritis. If a more detailed examination of the vagina or rectum is needed the client should be referred to an experienced nurse (Addison, 1995).

Vital signs (temperature and blood pressure) should be taken and urinalysis performed to check for conditions such as diabetes mellitus or urinary tract infection. If there is any indication of infection, a specimen of urine should be sent for culture to check for infective organisms.

▶ *Residual Volume*

A postmicturition residual volume of urine should be determined using either a nélaton catheter or ultrasound scanner as a non-palpable bladder does not mean an empty bladder. It is important to determine the residual volume on initial assessment as the symptoms of a client with an increased residual volume may mimic the symptoms of detrusor instability or stress incontinence. The wrong treatment may then be commenced and could cause damage, for example giving drug therapy to alleviate bladder spasm for a client with a high residual volume could result in a high-pressure bladder reflux and hydronephrosis.

▶ Charting

Following the physical examination a chart should be filled in, usually by the patient or a carer if this is not possible. The chart is the most useful nursing tool in assessing incontinence and has two main uses – as part of a baseline assessment and as a record of progress during treatment (Norton, 1986, p. 40). For accurate assessment the nurse must decide what information is needed – a record of times of voiding and episodes of incontinence or a frequency volume chart where the amount passed is recorded so that bladder capacity can be assessed as well. The fluid intake may also need monitoring if the nurse needs to assess whether the client is drinking enough (Figure 3.3.12).

▶ PROMOTING URINARY CONTINENCE

The main objective of nursing care is for a person to regain continence (Roe and Williams, 1994). Once the assessment has been completed the nurse will have a picture of the problems causing and being caused by incontinence and an action plan can be formed. This plan will depend on the type of incontinence and the client's physical, psychological and social ability to participate in this plan (Figure 3.3.13).

▶ Stress Incontinence

If a client has genuine stress incontinence, strengthening of his or her pelvic floor muscles will help the client regain or improve bladder control. This can be achieved by pelvic floor muscle exercises and/or electric stimulation (i.e. pelvic floor muscle re-education programme) (Laycock, 1992). Pelvic floor exercises are safe with no known risks (Roe and Williams, 1994) and should be a life-long habit for all women that should be started at school (Bonner, 1996)

Research has shown that in motivated women with no obvious prolapse experiencing small to moderate leakage of urine there is an 80% success rate using pelvic floor exercises (Norton, 1986a). Pelvic floor exercises can also be used for men following prostate surgery (Roe and Williams, 1994). Men can check that they are using the correct muscles by cupping a hand under the scrotum while exercising: the scrotal sac will rise and fall slightly with each contraction.

Figure 3.3.12: Charting.

1 BLADDER CHART
- Showing stress incontinence

Week commencing: 4/3/97   Name: A. Smith

Please tick in the **plain** column each time you pass urine

Please tick in the **shaded** column each time you are wet

Special instructions: *Chart for one week*

This chart shows near normal bladder frequency and wetting on exertion (ie getting out of bed) and coughing no nocturnal enuresis. Put E if leaking on exertion

	Monday		Tuesday		Wednesday		Thursday		Friday		Saturday		Sunday	
Midnight															
1am															
2															
3															
4															
5															
6			✓E	✓	✓		✓						✓		
7	✓E										✓		✓E		
8	✓		✓E		✓		✓		✓		✓E		✓	✓E	
9	✓	✓E	✓E		✓				✓		✓		✓	✓E	
10	✓				✓				✓		✓		✓		
11	✓		✓E		✓E		✓E		✓E		✓		✓	✓E	
Noon	✓				✓						✓		✓		
1pm			✓E		✓E		✓		✓		✓		✓		
2	✓E		✓E		✓				✓		✓		✓		
3	✓E		✓E		✓E		✓E		✓		✓		✓	✓E	
4	✓		✓		✓E		✓E		✓		✓		✓		
5	✓E		✓		✓E		✓E		✓		✓E		✓	✓E	
6	✓				✓						✓		✓		
7	✓		✓		✓E		✓E		✓		✓				
8	✓		✓E		✓E		✓E		✓		✓E		✓		
9	✓		✓		✓		✓		✓		✓		✓		
10			✓		✓										
11	✓E		✓E		✓E	✓	✓E	✓	✓E	✓	✓E		✓E	✓	
Totals	7	5	8	7	8	6	6	8	8	3	10	5	7	5

Compare with chart 3

2 BLADDER CHART
- Showing effect of pelvic floor exercises on stress incontinence

Week commencing: 17/6/97   Name: A. Smith

Please tick in the **plain** column each time you pass urine

Please tick in the **shaded** column each time you are wet

Special instructions:

After treatment of good fluid intake and pelvic floor exercises and suggestions to prevent constipation

	Monday		Tuesday		Wednesday		Thursday		Friday		Saturday		Sunday	
Midnight															
1am															
2															
3															
4															
5															
6			✓		✓						✓				
7	✓												✓		
8	✓		✓		✓		✓				✓		✓		
9	✓		✓		✓		✓		✓		✓		✓		
10	✓				✓		✓								
11	✓		✓		✓				✓		✓		✓		
Noon	✓		✓		✓		✓				✓		✓		
1pm	✓		✓		✓		✓		✓		✓		✓		
2	✓		✓		✓						✓				
3	✓		✓		✓		✓		✓		✓		✓		
4	✓		✓		✓		✓		✓		✓		✓		
5	✓		✓		✓				✓		✓				
6	✓		✓		✓		✓				✓		✓		
7	✓		✓		✓		✓		✓		✓		✓		
8	✓		✓		✓		✓		✓				✓		
9			✓		✓		✓		✓		✓		✓		
10	✓		✓		✓										
11			✓		✓		✓		✓		✓		✓		
Totals	7		7		8		7		6		7		7	1

3 BLADDER CHART

Week commencing: 3/5/97   Name: B. Green

Please tick in the **plain** column each time you pass urine

Please tick in the **shaded** column each time you are wet

Special instructions: *Chart as above plus measuring volume of void.*

This chart shows frequency, small bladder volume during day and some incontinence. - ie unstable bladder. Treatment: Increase fluid intake, decrease caffeine, bladder training and possibly medication

	Monday		Tuesday		Wednesday		Thursday		Friday		Saturday		Sunday	
Midnight															
1am															
2															
3					50										
4															
5															
6	300		350		250										
7							✓								
8	150		100		100										
9	50		60		80										
10	40		20		60										
11			60												
Noon		✓	40												
1pm	100		100		120										
2	30		30		40										
3	50		50												
4		✓	50		40		✓								
5	100		20		100										
6	60														
7	30		80		30										
8	50		10		70										
9	60		30		20										
10															
11	100		100		100										
Totals Vol.	13 1170	2	14 1050	3	13 1040	2									

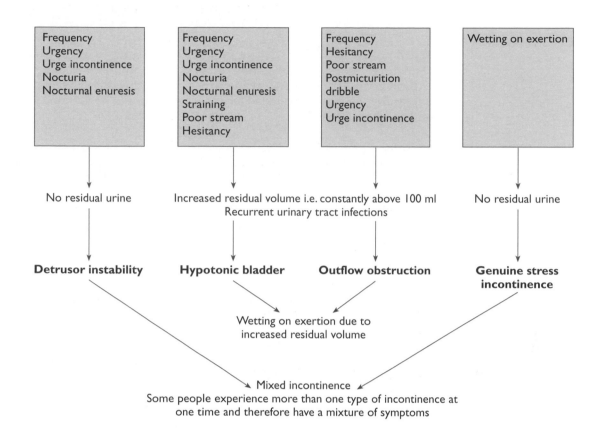

Figure 3.3.13: Flow chart for identifying the type of incontinence from the symptoms.

> Imagine yourself at a time when you feel anxious, for example awaiting an interview or driving test.
>
> • *Did you feel the need to pass urine on numerous occasions even though you only went ten minutes before?*
>
> • *How did you feel during the interview?*
>
> • *Did you need to pass urine after the interview?*
>
> • *How do you think an individual whose bladder is perma-nently in this state could retrain their bladder to a more normal pattern?*

Other treatments

Electrical stimulation involves the passage of electrical pulses between conductive electrodes applied in such a way that specific nerves and tissues are stimulated, helping to strengthen pelvic floor muscles. A 50% improvement in treatment is found with combined electrostimulation and pelvic floor exercises (Blowman *et al.*, 1991). Vaginal cones are weights the size of a tampon used to improve pelvic muscle tone. Once introduced into the vagina the pelvic floor contracts automatically to hold them in place. A well planned regimen using these cones will give a 60% improvement (Paettie *et al.*, 1988).

Detrusor Instability

Bladder training

Bladder training is used to promote continence in clients with frequency and urge incontinence. This treatment will restore the client's confidence in the bladder's ability to hold urine and to re-establish a more normal pattern. One method is to ask the client to 'hang on' between visits to the toilet for longer than they have been 'holding on' recently (Fader and Norton, 1994). It is thought that this improves the central nervous control of micturition (Kennedy, 1992). The client's goal should be to hold urine for approximately three hours. A sustained effort over a long period of time is necessary so the client will need support and encouragement (Moody, 1990). (For further information see Chiarelli (1992) and Roe and Williams (1994).)

▶ Fluid intake

When helping a patient with an unstable bladder you must always explain the importance of a good fluid intake in keeping the bladder properly expanded and preventing urine from becoming concentrated. Drinks containing caffeine cause bladder spasm and should be avoided (Creighton and Stanton, 1990).

▶ Drugs

Drug treatment in combination with bladder retraining will help promote continence in clients with an unstable bladder. They reduce the spasms of the detrusor muscle that cause urgency and urge incontinence by either decreasing parasympathetic action or increasing sympathetic action. Anticholinergic drugs have the first of these actions as they antagonize the parasympathetic neurotransmitter acetylcholine, for example oxybutynin. Tricyclic drugs have the second of these actions by prolonging the action of the sympathetic neurotransmitter, noradrenaline, for example imipramine. Imipramine is sometimes used for nocturnal enuresis, as is artificial antidiuretic hormone (desmopressin), which acts by reducing the volume of urine produced by the kidney and so when taken at night controls bedwetting (Table 3.3.4).

When in your mental health allocation, you will find tricyclic drugs used for patients with depression, reduction of bladder contractility may be a side effect, resulting in retention of urine. Other drugs used in the mental health branch of nursing also have this effect.

Drug treatment for outflow incontinence is limited, but alpha blockers block the noradrenaline action of the sympathetic innervation at the bladder neck, so reducing the sphincter resistance to the urine flow, for example indoramin. The use of intermittent catheterization has, however, reduced the need for drug therapy for hypotonic bladder (see Table 3.3.4). There are more specific drugs for enlarged prostate (see Table 3.3.4).

Oestrogen therapy can be used in menopausal and postmenopausal women to help stress incontinence. It increases the activity of alpha receptors in the lower bladder and sphincters to work more effectively and prevent leaking (Miodrag *et al.*, 1988).

DECISION MAKING

Drugs are useful in the promotion of continence, but there are medications that may influence bladder function in some way and cause incontinence. The nurse should be aware of this. Below is a list of drug categories that may affect continence. Using the *British National Formulary* (British Medical Association and Royal Pharmaceutical Society of Great Britain, 1997), look up examples of these drugs and their side effects. From this information work out how they cause continence problems.

- *Drugs used for people with heart problems: diuretics, digoxin, beta blockers.*
- *Drugs used for people with mental health problems: antidepressants, sedatives.*
- *Other drugs: antiparkinsonism drugs, smooth muscle relaxants, analgesics especially those used for the terminally ill, alcohol and caffeine.*

▶ *Toileting*

Toileting can be used in areas where incontinence has been found to be related to the behaviour of the client, and for those who are unable to ask to be taken to the toilet or are reliant on others to take them. It is useless to toilet a patient every two hours without having a prior knowledge of their voiding habits. For example a client may not require the toilet as often in the morning if he or she has not taken much fluid, but perhaps after lunch it may be essential to toilet him or her hourly for a few hours. Those clients on diuretic therapy will have differing toileting needs.

Charting is a very good method of ensuring the correct toileting pattern

Drug	Dose	Side effects
For detrusor instability		
Anticholinergic (antagonizes the parasympathetic action)		
Oxybutynin (has anti-spasmodic action as well)	2.5–5.0 mg bd–tds Start with minimum dose for the elderly	Dry mouth with foul taste Constipation
Tricyclic (prevent re-uptake of nor-adrenaline)		
Imipramine	50–75 mg nocte For nocturnal enuresis only use for 3 months at a time	Dry mouth Blurred vision Postural hypotension
Synthetic antidiuretic hormone		
Desmopressin Desmotabs	20–40 μg nasally 200–400 μg nocte orally	**Do not use if client has water retention**
For outflow incontinence		
Alpha Blockers (Block action of noradrenaline)		
Indoramin	20 mg nocte to 20 mg bd	Headache Drops blood pressure
Tamsulosin	0.4 mg daily	Minimal as drug is prostate specific
5 Alpha reductase inhibitors (androgen deprivation, shrinks benign hyperplastic tissue of prostate)		
Finasteride	5 mg daily	Decreased libido
For stress incontinence		
Oestrogens (increase the receptability of alpha receptor especially in the urethral sphincter)		
Oestrogen supplement therapy may be given: *Orally*, given cyclically with progesterone if the client has a uterus (this prevents endometrial stimulation) *Transdermally* (patches), again progesterone is added if uterus is still present *Topically*, administered as vaginal cream or pessaries		

Table 3.3.4 Drug treatment for incontinence.

is found and toileting is carried out at the necessary times. The individual needs to be encouraged to go to the toilet to pass urine either at the same time as they passed urine on the previous days or when they were incontinent of urine. Rigid regimens such as everyone is toileted after meals are best reserved for those people, usually the very demented, for whom all efforts at retraining have failed and where incontinence is intractable. Mass toileting is not only degrading, but ineffective. It does not take into account individual patterns of micturition and cannot lead to a restoration of independent continence. It may actually encourage clients to void before their full bladder capacity has been reached and could therefore impair normal bladder function.

▶ Nocturnal Enuresis

Children with nocturnal enuresis will need a specialized type of training. They should be assessed and a frequency–volume chart should be completed for approximately one week to determine if there are any medical problems and unusual voiding patterns. The principles of treatment include the following (Dobson, 1996):

- adequate fluid balance;
- avoidance of drinks containing caffeine, for example coffee, coca cola, and drinking chocolate, and avoidance of fizzy drinks, especially before bedtime;
- special charts, which award stars for each dry night, or for younger children, a colour chart where the reward is colouring part of a picture;
- buzzer alarms to wake the child, alerting them to the need to void;
- drug therapy (e.g. desmopressin, oxybutynin, imipramine).

Throughout the treatment, a positive attitude from the parents is essential to prevent negative feeling being transferred to the child (Dobson, 1996).

Sines (1996) suggests that parents of a child with learning disabilities begin toilet training at the same time as a normal child despite the fact that the child may be developmentally slow. It is often other factors, for example difficulties in walking, balance and dexterity that hamper the client gaining continence. The process of normalization and establishing the social role of a client is easier if the client has achieved continence (Boulter, 1995). Individual learning programmes can be introduced using the principles of behaviour modification. The programme may need to be broken into a series of smaller skills tailored to the client (Turner, 1988) and a suitable reward planned (Maleham, 1993). Full involvement of the clients, their carers, and key workers ensures a consistent approach to the plan (Boulter, 1995).

▶ ASSESSING FOR FAECAL INCONTINENCE

This assessment will follow a similar pattern to that discussed for urinary incontinence, especially the questions relating to mobility, environment, dexterity, psychological factors, fluid intake and diet. Those areas that differ are discussed below.

▶ *Main Complaint*

The following key issues are important:

- discover what term the client uses for defecation, and also what he or she understands by diarrhoea and constipation – people vary enormously in what they consider as a normal bowel action, both in terms of frequency and consistency (Alderman, 1988b);
- the client's normal defecation pattern should be noted – the frequency of passing stool, at what time of day and if there are any associated habits (e.g. reading the newspaper, smoking a cigarette);
- the client's perspective of the problem.

▶ *Defecation History*

This needs to include:

- a description of the faeces from the patient;
- nursing observation of the stool when possible;
- consistency of the stool – soft, loose;
- the shape of the stool – ribbon or sausage or pellet like;
- amount;
- ease of passing stool;

- does the client get rectal sensation of the need to defecate;
- does the client need to strain or is there pain on passing faeces;
- has the client noted any differences in the stool – a change in colour or consistency – or in the normal eliminating pattern (a black stool indicates gastrointestinal bleeding, pale stool indicates bilary problems, excess pus or mucus indicates inflammation, for example ulcerative colitis or Crohn's disease, altered bowel function may be due to a tumour).

Faecal Incontinence History

This needs to include:

- a description of how bad the incontinence is (light soiling, liquid stool etc.);
- how often the incontinence occurs;
- whether the client is aware that it is happening;
- whether the incontinence is due to urgency, and not being able to reach the toilet in time;
- whether the incontinence is associated with urinary incontinence;
- any foods that may cause constipation, diarrhoea, wind or stomach cramps;
- any foods that relieve the incontinence.

Medication History

A list of the client's drugs should be made as they may be responsible for constipation or diarrhoea. Details of any drugs taken for a bowel problem, particularly laxatives, must be taken, noting whether there is any laxative abuse as the colon may have become resistant to their effect or even atonic (Curry, 1992)

Physical Examination

The perineum should be observed for signs of prolapse or haemorrhoids. A rectal examination will show if the rectum is empty or full of hard, soft or loose stool. This nursing assessment will give a good picture of the problem and following the doctor's examination can be used to plan the management of the client. A good example of an assessment chart summarizing the above points can be found in *Faecal Incontinence* by Irvine (1996).

MANAGEMENT OF FAECAL INCONTINENCE

If the incontinence is due to impaction of faeces, the aim of treatment is twofold:

- first, to empty the rectum and colon;
- second, to avoid constipation and keep the rectum empty (Roe and Williams, 1994).

Emptying the rectum from below is carried out by giving daily enemas, either phosphate or micro enemas. Softener laxatives (Table 3.3.5) may be prescribed to treat the impaction from above, but care should be taken in the elderly if their faecal loading is soft to prevent an exacerbation of the problem (Barrett, 1992). Sodium picosulphate is a very strong

Name	Dose	Starts working after:	Action	Side effects and contraindications
(a) Osmotic Laxative				
Lactulose	10–15 ml bd	up to 2 days	It attracts water as it passes through the gut, softening the stool	Nausea and vomiting and problems with flatus
Fletchers' Phosphate Enema	1 × 128 ml enema	30 minutes	Increases water content causing rectal distension which stimulates motility	Local irritation. Avoid long term use. Contra-indicated in Hirschsprungs disease
Micro enemas (sodium citrate) e.g. Micolette, Micralax, Relaxit	30 minutes		Allows water to penetrate and soften the stool thus stimulating defecation	Local irritation, avoid long term use. Contra-indicated in inflammatory bowel disease
Stool softeners				
Docusate sodium	up to 5 × 100 mg capsules daily in divided doses	24 hours plus	It changes the surface tension of the stool allowing water to enter and soften it. This also has a stimulant effect	Abdominal cramps. Do not use over a long period of time, or in intestinal obstruction
Fletchers' Enemette (docusate sodium enema)	5 ml	20–30 minutes	As above	As above
Stimulant Laxative				
Senna	2–4 tablets nightly	24 hours plus	Increase rectal motility, i.e. increases peristalsis	Abdominal cramps, may colour the urine red. Do not use in intestinal obstruction
Danthron (Co-danthramer)	1–2 capsules nightly or suspension 5–10 ml at night	6–12 hours	As above	Abdominal cramps. May colour urine red. May cause cancer thus only use in elderly, or the terminally ill
Biscodyl tablets	10 mg nightly	10–12 hours	Increases rectal motility	Abdominal discomfort. Avoid prolonged use. Do not take at the same time as antacids
Biscodyl suppositories	10 mg in the morning	20–60 minutes	As above	
Bulking agents				
Bran		Up to 4 days	This attracts water increasing faecal mass and thus stimulating peristasis	Flatulence, abdominal distension, intestinal obstruction. **Adequate fluids are essential**
Ispaghula husk e.g. Fybogel Regulan	1 sachet bd 1 sachet 1–3 times a day	As above	As above	As above
(b) Anti-diarrhoeal agents				
Codeine phosphate	15–30 mg tds-qds		Stimulates opium receptors to decrease the gastro intestinal transit time	Short term use only. May produce morphine-like dependence. Not recommended for children
Loperamide	2 mg capsules after each loose stool up to 8 mg max		Synthetic opiate inhibits relaxation of the anal spincter thus retaining liquid stool	Short term use only. Do not use in liver disease, inflammatory disease, and children under 12 years

Table 3.3.5 Drug therapy for faecal incontinence: (a) in treating constipation and (b) in treating diarrhoea.

DECISION MAKING

Many people use laxatives, which they can buy over the counter in the chemist shop or even in the supermarket. You are asked for some health advice about their use.

- *Find out more about the different broad categories of laxatives and their action on the lower bowel.*
- *Decide which laxative would be appropriate if the stools are hard and which would be appropriate if the stools are soft.*

stimulant laxative that can be used to clear the bowel, but its strong action can cause incontinence until the bowel is clear, causing some clients distress. Occasionally manual evacuation is suggested, but this must only be used as a last resort by an experienced practitioner. There are serious risks associated with this procedure, for example stimulation of the vagus nerve causing dysrhythmias, stretching the anal sphincter, perforation of the colonic wall (Addison, 1995).

Simple improvement to a client's lifestyle may be enough to keep the bowel empty. The nurse has an important role in educating the patient, explaining the importance of a good fluid intake (2000 ml/day) and the dietary intake of roughage. The client should not eat too much bran without a good fluid intake as this may increase faecal loading in the elderly (Ardron and Main, 1990). The ways in which the client could increase their exercise can be discussed. A regular laxative may be needed, but must be used appropriately.

Those people who are unable to identify when their rectum is full are managed by planned constipation and evacuation. Constipation is drug induced using codeine phosphate or loperamide, and the bowel is then evacuated by laxatives or enemas. The nurse's role is to ensure that a regimen that fits the client's lifestyle is developed. Some paraplegic patients are able to recognize when they have a full rectum by non-rectal signs, for example increased heart beat, sweating, or flushing, and can remain continent if they can reach a toilet in time.

Restoring the anorectal angle to improve incontinence can be a more difficult problem, and surgery may be needed. Strengthening the pelvic floor by exercises concentrating on the anal area can be of some help as can electrical stimulation. Treatment of diarrhoea causing incontinence can be treated by drugs if investigations show this is appropriate (see Table 3.3.5)

▶ MANAGEMENT OF INCONTINENCE

There are clients who despite all efforts to regain continence never achieve it and clients who are too ill or frail to benefit from or indeed manage the treatment programmes recommended.

The aim of management should then be to ensure that the client keeps their dignity and self-esteem and that the client is socially acceptable by using pads, sheaths or catheters (Norton, 1986). All aids must prevent leakage of urine, faeces or any smell, be discreet under clothing and be comfortable to wear.

▶ *Absorbent Products*

These fall into three designs:

- ▶ body worn pads (all in one or fitted with pants);
- ▶ pads built into the gusset of normal style pants;
- ▶ pads placed on the bed or chair (Figure 3.3.14).

All these products may be disposable or reusable (White, 1995).

There is a range of pads, those absorbing small amounts (up to 80 ml) to suit mild stress incontinence or dribbling to those absorbing large amounts (up to 1000 ml) for heavy incontinence (White, 1995).

Pad type depends upon patient preference: older people may prefer the safety of large pads, younger patients may choose a slimmer one because

Figure 3.3.14: Types of disposable body worn pads.

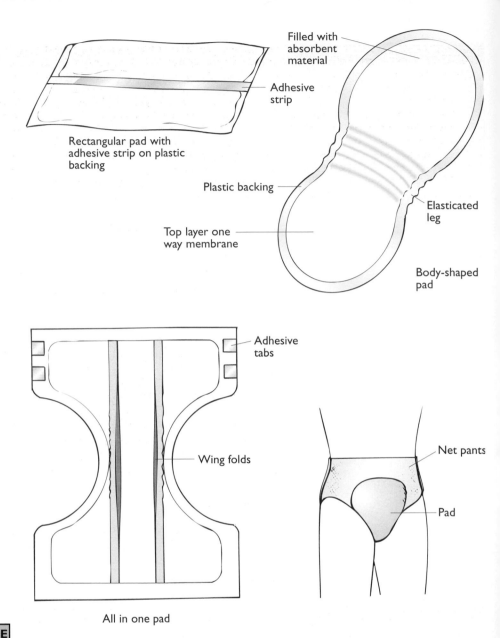

Rectangular pad with adhesive strip on plastic backing

Filled with absorbent material

Adhesive strip

Plastic backing

Top layer one way membrane

Elasticated leg

Body-shaped pad

Adhesive tabs

Wing folds

Net pants

Pad

All in one pad

RESEARCH BASED EVIDENCE

Clancy and Malone-Lee (1991) researched the absorbency of pads and showed that the construction of the pad and the way the pad is held in position are essential in preventing leakage of excreta.

Le Lievre and Addison (1995) surveyed the nursing knowledge and research on skin care of the incontinent client showing the complex nature of skin care. Measures to prevent overhydration of the skin, what sort of creams should be used, and if and when they were appropriate were discussed (see also Chapter 2.4 on skin integrity and Chapter 3.1 on personal hygiene).

of the appearance, and many men dislike pads, preferring alternative aids and sheaths.

Before applying a pad, the client should empty their bladder, even when wet, as contraction of the bladder maintains bladder tone and prevents residual volumes building up. Pads should be applied front to back, preventing contamination of the urethra by bowel flora. They must also be folded to form a valley shape to channel urine towards the most absorbent part of the pad.

Manufactures claim that reusable products, which are environmentally friendly, less bulky than disposables, easier to apply, can be washed frequently and are more cost-effective than disposables (McKibben, 1995), They also look like normal underwear, which is preferred by some clients. However, they are not suitable for faecal incontinence or heavy urinary incontinence.

'Disposable underpads or bedpads are possibly one of the least effective and most misused of all items that nurses use' (Norton, 1986, p. 257).

Disposable pads were designed to protect chairs and beds, and well applied body worn pads render these redundant. However, reusable bed or chair pads (Kylie sheets) are still widely used in residential homes and the community. They are thick and highly absorbent and suitable for heavy urinary (but not faecal) incontinence.

▶ *Sheaths*

Sheaths or condom urinals are often used by men in preference to pads. They are made of latex or silicone in different sizes, according to the diameter of the penis. Fitting correct sized sheaths is important as a device that is too small can restrict the blood flow to the penis, while one that is too large will fall off when urine is passed. The sheath is held in place by an adhesive which may line the sheath or be a separate coating. The sheath is then connected to a drainage bag. This type of aid is unsuitable for men with a small or retracted penis, symptomatic urinary tract infection or outflow obstruction.

▶ *Catheters*

A catheter is a hollow tube used for draining urine. Three types of catheter are used in practice – intermittent, indwelling and suprapubic.

▶ Intermittent catheters

According to O'Hagan (1996), the biggest single advance in the management of neurogenic voiding difficulties has been the introduction of intermittent catheterization. An intermittent catheter is a simple plastic tube with inlet holes at the tip and no balloon (i.e. a nélaton catheter), which is introduced periodically into the bladder to remove residual volumes greater than 100 ml in clients experiencing problems of overflow incontinence or recurrent urinary tract infection.

Intermittent catheterization is used in all areas of nursing where patients have problems with residual volumes of urine, for example for people with spinal injury or peripheral neuropathy, children with spina bifida, the elderly with hypotonic bladder tendencies and postoperatively.

The frequency of catheterization varies with each individual. Some people's residual volume of urine builds up slowly over a week, needing catheterization once or twice a week; others are frequently in retention and may need to catheterize 4–6 times a day. The timing of catheterization should aim to regain and maintain continence, avoid urinary tract infection and keep bladder volume below 400 ml (including the amount voided and the residual volume) (Alderman, 1988a).

Many clients self catheterize. To do this they must have a reasonable degree of manual dexterity, an ability to understand the procedure and motivation. However, if necessary the procedure can be performed very successfully by a carer. If a client or carer is using intermittent catheterization at home the infection rate is very low, but it is higher when carried out in hospital by nurses (Winder, 1992).

▌ Indwelling catheters

Indwelling (or Foley) catheters may be used for a client with chronic incontinence after all alternative methods of management have been unsuccessful or are inappropriate. Once this method has been decided it is imperative to prevent complications, for example infection, tissue damage and encrustation and blockage (Getliffe, 1997). This is achieved by assessing the client to ensure that the correct catheter size and type with a suitable drainage system is used (Figure 3.3.15). The length of time a catheter will be *in situ* will determine the most appropriate catheter material – either latex or Teflon-coated latex for short-term catheterization, while silicone or hydrogel-coated catheters are used for long-term catheterization. Catheters come in two lengths for males and females and with differing diameters, which are measured in Charrières (ch) (0.3 mm = 1 ch). Size 10–12 ch should be used for female clients, 12–14 ch for males and 6–10 ch for children. The smallest catheter possible should be used as one that is too large can cause bladder irritability, occlude urethral glands and cause ulceration of the bladder or urethra or strictures (Getcliffe, 1993). The catheter is held in place by a catheter balloon, volumes 5 ml, 10 ml and 30 ml: a smaller balloon minimizes bladder spasms and reduces residual volumes left in the catheterized bladder (Norton, 1986). A 10 ml balloon is used for most adults.

The most suitable drainage system selected for a client using a catheter for incontinence is a body worn drainage bag with a capacity of 350 ml to 750 ml as it will allow more independence (Getliffe, 1993).

▌ Suprapubic catheters

Suprapubic catheterization is becoming a more popular alternative to an indwelling catheter. The catheter (usually a Foley type size 16 ch) is inserted through a small cut in the abdominal wall just above the pubic bone and drains into an ordinary catheter bag (Iacovou, 1994). This method is used for urethral scarring, urinary retention, lifetime catheterization for incontinence and clients who wish to be sexually active.

▌ Catheter management

The natural defences against urinary tract infection (a common complication of catheterization) include the tightly closed folds of the urethra and the bladder's flushing action caused by regular emptying. The invasive nature of catheterization compromises these defences and bacteriuria is an inevitable consequence (Roe, 1992). Microorganisms gain entry to the bladder during catheterization by migrating along the catheter lumen from the collection bag and via the periurethral route between the mucosa and the catheter. To prevent this, catheterization must be aseptic, and once *in situ* the drainage system is closed, allowing free drainage but no bacterial entry unless broken (Garibaldi *et al.*, 1974) (see Figure 3.3.15).

All clients with catheters are encouraged to have a fluid intake of approximately 2000–3000 ml/day (Roe and Williams, 1994). Clients prone

• **Review your knowledge of catheter care using this textbook, other nursing texts and the following references – Crow et al. (1988), Barnett (1991), Falkiner (1993), Getliffe (1997).**

• **Reflect on your experience of caring for patients with catheters in the clinical areas where you have worked.**

• **Using the information gained above and illustrated in Figure 3.3.15, audit how well catheter care is managed in these clinical areas.**

Figure 3.3.15: Closed urinary drainage system.

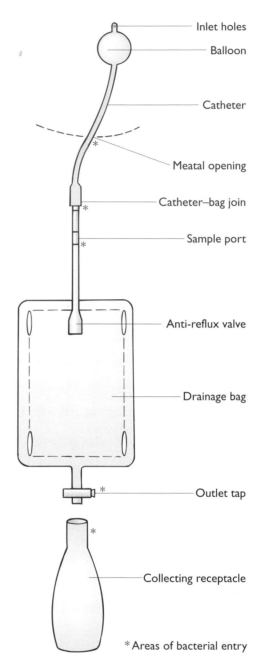

Inlet holes
Balloon
Catheter
Meatal opening
Catheter–bag join
Sample port
Anti-reflux valve
Drainage bag
Outlet tap
Collecting receptacle

*Areas of bacterial entry

DECISION MAKING

Until recently Ethel and Arthur Harris have led a very eventful life, for example travelling, entertaining friends and bowling. However, Arthur was then diagnosed as having prostatic cancer and has become ill quite quickly. Although Ethel has had a lot to come to terms with, she has decided to care for Arthur at home for as long as possible, but finds that she is unable to cope with the laundry as Arthur has recently become incontinent of urine. After a thorough assessment the district nurse, Ethel and Arthur have decided that an indwelling catheter would make life a lot easier. To help Ethel continue to care for Arthur at home she will need to feel confident in managing his catheter. The nurse will need to educate and support her in this.

- *Develop an educational programme for Ethel to help her cope with managing Arthur's continence care.*
- *Decide on what the priorities might be in care bearing in mind Arthur's prognosis.*

RESEARCH BASED EVIDENCE

Up to 50% of long-term catheterized patients experience blocking of their catheters due to encrustation. Getliffe (1994) researched this problem, finding that patients could be classified as 'blockers' or 'non-blockers' and recommended the identification of 'blockers' so that they could be assessed for the pattern of their 'catheter life'. By doing so, recatheterization could be planned before blocking and a suitable bladder washout regimen could be instigated.

to urinary tract infection may benefit from drinking cranberry juice as a preventive measure (Avorn *et al.,* 1994). Further complications associated with long-term catheterization and their management are listed in Table 3.3.6.

Problem	Cause	Action
Catheter not draining urine	Kink in tubing	Check tubing and reposition as necessary
	Drainage bag positioned above bladder	Reposition drainage bag below the bladder
	Drainage bag too full	Empty regularly as per procedure
	Inadequate fluid intake	Increase to approximately 10 drinks per day
	Constipation	Clear constipation (see text)
	Encrustation/blocked catheter	See below
Urine bypassing catheter (a) While catheter is still draining	Detrusor spasm due to:	
	Too large a catheter	Recatheterization with smaller catheter
	Too large a balloon	Recatheterization using catheter with smaller balloon
	Concentrated urine	Increase fluid intake
		Anticholinergic medication
		Bladder washouts not recommended
(b) When there is no drainage from the catheter	Debris	Intermittent bladder washouts
	Encrustation	Change catheter and observe tip for encrustation
		If this is an ongoing problem planned catheter changes should be adopted, see research based evidence
Bladder expelling the catheter	Balloon deflation	Replace catheter
	Detrusor spasm	Anticholinergic medication
	Poor support of drainage system	Check tapes etc. holding the catheter bag
	Self removal by client	Check for pain and discomfort
	Inflamation around catheter	Remove to allow inflammation to subside, check catheter material
Haematuria	Trauma	Monitor by observation, if bleeding becomes heavy seek medical advice immediately
	Infection	Urinalysis, urine sample for culture

Table 3.3.6 Some complications of catheterization.

PROFESSIONAL KNOWLEDGE

It is important to focus on the resources available to people with continence problems, the most significant being the Continence Advisory Service and its network of specialist nurses. In this part of the chapter there will be a discussion of the various roles of the specialist nurse in providing a quality service.

▶ THE CONTINENCE ADVISORY SERVICE

The attitudes of health professionals to continence and incontinence have changed dramatically over the last 30 years. By looking at the development of the continence advice service offered in the UK, reportedly the most comprehensive in the world (International Continence Society, 1993), the role of the hospital based and community nurse in promoting continence can be seen.

In 1974 the Disabled Living Foundation appointed the first continence advisor and by 1994 there were 400 (Beadle, 1996). During the 1970s awareness of the magnitude of the problem and the needs of the incontinent client grew, and through the 1980s, the aim of clinical practice changed from coping with incontinence to promoting continence. By the 1990s government policies recognized the need for a continence advisory service (White, 1997) This service has grown in a patchy fashion as no formal qualifications are necessary and there is no universal job description for a continence advisor post. The role often reflects the needs of

RESEARCH BASED EVIDENCE

Rhodes and Parker (1995) conducted a survey to provide basic quantitative information from continence advisors in the UK in order to ascertain their role. Continence advisors were found to have four main functions: education, management, clinical practice and research – too much for a single person to cover. In some areas this was resolved by forming a continence advisory team, whereas in other places the advisor had to relinquish part of the role, often the clinical and teaching role. The authors concluded that the increasing demands of the role would in the future require a multitiered service of a continence manager plus continence advisors and/or link resource nurses.

- **Investigate the Continence Advisory Service within the scope of your practice placements.**
- **Find out how it is managed and the range of services available to both institutional and community clients and patients.**
- **Compare the service available locally with the standards proposed in the Charter for Continence.**

RESEARCH BASED EVIDENCE

Cheater (1992a) studied the education, preparation and knowledge of nurses in continence promotion. She found that nurses irrespective of grade had insufficient knowledge on which to base good nursing practice and that both pre and postregistration education in continence care tended to be palliative with little thought to promoting continence.

the unit that funds them, for example urology, health care of the elderly or community services. The advisory service may be purely hospital or community based or run as a district service covering both (Rhodes and Parker, 1995). The formation of trusts in the UK in the 1990s, which separate hospital and community in some areas, may cause further fragmentation of the service.

Government policy has also helped to increase the profile of continence promotion. The white papers *Working for Patients* (Department of Health, 1989a) and *Caring for People* (Department of Health, 1989b) encourage the service to be part of an overall quality assurance programme (Roe, 1992). A review of these policies in 1991 found incomplete implementation of government policy and the *Agenda for Action for Continence Services* (Department of Health, 1991) was issued which identified the need for a seamless service from hospital to home (White, 1996). This was backed by the 1995 report of the Royal College of Physicians. In March 1995, a *Charter for Continence* was produced by the Association for Continence Advice (Figure 3.3.16) to state the standards of care clients should expect. A charter for children with bedwetting and daytime wetting and their families has also been drawn up by the Enuresis Resources and Information Centre (ERIC).

▶ EDUCATION FOR CONTINENCE PROMOTION

The first two points of the Association for Continence Advice continence charter emphasize there must always be individual assessment and care that is non-judgemental as has already been discussed. Other elements of the charter can be achieved by knowledgeable nurses and care professionals, with the continence advisor taking a key role. This role encompasses education of nurses, carers and the public, providing a consultation and information service, and clinical practice management and research (Rhodes and Parker, 1995).

'The prevalence of incontinence both urinary and faecal is such that it is impossible for all patients to be seen by an advisor' (Association for Continence Advice, 1993). 'Most continence management is within the scope of all nurses' (Beadle, 1996). Thus a scheme is needed with the clinical nurse specialist advising on difficult cases and teaching nurses so they can assess and treat the others, for example a link nurse system. This consists of a group of interested nurses from all areas of clinical practice headed by the continence advisor and provides a vehicle for the dissemination of knowledge and information and the introduction of new research-based skills.

Concern about the lack of education to promote continence was voiced by the Association for Continence Advice (1993) and the Royal College of Physicians (1995), not just in nursing, but for most health professionals. The English National Board (ENB) courses such as *Introduction to Promotion of Continence* are suitable for all nurses, and a longer programme is available for the specialist continence advisor. The National Vocational Qualification (NVQ) level three course in caring includes continence as part of its programme of training.

▶ QUALITY ASSURANCE OF CONTINENCE CARE

If the continence service is to be part of a quality assurance plan it must be prepared to be audited. For this to become a reality, all continence

Figure 3.3.16: Charter for continence.

CHARTER FOR CONTINENCE

The Charter for Continence presents the specific needs and rights of people with bladder or bowel problems. It outlines the resources available and the standards of care that can be expected.

As a person with bladder or bowel problems you have the right to:

▶ Be treated with sensitivity and understanding.
▶ Become continent if achievable.
▶ Receive a thorough individual assessment of your condition by a doctor or nurse knowledgable in this aspect of care.
▶ Request specialist advice about continence care.
▶ Be provided with a clear explanation of your diagnosis.
▶ Participate in a full discussion of treatment options, their advantages and disadvantages.
▶ Be provided with full, impartial information on the range of products which are available and how to obtain them.
▶ Expect products to have clear instructions for use.
▶ Receive regular reviews of treatment and be given the opportunity to change treatments if your condition has changed.
▶ Be made aware of any treatments or products as they become available.
▶ Be provided with a personal contact point able to give you on-going advice and support.

Developed by:
The Continence Foundation, InconTact, Association for Continence Advice (ACA), the RCN Continence Care Forum, the Enuresis Resource and Information Centre (ERIC), the Spinal Injuries Association and the Multiple Sclerosis Society.

Produced by an educational grant from Bard Limited.

March 1995

• *Find out if there is a 'link nurse' scheme in operation in your area and if there is a continence link nurse. What is the scope of his or her role?*

• *Find out if there are standards for continence promotion in your practice area. If available, how often are these standards monitored?*

advisors need to produce local standards and policies reflecting the quality of care delivered. These standards should encompass all practice areas. At ward level it could be a simple statement such as 'a registered nurse will complete an assessment using the locally recognized assessment form and plan the intervention or referral for that client' (Baker and Roe, 1992). To achieve such a standard, the continence advisor will need to ensure that suitable local forms are compiled and that education is available for the nurses, but the individual nurse must also be responsible for enhancing his or her knowledge to assess and care for these clients (see Boulter, 1997).

▶ COST-EFFECTIVENESS IN CONTINENCE CARE

The continence advisor also has responsibilities for budgeting, part of which is controlling expenditure on continence products (Beadle, 1996), which fall into four categories:

▶ products to promote continence (e.g. raised toilet seats);
▶ products to treat incontinence (e.g. electrostimulators);
▶ products to contain incontinence (e.g. absorbent pads);
▶ products to manage the effects of incontinence (e.g. deodorizers).

These products can be obtained by various methods such as by private purchase from a pharmacy or supermarkets, from the drug tariff (FP10) prescribed by the general practitioner, from health authority supplies or from joint NHS and social services. The products available on drug tariff are the same throughout the country, but the products obtained from the other sources may vary from area to area depending on clinical trials, preference of clients and cost.

Ideally, only products that have been researched thoroughly should be chosen, but lack of good research on products makes this impossible, so individuals should be guided by a knowledgeable nurse and information from NHS supplies and the DoH. The manufacturers do sponsor research, but this may not give a true picture (Baker and Roe, 1992). They can, however, be a good resource for product information, for example instruction booklets and videos. All products should conform to British or international standards where they exist.

Each individual NHS trust can choose the products that suit their requirements, but this choice may not be the same as that of the individual consumer as resources are not always available to cope with demand (White, 1997). This can be an advantage, but can cause problems for the clients, for example when being discharged into the community from hospital where the product that has been used in hospital is unavailable, and vice versa. Therefore good liaison between the hospital and the community is essential.

▶ RESEARCH INTO CONTINENCE CARE

Finally, research is a key function of continence advisors as they are in a position to collect data on for example the effectiveness of products and quality of care. However, there remains an urgent need for well-designed multidisciplinary research studies (Beadle, 1996). Rhodes (1995) found that continence advisors found difficulty in fulfilling this role. Baker and Roe (1992) suggest that this may be due to a lack of research training or because managers do not recognize research as an essential part of the continence advisor's role.

A well-run continence advice service backed by knowledgeable nurses will provide a client with continent problems with the rights stated in the *Patient's Charter* (NHS, 1989).

DECISION MAKING

Choose one area of this chapter that has interested you.
- *List the knowledge and skills needed to ensure good patient care in this area.*
- *Using one of your clinical placements assess the knowledge of the different grades of staff using your list.*

Now put yourself in the position of the continence link nurse and describe your action either:
- *In an area where you feel that nursing practice is at a good standard – how would you ensure that the staff are updated with new developments? or;*
- *In an area where knowledge and skills are not up to date – decide what you need to introduce or improve; how would you disseminate your knowledge and skills to improve standards in this area? what improvement would you expect in client or patient care and how could you monitor this to evaluate your education?*

REFLECTIVE KNOWLEDGE

To be an effective decision maker in relation to continence care, the nurse needs knowledge and skills in the area of continence promotion and the management of incontinence. An understanding of the altered physiology, the psychosocial pressures and the many possible causes for both urinary and faceal incontinence in all age groups is a prerequisite to making an accurate and sensitive assessment of the adult or child who has problems in maintaining continence. A knowledge of the resources available, both physical and human, is essential in order to provide quality care and a cost-effective service. Under the guidance of specialist nurses and the continence advisory service, all nurses with the requisite knowledge and skills from all branches of nursing can provide good standards of care for their clients. Sensitivity to each individual client's need for support and privacy is essential in this area of nursing practice. All nurses have a responsibility to update their knowledge and skills in continence care.

▶ REFLECTION AND CONSOLIDATION

Reflective exercises have been provided throughout the chapter. By completing these exercises and also keeping a reflective journal of your practice learning you will build up your knowledge base and expertise.

▶ CASE STUDIES

In this final part of the chapter, case studies are presented with related decision-making questions in order for you to consolidate the knowledge you have gained from this chapter and your experiences in the practice setting.

▶ CASE STUDY: ADULT

Mrs Macdougal is a 55-year-old teacher with three children. On many occasions while at work she has been left in an embarrassing situation on carrying out simple everyday jobs such as lifting books, writing on the board and running for the bell as she has found she has been unable to stop herself passing urine. Feeling embarrassed she has not mentioned the problem to her husband as he works abroad and only returns home every 12 weeks. She finally decides to visit her doctor after her husband's last visit as she found intercourse very uncomfortable and on one occasion when having sex she passed a small amount of urine. This was not enough for her husband to notice, but left her feeling ashamed and dirty. It also marred the visit, making her husband feel very confused.

■ **Using the assessment tool described in the chapter try and identify Mrs Macdougal's problems.**

■ **A frequency/volume chart showed that Mrs Macdougal was passing urine approximately 13 times a day. She passed between 100–200 ml** each time and was incontinent 2–3 times a day on exertion. Using this information and the problems you have identified, decide on an action plan for this lady.

▶ CASE STUDY: LEARNING DISABILITIES

Tom Simpson is 26 years old and has mild learning disabilities. He lives at home with his widowed mother. He is six feet tall and although he likes his food he is not overweight. Three days a week he is picked up by taxi and taken to a day centre. A midday meal is provided at the day centre, but Tom is rather fussy and will only eat chips with either fish fingers or beef-burgers. He takes the rest of his meals at home. Recently he has been rather difficult and will only eat toast or cheese sandwiches and drinking only small amounts of coca cola. Tom's main interest is collecting Matchbox cars and taking the dog for a walk with his mum. Unfortunately four months ago the dog was killed on the road. Tom's mother does not want to replace it as she suffers from arthritis and was finding it diffi-cult to care for the dog. Recently Tom has been messing his pants faecally. When this was investigated he was found to be faecally impacted with overflow and this has now been resolved by the community nurse.

- ■ Review how the community nurse might have dealt with the immediate problem of the incontinence.

- ■ Plan how you could prevent this incontinence occurring again by adapting Tom's lifestyle.

- ■ Debate the long-term support Tom might need should his mother not be able to care for him in the future.

▶ CASE STUDY: MENTAL HEALTH

Mrs Greenwood, aged 83 years, suffers from senile dementia and lives in a residential home. She is confused, but not aggressive and tends to wander. Over the last three months, she has been wandering much more than before and appears very anxious. Her general practitioner has prescribed medication to calm her down. Yesterday she became abusive and hit her grandson when he visited. The carers in the home have noticed that Mrs Greenwood is sometimes wet during the day.

- ■ Using an assessment tool, decide what Mrs Greenwood's presenting problem is.

- ■ Remembering that Mrs Greenwood may not be able to give a full history, plan how you would involve the carers and list what non-verbal cues may give you information about her toileting pattern.

- ■ Using the above information, what would be the factors causing Mrs Greenwood's incontinence?

■ Suggest ways these problems could be better managed or resolved.

■ What would you need to teach the carers from the residential home to ensure this improved management is continued?

CASE STUDY: CHILD

Matthew, aged eight years, is a persistent bedwetter who has never been dry before, but would like to be. Mum has coped very well up to now and never asked for any help, but as Matthew now has a chance to go to cub camp, she feels it is time for her son to get some form of treatment. Mum herself remembers having the same problem as a child, but Amy his six-year-old sister was dry at night by four years of age. She often teases her brother about his wetting. Matthew is beginning to show behavioural problems.

■ Identify the key points you would note in the assessment?

■ What treatment options may be available for Matthew?

■ What advice or explanation would you give to Matthew's mother?

▶ ACKNOWLEDGEMENTS

Thanks to Emma Cook, Nottingham Community Health Trust; Anita Counsell, Nottingham City Hospital NHS Trust and Nottingham Health Care NHS Trust.

▶ ANNOTATED FURTHER READING

BARRETT, J.A. (1993) *Faecal Incontinence and Related Problems in the Older Adult.* London. Edward Arnold.
A textbook that thoroughly explores the problem of faecal incontinence.
CHIARELLI, P. (1992) *Womens Water Works.* Dereham. Neen Health Care Books.
This is a self-help book written for motivated clients. It also provides nurses with good information about female continence problems and a good description of conservative treatments that can help when educating clients. There is a good description of bladder training regimens in Chapter 7.
CHIARELLI, P., MARKWELL, S. (1992) *Lets Get Things Moving (Overcoming Constipation).* Dereham. Neen Health Care Books.
Similar style to the previous book, but covering the problems of constipation.
COLBURN, D. (1994) *The Promotion Of Continence In Adult Nursing.* London. Chapman.
A good textbook that covers ways of promoting continence and managing incontinence in the adult. Particularly useful for adult branch students.
GETLIFFE, K., DOLMAN, P. (1997) *Promoting Continence.* London. Baillière Tindall
A fuller explanation of audit can be found in Chapter 11 (Quality Assurance in Continence Care) of this very informative book. A full discussion on catheters and their drainage systems is found in Chapter 8. Chapter 5 (Mainly children: childhood enuresis and encopresis) is useful for Child Branch students.
NORTON, C. (1996) *Nursing For Continence,* 2nd edition. Beaconsfield. Beaconsfield Press.

This book covers most areas of incontinence. There are chapters suitable for child branch (Chapter 5) and learning disabilities branch (Chapter 4) and continence care for people with physical disabilities (Chapter 13)

ROE, B.H. (1992) *Clinical Nursing Practice. The Promotion and Management of Continence*. Hemel Hempstead. Prentice Hall.

A good book covering all aspects of both urinary and faecal incontinence. Well researched and provides many useful references.

ROE, B., WILLIAMS, K. (1994) *Clinical Handbook for Continence Care*. London. Scutari Press.

A short clear overview of continence problems. There are simple descriptions of bladder training schemes in Chapter 2.

STOKES, G. (1987) *Incontinence and Inappropriate Urination (Common Problems with the Confused Elderly)*. Bicester, Oxon. Winslow Press.

This book is useful for all nurses who are caring for confused or demented clients, giving an overview of incontinence they may suffer and ways of assessing, promoting continence and managing incontinence.

WHITE, H. (1995) In control with incontinence aids. *British Journal of Nursing* **4(6)**: 334–338.

The designs for absorbent pads are fully discussed in this article

▶ REFERENCES

ANDERSON, J. (CHAIRMAN), ABRAMS, P., BLAIVAS, J.G., STANTON, S.L. (1988) The standardization of terminology of the lower urinary tract function. *Scandinavian Journal of Nephrology, Supplementation* **114**: 5–19.

ADDISON, R. (1995) *Continence Care Forum – The Role Of The Nurse In Digital Examination of The Rectum And Manual Removal Of Faeces*. London. Royal College of Nursing.

ALDERMAN, C. (1988a) DIY catheters freedom. *Nursing Standard* **2**: 25–26.

ALDERMAN, C. (1988b) Faecal incontinence. *Nursing Standard* **2(29)**: 32–34.

ARDRON, M.E., MAIN, A.N.H. (1990) Management of constipation. *British Medical Journal* **300**: 1400.

ASSOCIATION FOR CONTINENCE ADVICE (ACA) (1995) *Sexuality and Incontinence: Professional Issues*. London. Association for Continence Advice.

AVORN, J., MONANE, M., GURWITZ, J.H., GLYNN, R.J., CHOODNOVSKIY, I., LIPSITZ, L.A. (1994) Reduction of bacteriuria and pyuria after ingestion of cranberry juice. *Journal of the American Medical Association* **271(10)**: 751–754.

ASSOCIATION FOR CONTINENCE ADVICE (ACA) (1993) *Guidelines for Continence Care*. London. Association for Continence Advisors.

BAKER, K.E.M., ROE, B.H. (1992) Setting up a continence advisory service. In Roe B.H. (ed.) *Clinical Nursing Practice. The Promotion and Management of Continence*. pp. 220–230. Hemel Hempstead. Prentice Hall.

BARNETT, J. (1991) Preventive procedures. *Nursing Times* **87(10)**: 67–69.

BARRETT, J. (1992) Faecal incontinence. In Roe B.H. (ed.) *Clinical Nursing Practice. The Promotion and Management of Continence*. pp. 196–219. Hemel Hempstead. Prentice Hall.

BAYLISS, H. (1996) Incontact public education programme main findings. *ACA Newsletter* **Summer**: 21–22.

BAYLISS, V. (1996) Female urinary incontinence. In Norton, C. (ed.) *Nursing for Continence*. 2nd edition, pp. 123–150. Beaconsfield. Beaconsfield Publishers.

BEADLE, J. (1996) Continence is everybody's business. In Norton, C. (ed.) *Nursing for Continence*. 2nd edition, pp. 365–382. Beaconsfield. Beaconsfield Publishers.

BENDALL, M.J. (1989) Faecal Incontinence. Wallace Teaching Pack. No. 9. Teaching pack for continence advisors. Colchester. Wallace.

BLACKWELL, C. (1989) *A Guide to Enuresis UK*. Enuresis Resource and Information Centre.

BLISS, J., WATSON, E. (1992) A basis for change. *Nursing Times* **88(13)**: 69–70.

BLOWMAN, C., PICKLES, C., EMERY, S. (1991) Prospective double blind controlled trial of intensive physiotherapy with and without stimulation of the pelvic floor, in the treatment of genuine stress incontinence. *Physiotherapy* **77(10)**: 661–664.

BONNER, L. (1996) *Pelvic Awareness Training Package*. (Oral Abstract presented at A.C.A. Conference.) Association of Continence Advice.

BOULTER, P. (1995) Increasing independence. *Nursing Standard* **10(4)**: 18–20.

BOULTER, P. (1997) What is audit. In Getliffe, K., Dolman, P. (eds) *Promoting Continence*. pp. 410–434. London. Baillière Tindall.

BRITISH MEDICAL ASSOCIATION AND ROYAL PHARMACEUTICAL SOCIETY OF GREAT BRITAIN (1995) *British National Formulary*. London. BMA and RPSGB

BROCKLEHURST, J.C. (1984) Urinary incontinence in the elderly. *The Practitioner*. **228**: 275–282.

BROOMFIELD, J.W., DOUGLAS, J.W.B. (1956) Bedwetting: Prevalence amongst children aged 4–17. *Lancet* **1**: 850–852.

CARDOZO, L., CUTNER, A., WISE, B. (1993) *Basic Urogynaecology*. Oxford. Oxford Medical Publications.

CHEATER, F.M. (1992a) Nurses education preparation and knowledge concerning continence promotion. *Journal of Advanced Nursing* **17**: 328–338.

CHEATER, F.M. (1992b) The aetiology of urinary incontinence. In Roe B. (ed.) *Clinical Nursing Practice. The Promotion and Management of Continence*. pp. 20–40. Hemel Hempstead. Prentice Hall.

CHIARELLI, P. (1992) *Womens Waterworks – Curing Incontinence*. Dereham. Neen Health Care Books.

CHIARELLI, P., MARKWELL, S. (1992) *Lets Get Things Moving, Overcoming Constipation*. Dereham. Neen Health Care Books.

CLANCY, B., MALONE-LEE, J. (1991) Reducing the leakage of body worn incontinence pads. *Journal of Advanced Nursing* **16**: 187–193.

COLBORN, D. (1994) *The Promotion of Continence in Adult Nursing*. London. Chapman and Hall.

CONCISE OXFORD DICTIONARY (1978) Oxford. Clarendon Press. p. 546.

CREIGHTON, S., STANTON, S.I. (1990) Caffeine: does it affect your bladder? *Journal of Urology* **66**: 613–614.

CROW, R., MULHALL, A., CHAPMAN, R.G. (1988) Indwelling catheterisation and related nursing practice. *Journal of Advanced Nursing* **13**: 489–495.

CUNNINGHAM, S., NORTON, C. (1993) *All Mod Cons. Public In-Conveniences; Suggestions for Improvements.* London. The Continence Foundation.

CURRY, T. (1992) Drugs and Constipation; a View from Pharmacy. *Prescriber* **May**: 53–55.

DEPARTMENT OF HEALTH (1989a) *Working for Patients.* London. Her Majesty's Stationery Office.

DEPARTMENT OF HEALTH (1989b) *Caring for People.* London. Her Majesty's Stationery Office.

DEPARTMENT OF HEALTH (1991) *An Agenda for Action on Continence Services.* London. Her Majesty's Stationery Office.

DIOKNO, A.C., SANDO, L.P., HORRIDANDER, J.B., LAPIDES, J. (1983) Fate of patients started on clean intermittent self catheterisation therapy ten years ago. *Journal of Urology* **129**: 1120–1122.

DOBSON, P. (1996) Childhood enuresis. In Norton, C. (ed.) *Nursing for Continence* (2nd edition). pp. 102–118. Beaconsfield. Beaconsfield Publishers.

EISBERG, H. (1995) Assignment of dominant inherited nocturnal enuresis (ENURI) to chromosome 13q. *Nature Genetics* **10(3)**: 354–356.

FADER, M., NORTON, C. (1994) *Caring for Continence, a Care Assistant's Guide.* London. Better Care Guides. Hawker Press.

FALKINER, F.R., WILSON, M. (1994) The insertion and management of indwelling urethral catheters – minimising the risk of infection. *Journal of Hospital Infection* **25**: 79–90.

FENELEY, R.C.L. (1986) Normal micturition and its control. In Mandelstam (ed.) *Incontinence and its Management.* Kent. Croom Hall.

GARIBALDI, R.A., BURKE, J.P., DICKMAN, M.L., SMITH, C.B. (1974) Factors predisposing to bacteruria during indwelling catheterisation. *The New England Journal of Medicine* **29 (5)**: 215–219.

GETLIFFE, K. (1993) Informed choices for long term benefits, the management of catheters in continence care. *Professional Nurse* **9(2)**: 122–126.

GETLIFFE, K.A. (1994) The characteristics and management of patients with recurrent blockage of long term urinary catheters. *Journal of Advanced Nursing* **20**: 140–145.

GETLIFFE, K. (1996) Care of urinary catheters. *Nursing Standard* **11(11)**: 47–50.

GETLIFFE, K. (1997) Catheters and catheterisation. In Getliffe K., Dolman, P. (eds) *Promoting Continence.* pp. 281–342. London. Baillière Tindall.

HAGGAR, V. (1995) Strong developments. *Nursing Times* **91(33)**: 53–55.

HINCHLIFF, S. (1988) The acquisition of nutrients. In Hinchliff, S. and Montague, S. (eds) *Physiology for Nursing Practice.* pp. 395–440. London. Baillière Tindall.

HINCHLIFF, S., MONTAGUE, S. (1988) *Physiology for Nursing Practice.* p. 538. London. Baillière Tindall.

HERBERT, R.A. (1991) The biology of human aging. In Redfern, S. (ed.) *Nursing Elderly People.* p. 47. Edinburgh. Churchill Livingstone.

IACOVOU, J.W. (1994) Suprapubic catheterisation of the urinary bladder. *Hospital Update* **March**: 159–161.

INTERNATIONAL CONTINENCE SOCIETY (1993) Workshop: Continence Organizations Worldwide. *International Continence Society 23rd Annual Meeting.* Rome. September.

IRVINE, L. (1996) Faecal incontinence. In Norton, C. (ed.) *Nursing for Continence* (2nd edition). pp. 226–254. Beaconsfield. Beaconsfield Press.

KALVIN, I., MACKEITH, R.C., MEDOWS, S.R. (eds) (1973) *Bladder Control and Enuresis.* London. Heinmann Medical Books.

KENNEDY, A.P. (1992) Bladder re-education for the promotion of continence. In Roe B.H. (ed.) *Clinical Nursing Practice. The Promotion and Management of Continence.* pp. 77–93. Hemel Hempstead. Prentice Hall.

LAYCOCK, J. (1992) Pelvic floor re-education for the promotion of continence. In Roe B.H. (ed.) *Clinical Nursing Practice. The Promotion and Management of Continence.* pp. 95–127. Hemel Hempstead. Prentice Hall.

LE LIEVRE, S., ADDISON, R. (1995) *Continence Care Forum. Incontinence and Skin Care.* London. Royal College of Nursing.

LEWIS WALL, L. (1994) Anatomy and physiology of the pelvic floor. In Laycock J., Wyndale, J.L. (eds) *Understanding the Pelvic Floor.* Dereham. Neen Health Books.

MALEHAM T (1993) A dry run. *Nursing Times* **89(30)**: 66–67.

MALONE-LEE, J. (1989) *Anatomy and Physiology of the Lower Urinary Tract; Continence Information Pack.* Sponsored by H. G. Wallace Ltd and SimmsSmiths Industries Medical Systems.

MCKIBBEN, E. (1995) Pad use in perspective. *Nursing Times* **91(24)**: 61–62.

MIODRAG, A., CASTLEDEN, M., VALLANCE, T. (1988) Sex hormones and the urinary tract. *Drugs* **36**: 491–504.

MITTENESS, L.S. (1992) Social aspects of urinary incontinence in the elderly. *AORN Journal* **56(4)**: 731–737.

MOODY, M. (1990) *Incontinence: Patients Problems and Nursing Care.* Oxford. Heinemann.

MOHIDE, A.E. (1992) The prevalence of urinary incontinence. In Roe B.H. (ed.) *Clinical Nursing Practice. The Promotion and Management of Continence.* pp. 1–16. Hemel Hempstead. Prentice Hall.

NEWMAN, J.L. (1962) Old folks in wed beds. *British Medical Journal* **I**: 1824–1827.

NORTON, C. (1986) *Nursing for Continence.* Beaconsfield. Beaconsfield Press.

NORTON, C. (1991) Eliminating. In Redfern S. (ed.) *Nursing Elderly People.* Edinburgh. Churchill Livingstone.

NORTON, C. (1996) *Nursing for Continence,* 2nd edition. Beaconsfield. Beaconsfield Press.

O'HAGAN, M. (1996) Neurogenic bladder dysfunction. In Norton, C. (ed.) *Nursing for Continence* (2nd edition). pp. 170–191. Beaconsfield. Beaconsfield Press.

PEATTIE, A.B., PLEVNIK, S., STANTON, S.L. (1988) Vaginal cones, a conservative method of treating stress incontinence. *British Journal of Obstetrics and Gynaecology* **95(10)**: 1049–1053.

RHODES, P. (1995) The postal survey of continence advisors in England and Wales. *Journal of Advanced Nursing* **21**: 286–294.

RHODES, P., PARKER, G. (1995) The role of the continence advisor in England and Wales. *International Journal of Nursing Studies* **32(5)**: 423–433.

ROBBINS, B. (1985) The psychology of incontinence. *Journal of District Nursing* **16**: 36–37.

ROE, B., WILLIAMS, K. (1994) *Clinical Handbook for Continence Care.* London. Scutari Press.

ROE, B.H. (1992) Use of indwelling catheters. In Roe B.H. (ed.) *Clinical Nursing Practice. The Promotion and Management of Continence.* Hemel Hempstead. Prentice Hall. pp. 177–191.

ROYAL COLLEGE OF PHYSICIANS (1995) *Incontinence Causes and Management and Provision of Services.* London. Royal College of Physicians.

SANDFORD, J.R.A. (1975) Tolerence of debility in elderly dependents by supporters at home: its significance for hospital practice. *British Medical Journal* **3**: 471–473.

SIMMONDS, J.F. (1977) Enuresis: A brief survey of current thinking with respect to pathogenesis and management. *Clinical Paediatrics* **16**: 79–82.

SINES, D. (1993) Helping people with mental handicap. *Nursing Times* **79(33)**: 52–55.

SINES, D. (1996) Acquiring continence – supporting people with learning disabilities. In Norton, C. (ed.) *Nursing for Continence* (2nd edition). pp. 317–334. Beaconsfield. Beaconsfield Press.

SMITH, N.K.G., MORRANT, J.D. (1990) Post operative urinary retention in women: management by intermittent catheterisation. *Age and Ageing* **19**: 337–340.

SOBATA, A.E. (1984) Inhibition of bacterial adherence by cranberry juice; potential use for the treatment of urinary tract infection. *Journal of Urology* **131**: 1013–1016.

STOKES, G. (1987) *Incontinence and Inappropriate Urination (Common Problems with the Confused Elderly)*. Bicester, Oxon. Winslow Press.

TURNER, A.F. (1988) Incontinence in people with mental handicap. *Professional Nurse* **3(9)**: 348–352.

THOMAS, T., PLYMAT, K., BLANIN, J., MEAD, T. (1980) Prevalence of urinary incontinence. *British Medical Journal* **281**: 1243–1244.

WELLS, M. (1996) The development of urinary continence and the causes of incontinence. In Norton, C. (ed.) *Nursing for Continence* (2nd edition). pp. 12–16. Beaconsfield. Beaconsfield Press.

WHITE, H. (1995) In control with incontinence aids. *British Journal of Nursing* **4(6)**: 334–338.

WHITE, H. (1997) Incontinence in perspective. In Getliffe, K., Dolman, P. *Promoting Continence*. pp. 1–22. London. Baillière Tindall.

WINDER, A. (1992) Intermittent catheterisation. In Roe, B. (ed.) *Clinical Practice. The Promotion and Management of Continence*. Hemel Hempstead. Prentice Hall.

WINDER, A. (1996) Assessment and investigations of urinary incontinence in Norton, C. (ed.) *Nursing for Continence*, 2nd edition. Beaconsfield. Beaconsfield Press.

WONG, D.L. (1993) *Essentials of Paediatric Nursing*, pp 349–352. London. Mosby.

3.4 Mobility

D. Nichol

KEY ISSUES

■ SUBJECT KNOWLEDGE
- the meaning of mobility
- biological components of human mobility
- movement and exercise
- developmental changes in mobility
- the physical effects of immobility
- the psychosocial effects of immobility

■ PRACTICE KNOWLEDGE
- multidisciplinary assessment of mobility
- implementing mobility care
- aspects of implementation of care

■ PROFESSIONAL KNOWLEDGE
- nursing responsibilities in mobility care
- implications of the *Disability Discrimination Act 1995*
- facilities for mobility care

■ REFLECTIVE KNOWLEDGE
- using mobility aids and appliances
- experiencing and understanding the difficulties of mobility impairment
- case studies in decision making related to the immobile client in all branches of nursing

▶ INTRODUCTION

Mobility is a relative term. It is most frequently used in the context of nursing to refer to physical mobility. Most of us take this for granted. We get up in the morning without thinking about what we are doing and without restrictions or limitations, and our expectation is that full mobility will continue. For most of us this is true, but for some mobility requires great effort, and for others it is impossible without assistance or impossible even with assistance. The groups of people who have difficulty mobilizing will be the focus of attention in this chapter, and the aim is to gain a greater appreciation and understanding of those less physically able than ourselves. By doing this, the future may be brighter for these people, as we may then start to wake up in the morning and think about what we have and not take our mobility for granted. Mobility and its maintenance, no matter what branch of nursing you work in, takes up a large proportion of nursing time and daily decision making for providing the most effective care.

▶ OVERVIEW

▶ Subject Knowledge

The biological section includes relevant anatomy and physiology of the musculoskeletal and nervous systems and the physical effects of exercise and immobility. The psychosocial section considers the developmental aspects of mobility and the psychosocial effects of immobility as well as the related attitudes, both societal and individual, towards the mentally and physically impaired.

▶ Practice Knowledge

This part involves a multidisciplinary assessment of the extent and risks of immobility for both the mentally and physically impaired. It identifies several assessment tools and appropriate aids for different situations and environments. Planning the intervention of mobility assistance and its implementation and evaluation for effective care in all branches of nursing are also covered.

▶ *Professional Knowledge*

Issues surrounding the nurse's accountability in mobility care are explored. There is a review of our responsibilities in relation to our knowledge of health promotion and advice for the immobile. Also included is knowledge of the political arena relating to policies aimed at supporting the disabled and proactive intervention in policies such as the *Disability Discrimination Act* of 1995.

▶ *Reflective Knowledge*

In this section you are encouraged to carry out exercises to experience and appreciate some of the problems associated with immobility. Exploration and discussion through the use of case study and decision making exercises will also be of great value if you participate.

On pp. 444–446 there are four case studies, each one relating to one of the branch programmes. You may find it helpful to read one of them before you start the chapter and use it as a focus for your reflections while reading.

SUBJECT KNOWLEDGE

After outlining some definitions of mobility and demographic trends related to immobility the first part of Subject Knowledge will focus on an overview of anatomy and physiology related to mobility, including that of the musculoskeletal system and the microscopic structure of bone, joints and muscles and how they function in mobility. The physical effects of immobility will also be addressed.

▶ DEFINITIONS

Mobility is described by The Chambers Dictionary as 'Quality or power of being mobile; freedom or ease of movement' (Schwarz, 1995) and by Collins English Dictionary as 'The ability to move physically: a handicapped person's mobility may be limited' (Makin, 1991). Mobilization, on the other hand, is seen as the rendering of a fixed part movable (Weller, 1989). Physical definitions, however, have more than physical effects and consequences. Immobility in a mobile world can affect not only physical health, but also psychological and social health. Our ideas of an optimum level of mobility change over time and are not necessarily the same in all cultures at the same point in time. Increasingly in developed countries, full mobility is seen as the norm and something to aim for and achieve. Anything less is seen as a failing or an abnormality. Under such circumstances, it is not surprising that anything less than full mobility can have devastating effects.

According to the Office of Population Censuses and Surveys (1995, p. 111) 8% of people in Britain reported having mobility difficulties, and this figure increased with age. It was seen as a problem by 30% of those aged 16–74 years and 80% of those aged at least 75 years. Of the 8% total, 7% considered that their mobility difficulties were permanent. Over 50% were restricted both indoors and outdoors.

With an increasing elderly population, it can be suggested that mobility problems will continue to increase in future years. The implications of increased immobility will mean a further need for resources that are already limited. Given this potential situation we may see major changes in the attitudes towards and effects upon the immobile population. These effects can be both negative and positive. A negative perspective views the increased need for government funding as a drain on limited resources. On the positive side, the greater number of immobile people may bring about changes because they become a more visible part of society and therefore possibly more powerful and acceptable to the able-bodied. However, we must not consider the immobile within a unidimensional context: although many are elderly, they are also women, children, unemployed, members of ethnic minorities and from different classes. Webb and Tossell (1991, p. 95) suggest that people can experience multiple marginalization through being a member of many disadvantaged groups at the same time. They may suffer from what has been referred to as triple jeopardy (Norman, 1985), for example from being elderly, disabled and black. We therefore cannot view mobility or immobility in isolation from the other influences upon us and the environment we share. Before we can understand abnormal mobility or immobility, however, we first need to understand the physical dimension.

Biological

▶ THE MUSCULOSKELETAL SYSTEM

To be physically mobile, you need bones, muscles, tendons, ligaments, joints and nerves. Each of these shall be considered in turn, but it must be remembered that although an impairment of one element can affect mobility, it can also affect the other elements.

The skeleton has five functions (Table 3.4.1) and the skeletal system is comprised of two types of connective tissue, bone and cartilage. The body is made up of 206 bones and microscopically consists of two types of bone: compact and cancellous.

Support	Provides a framework for soft tissue and attachment of muscles
Protection	Protects internal organs from external injury (e.g. the ribs and sternum protect the heart and lungs)
Movement	Muscles are attached to the skeleton and act as levers to produce movement
Storage of minerals	Minerals are stored in bone, which acts as a reservoir, ready for distribution when required (e.g. calcium and phosphorous)
Blood cell production	Red marrow in cancellous bone produces blood cells in the process known as haemopoiesis – mainly red blood cells, but some white cells and platelets are also produced

Table 3.4.1 Functions of the skeleton. (From Tortora and Anagnostakos, 1987, p. 120.)

▶ MICROSCOPIC STRUCTURE OF BONE

▶ *Compact Bone*

Compact bone (Figure 3.4.1) is also referred to as Haversian bone in which nerves and blood vessels enter through the structure of Volkmann's canals, leading to the central canals within the compact structure, called

Figure 3.4.1: Microscopic structure of bone.

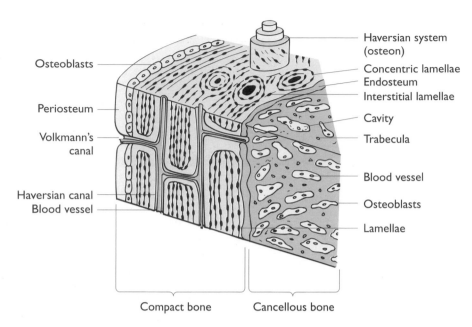

Haversian canals. These canals are surrounded by concentric rings of lamellae, a hard calcified substance. Between these lamellae are small spaces known as lacunae, which contain osteocytes, the mature bone cells. Leading from the lacunae, in all directions, are tiny canals called canaliculi. Together these components are known as an osteon and they serve to ensure that each part of the bone receives nutrients and that waste products are disposed of.

Cancellous Bone

Cancellous bone or non-osteon bone is sponge-like in appearance due to its internal meshwork structure of trabeculae (see Figure 3.4.1). Between the spaces of this arrangement lie red bone marrow in which blood cells are produced. Two types of cells lie on opposite surfaces of the trabeculae:

▶ first, osteoblasts, which are responsible for laying down new bone;
▶ second, osteoclasts, which incorporate a phagocytic action to absorb bone.

This particular arrangement is designed rather like the external scaffolding of a new building.

The skeletal system consists of five types of bone:

▶ long bones;
▶ short bones;
▶ irregular bones;
▶ flat bones;
▶ sesamoid bones.

▶ JOINTS

These occur where two or more bones meet and they are said to have the following functions (Goodinson, 1988, p. 243):

▶ to aid movement of different parts of the body;
▶ to aid stability on movement;
▶ to aid the maintenance of body posture.

DECISION MAKING

In your anatomy text, notice how, on the gross structure of the bony matrix of cancellous bone, a regular pattern is formed.

- *Why do you think it is arranged in this way?*
- *How do you think this knowledge might help with your decision making in nursing practice?*

DECISION MAKING

At this point, look at your anatomy and physiology textbook to identify the location of the five types of bone (McLaren, 1996).

- *Why do you think they are arranged into such shapes and structures?*
- *When these different bones are fractured, why do they heal at different rates and why is it important for the nurse to know this?*
- *What effect does age have on the healing rates of bone?*

There are many different types of joints in the body and not all are moveable or concerned with movement. So again for the sake of brevity and to concentrate upon our main concern of mobility, only synovial joints will be considered. (For a full description of bones and joints see McLaren, 1996, pp. 302–304.)

▶ *Synovial Joints*

These joints are fundamental to full mobility and are termed 'freely movable' or 'diarthroses'. They are enclosed within a fibrous capsule of connective tissue. Articular or hyaline cartilage lines the ends of the bones. The stability of these joints is enhanced by the presence of ligaments, which are attached between one bone and the other. Joint stability is also aided by the adjacent muscles, which are attached via tendons to bones. The nerve supply to joints comes from the surrounding muscles.

The joint capsule is lined with synovial membrane containing microscopic villi, which secrete synovial fluid to lubricate and nourish the articular surfaces. All synovial joints have a similar structure to one another, but they vary in terms of their shape and range of movement.

▶ RANGE OF MOVEMENTS

To be effective in care and protect our patients we need to know the extent of movement and the limitations that exist. Therefore it is important to know the normal range of movements (Figure 3.4.2) as given below:

- ▶ flexion;
- ▶ extension;
- ▶ circumduction;
- ▶ eversion;
- ▶ pronation and supination;
- ▶ abduction and adduction;
- ▶ dorsiflexion and plantar flexion;
- ▶ rotation;
- ▶ protraction and retraction;
- ▶ opposition (McLaren, 1996, p. 309).

Movement at synovial joints is limited by the shape of the articulating bones and the structure of extracapsular (and sometimes intracapsular) ligaments. Other limiting factors are the strength and tension of adjacent muscles. There are basically six types of synovial joints:

- ▶ ball and socket joint;
- ▶ hinge joint;
- ▶ pivot joint;
- ▶ gliding joint;
- ▶ saddle joint;
- ▶ ellipsoid joint.

It is important that nurses learn about synovial joints so that they can identify normal movement and the range that exists.

The knee joint is referred to as a hinge joint, but the classification given to some joints is not always a full and accurate description. This led to the problem of loosening with the older varieties of artificial knee joints that were inserted in the past. They were designed to act only in

---

DECISION MAKING

If a child sustains a fracture of the distal (lower) part of the tibia following a fall while playing:

- *What knowledge do you as a nurse need to know about the structure, function and movement of this bone and surrounding bones and joints?*
- *What advice would you give to the parents in relation to their child's mobilization, joint movement and bone healing?*

There are the many different types of joints.

- *Use your anatomy and physiology textbook to discover more detail.*
- *Try to gain access to a skeleton within your school or department and attempt the movements identified above on the skeleton.*
- *Attempt some of the common movements yourself.*
- *Note the range that you may go through in a gym or exercise class when doing a 'warm up' or 'cool down' stretch.*

Circumduction:
A combination of movements that makes the body part describe a circle.

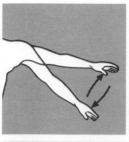

Rotation:
The pivoting of the body part around its axis, as in shaking the head. No rotation of any body part is complete (i.e. 360 degrees).

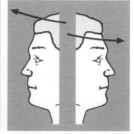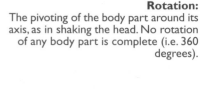

Protraction:
The protrusion of some body part, e.g. the lower jaw.

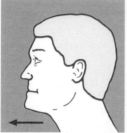

Retraction:
The opposite of protraction.

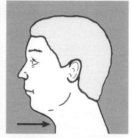

Abduction:
A movement of a bone or limb away from the median plane of the body. Abduction in the hands and feet is the movement of a digit away from the central axis of the limb. One abducts the fingers by spreading them apart.

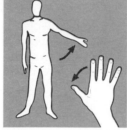

Adduction:
The opposite of abduction, involving approach to the median plane of the body or, in the case of the limbs, to the central axis of a limb.

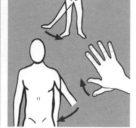

Inversion:
An ankle movement that turns the sole of the foot medially. Applies only to the foot.

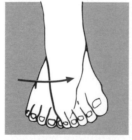

Eversion:
The opposite of inversion. It turns the sole of the foot laterally.

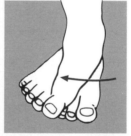

Supination:
The opposite of pronation. When the forearm is in the extended position, this movement brings the palm of the hand upward .

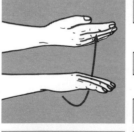

Pronation:
A movement of the forearm that in the extended position brings the palm of the hand to a downward position. Applies only to the forearm.

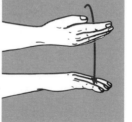

Extension:
The opposite of flexion, it increases the angle between two movably articulated bones, usually to a 180-degree maximum. If the angle of extension exceeds 180 degrees (as is possible when throwing back the head), this action is termed hyperextension.

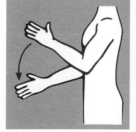

Flexion:
The bending of a joint; usually a movement that reduces the angle that two movably activated bones make with each other. When one crouches, the knees are flexed.

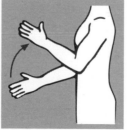

Figure 3.4.2: Types of movement of synovial joints. (Redrawn from Hinchliff *et al.*, 1996, p. 309.)

If you sit on a chair and then flex and extend your knee, the movement created is that of a hinge. If you now stand with your foot firmly fixed to the floor, try (within your limitations) to rotate at the knee joint. Notice how there is some rotational movement, but bear in mind that the ankle joint is also rotating.

a hinge movement and did not take into account the rotational forces exerted on the knee.

▶ MUSCLES

For stability to be maintained and movement to occur, muscles need to work effectively. These skeletal muscles consist of very specialized cells that allow contraction. The muscle contractions not only allows movement, but also maintains body posture. Another function of skeletal muscle is to produce heat. It has been stated that only 25% of the energy generated by skeletal muscle is used for mechanical work as the remainder is dissipated as heat to help maintain body temperature (Goodinson, 1988, p. 205).

To move, then, skeletal muscles require a great deal of energy. The nutritional aspects, especially sugar and carbohydrate intake are therefore of paramount importance. The full potential of mobility improvement or maintenance cannot be reached if this area is neglected and patients lack energy.

To aid movement, skeletal muscles are arranged around an origin and an insertion (Figure 3.4.3). The origin is usually the least moveable end of the muscle and the insertion the most moveable. The ends of muscles terminate in a cord of connective tissue, a tendon. This is inserted into the periosteum (covering) of the underlying bone. As a general rule, the nearest (or proximal) tendon is the origin and the one furthest away (distal) is the insertion.

Skeletal muscles are striated (striped) in appearance and are under voluntary control. They are surrounded by sheets of fibrous connective tissue called fascia. The deep fascia is said to facilitate free movement and carries blood vessels and nerves. It also fills the spaces between muscles and sometimes provides the origins of muscles (Tortora and Anagnostakos, 1987, pp. 120, 195).

▶ Blood and Nerve Supply of Muscles

Skeletal muscles are extremely well supplied by blood vessels and nerves. Each muscle is supplied by at least one nerve that contains motor and sensory fibres. Information is relayed from the cerebral cortex of the brain

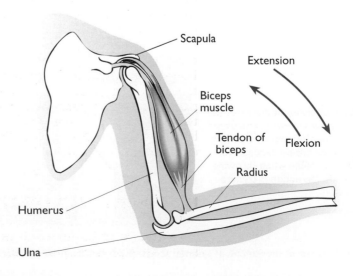

Figure 3.4.3: Biceps muscle of arm. Label the origin and insertion.

via the pyramidal tracts to the anterior horn of the spinal cord (the upper motor neuron) and impulses then travel from the anterior horn of the spinal cord to the muscle fibres (lower motor neuron).

Where muscles and nerves meet is termed the neuromuscular junction. At this point the end of the lower motor neuron is flattened and referred to as the motor end-plate. The chemical transmitter acetylcholine is released when a nerve impulse reaches the motor end-plate. The acetylcholine becomes attached to the muscle receptors and allow impulses to cross the gap between the nerve and muscle – hence body movement! The enzyme cholinesterase is released from vesicles near the end-plate receptors and stops the action of acetylcholine (Judd, 1989a).

There are sensory nerve fibres in these muscles and tendons and some are referred to as proprioceptors. These detect information about body movement and position and relay this information to the central nervous system. Some sensory nerve fibres respond to the stimuli of inflammation, ischaemia (lack of blood supply), compression and necrosis (death of tissue).

The blood supply to voluntary muscles is also extremely good. A great deal of energy is required during muscle stimulation and a good blood supply is needed to provide oxygen and nutrients and to remove waste products. A vast network of blood capillaries is therefore distributed within the muscle fibres for this purpose.

You may have noticed how marathon runners are given regular supplies of glucose drinks; this is not only to prevent dehydration, but also to combat the effects of muscle fatigue. This is a condition in which there is diminished availability of oxygen and it results from the toxic effects of waste products such as carbon dioxide and lactic acid.

Nurses should be able to understand the anatomical components involved and the physiological processes that occur when a patient's mobility is affected by paralysis, stiffness or fatigue. Without this knowledge we cannot understand the changes taking place and are therefore unable to make appropriate decisions in nursing care.

> Try to exercise your fingers or grip something tightly over a long period of time. When you feel fatigued, attempt to write neatly. What is your observation?

▶ BODY LEVERS

In order for movement to take place a system of levers is used incorporating the structures of muscles, bones and joints. Muscles cross at least one joint between the origin and insertion and movement is produced through a system of levers. These levers are the means of transmitting energy through muscular contraction to move different parts of the body. All levers have a fulcrum, an effort arm and a resistance arm and are classified according to the differing arrangement of these. What is also important in the application of nursing is that by shortening the resistance arm, less effort is required to lift a large weight (i.e. bringing the patient closer to your body reduces the muscular effort required by you to lift him or her). (For a full description and explanation of the different body levers, see McLaren (1996, pp. 302–304) and see also Chapter 1.2 on handling and moving.)

▶ EXERCISE AND ITS EFFECTS

To maintain or improve our health, we all need to exercise. It has been stated that physical performance and fitness are determined by:

▶ an individual's capacity for energy output;
▶ neuromuscular function;
▶ joint mobility;
▶ psychological factors (e.g. motivation) (Herbert and Alison, 1996).

The capacity and extent of physical fitness is determined mainly by the above. The integrity of the involved systems such as the respiratory and cardiovascular systems is vital, therefore, to the overall result. Oxygen and nutrients are needed during exercise to maintain muscular activity. There is also a need to increase the removal rate of carbon dioxide, heat, water and metabolic waste products. It follows, then, that increased cardiac output is required via the coordination of the autonomic nervous system.

Vasodilation and increased blood flow occur during exercise and peripheral resistance in muscles falls as a result. To maintain total peripheral resistance at adequate levels there is therefore a compensatory vasoconstriction, especially in the gastrointestinal tract and kidneys. Venous return to the heart increases, which results in an increased stroke volume. This in turn leads to an increased systolic blood pressure. Excess heat generated through muscular activity during exercise is removed via the blood and causes sweating and flushing of the skin to facilitate heat loss through convection and evaporation (Herbert and Alison, 1996).

Some of the benefits obtained through regular exercise are:

▶ an increased metabolic rate and prevention of obesity;
▶ improved muscular and ligament strength;
▶ prevention of disuse osteoporosis;
▶ improved cardiovascular function;
▶ maintenance of normal blood glucose levels;
▶ reduction of stress and anxiety;
▶ increased feeling of wellbeing.

(For a full discussion of the physiological effects and benefits of exercise on the body, see Hinchliff *et al.*, 1996, Sections 3 and 4.)

▶ THE PHYSICAL EFFECTS OF IMMOBILITY

In Britain in 1993 7% of the population reported permanent difficulties with mobility (Office of Population Censuses and Surveys, 1995, p. 111); not surprisingly the majority of these were aged 65 years and over. There is also a trend towards reduced activity in childhood. However, there are long-term effects of immobility or reduced mobility.

The causes of immobility have been identified by Judd (1989, p. 9) as:

▶ changes in the nervous system with resulting lack of muscle stimuli;
▶ changes in muscle tissue, which can lead to permanent contraction (spasticity) or permanent relaxation (flaccidity);
▶ changes in joints that can prevent movement of the articular surfaces.

Restricted mobility or a full loss of mobility can in turn affect other body systems resulting in:

▶ cardiovascular changes;
▶ respiratory changes;
▶ metabolic and hormonal changes;

RESEARCH BASED EVIDENCE

The rising trend in sporting activities among the able-bodied in Britain is demonstrated in research undertaken by the Office of Population Censuses and Surveys. In the 1993 report it was identified that participation in sports such as keep fit, yoga and cycling had markedly increased since 1987. This was true for men and women of all ages (Office of Population Censuses and Surveys, 1995, p. 137).

RESEARCH BASED EVIDENCE

The trend towards reduced activity in childhood was identified in research by the director of the Coronary Prevention in Children Project. A worrying low level of physical activity among British school children was revealed and suggests that there may be long-term effects such as high blood pressure, elevated blood cholesterol levels and coronary heart disease (Armstrong, 1993).

Reflect on your practice placements and using the above broad classifications (Judd, 1989):

- *Review the reasons why some of your clients had difficulty with mobility.*

- *Decide whether the degree of immobility was temporary or permanent.*

- *From knowledge of the anatomy and physiology of movement review the rationale for the patterns of care and treatment you have seen to improve mobility or overcome the effects of immobility.*

> gastrointestinal changes;
> muscular changes;
> skeletal changes;
> other changes.

Cardiovascular Changes

There can be a shift in fluid and electrolyte balance with a resulting loss of potassium and sodium. Also, confinement to bed for periods longer than one week results in a breakdown of fibrin and a shortened blood clotting time. This increases the risk of thrombosis, especially in the lower limbs. The immobile person can also be more susceptible to infections, which may possibly be due to muscular inactivity interfering with transportation of lymph.

Respiratory Changes

If, through immobility, recumbency (lying down) is increased, then the pressure of the abdominal contents pushing on the diaphragm can reduce lung volume. Stress is placed upon the muscles of inspiration, leading to inefficient respiratory muscular action. After approximately three weeks of bed rest, 26% less oxygen is taken in by the body (Heebink, 1981). A decrease in the efficiency of the muscles of respiration can lead to an inability to cough effectively. This can result in an accumulation of mucus, creating the perfect medium for the growth and multiplication of bacteria.

Tidal volume (the amount of gas passing in and out of the lungs with each respiration) remains the same in recumbency and there is little effect upon lung function, for those aged 61 years and over. However, gaseous exchange is impaired for those aged 35–61 years (Tyler, 1984).

Metabolic and Hormonal Changes

Following approximately 4 weeks of immobilization and bed rest, there is some disruption in the cyclic rhythm. This leads to changes in the peak times for insulin (i.e. peaking of serum insulin in the evening despite food taken at meal times). The activity of the pancreas and the ability to take sugar is also reduced. Adrenaline peaks in the afternoon instead of early morning before awakening.

Aldosterone normally peaks at midday, but following long periods of bed rest, it ceases to peak at this time and instead the morning levels remain the same or slightly elevated.

Because the energy required through inactivity is decreased, the basal metabolic rate decreases unless an infection is present. One result of a reduced basal metabolic rate is an increase in the amount of body fat, which also results from the loss in body mass through protein breakdown.

There is an increased excretion of calcium via the kidneys after approximately 4 days' immobilization due to bone reabsorption giving rise to osteoporosis. This can result in increased blood levels of calcium (hypercalcaemia) because the kidneys are unable to cope with such large amounts.

Long periods of immobility can also result in increased nitrogen excretion because nitrogen breakdown exceeds nitrogen intake.

▶ *Gastrointestinal Changes*

A decrease in gastrointestinal function can be seen following a three-day period of bed rest when the stomach tends to secrete less gastric juice. A decreased intake of food due to inactivity and lowered basal metabolic rate can lead to constipation. Diarrhoea can also result from faecal overflow due to the impaction of faeces. This, in turn, can lead to further electrolyte imbalance and dehydration.

▶ *Muscular Changes*

It is not surprising that reduced muscular activity leads to a decrease in strength. This can be identified through girth measurements of the limbs and a decreased exercise tolerance, which presents as fatigue. These detrimental changes can lead to an increased risk of falling, injury and further immobility.

▶ *Skeletal Changes*

Impaired mobility can give rise to changes in calcium metabolism. Bone reabsorption occurs, with a resulting decrease in bone density and disuse osteoporosis. When joints remain immobilized or if there is limited mobility for long periods of time contractures and stiffening of those joints can ensue. One common and severely debilitating contracture is seen in the ankle and referred to as a foot drop. The abnormalities of muscles, tendons and ligaments around an inactive joint can lead to structural joint abnormality, stiffness and pain.

DECISION MAKING

A 75-year-old nursing home resident has suffered from senile dementia for many years. She is gradually losing her full mobility and can now only walk with the aid of two nurses. It appears very difficult to make her understand the importance of exercise or for her to understand the physiotherapists' and nurses' instructions.

- *How might the multidisciplinary team plan to deal with this problem?*
- *What additional care will be needed in order to prevent or reduce some of the complications of immobility outlined in this section?*

▶ *Other Changes*

Other effects of immobilization can also be devastating, such as those on the skin, urinary system and sleep. These are discussed in Chapter 2.4 on skin integrity, Chapter 3.3 on continence and Chapter 4.4 on sleep and rest, respectively.

▶ DEVELOPMENTAL ASPECTS OF MOBILITY

We cannot look at the developmental aspects of mobility solely from a physical viewpoint. We must understand that mobility does not occur in isolation from the rest of society, our recent and distant history and sociocultural and personal influences. All these factors will affect what we value, think and feel about the subject of mobility or lack of it.

From the moment babies are born they are assessed against the criteria of normality. Various observations and recordings are undertaken, and comparisons made on the basis of present day knowledge and ideals. Tests to assess motor skills may have a bias towards those of developed countries and children from for example an Asian culture may not respond to the so-called normal pattern (Miller *et al.*, 1984). This is not to say that they have delayed motor development or abnormal development, but simply that they are being judged using irrelevant or inappropriate criteria. However, if mobility is not restricted or discouraged, infants will gain voluntary control of their movements at approximately four months

RESEARCH BASED EVIDENCE

Wyn Williams and Nolan (1993) looked at different research data relating to falls. One study identified that 70% of all accidental home deaths in the UK occurred in those over 65 years of age, with the vast majority occurring in those aged 75 years or over. Approximately 300 000 people over 65 years of age required hospital treatment each year for non-fatal injuries (Consumer Safety Unit, 1990).

of age, although accurate and deliberate fine movements can take up to three years to develop.

Two of the most distinctive human capabilities are those of grip and the ability to walk in an upright position on two legs (Papalia and Wendkos Olds, 1989). By the age of three or four years, most children can balance on one foot for a second or so and can hop, run and jump. By the time they reach the age of five years they are able to use advanced motor skills that enable them with practice, to dance, dress themselves and use the fine motor movements that will improve with age to equip them for adulthood.

Adolescence brings the same body changes for the disabled as for anyone else. It brings the same sexual urges, yet young people who are disabled may feel frustrated and inadequate because they are mentally alert, but physically trapped. If the physical, psychological and social environment is deficient these milestones may be delayed or not achieved and lead to immobility. But even in health, the ageing process of later life can result in a decreased range of joint movements. Muscular strength and mass may be reduced and coordination diminished. This can lead to an unstable balance and an increased risk of falling (Masterson, 1995).

Psychosocial We live in a society of able-bodied people and conduct the greater part of our lives surrounded by and affected by people who are fully mobile. As nurses we need to appreciate what effects immobility has on society and to consider what can be done to change and improve the situation.

At the outset of this chapter it was stated that we live in a mobile world – a world in which immobility or impaired mobility is seen as abnormal and undesirable. This is particularly true in developed countries. As the elderly (aged 65 years and over) experience significantly more mobility problems than younger people (Office of Population Censuses and Surveys, 1995, p. 82), we cannot disassociate the other influences and effects such as stigmatization upon the elderly. The child is also expected to achieve certain goals in relation to mobility. From birth to adulthood these goals are stressed not only by health professionals, but also the community. We need only to look at our own community to see what an alien environment it is for the disabled and the immobile. Steps, for example, create boundaries for the immobile person. They limit access, further limit their movement and make their world much smaller than it should be.

Schools are designed with the expectation that the child is fully mobile. The disabled child is therefore expected to attend a special school. Where segregation occurs, the notion of normality is brought about through experience and socialization. In a society where therapeutic abortions are an acceptable practice, the incidence of physical and mental abnormalities decline. On the one hand this may produce benefits, such as fewer disabled children, but on the other if children see and associate only with those who are fully mobile, then this image – that normality is not being disabled – is enhanced and becomes (for the able-bodied) the norm. As these ideas form the majority ideas, so the immobile and disabled become increasingly marginalized in our society.

In the past, and to an extent today, institutions for the immobile were designed to house disabled people for most of their lives. This served to increase the marginalization and as French (1994) states 'By the 1950s and 1960s disabled people, whether they were in institutions or not, were so separated from the community that they were practically invisible'.

Professional experts and others such as bureaucratic decision makers become the voice of the disabled, but is it the words of the disabled they are speaking? Most health professionals require full mobility to be able to train and most have little practical experience and appreciation of the physical and emotional effects of disability on the disabled person. It has been said (Open University, 1985) that the non-disabled make the decisions that affect the disabled. This does not allow them an active role in the decision-making process and so they are unable to change or control their lifestyle or environment.

It is not suggested that institutionalization (Goffman, 1961) is the result or that institutionalization can only occur in an institutional setting. Apathy and withdrawal, which are seen as major components of institutionalization, can be observed elsewhere and it has been stated that patients who have never been in an institution can be profoundly institutionalized (Bowers, 1991).

Our perception of a person can be influenced by social stereotypes and prejudice. An understanding and awareness of the perceptual processes and of the attitudes that each of us hold can lead to improved care of patients with mobility problems (Davis and Kenyon, 1981; Goffman, 1990). By realising that these components can affect the care given and received, we may more easily recognize the problems that exist and therefore be more able to devise ways to prevent an occurrence, or alternatively, counteract the effects upon us, our clients, patients and significant others.

The elderly now account for over 21% of the population in the UK and for over 50% of the health care budget. Increasingly they are seen as dependent upon and a burden to society (Bond *et al.*, 1993). Since industrialization there has been the notion that this group of people on reaching a certain chronological age (presently 65 years) become unproductive and are a drain on limited resources. The majority, however, do not require hospitalization or residential care and in fact 93% live in private households (Jones, 1994). Nevertheless a significant proportion over the age of 75 years require some assistance to aid their mobility. So not only is the notion of immobility associated with this section of the population, but also the combined effect of being elderly and immobile. This is what has been previously described (Webb and Tossell, 1991, p. 95) as multiple marginalization where these inequalities exist that only serve to compound a difficult situation and existence.

Although many elderly people have a chronic illness, illness is not the same as reduced ability (Kastenbaum, 1979), but ironically we have seen that in the last century medicalization of immobility has served to enhance these negative attitudes. Nurses are part of society and these ideas can influence their judgement and care. Many health professionals may consider the elderly to be unsuitable for therapy. This can be based on the false belief that the elderly are inflexible, rigid or unable and unwilling to change. Recent research has shown otherwise. Nevertheless negative attitudes still persist and serve to perpetuate the myths we identify as negative stereotypes.

Negative stereotypes can lead to prejudice, aimed not only at the elderly, but also at those with mobility problems. What is termed 'mobilism' is based on the now widely quoted reference of Comfort (1977) in which 'ageism' is identified as 'The notion that people cease to be people, cease to be the same people or become people of a distinct and inferior kind, by virtue of having lived a specific number of years'. So mobilism can be seen as 'The notion whereby people are seen as different and inferior simply through having a permanent or temporary, partial or complete, loss of physical mobility'.

DECISION MAKING

Reflect on a practice placement where there were disabled clients.

- *Try to identify how professional carers, clients and relatives may have perceived the situation differently.*
- *Analyse the situation and decide on whose needs received priority in the design and organization of the client's day.*
- *What changes would you make to alter the situation if you had the power to implement your decisions.*

RESEARCH BASED EVIDENCE

Buckwalter et al. (1993) have identified that the elderly can be responsive to cognitive and behavioural interventions including psychodynamic approaches. They looked at several methods by which nurses can confront their own values, beliefs and convictions about ageing to highlight possible sources of conflict that may interfere with the delivery and quality of care.

Try to observe a carer assisting a disabled person or pushing a disabled person in a wheelchair in a public setting.

- *Notice their interactions with others.*
- *Do others concentrate upon the carer or the disabled?*
- *Notice if there is any lack of interaction.*
- *Notice if there is any* *inappropriate interaction such as staring.*
- *Recall honestly how you feel and react when you meet a disabled person, particularly of your own age, in a social setting.*
- *How could knowledge gained from this chapter affect your attitude and feelings in future?*

Think of disabled groups throughout the life span from birth to old age. From your personal experience and from your learning based on material in this chapter:

- *Identify different ways in which each of the groups you select may be marginalized and analyse the* *factors in society that can contribute to such marginalization.*
- *Discuss with your fellow students the issues involved in helping to overcome such marginalization*

(See Webb and Tossell, 1991, Chapters 1 and 5.)

Stigmatization can therefore occur because of people's fears, ignorance or embarrassment. It is based upon a simplistic stereotypical view that involves perceived negative attributes about other people. This results in the labelling of such people (Taylor and Field, 1993). These labels are not a true reflection of reality, for example those with mobility problems can also be perceived as having mental problems or learning difficulties.

The effects of inappropriate interactions on the disabled can be devastating and the mass media plays its part in enhancing this negative image. It can lead to a loss of self esteem and result in withdrawal from social life (Figure 3.4.4) (Taylor and Field, 1993).

Society in many respects assists in withdrawal by encouraging the permanently immobile to seek refuge in specific centres and homes. The point here is not to denigrate the valuable work done in such places, but to increase awareness of the consequences of such actions and policies.

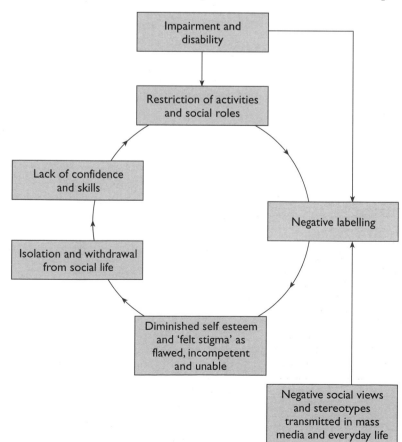

Figure 3.4.4: Negative feedback between stigmatization, self esteem and participation in social activities. (From Taylor and Field, 1993, with permission of Blackwell Science Ltd)

Most of us have little appreciation of what is involved in any disability – the frustration of a lifetime of hardship and inequalities that many disabled people have to face, of having to depend upon others for what may be seen by the able-bodied as a natural right or ability. What is surprising is that more disabled people do not resort to violent or illegal means to air their grievances. Immobility and ill health in general can have major consequences and effects on patients. By studying the psychological and sociological aspects of mobility and immobility we can gain a much greater insight into the associated problems.

PRACTICE KNOWLEDGE

Considering the variation in the role of the nurse in the differing contexts of immobility, a specific nursing model will not be referred to, but the nursing process, which involves assessment, planning, implementation and evaluation of nursing care, will form the basis for the organization of this section.

▶ MULTIDISCIPLINARY ASSESSMENT OF MOBILITY

Both inside and outside the hospital environment, the care surrounding immobile patients involves much more than nursing care. Although some of these carers may not specifically be concerned with mobility, they may contribute towards it. There is a move in health care towards a multidisciplinary approach to assessment, including the use of single documentation for all. On a nationwide basis this is at an early stage and not yet widespread.

For the multidisciplinary team there are various tools available to assess levels of mobility, the most common element being a focus on the client being able to achieve the activities of daily living (ADL). The Barthel ADL scale (Mahoney and Barthel, 1965) is used extensively as an overall assessment of levels of dependency on a 0–20 point scale. Other tools have been developed to suit the particular disability (Wade *et al.*, 1985), the degree of muscle strength (Medical Research Council, 1976) or body part that is immobilized (Robinson and Schmidt, 1981; Stewart *et al.*, 1990).

Alongside the multidisciplinary assessment tools for mobility mentioned above, other tools may be appropriate because of the effects overall on mobility. These tools may, for example, be in the form of pain scales or risk calculators for pressure areas (see Chapters 2.3 and 2.4, respectively, for a full description). If a patient is in pain then this will directly affect their level of mobility. Complications of mobility can also be the cause of pain and lead to further immobility. The immobile patient is at risk from pressure sores and if these develop, then again further immobility can result. Any aid in the detection and awareness of complications and risk factors can only help to promote effective practice.

Mobility, then, in relation to a nursing diagnosis may be seen as 'impaired physical mobility' or 'activity intolerance'. It may also be identified as 'limited strength' or 'limited muscle power' or even 'paralysis'. The medical diagnosis will vary and may be one of osteoarthritis, cerebral palsy or stroke, and although a knowledge of the aetiology is important, nevertheless, there is no specific requirement to identify the medical diagnosis in the nursing care plan.

Assessment can identify the degree of weakness or impairment and to do this it will necessarily involve the nurse's personal experience and professional knowledge in the use of skills in observation and

Range of movement
Gait
Tolerance to exercise and activity
Body alignment
Balance

Table 3.4.2 Elements within an assessment of mobility. (Adapted from Masterson, 1995.)

communication and of specific mobility assessment tools. A full assessment by the nurse may seem unrealistic in a busy placement area, so it is important therefore to incorporate the multidisciplinary approach. The cooperation and involvement of the occupational therapist, physiotherapist and others are necessary for effective holistic care.

Another difficulty is that nurses frequently attempt an assessment based upon verbal information alone. This can be due to the fact that patients are initially assessed during an acute phase of an illness where an accurate and full assessment cannot be made. The nursing process, though, is a cyclical process and the element of reassessment is a vital component.

Many elements of mobility must be incorporated within the assessment process (Table 3.4.2). Batehup and Squires (1991) have suggested that an assessment should include gait, initiation of mobility, turning and stopping. In hospital we are inclined to make such assessments on non-slip, non-carpeted floors, but it is important when considering discharge to make such an assessment under conditions similar to those at home or ideally, in the patient's own home. There is a need therefore to consider the environment in which the assessment takes place. An alien or unfamiliar environment may result in a different assessment than one which is performed in an acceptable and conducive environment.

Specific mobility assessment should also be made in various positions (i.e. sitting down, standing and in recumbency) if the patient is able. This will provide an overall picture so that future and present needs can be met. One must remember, however, that problems with mobility can be affected by psychological differences, which will affect a person's beliefs and motivation for mobilizing; on the other hand, children may also be at different developmental stages and operate at different levels of understanding.

▶ MANAGEMENT OF MOBILITY CARE

Before the implementation of care, information obtained through the many forms of assessment is reviewed by the multidisciplinary team and the client. Goals are set that are realistic to achieve. These goals can be short term or long term depending upon the cause and degree of immobility, any concurrent condition of the client that will limit mobility, the environmental circumstances and the degree of motivation and support for the client. Many clients, even after orthopaedic surgery, which renders them temporarily immobile, can be assisted in their own homes by members of the multidisciplinary team.

In the decision making about care programmes it is worth considering the previously identified areas (Table 3.4.2), as a part of our assessment above. These include:

> ▶ range of movement;
> ▶ gait and body alignment;
> ▶ balance;
> ▶ exercise and activity.

Each will be considered in turn.

▶ *Range of Movement*

Muscles with full strength will have little benefit to patients if their joints are stiff from lack of movement. In certain instances such as joint replacement or ligament repair, flexion or extension may have to be limited for a time, but on the whole if a joint is allowed to be moved then this should be encouraged. Active joint movements not only increase and maintain the range, but also help maintain muscle strength and joint stability. These elements are essential for mobility.

If a joint is not moved then a fixed flexion deformity can occur. This is abnormal shortening of muscle tissue that becomes resistant to stretching and can lead to permanent disability due to fibrosis of the muscle or joint (Weller, 1989). The aim in mobility therefore is to prevent such an occurrence as this will severely hamper the rehabilitation process. It takes only a few seconds to remind patients to move their knees, ankles or hips, whether they are confined to bed or not. Remember though that a part of the patient's limb may need support to achieve a full range of movements comfortably.

▶ *Gait and Body Alignment*

Gait is the style and manner of walking and an observation of the patient's gait can be made at anytime while he or she is walking. Normal walking consists of two basic movements:

> ▶ the stance, in which one leg bears most of the body weight at one point in the movement;
> ▶ the swing, in which the foot does not touch the ground and the weight is taken on the opposite side.

There can be many styles of walking, most of which present no problem. Problems, however, can occur when the style of gait and alignment gives rise to or arises from instability. When an unstable gait or alignment has been diagnosed, it should be corrected. Occasionally it may not be possible to correct an unstable gait, for example for a client with spina bifida or cerebral palsy. Care should focus on preventing further damage and maintaining maximum function for as long as possible.

The age of a person is important, for example, a normal child's gait is not the same as that of an adult. However, abnormal gaits can be similar in both the child and the adult.

Although there are many different types of gait, body alignment and balance, the cause of instability can be multifactorial. The programme of implementation may involve, for example, the reduction of a patient's pain through the administration of analgesia or the application of local heat or cold substances. Programmes may also need to take poor eyesight into account. This is especially relevant in the elderly as some deterioration of eyesight is a natural part of growing old. In fact longsightedness (presbyopia) may begin to develop around the age of 40, so it is important therefore to initiate checks on a patient's eyesight if there is any doubt. Rooms that may seem adequately lit to us, may be inadequate for those with some visual impairment.

▶ *Balance*

Balance, or the state in which the body is in equilibrium, is an important factor in mobility. Balance is a very complex area and depends upon the integrity of:

▶ the central nervous system;
▶ the musculoskeletal system.

It relies upon the adequate functioning of:

▶ vision;
▶ the vestibule (the cavity in the middle of the bony labyrinth or inner ear);
▶ proprioceptive efficiency;
▶ tactile input, especially to the feet and hands;
▶ integration of all stimuli by the central nervous system;
▶ visuospatial perception;
▶ effective muscle tone;
▶ muscle strength;
▶ joint flexibility (Galley and Forster, 1987).

Any damage to one or all of the above factors needs be taken into account before, during and after mobilization. The ear, for example, is the organ of balance, so any deterioration in function can lead to an increased number of falls (Windmill, 1990). In such circumstances hearing tests and appropriate aids can improve and maintain a person's balance, thus preventing further falls and immobility.

▶ *Mobility Aids*

When using walking aids Ogden (1992) has identified five points for consideration. These are:

▶ is there space available for the aid?
▶ does the person have the ability to use the aid appropriately?
▶ is the aid to be used indoors, outdoors or both?
▶ is public or private transport required to accommodate the aid?
▶ do stairs or steps need to be negotiated?

Most mobility aids such as walking frames, sticks or crutches (Figure 3.4.5) are initially ordered by the physiotherapist and mobility commenced with their assistance. This is especially so for hospitalized patients, but nurses in the community are frequently the care workers who evaluate progress following a patient's discharge. There are community physiotherapists and occupational therapists, but because of resourcing difficulties they are often unable to evaluate all patients discharged with a mobility aid. Nurses may then undertake a formal or informal assessment of mobility. Although nurses may not have the relevant expertise to make the necessary adjustments or changes to equipment, a referral can be made to the appropriate person or department.

Walking aids need to be in good working order. For example walking aids have a ferule or ferules at their base, which are usually made of rubber and add to the stability of the equipment by providing a larger point of contact with the ground or floor. Ferules also help prevent slipping on shiny or wet surfaces. If mobility aids are required for long periods, these ferules need to be regularly checked for wear.

If aids incorporate the use of screws and bolts, these may have to be tightened for safe operation. If patients are able they or their carers can

Figure 3.4.5: Walking aids. (a) Axilla crutch. (b) Elbow crutch. (c) Gutter frame. (d) Waist high frame. (e) Sticks. (Courtesy of Coopers Healthcare PLC.)

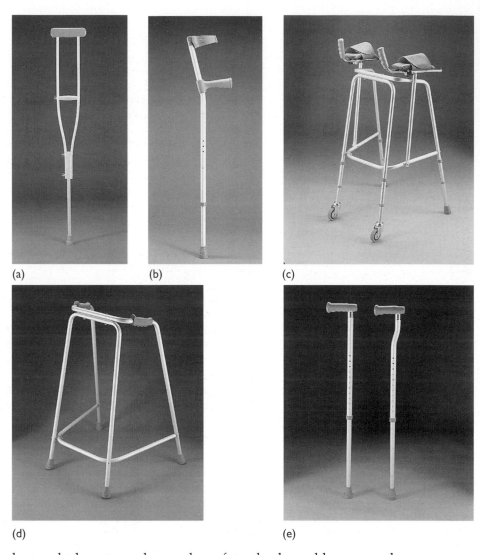

(a)   (b)   (c)

(d)   (e)

be taught how to make regular safety checks and how to make any necessary adjustments to their equipment. While evaluating the patient's overall mobility problem, the nurse may also need to evaluate the patient's dexterity and their effectiveness in checking all aspects of appliance safety.

If nurses prescribe, administer and initiate walking with mobility aids then they should ensure that the correct size has been ascertained, and be aware of their responsibilities under the *Consumer Protection Act* of 1987. Crutches, for example, cannot be given to patients without proper advice on their use and maintenance (Chartered Society of Physiotherapists, 1988a,b). In the absence of physiotherapists, nurses continue to mobilize patients with mobility aids. They therefore need not only a working knowledge of the equipment, but also an understanding of some of the basic principles involved to provide accurate and effective care. Judd (1989, p. 166) has identified two such principles as:

- the wider the base and weightbearing area of the aid, the greater the stability;
- the higher the patient takes their weight, the more stable they will be.

It is seen, therefore, that patients using gutter frames are more stable than those using the more common waist high frames, and those using axillary crutches are more stable than those using elbow crutches. To

---

DECISION MAKING

Make a list of the mobility aids you know about or have seen in use in your practice placements.
- *Identify a client with a specific mobility problem.*
- *Decide on what aid you would use and give reasons for your choice.*

enable appropriate assessment, evaluation and documentation there is also a need to be aware of the different gait patterns associated with such mobility aids (Figure 3.4.6). The different points of the frame, footsteps and crutches shown in Figure 3.4.6 refer to the number of weightbearing areas that touch the ground or floor. It is important that in the absence of the physiotherapist the nurse can recognize when the equipment is used correctly and incorrectly. Axillary crutches, for example, are not designed so that the patient's weight is taken through the axilla. The crutches serve to stabilize the body by giving added support to the sides, while the weight is taken through the hands, wrists and arms. Using the axilla to take weight would only encourage a crutch palsy, which is caused by pressure on the brachial plexus. Crutches, therefore, need to rest two or three fingerwidths below the axilla. Patients should continue to maintain a proper and safe technique while ascending and descending stairs (Figure 3.4.7).

Besides walking with or without aids, another part of managing poor balance is to ensure safety to and from the sitting position. Batehup and Squires (1991) see the prerequisites for this as a suitable chair (i.e. one that is at an appropriate height with appropriate arms and with a correct angle of the back and seat) and good technique, which can be facilitated by the carer. One such technique, used in the rehabilitation of stroke patients, is the Bobath method. The main principle is that the damaged body should be retrained in natural patterns of movement that are symmetrical. The aim is also to break the automatic patterns of spasticity associated with these patients (Holmes, 1988). If we concentrate upon the stronger side of the body to compensate for the weaker side then we may inadvertently encourage further weakness and loss of mobility to the affected side.

During your practice placements, observe how clients with problems with mobility are assisted or instructed to move from lying to sitting to standing.

- *Note the rationale for the specific methods used and relate these to the knowledge gained from this chapter.*
- *Monitor your own technique or get a member of the multidisciplinary team to assess your ability in this area (see Chapter 1.2).*

Figure 3.4.6: Gait patterns with a walking frame and with crutches. (From Judd, 1989, pp. 168–169, with permission)

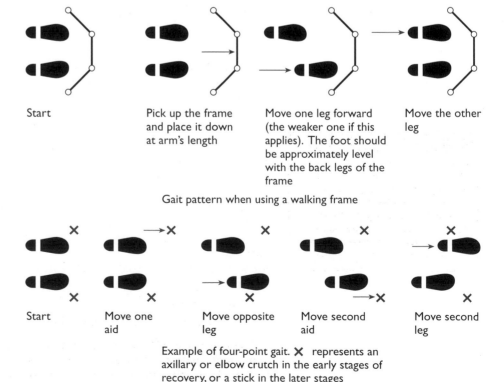

Start

Pick up the frame and place it down at arm's length

Move one leg forward (the weaker one if this applies). The foot should be approximately level with the back legs of the frame

Move the other leg

Gait pattern when using a walking frame

Start

Move one aid

Move opposite leg

Move second aid

Move second leg

Example of four-point gait. ✗ represents an axillary or elbow crutch in the early stages of recovery, or a stick in the later stages

Figure 3.4.7: Ascending and descending stairs using crutches. (From Judd, 1989, pp. 168–169, with permission.)

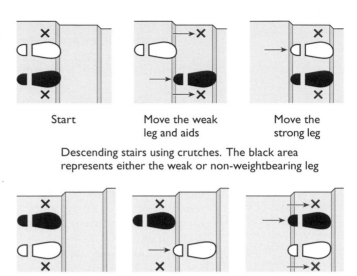

Descending stairs using crutches. The black area represents either the weak or non-weightbearing leg

Ascending stairs using crutches. The black area represents either the weak or non-weightbearing leg

▶ *Exercise and Activity*

Exercise is the undertaking of physical exertion with the main aim of improving fitness and health. Exercise and activity are fundamental to mobility and there are many different types of exercise. These have been described by Brunner and Suddarth (1989) as:

▶ passive – exercises that are usually carried out by the physiotherapist or the nurse without the assistance of the patient;
▶ active assisted – exercises performed by the patient, but with assistance from the physiotherapist or nurse;
▶ active – exercises undertaken by the patient without any assistance.
▶ resisted – exercises performed against manual or physical resistance.
▶ isometric or static – exercises carried out by the patient where muscles are alternately contracted and relaxed while that part of the body remains in a fixed position.

The reason for undertaking a particular exercise will depend on the diagnosis and the intended outcome. The patient, for example, may have a knee injury immobilized in a splint and have developed muscle wasting and weakness. In this case, static exercise of the quadriceps muscles may be required to regain muscular strength to achieve stability upon walking.

It is not always the case that passive movements are undertaken because the patient cannot perform active movements themselves; sometimes they are undertaken to prevent damage through overexertion. However, the nurse or physiotherapist needs to be aware that their efforts can be too vigorous during passive movement and can cause damage that can hinder progress.

If a programme of exercise and mobility is implemented, this should be agreed between the health care team and the patient, and the patient should be capable of the initial activity of standing and balancing. To achieve the latter, as discussed in the previous section, some mobility aid may be required.

Many of the aids you may have identified will be those that promote or extend one's ability to exercise and increase activity. Exercise tolerance, though, should not only imply the extent to which exercise can be

---

RESEARCH BASED EVIDENCE

A study undertaken by Jirovec (1991) looked at the impact of a daily exercise regimen on mobility and balance in patients who were cognitively impaired, and residing in community nursing homes. The results indicated that residents were able to walk significantly further following the exercise regimen. It also had the added benefit of reducing the incidence of urinary incontinence.

undertaken without a mobility aid as frequently patients are unable to exercise effectively without such aids.

It has been suggested by Banyard and Hayes (1994), in relation to successful skills training, that there are two key features:

▶ guidance – which tells us what to do;
▶ feedback – which tells us how successful we have been.

When planning an exercise programme, it is important to ensure that patients, whatever their age, are able to understand what is required, and what is about to be performed. Feedback will involve different means for different people and for different ages. Galley and Forster (1987) identify the aims in planning any exercise programme as:

▶ to motivate to improve morale;
▶ to relieve symptoms, particularly the presence of pain and oedema;
▶ to regain all possible function;
▶ to provide a foundation for forward planning;
▶ to set up a programme for independent working to note any restrictions and special precautions, whether local or general;
▶ if possible, to prevent further disability;
▶ to maintain or improve all unaffected functions;
▶ to maintain or gain any physical fitness.

Patients are individuals and need to be considered as such. Implementing any exercise programme will involve unique demands on a patient's body: demands upon their muscles, ligaments, joints and other body systems. An ill child will not be able to tolerate exercise in the same way or to the same extent as a fit child, nor will a fit child tolerate the same programme as a fit adult. Different methods and ways to motivate different people are often required in conducting exercise programmes. Remember that exercise can also be used as a form of relaxation and psychotherapy and be beneficial to patients with severe mental health problems.

All decision making for nursing practice knowledge requires a thorough assessment and an ongoing evaluation of the progress of the client in maintaining his or her mobility within the nursing process cycle.

RESEARCH BASED EVIDENCE

Research by Adams (1995) describes a 12-week exercise programme undertaken by a young schizophrenic patient in which it was identified that this not only improved physical fitness, but also reinforced self confidence and a positive body image and nurtured emotional and psychosocial skills.

DECISION MAKING

Imagine that you are about to conduct an exercise programme for a client group from within each of the branches of nursing (adult, child, learning disabilities, mental health).

• **Reflecting on the specific needs of clients within your selected branch, identify what you would do to encourage, maintain or improve function and mobility.**

• **If you can, with your fellow students, compare the different approaches that will be needed for different client groups in differing contexts of care.**

PROFESSIONAL KNOWLEDGE

The section that follows will concentrate upon the increased responsibilities placed upon nurses in recent years. It looks at our own knowledge base, and the political and societal changes in relation to mobility. With these in mind, it also suggests ways forward that may benefit our clients and patients.

As registered nurses, we are responsible professionals and as such are accountable to our clients. If we are working in areas that involve a great deal of assisted patient mobility or the use of mobility aids then we have a duty to maintain our expertise and update our knowledge in the field. If we are unsure of our responsibilities or our skills, then we need to ascertain who is responsible, or ensure updating takes place. If the responsibility for mobility lies with others such as the community physiotherapist then we must ensure that patients are referred to the appropriate person

Much has been discussed and written over the past few years about the positive aspects of promoting exercise for health. What we also see though, in a system of limited NHS resources, is the increased cost of treatment for individuals who have sustained injuries due to inaccurate or overexercising.

- *Where do you think the nurse's responsibilities lie if this trend continues?*

RESEARCH BASED EVIDENCE

In the USA, Kilbury et al. (1992) researched areas that created barriers to equal opportunities and full social participation for the disabled following The Americans with Disabilities Act *of 1990 (US Congress, 1990). The researchers looked at the potential impact of the legislation and it was seen as the catalyst for enabling improved attitudes and also the stimulus for the development of further related legislation.*

or department. We must also ensure that local and national policies and procedures are adhered to, therefore enabling effective patient safety and comfort.

Nurses also need to become more proactive in the fight for greater patient rights. We may need to pinpoint, for example, inadequacies of the 1990 *National Health Service and Community Care Act* or the *Chronically Sick and Disabled Persons Act* of 1970. This latter legislation has been said to encourage the medicalization of disability, with an over-reliance on the expert medical assessor or doctor. The social security system also forces the disabled to emphasize their inabilities to obtain benefit (Morris, 1993).

However, disabled people are usually legislated for by the able-bodied and the legislators cannot wholly appreciate the problems that exist for the disabled or immobile.

▶ *Disability Discrimination Act (1995)*

New laws relating to the above *Disability Discrimination Act* will be introduced between 1996 and 1997. The aim is to end discrimination within the area of disability. The Act defines disability as 'A physical or mental impairment which has a substantial and long term adverse effect on a person's ability to carry out normal day-to-day activities' (Minister for Disabled People, 1996).

To assist in the implementation of the Act, two new independent bodies have been set up. These are the National Disability Council for England, Scotland and Wales, and the Northern Ireland Disability Council. They are charged with advising government on disability issues and ensuring operation of the Act. However, the advice they give government must be accompanied by an outline of the cost and an identification of the envisaged benefits. The councils are also required to formulate a code of practice for submission to government, but cannot investigate individual disability discrimination complaints.

The Act introduces new rights in relation to:

- ▶ employment;
- ▶ access to services and goods;
- ▶ buying and renting of land or property;
- ▶ education;
- ▶ public transport.

Schools and further and higher education establishments, for example, have to take into consideration the needs of disabled students. However, certain exemptions apply to Northern Ireland and Scotland, as provision had already been made in other Acts.

Public transport regulations, within the Act, are designed to ensure safety, comfort and accessibility for the disabled. Although again exceptions can apply to taxis if it is considered inappropriate or that the numbers of taxis would substantially diminish as a result of alterations. Trains and trams, too, can also be exempt in some circumstances.

Other areas such as access to goods, facilities, services and employment also go some way to improve the present situation; however, concern relates to the many exceptions within all areas identified. Unlike the *Race Relations Act* (1976) and the Equal Opportunities Commission,

Reflect on the facilities available in your local community and on the difficulties that a person with limited mobility or who is wheelchair bound may have.

- *What role can the nurse play in effecting political change towards improved conditions?*

it has been stated that there are no powers to police the *Disability Discrimination Act* and that individuals with a grievance can only turn to industrial tribunals or small claims courts (Taylor, 1995). This may lead to criticism that the Act lacks teeth for effective change. As nurses, and patient and client advocates, we have a duty and responsibility to protect the interests of our patients and clients. We need to be proactive to ensure improvements, even if this means legitimate pressure brought to bear upon central and local government so that the present law is made effective and future amendments can be made.

▶ FACILITIES

In their roles as health promoters nurses need to be aware of what facilities are available in the community and where they and their patients can obtain expert help and advice. One such facility is the Disabled Living

Figure 3.4.8: How to get equipment for disability. (Reproduced with permission from Mandelstam, 1993.)

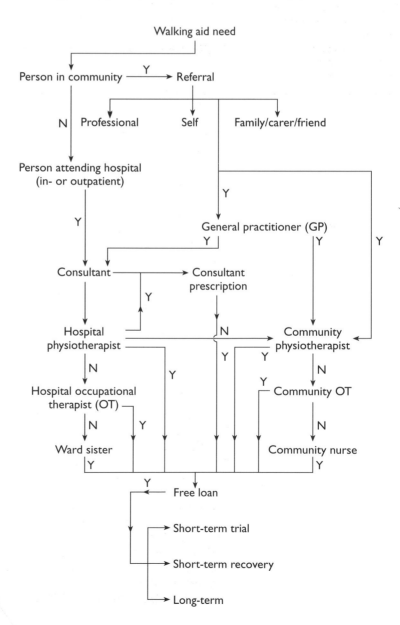

Centre. There are 39 of these, situated in towns and cities throughout England, Wales and Scotland. They are financed through different means such as charities, health authorities, social services, donations or a combination of these. They can be accessed by anyone, for example patients, relatives, significant others, voluntary carers, voluntary organizations and health professionals. The centres give expert physiotherapy and occupational therapy advice on a wide range of disability equipment. This advice is unbiased and the equipment is available for trial. Assessments are also made as to the suitability of the equipment for individual patient or client use. The staff are also an invaluable source of information about the many different aspects of mobility and mobility aids. They can facilitate negotiations between patients and the relevant mobility or disability departments. They can also give patients the appropriate contact address or telephone number for financial aid or physical or psychological care.

These centres also assess new equipment and provide training and advice for professional and non-professional carers. They can also advise patients or carers about where or whom to obtain equipment from (Figure 3.4.8). Overall, the centres are an invaluable facility for people with permanent or temporary mobility problems, yet many people, including health professionals, are not aware of their existence.

Are you aware of any Disabled Living Centre or Mobility Centre in your area? Are you aware of the services they provide? Are you aware of why they are provided? Have you visited any of these centres?

- *If the answer to any of these questions is 'no' make positive steps to discover the answers.*

This chapter began by looking at the meaning of mobility. It was seen mainly from a physical perspective, especially since most of us take full mobility for granted. To understand the full scope of this area of nursing practice, we looked not only at the anatomical, physiological and developmental functioning of mobility, but also at the psychological, social and environmental effects of immobility.

Nurses deal with mobility problems 24 hours a day and need to maintain their knowledge and skills in this area of nursing practice in order to make informed and effective decisions in the administration of quality care for their clients.

▶ EXPERIENTIAL EXERCISES

Throughout this chapter you have been asked to carry out different exercises that were aimed at increasing your knowledge and awareness of mobility, immobility, and the problems that exist. We shall now concentrate upon a variety of practical exercises that are designed to be undertaken in or around the formal classroom setting and in the community.

▶ *Mobility Appliances*

It is important that the person conducting these exercises is fully trained in the use of all the appliances used so that the correct advice about and practice of the techniques can be taught before the students embark.

At the outset the facilitator should stress that safety is of paramount importance in the exercises described below and should not be compromised. Students should also make the most of these experiences, which may therefore involve:

- asking for directions;
- obtaining money from a bank or cashpoint;
- making a purchase at a shop;
- having refreshments in a cafe;
- sitting in a public area.

▶ *Elbow Crutches and Axillary Crutches*

Once proper instruction has been given, and the students have been assessed as competent, they should be asked to venture into both the hospital and town or city to:

- experience what practical difficulties exist;
- identify if planners and architects have made adequate or inadequate provision for anyone using crutches;
- experience how users of crutches are perceived and treated by the general public.

Two students will need to work together. One student will use the crutches and the other will identify (in writing) the findings. This demonstrates the first problem; the difficulty of using crutches and writing at the same time! Both students should have equal opportunity to practice both skills. To gain a better appreciation this should ideally be conducted over one day and group discussion take place the following day.

REFLECTIVE KNOWLEDGE

▶ *Wheelchairs*

The process of this exercise is undertaken in the same way as the previous one, with the same three questions to be answered. However, there are two methods here:

- ▶ the three-student method – one student sits in the wheelchair, one assists and the third student observes and records any interactions with the public, and the difficulties encountered;
- ▶ the two-student method – one student uses the wheelchair independently and the other student records the interactions and difficulties.

With both methods, each team should discuss between them the whole experience so that additional points can be made before feeding back to the whole group.

▶ *Obstacle Audit*

One simpler but less effective method is where students work in pairs and are initially given guidance about what obstacles to effective mobility might be. Each pair then go out into the community and hospital where they identify, in writing, a list of obstacles to effective mobility. If facilities are available, a video camera is a useful aid to this exercise.

When the practical exercise is complete, the students return to the classroom setting where a full discussion takes place. This should include:

- ▶ the items identified;
- ▶ the difficulties that may be encountered;
- ▶ suggested reasons why changes or adaptations have not been made.

One might expect that hospital planners, and managers would have looked closely at such difficulties. They may have rectified the situation according to the needs of their clients and patients with mobility problems. However, this is not always the case, so again, we need to ask why and what is being done?

▶ CASE STUDIES

The following case studies are included to help you consolidate knowledge gained from the chapter and your practice experience.

▶ CASE STUDY: ADULT

Mrs Margaret Messenger is an 85-year-old widow. She owns her own home and claims to be fiercely independent, but due to arthritis in her hips, she finds it difficult to climb the stairs. Her daughter is concerned that because of her worsening mobility she will fall and sustain serious harm and has tried to persuade Mrs Messenger to move into a rest home, but her mother refuses. Mrs Messenger does manage to visit the local shops for her daily needs, but with winter approaching, the threat of falling is ever increasing. Mrs Messenger's daughter contacts her mother's general practitioner for help and so the district nurse is asked to assess the situation.

- What facilities and personnel are available to alleviate the situation?

- If, as the district nurse, you are called in to make an assessment, how would you approach it?

- How would you deal with the conflict of interests between the mother and the daughter?

- What options are open to the nurse?

- Can the nurse deal with all eventualities that may result from the assessment?

- We are obliged to act in the best interests of our patients (UKCC, 1992), but on the one hand, there is the aspect of safety and on the other, the patient's psychological wellbeing. Would a compromise be in order, and if so, what would it be?

▶ CASE STUDY: MENTAL HEALTH

Mr Roy Thorne lives in a bungalow with his wife, Dianne. He is a 60-year-old man who has suffered from bouts of depression for the last ten years. Roy's problem is compounded by the fact that he suffered a stroke six years ago, which has left him with a permanent weakness down the left side of his body. However, he does manage to walk short distances with the aid of a stick, but requires help to get in and out of his chair. His long illness has taken its toll on Dianne's physical and psychological condition and wellbeing. Roy attends a psychiatric day centre three times a week, but his depression and mobility have not improved.

- Do you think that Roy's mobility problems have any bearing on his state of mind?

- Would it mean that if Roy's mobility improved his mental health would do likewise?

- If it is identified that Roy lacks the motivation to improve his mobility and state of mind, what can be done?

- Student nurses today undergo a shared Common Foundation Programme for the first 18 months of the course, regardless of the chosen branch. Does this overall experience equip a qualified mental health nurse to undertake Roy's full mobility care?

▶ CASE STUDY: LEARNING DISABILITIES

Paul Brown is a 12-year-old boy who suffers from severe brain damage following a road traffic accident two years ago. He lives with his parents and his 14-year-old sister. Paul is now unable to talk coherently or walk. His arms and legs have developed flexion contractures over the last year. Paul's mother, Elaine, is the main carer in the family and she is worried that what little mobility Paul has, he is about to lose. He is attending the local physiotherapy department twice a week. Elaine does not want Paul to be placed in a permanent care facility.

■ **Is it inevitable that full mobility will be lost?**

■ **How do you think that the family can help?**

■ **Who else can help them, and how?**

■ **It has been suggested that significant improvements have been made as a result of research findings surrounding the care of the severely disabled child (Beresford, 1994). What is your experience in practice?**

■ **Should the severely mentally and physically disabled be encouraged to mix with the able-bodied? What are the reasons for your answer?**

▶ CASE STUDY: CHILD

Laura Davis is a six-year-old girl who fell and fractured her right tibia while climbing a tree. She was taken to the accident and emergency department and immobilized in a long leg plaster of Paris. She was then taught how to use crutches and she and her parents returned home with instructions not to take any weight on her right leg. Two days later, Laura's leg felt pain free and so she began to take her full weight upon it. Despite her parents efforts to prevent this, Laura continues to defy their instructions and says her leg is better and does not need crutches. They return to the hospital for a routine check, where Laura's mother explains this to the nurse.

■ **It is evident that Laura still requires full weight relief on her right leg. What can you do to encourage this?**

■ **What advice can be given to Laura's parents?**

■ **What skills would you use to ensure compliance?**

■ **In most cases we as nurses would encourage full mobility, yet here we are expected to limit this. Ensuring compliance and limiting mobility at this stage will probably result in Laura's full mobility in the future. If all patients with mobility problems who do not comply were to be admitted into hospital, extra resources would be required. Discuss whether hospital admission is the solution or not.**

▶ ANNOTATED FURTHER READING

DAVIS, P.S. (1994) *Nursing the Orthopaedic Patient*. pp. 69–101. London. Churchill Livingstone.
An excellent chapter entitled Why Move, which encompasses the practical problems of immobility.
JONES, L. (1994) *The Social Context of Health and Health Work*. pp. 330–587. London. Macmillan.
These five chapters include material that bears an important relationship to mobility, immobility and nursing care. Topics such as ageing, disability,

differing health beliefs, professional power and control, and the politics of health care are discussed.

JUDD, M. (1989) *Mobility: Patient Problems and Nursing Care*. Oxford. Heinemann Nursing.

Few textbooks solely concentrate on the subject of mobility in nursing. This does, and is therefore a valuable reference.

MANDELSTAM, M. (1993) *How To Get Equipment for Disability*. London. Jessica Kingsley Publishers and Kogan Page for The Disabled Living Foundation.

This useful guide identifies what equipment is available, how to obtain it and who is responsible.

MASTERSON, A. (1995) Mobility and immobility. In Heath, H.B.M. (ed.) *Potter and Perry's Foundations in Nursing Theory and Practice*. pp. 481–584. London. Mosby.

This chapter includes many concise details on mobility related to nursing theory and practice.

McLAREN, S.M. (1996) Mobility and support. In Hinchliff, S.M., Montague, S.E., Watson, R. *Physiology for Nursing Practice*. pp. 261–319. London. Baillière Tindall.

An excellent modern text that includes the physiology of mobility, related problems and application to nursing. Excellent colour diagrams supplement the text.

MINISTER FOR DISABLED PEOPLE (1996) *The Disability Discrimination Act*. Booklets DL60, DL70, DL80, DL90, DL100, DL110 and DL120. HSSS JO3–6299JP.100m.

A government reference source describing concisely all parts of the *Disability Discrimination Act*.

MULLEY, G. (ed.) (1989) *Everyday Aids and Appliances*. London. British Medical Journal.

MULLEY, G. (ed.) (1991) *More Everyday Aids and Appliances*. London. British Medical Journal.

Both texts are important for those embarking on a nursing career that involves substantial mobility assistance.

TAYLOR, S., FIELD, D. (1993) *Sociology of Health and Health Care*. pp. 79–132. London. Blackwell Scientific Publications.

These two chapters concentrate upon the experience of health and illness in a social context – an important dimension.

WILSON–BARNETT, J., BATEHUP, L. (1988) *Patient Problems: A Research Base for Nursing Care*. pp.182–203. Harrow. Scutari Press.

The chapter entitled Mobility Problems is a detailed text structured within the nursing process approach.

▶ REFERENCES

ADAMS, L. (1995) How exercise can help people with mental health problems. *Nursing Times* **91(36)**: 37–39.

ARMSTRONG, L. (1993) Promoting physical activity in schools. *Health Visitor* **66(10)**: 362–364.

BANYARD, P., HAYES, N. (1994) *Psychology, Theory and Application*. p. 298. London. Chapman Hall.

BATEHUP, L., SQUIRES, A. (1991) Mobility. In Redfern, S.J. (ed.), *Nursing Elderly People* (2nd edition). pp. 135–136. London. Churchill Livingstone.

BERESFORD, B. (1994) *Positively Patients, Caring for a Severely Disabled Child*. pp.1–4. London. Her Majesty's Stationery Office.

BOND, J., COLEMAN, P., PEACE, S. (eds) (1993) *Ageing in Society: an Introduction to Social Gerontology*. London. Sage.

BOWERS, L. (1991) Don't blame the institution. *Nursing Times* **87(22)**: 32–34.

BRUNNER, L.S., SUDDARTH, D.S. (1989) *The Lippincott Manual of Medical–Surgical Nursing* (2nd edition). pp. 17–18. London. Harper Row Publishers.

BUCKWALTER, K., SMITH, M., MARTIN, M. (1993) Attitude problem. *Nursing Times* **89(5)**: 55–57.

BYERS, D., PARKER, M. (1992) Early rehabilitation for the patient with a hip fracture. *British Journal of Occupational Therapy* **55(9)**: 351–354.

CHARTERED SOCIETY OF PHYSIO-THERAPISTS (1988a) The Consumer Protection Act 1987, Implications for physiotherapists. *Physiotherapy* **74(4)**: 175–176.

CHARTERED SOCIETY OF PHYSIO-THERAPISTS (1988b) The Consumer Protection Act 1987 – Update. *Physiotherapy* **74(10)**: 530.

COMFORT, A. (1977) *A Good Age*. London. Mitchell Beasley.

CONSUMER SAFETY UNIT (1990) *Home and Leisure Accident Research: 12th Annual Report, 1988 data*. London. Department of Trade and Industry.

DAVIS, H., KENYON, P. (1981) Psychology: its relevance to the practice of physiotherapy. *Physiotherapy* **67(3)**: 67–69.

FRENCH, S. (1994) In whose service? A review of the development of the services for disabled people in Great Britain. *Physiotherapy* **80(24)**: 200–204.

GALLEY, P.M., FORSTER, E.L. (1987) *Human Movement, an Introductory Text for Physiotherapy Students* (2nd edition). pp. 139, 179. London. Churchill Livingstone.

GOFFMAN, E. (1961) *Asylums: Essays on the Social Situation of Mental Patients and Other Inmates.* New York. Doubleday.

GOFFMAN, E. (1990) *Stigma: Notes on the Management of Spoiled Identity.* Harmondsworth, Middlesex. Penguin.

GOODINSON, S.M. (1988) Mobility and support. In Hinchliff, S., Montague, S. *Physiology for Nursing Practice.* pp. 205, 243–263. London. Baillière Tindall.

HEEBINK, D.M. (ed.) (1981) Effects of bedrest on physical condition. *Respiratory Care* **26**: 1278–1280.

HERBERT, R.A., ALISON, J.A. (1996) Cardiovascular function. In Hinchliff, S.M., Montague, S.E., Watson, R. (eds) *Physiology for Nursing Practice,* 2nd edition. pp. 445–447. London. Baillière Tindall.

HINCHLIFF, S.M., MONTAGUE, S.E., WATSON, R. (1996) *Physiology for Nursing Practice,* 2nd edition. London. Baillière Tindall.

HOLMES, P.A. (1988) World turned upside down. *Nursing Times* **84(6)**: 42.

JIROVEC, M.M. (1991) The impact of daily exercise on the mobility, balance and urine control of cognitively impaired nursing home residents. *International Journal of Nursing Studies* **28(2)**: 145–151.

JONES, L. (1994) *The Social Context of Health and Health Work.* p. 331. London. Macmillan.

JUDD, M. (1989) *Mobility: Patient Problems and Nursing Care.* pp. 3–4. Oxford. Heinemann Nursing.

KASTENBAUM, R. (1979) *Growing Old.* London. Harper Row.

KILBURY, R.F., BENSHOFF, J.J., RUBIN, S.E. (1992) The interaction of legislation, public attitudes and access to opportunities for persons with disabilities. *Journal of Rehabilitation* **58(4)**: 6–9.

MAHONEY, F.I., BARTHEL, D.W. (1965) Functional evaluation: the Barthel Index. *Maryland State Medical Journal* **14**: 61–65.

MAKIN, C. (ed.) (1991) *Collins English Dictionary* (3rd edition). p. 1003. Glasgow. Harper Collins.

MANDELSTAM, M. (1993) *How to Get Equipment for Disability.* p. 142. London. Jessica Kingsley Publishers and Kogan Page for The Disabled Living Foundation.

MASTERSON, A. (1995) Mobility and immobility. pp. 485, 488. In Heath, H.B.M. (ed.) *Potter and Perry's Foundations in Nursing Theory and Practice.* London. Mosby.

McLAREN, S.M. (1996) Mobility and support. In Hinchliff, S.M., Montague, S.E., Watson, R. (eds) *Physiology for Nursing Practice,* 2nd edition. pp. 309–319. London. Baillière Tindall.

MEDICAL RESEARCH COUNCIL (1976) *Aids to the Examination of the Peripheral Nervous System.* London. Her Majesty's Stationery Office.

MILLER, V., ONOTERA, R.T., DEINARD, A.S. (1984) Denvir Development Screening Tests: Cultural variations in southeast Asian children. *Journal of Paediatrics* **104(3)**: 481–482.

MINISTER FOR DISABLED PEOPLE (1996) *The Disability Discrimination Act, Definition of Disability.* p. 2. DL60, HSSS JO3–6299JP.100m.

MORRIS, J. (1993) *Independent Lives, Community Care and Disabled People.* p. 13. London. The Macmillan Press Ltd.

NORMAN, A. (1985) *Triple Jeopardy: Growing Old in a Second Homeland.* London. Centre for Policy on Aging.

OFFICE OF POPULATION CENSUSES AND SURVEYS (1995) *1993 General Household Survey No. 24.* London. Her Majesty's Stationery Office.

OGDEN, B. (1992) Moving and lifting. In Brown, H., Benson, S. (eds) *A Practical Guide to Working with People with Learning Disabilities.* pp. 123–146. London. Hawker Publications.

OPEN UNIVERSITY (1985) *Birth to Old Age, Health in Transition.* p. 170. Milton Keynes. The Open University Press.

PAPALIA, D.E., WENDKOS OLDS, S. (1989) *Human Development* (4th edition). p. 105. New York. McGraw Hill.

POMEROY, V. (1990) Development of an ADL orientated assessment of mobility scale suitable for use with elderly people with dementia. *Physiotherapy* **76(8)**: 446–448.

PRYOR, G.A., WILLIAMS, D.R.R. (1989) Rehabilitation after hip fractures. *Journal of Bone and Joint Surgery (Br)* **71B(3)**: 471–474.

ROBINSON, J.L., SCHMIDT, G.L. (1981) Quantitative gait evaluation in the clinic. *Physical Therapy* **61**: 351–353.

SCHWARZ, C. (ed.) (1995) *The Chambers Dictionary.* p. 1077. Edinburgh. Chambers Harrap Publications.

STEWART, D.A., BURNS, J.M.A., DUNN, S.G., ROBERTS, M.A. (1990) The two minute walking test: a sensitive index of mobility in the rehabilitation of elderly patients. *Clinical Rehabilitation* **4**: 273–276.

TAYLOR, A. (1995) Debilitating discrimination. *Nursing Times* **91(44)**: 38–40.

TAYLOR, S., FIELD, D. (1993) *Sociology of Health and Health Care.* pp. 127, 128. London. Blackwell Scientific Publications.

THAPA, P.B., GIDEON, P., FOUGHT, R.L., KORMICKI, M., RAY, W.A. (1994) Comparison of clinical and biomechanical measures of balance and mobility in elderly nursing home residents. *Journal of American Geriatrics Society* **42(5)**: 439–500.

TORTORA, G.J., ANAGNOSTAKOS, N.P. (1987) *Principles of Anatomy and Physiology* (5th edition). pp. 120, 195. London. Harper and Row.

TYLER, M. (1984) The respiratory effects of body positioning and immobilisation. *Respiratory Care* **19**: 472–483.

UKCC (1992) *Code of Professional Conduct.* London. UKCC.

US CONGRESS (1990) *Public Law 101–336: The Americans with Disabilities Act,* Washington DC: 101st Congress.

WADE, D.T, LANGTON–HEWER, R., SKILBECK, C.E., DAND, R.M. (1985) *Stroke: A Critical Approach to Diagnosis, Treatment and Management.* London. Chapman and Hall.

WEBB, R., TOSSELL, D. (1991) *Social Issues for Carers, a Community Care Perspective.* London. Edward Arnold.

WELLER, B.F. (ed.) (1989) *Baillière's Encyclopaedic Dictionary of Nursing and Health Care.* pp. 221, 602. London. Baillière Tindall.

WINDMILL, V. (1990) *Ageing Today, a Positive Approach to Caring for Elderly People.* p. 6. London. Edward Arnold.

WYN WILLIAMS, M., NOLAN, M. (1993) Prevention of falls among older people at home. *British Journal of Nursing* **2(12)**: 609–613.

3.5 Death and Dying

L. Wilson

KEY ISSUES

■ SUBJECT KNOWLEDGE

▷ different forms of death from death of the cell through to cortical and brain stem death
▷ concept of ontological death and the 'near death experience'
▷ differing cultural perspectives on death
▷ the grieving process and coping with loss

■ PRACTICE KNOWLEDGE

▷ breaking bad news
▷ physical signs of an approaching death
▷ the management of care of the dying patient

■ PROFESSIONAL KNOWLEDGE

▷ trends in the location of death in today's society
▷ issues in the professional coping with death
▷ the impact of the living will or advance directive
▷ euthanasia
▷ the role of the coroner in certain deaths

■ REFLECTIVE KNOWLEDGE

▷ personal fears and misgivings about own death and that of others
▷ consolidate knowledge through case study exercises

▷ INTRODUCTION

Death is a unique experience for each person and unlike certain other nursing and medical interventions where we can improve on our initial care, we have no second chance in this situation. It is vital that as nurses we never treat the death event as a routine experience. The care of dying people is an issue within the care of clients in a broad spectrum of settings.

As an introduction to the subject of death and dying, it is essential that we are able to differentiate between palliative care and terminal care:

▷ palliative care or palliation is a broad band of care of indeterminate length that should start from the moment a patient is diagnosed as having a disease for which there is no cure, and the focus of the care of the client moves from curing to caring (i.e. symptom relief as opposed to curative treatment);
▷ terminal care is the management of the end of life (i.e. the last hours or days before death).

It has been argued that health professionals have difficulty managing patients who require palliative care, partly because of the conflict in cure versus care. Virginia Henderson (1966) in her definition of nursing identified the management of the dying patient as a key part of the nurse's function, carrying equal weight with the curative element. As medicine is very much concerned with cure, a dying patient is often seen as a failure and this may lead to treatment being offered that is no longer of benefit to the individual (Cassell, 1974). The registered nurse is often in a position to help junior medical staff cope with the loss of the patient and handled sensitively, the nurse can have a marked influence on the subsequent management of such patients.

This chapter will enable you to consider many of the issues surrounding death and dying and to empower you to make sound, well considered nursing decisions as you progress through your career.

▶ OVERVIEW

▶ *Subject Knowledge*

In the biological part, the definitions of death, what it is and how it may impinge on the art of nursing are explored. The physical manifestations of death, the life cycle of the cell and types of death are addressed. In the psychosocial part societal and cultural attitudes to death are explored, the determinants and processes of grieving are examined, and finally the stages in the dying process are outlined.

▶ *Practice Knowledge*

The role of the nurse in managing the care of the dying is discussed. Care needed by relatives is introduced.

▶ *Professional Knowledge*

In this part we discuss the role of the coroner, managing the death, the necessary formalities and the legal and ethical problems associated with the dying individual.

▶ *Reflective Knowledge*

Here you are asked to explore your own personal responses to death and dying. You have an opportunity to consider four case studies using your personal experience and the chapter content.

On pp. 472–473 there are four case studies, each one relating to one of the branch programmes. You may find it helpful to read one of them before you start the chapter and use it as a focus for your reflections while reading.

SUBJECT KNOWLEDGE Biological

What is death? On a microscopic level, cells in our body are dying and renewing constantly from the time we are born. At this stage it is therefore probably helpful to consider the life cycle of the cell from its inception to its death.

▶ CELL LIFE AND DEATH

Normal cells undergo orderly regular periods of mitosis (cell reproduction) and normal cell growth occurs in two phases in man and animals:

- ▶ the first phase of growth is from birth to maturity where the total number of cells is constantly increasing as the person or animal gets bigger and grows to full size;
- ▶ the second phase of growth is from maturity to death when the number of cells produced equals the number of cells that die as overall body size remains relatively constant.

In adults, whether cell growth is fast or slow, the overall number of cells normally does not increase (Sinclair, 1989).

Cells are created either by the process of:

- ▶ mitosis, where the parent cell reproduces itself to produce two daughter cells identical to the parent cell;

▶ or meiosis, which occurs only in spermatozoa or egg cells where each daughter cell has the haploid number of chromosomes.

Some cells are incapable of replacement, for example heart cells and neurones, while others have a limited ability to replicate. The lifespan of a cell varies according to its cell type. A neurone does not reproduce in a lifetime whereas an epithelial cell in the gut wall may reproduce every day. Tissues composed of relatively undifferentiated cells, for example bones and the liver, are able to regenerate themselves easily. At the other extreme, a cell can become so specialized that it cannot reproduce itself, for example the erythrocyte (Montague and Knight, 1996). There is normally strict control over the rate of growth of cells in any body tissue by the integrated actions of hormones and growth factors. Loss of such control leads to tumour growth. In cancer, the life cycle of the cell is somewhat different. Apparent spreading of a malignant disease is generally due to the increased life span of cells rather than the proliferation of cancer cells. Priestman (1989) points out that only 50–60% of cancer cells die during the span of the disease.

When a cell is injured or is dying, the lysosomes (Greek: lysis, dissolution; soma, body) release their enzymes and the cell is broken down. Lysosomes are vital for phagocytosis to occur and large numbers of them are present in leucocytes. Lysosomes are sometimes thought of as the trigger for cell suicide.

A regulated change occurs as we advance in chronological age and is referred to as the normal ageing process. Normal life expectancy, which refers to the average length of survival of a species, is determined by environmental factors, whereas life span denotes the maximum age reached and appears to depend upon genes (Montague and Knight, 1996). Although life expectancy can improve when the environment improves, life span for an individual may remain unchanged. Several theories have been proposed to explain how cellular ageing occurs (Cunningham and Brookbank, 1988; Brookbank, 1990), but none are conclusive (see Annotated Further Reading). Generalized changes with ageing involve all organ systems resulting in a loss of reserve function, which will eventually lead to total system failure and death. The rate at which this occurs naturally varies with each individual. However, if there is acute damage to organs at any age, as in multiple trauma, which leads to shock and loss of circulation to vital tissues, then multiple organ failure becomes a feature in the dying process of that individual (Viney, 1996).

▶ CARDIORESPIRATORY DEATH

Most people regard death as cardiorespiratory death, that is the heart and lungs are no longer functioning. Until the advent of resuscitation and ventilation of patients this was death. However, one of the universal truths about death is that it is irreversible and resuscitation meant that this was no longer necessarily the case. The majority of people who die will still, however, be judged against the cardiorespiratory criteria outlined in Table 3.5.1.

▶ BRAIN STEM DEATH

With the advent of ventilation, it has become necessary to devise an alternative method of diagnosing death as the patient on life support will

Cessation of respiration
Absent heart and pulse sounds
Lack of spontaneous activity
Absence of reflexes and response to stimuli
Dilated fixed pupils
Persistent distortion of the pupil and eyeball on pressure
Segmentation of blood in the retinal arteries when viewed by ophthalmoscope
Rigor mortis

Table 3.5.1 Criteria for cardiorespiratory death.

Fixed pupils
Absent corneal reflex
Absent vestibulo-ocular reflexes: no eye movements during or after slow injection of ice cold water into each ear
No motor cranial nerve responses
No gag reflex or response to bronchial stimulation by catheter
No respiratory effort off the respirator with the $P_{CO_2} > 6.7$ kPa

Table 3.5.2 Criteria for brain stem death. (From Hinds and Watson, 1996.)

have a maintained heart beat and lung function. The criteria to establish brain stem death (Table 3.5.2) were devised to provide clear parameters for clinical staff when making decisions about discontinuing life support (Pallis, 1983; Pallis and Harley, 1996).

Brain stem death was identified and discussed by the Conference of Medical Colleges and Faculties of the United Kingdom in 1976 (Jennett, 1982) and Hinds and Watson (1996) speak of it as 'If the brain stem is destroyed, consciousness is lost and spontaneous respiration ceases. Independent existence is then impossible, and in the absence of therapeutic intervention cardiac arrest rapidly supervenes'. The criteria by which brain stem death can be diagnosed have been the subject of debate and review since brain stem death was recognized and identified as a specific form of death (Pallis, 1983; Fisher, 1991; Norton, 1992; Day, 1995). Doctors must ensure that the individual being tested for brain stem death is not under the effect of any paralyzing drugs such as vecuronium bromide and atracurium besylate, which may be used to sedate patients while they are ventilated. These drugs act by competing with acetylcholine at the receptor site at the neuromuscular junction. The action of these muscle relaxants can be reversed with anticholinesterases such as neostigmine (British Medical Association and Pharmaceutical Society, 1997). Likewise the patient who has overdosed on barbiturates, which is now rare, requires a careful assessment to ensure that the sedative effects of the drug do not mask the patient's reaction to the brain stem death criteria. The same caution applies if barbiturates have been used to treat intractable cerebral oedema (Louis *et al.*, 1993) and sufficient time should be given after the cessation of treatment before undertaking the brain stem tests. Similar problems arise with clients suffering from myxoedema and hypothermia as their reactions will be very sluggish and may even be imperceptible. A number of other endocrine and metabolic disorders also need to be excluded and these are clearly identified within the guidelines available at your hospital, which will be based on the national guidelines.

The patient must be maintained at a temperature of at least 35°C. The brain stem death tests are carried out by two medical practitioners, one of whom is the anaesthetist or physician in charge of the case while the

Find out if your practice placement areas have got a copy of any local guidelines for diagnosing brain stem death.

- *Compare these local guidelines with what has been outlined in this chapter.*

- *Reflect on what relatives feelings might be if their relative is diagnosed as dead and yet the body remains ventilated.*

- *Discuss with your peers how you feel and how health care professionals cope with these situations.*

other must not be involved with either the care of the patient or the transplant team if an organ transplant is being considered. The brain stem tests are carried out once and then repeated 4–48 hours later. If both tests are negative the ventilator support maintaining respiratory function is discontinued.

▶ CORTICAL BRAIN DEATH

The concept of cortical brain death was first proposed in the USA with the Nancy Cruzan case and subsequently in the UK with the Tony Bland case (Jennett and Dyer, 1991), in which the patients were in a 'persistent vegetative state' and had suffered irreversible cortical brain damage, which had destroyed the higher senses. This situation does not mean, however, that the patient's death is imminent. With feeding and skilled nursing management such an individual can exist for many years. It is difficult to class this as living as this suggests a life of which one is aware. The fact remains that unlike brain stem death, the life of these patients can be sustained. The ethical dilemmas related to the concept of cortical brain death are discussed more fully later in the Professional Knowledge part of this chapter.

▶ ONTOLOGICAL DEATH

A highly controversial notion is that of ontological death. Philosophers in the USA have suggested that once the personhood of an individual has been irretrievably destroyed, they are to all intents and purposes dead and can be used as donors. Personhood concerns the essence of the individual not the biological being – it is consciousness, recognition of self as an entity, reasoning, moral coding and the many other attributes we associate with being 'ourselves'. Loss of personhood is seen as loss of the self. This theory would have significant repercussions for the severely handicapped, dementing and other vulnerable individuals.

▶ THE NEAR DEATH EXPERIENCE

Throughout history, individuals have described experiences of having glimpsed the hereafter; one of the more interesting descriptions can be found in the *Book of Revelations* in the *Bible* (Chapter 21), which theologians believe must have included this phenomenon. Cole (1993) cites an American opinion poll that suggests that near death experiences (NDEs) are not rare occurrences. Some 38–50% of those who come close to death recount experiences consistent with an NDE.

Physiologists have claimed that such experiences can be replicated in the laboratory by the use of mind altering drugs and brain stimulation. Blackmore (1988) gives a detailed breakdown of the process, but does not, however, totally explain why only some patients experience an NDE. The salient features of any NDE are similar regardless of culture, age, sex, educational background, financial status or psychiatric history (Osis and Haraldsson, 1986). A study by Sabom (1982) reinforces these findings and highlights the concern of those who have had this kind of experience that they are not believed. According to Ring (1980) the features of an NDE are:

- **Have you or any of your relatives or friends experienced what has been described above as an NDE?**
- **Were you or they able to describe their experiences to others?**
- **What was the reaction of others to your or their experience?**
- **Reflect on what your reactions and feelings are about this phenomonon?**
- **How might your reactions influence your response and decision making if confronted with a patient who recounts an NDE to you?**

- an initial phase linked to feelings of extraordinary peace, calm, warmth and comfort;
- separation from the physical body with a bird's eye view of the body – the so-called 'out of body experience';
- movement through a cylindrical dark space, which ends with a bright light;
- meeting a being of light, which is often the appropriate deity for the individual;
- emerging into a beautiful place such as a garden or a 'heaven-like' place where those who are already dead are encountered.

The vast majority of NDEs are described as joyous and not alarming. However, for a few the experience is very distressing, these same features creating a hell-like environment rather than the reassuring one described above. Given that at least 20% of patients undergoing a cardiac arrest procedure experience an NDE, nurses need to recognize their role in allowing patients to discuss what they have experienced.

The author's clinical experience suggests that patients worry that they will not be believed, or worse still that they are hallucinating, and feel a considerable sense of relief when they realize that they are not alone in what they have seen and felt. It may be worthwhile for the nursing care plan following a cardiac arrest with the subsequent survival of the patient to include the potential problem of the patient having had an NDE.

A change in behaviour may lead the nurse to suspect that the patient has had an NDE with the patient commonly becoming either agitated or conversely withdrawn and quiet. The patient should be encouraged, but never pressed, to talk about what happened and whether they saw or experienced anything while they were very ill. It is essential that anything confided by the patient is not dismissed, though it may appear extremely bizarre. These episodes may be interpreted as confusion on occasions. Children also have these experiences.

For information on grieving in children see Annotated Further Reading – Hill (1994).

DECISION MAKING

Schoenbeck (1993) discusses several cases gleaned from discussions with nurses. Mandy was ten years old and dying following an unsuccessful third bone marrow graft. 'Gowned masked and gloved, Stacey entered the isolation cubicle. The girls talked about old times – the years that they had known each other. Mandy told her friend she knew she would not get better, that she was going to die. Then Mandy spoke of something that Stacey didn't understand. Mandy said she had already left her body once and had gone through a tunnel. She said she came back to say goodbye and when she left this time she wouldn't return. She told Stacey that Jesus was waiting for her and that everything would be alright'. Mandy died the same night.

- **How could you support Stacey, another ten year old in the grieving process?**
- **Try to identify what support she would need.**
- **How significant do you think the account of Mandy's NDE will be in trying to help Stacey to grieve?**

Psychosocial   This part of Subject Knowledge will first briefly examine the common causes of death before exploring cultural attitudes to death. It will then discuss what is meant by an 'appropriate' death before finally outlining theories about the grieving and dying processes.

▶ THE CAUSE OF DEATH

The disease most feared by people is cancer, despite the many forms of the disease that are now curable or responsive to treatment (Open University, 1992). More people die in road accidents or of chronic obstructive airways disease (COAD) than die of cancer (Office of Population

Censuses and Surveys, 1991). Diseases that have a poorer prognosis do not inspire the same fear among the general public for many reasons. As health care professionals we can help to dispel some of the myths about cancer by informing ourselves, for example at five years after diagnosis 3% of people with COAD are still alive compared with 62% of patients with cancer of the breast (Cancer Research Campaign, 1988). It is always useful to be aware of local trends in illness as they are variable depending upon the cultural mix, the environment and employment patterns, as well as on the level of individual wealth or deprivation and on the health beliefs and attitudes of individuals.

The death of a child is extremely difficult to cope with, particularly as we know that most children recover from their accidents and illnesses much more rapidly than adults. However, children do die and the impact of their deaths is more acute than that for any other deaths (Hindmarch, 1993). The majority of deaths occur prenatally (26%) or neonatally (25%) (Office of Population Censuses and Surveys, 1991). In the early months of life, sudden unexplained deaths or 'cot deaths' (sudden infant death syndrome) cause extreme distress to parents who cannot understand why their child has died. Although in many cases, a cause can be found, in others there is no explanation. Reducing the risk by identifying factors that may be influential is the best that can be achieved at present (Hindmarch, 1993). Accidental death accounts for 19% of childhood deaths (Office of Population Censuses and Surveys, 1991) and occurs at all ages and from many causes. As with adults, coping with the diagnosis of cancer in a child is extremely difficult despite the recent improvements in prognosis. The uncertainty about the future health of the child causes a different kind of anguish, described by Eisenberg (1981) as the 'Damocles syndrome' (the sword of sorrow hanging over the family).

▶ ATTITUDES TOWARDS DEATH

Attitudes towards death and dying have changed dramatically this century, particularly in the years since World War II. With the improvement in infant mortality rate and increasing life expectancy, death is no longer a commonplace experience among the public. Rather than being an event for which families would gather at the bedside and the body would lie in the front parlour, many people have not had contact with a death. Care of the deceased is now left largely to the professional, namely undertakers. In effect, as long as you can pay, you need not have any contact with the body at all. The lack of familiarity with death makes people fearful and anxious about their own death and that of their family members.

We are confronted by horrific scenes of murder and carnage nightly on television and in graphic pictures in newspapers, to the extent that it no longer impinges on our consciousness, so–called 'compassion overload'. If it happened in front of us, doubtless we would be profoundly affected and would do all we could to help, but it is, in fact, removed from us and distant.

- *Reflect on your own views about how you would like to die if you had a choice.*
- *Discuss in a sensitive way with your parents and grandparents what they believe would be a 'good death'.*

DECISION MAKING

Rebecca Weinburger, aged 70 years, is terminally ill with breast cancer and is admitted to hospital for symptom control. Sadly she rapidly deteriorates and subsequently dies.

- *As this woman is a very Orthodox Jewess, what constraints and restrictions will be placed on gentile nursing staff in caring for her before she dies?*
- *How should her body be treated after death while it is still in your care?*

Our attitudes towards the type of death that is preferable have also changed. Our forefathers would have chosen a slow lingering death in preference to a sudden death because of the need to settle their affairs and gather everyone together. Surveys carried out now suggest that people would prefer to die in their sleep or suddenly (Open University, 1992). Attitudes are very much culturally determined and depend upon the beliefs that people have about for example the afterlife, retribution and reincarnation.

Knowledge of the customs and beliefs of ethnic or minority religions can provide great comfort to relatives and friends. Demonstrating an understanding and respecting their views facilitates the grieving process instead of making them angry or defensive. There are marked religious norms in relation to the grieving process. Whereas, in western culture, a dying individual is visited by close family and friends, within Asian groups, large numbers of visitors may arrive to pay their respects and wish to stay night and day. A dying Buddhist will often wish to forego pain relief and to lie on the floor to be near to Mother Earth and to meditate. Such behaviour can be interpreted as confusion and caring staff may put the patient back to bed several times because they do not understand the significance of what is happening. It is important to ask the patient or relatives for an explanation of any behaviour that you consider bizarre within your culture.

If a religion is cyclical, as in eastern religions (e.g. hinduism, buddhism), and individuals believe in a continuous series of lives, the death will only be a means of transfer to a new life. This belief may explain in part the more readily accepting manner in which death is approached by both the family and the client. Religious beliefs and references to the practice and customs of different ethnic groups are numerous and diverse and should be explored in depth (see Annotated Further Reading) (Green, 1989; Narayansamy, 1993, 1995; Praill, 1995).

It is useful to record a contact name and number for the religious representative of any patient from a minority group, as well as recording religious affiliation so that if the patient suffers an unexpected collapse the appropriate people can be contacted to provide support for both the patient and family. A knowledge of where people can find support is valuable for both the dying person and the dying person's friends and relatives. The aim of care must be to meet the holistic needs of the patient – physical, psychological, social and spiritual – if we are to make a significant contribution towards the patient's 'good death'. Sadly many of our standards of care for the dying patient fall far short of what we would personally find acceptable or desirable for ourselves or our relatives (Copp, 1994).

RESEARCH BASED EVIDENCE

In her article Palliative Care – Nursing Education, *Copp (1994)* looks at the efficacy of specialist education and its application to the care of dying patients. She cites studies that look at the stresses associated with the management of such patients. She particularly focuses on the skills and specific knowledge required to enable nurses to give good palliative care. Kuhse and Singer (1993) looking at voluntary euthanasia quote numerous nurses who feel that the palliative care offered to patients is lacking. The questionnaire was distributed to 1942 nurses at random and had a 49% reply rate. Although the emphasis of the research was euthanasia, it gave an interesting view of Australian perspectives on the dying process.

▶ AN APPROPRIATE DEATH

All of us have images in our heads of what we would consider to be the ideal way to die and have probably discussed this 'ideal' with relatives and friends in terms of 'wishes'. We can also think of things we would like to achieve before we die. These achievements become more acute

A 60-year-old woman attending day care at her local hospice explains that she has been coming for 18 months. The criterion for attendance is a projected life expectancy of less than six months. Most of her friends there have died and she had been very depressed by this until she realized that she was still alive and could get on with living. In her words 'I'm not dead yet so I had better get on with living'.

- *What communication skills would be necessary in order to help this woman decide what she most wants to achieve in her time before she dies?*
- *Investigate what support services may be available locally now that she has decided to make the most of the time she has left.*
- *Attend one of these support groups and analyse the key aims of the group and how they achieve these aims.*
- *How will completing this exercise help in your decision making in the future with a similar or comparable situation.*

and important when a person is given an estimate of how long he or she will live when diagnosed with an incurable disease. Weisman (1988) speaks of 'appropriate' death and suggests that certain criteria jointly constitute this for the individual. These criteria include:

- reducing, but not necessarily eliminating, conflict;
- making dying compatible with the dying person's own view of him or herself and his or her achievements;
- preserving or restoring relationships as much as possible;
- fulfilling some of the dying person's expressed aims.

Our expectations of when death is appropriate also affects the way in which we react to it. For an adult the death of a parent is seen as a great sadness, but is within the natural scheme of things – that is the elders leaving room for the new generation. The death of a child is a death of the future, the life that would have been rather than the life that has been. Sudden death in contrast to the expected death is particularly stressful because it challenges all our established coping strategies (Wright, 1996, Chapter 2.2). There are numerous factors influencing how we manage the unmanageable, and the overwhelming nature of sudden death needs to be brought down to manageable proportions, for example where a young mother has died, who will look after the children and who can collect them from school. The bereaved individual needs to work in small steps initially to cope. These coping strategies in relation to death are usually referred to in terms of the 'grieving process'.

▶ GRIEF

Grief and its expression are very individual phenomena and each person who is suffering must be helped in the ways most suited to his or her needs. Many studies have been carried out in order to investigate common patterns that contribute to grief as a concept and a reality (Parkes, 1975, 1987; Parkes and Parkes, 1984). Wright (1991) cites the determinants of grief as identified by Parkes (1975) in the Harvard Study. These determinants are listed in Table 3.5.3 and each is discussed in more detail.

Mode of death
Nature of the attachment
Who the person was
Historical antecedents
Personality variables
Social variables

Table 3.5.3 Determinants of grief.

RESEARCH BASED EVIDENCE

Stone (1995) surveyed surviving spouses of 35 people who had committed suicide and 31 people who had died a non-suicide death and reported that among the survivors of suicide, there was more illness after the death, stigma was associated with the death, spouses were blamed by friends and relatives, and spouses felt angry with the dead spouse and guilt about their own actions both before and after the death.

Research by Dunne et al. (1987) of responses of family members to the suicide of a family member found that family divisions, a pessimistic view of the future, and self destructive behaviours were frequently mentioned by survivors.

DECISION MAKING

Trevor Stevens was a 20-year-old chemistry student who had recently split up from his girlfriend, Rosemary. An exceptionally bright young man, he was also extremely reserved. He attempted suicide by ingesting 30 paracetamol tablets with whisky. He was not found for several hours and despite inpatient treatment died. Rosemary was not blamed initially, but within weeks of the funeral, Mrs Stevens could not be civil to her and the atmosphere at the inquest was very bitter. Rosemary continued to feel guilty and depressed and eventually needed professional help to come to terms with Trevor's death.
- *Reflect on the factors that may have compounded Rosemary's grief.*
- *Decide on which counselling approach might be appropriate in helping Rosemary come to terms with the situation (see Chapter 4.1).*

The Mode of Death

How a person dies can be extremely important, especially if the person is found dead and the death is unexpected. Questions such as did he or she suffer? was he or she involved in an accident? was it his or her fault? puzzle and concern grieving relatives for a long time afterwards. All of us wish to die in familiar surroundings and if death occurs in a strange environment it gives an added dimension to the grief. Suicide produces particular problems because those who are left look for reasons and apportion blame in order to try to make sense of what has happened. A suicide in adolescence is particularly hard to bear as it is difficult to accept that a young person with all of life's potential before them should choose to end it and suicide can be seen as a massive rejection of the parents who conceived and nurtured that life (Hindmarch, 1993).

The Nature of the Attachment

The natural peaks and troughs of any relationship will affect the way in which the death is perceived. The feelings will not be the same if the relationship was strong and supportive as those if the couple were ambivalent towards each other.

Who the Person Was

The unique position of the dead person in the family will affect the grief that is felt at their demise. The strong matriarch, the downtrodden wife, the domineering husband are but a few examples of the relative influence and position of the dead person within the family circle. The dependence upon the deceased may give some pointers as to the progress of grief. The death of a spouse may give the surviving partner freedom once again and may be seen as a good thing.

Historical Antecedents

How the bereaved individual has coped with crisis previously will have an effect on this bereavement. If he or she did not work the grief through in the past, the current problems may well be compounded and this will complicate the grieving process.

Personality Variables

Problems occur more readily if the bereaved person has had a particularly dependent and clinging relationship with the deceased or has been ambivalent towards the deceased.

Social Variables

Religious beliefs and responses of communities to grief may help or hinder the grieving process. Wright (1991) cites the case of a Jewish woman who had great difficulty coping with the death of her baby son because of the tradition of burial within 24 hours and her subsequent feelings of not being able to say goodbye.

THE GRIEVING PROCESS

The experience of grief can concern nurses who have had no previous experience of bereavement. However, reflect on an occasion when you have failed at something such as an important relationship or examination as the feelings are almost the same and you can provide suitable support by remembering this. Engel (1964) identified the stages of grief as follows:

▶ numbness and disbelief, often with a sense of unreality and slow motion;
▶ anger and guilt;
▶ depression and sadness;
▶ grief pangs;
▶ readaptation (resolution);

Engel (1964) takes the view that losing a loved one is as psychologically traumatic as being seriously injured oneself. He argues that normal grief reactions are a threat to one's mental health. In the same way that physical healing is necessary to help the body restore its equilibrium, thus a time is required to allow grieving to occur.

Stages in the grieving process apply equally to anticipatory (before the event) grief and the feelings experienced when a loved one actually dies. The reactions of relatives to a poor prognosis and the death of their loved one can be many and varied, ranging from frozen to histrionics. Judging the relative who does not appear unduly moved as coping well is often erroneous.

Grief in children, especially when grieving for a brother or sister, can get mixed up with feelings of guilt that something they have done has caused the illness and death. Relationships with parents can also be affected as children may blame the parents for their sibling's illness and death (Sourkes, 1987). There is a concurrent need to allow the grieving child space and time to question and talk about their feelings as well as for parents to share their grief with the child or children that remain (Cowlishaw, 1993).

Worden (1991) identified the tasks of mourning as being able to:

▶ accept the reality of loss;
▶ experience the pain of loss;
▶ adjust to the environment where the deceased is missing;
▶ move on with life.

According to Worden (1991) the first step is to accept the reality of the loss. Where a death has been anticipated and the family have observed the gradual decline in health of the significant person who is dying, the loss is an observable phenomenon. In the case of sudden death, particularly where there is no body, as in a major maritime disaster, accepting the loss can be extremely difficult. Parents bereaved through cot death often return to the hospital to see the baby several times to reassure themselves that it is their baby who has died. Parents may find it difficult to hand the baby over to the staff to be moved to the mortuary and hospital staff have said that they find it difficult to put the baby in the fridge without wrapping it in a blanket.

Worden (1991) also says that we need to experience the pain of the loss. As nurses and as fellow human beings, watching individuals who are suffering and not being able to stop the hurt is very difficult. However, severe psychological problems can result if someone is not allowed to grieve. Unresolved grief can lead to psychological disturbance and mental ill health. The pain is needed to allow healing. Large companies allowing three days' compassionate leave can suggest that the acute grief can be dealt with within this time frame. Parkes and Parkes (1984) suggest that

---

DECISION MAKING

Mrs James waved goodbye to her husband before taking the children to school. Mr James was then involved in a road traffic accident on his way to work and died instantly. Mrs Jones was vacuuming when the police arrived to give her the news. She said she would just be a moment and then continued her housework. She had to be told three times before the information started to impinge on her consciousness. Shock can have a delaying effect on grieving.

• *Using Engel's model for grieving (Engel, 1964) can you identify why Mrs James behaved as she did?*
• *What strategies could be used to support Mrs James while in this particular stage of grieving?*

DECISION MAKING

Mrs Feeney had been married for 37 years to Charles when he collapsed with a massive stroke and died. Mrs Feeney's daughter was very worried by the overwhelming nature of the grief and asked the general practitioner to call. He prescribed a course of antidepressants and Mrs Feeney remained on the tablets for several years, not feeling very much pleasure or pain. When Mrs Feeney became aware of the problems of tranquillizer addiction, she decided to try to stop and sought help from her general practitioner. He referred her to a community psychiatric nurse , who is now helping her with in-depth counselling and support as Mrs Feeney is now battling dependence and coping with her unresolved grief. She has had two short admissions to the psychiatric department.

- **How could Mrs Feeney have been helped to cope with her grief immediately after her husband's death?**
- **Debate the issue of prescribing drug therapy in order to help people cope with loss in any form.**
- **Explore the specific counselling approaches that the community psychiatric nurse could take in helping Mrs Feeney.**

---

two years is a realistic period of mourning. Although we recognize the needs of bereaved people to explore the loss, often many times over, it is very difficult to facilitate this and people cannot then share the distress they feel.

The third task in mourning involves adjusting to an environment in which the deceased is missing. Worden (1991) recognizes that the survivor does not always realize all of the roles performed by the deceased until some three months have elapsed from the time of the death. The survivor has to learn skills that were previously the responsibility of the deceased. Through doing this, the bereaved person may well restore the damage to their feelings of self worth.

Finally the survivor needs to 'relocate the deceased and move on with life' (Worden, 1991). The deceased will always be remembered and significant, but the time has now come to love and live again. Worden (1991) cites a case from Alexy (1982, p. 503) where a mother is talking about her dead son as a good example of 'moving on': 'Only recently have I begun to take notice of things in life that are still open to me. You know things that can bring me pleasure. I know that I will continue to grieve for Robbie for the rest of my life, and that I will keep his loving memory alive. But life goes on, and like it or not I am part of it. Lately there have been times when I notice how well I seem to be doing on some project at home, or even taking part in some activity with friends'.

DECISION MAKING

Mrs Monk was a 67-year-old widow who had multiple myeloma diagnosed for more than one year. She attended the ward for frequent blood transfusions, but appeared totally unwilling to explore what was wrong with her. Having asked several very leading questions to the students on the ward, the registrar decided to discuss her diagnosis with her. He explained frankly and clearly to her the type of illness she had, the likely prognosis and the treatment. She appeared to be very grateful to him and expressed this as he left. However, within 15 minutes, she was heard expressing serious doubts about his knowledge and competence. Mrs Monk knew, but had not been thrilled at having what she had already guessed confirmed.

- **Using Kubler Ross's model, can you identify which stage (if any) of the dying process Mrs Monk is expressing.**
- **Explore Kubler Ross's model in more detail and discuss how well it fits with your practice experiences to date.**
- **Can this model be applied to your personal experiences of loss of any kind?**

▶ THE DYING PROCESS

So far in this section we have focused on societal and cultural attitudes to death and on coping with grief. The focus has been on the bereaved and outside what the actual experience of dying might mean for the individual. In this section, the focus is on the dying process itself. One of the best recognized approaches to the dying process was devised by Kubler Ross (1975) (Table 3.5.4). She postulated a series of steps or stages through which dying people frequently pass. These stages do not apply to everyone and

Denial	'They can't mean me'
Anger	'Why should this be happening to me'
Bargaining	'What can I do to take this weight away from me'
Depression	'Everything is useless, I wish I were dead'
Acceptance	'Let me enjoy what time I have left'

Table 3.5.4 Stages in the dying process. (From Kubler Ross, 1975.)

are frequently not followed in a clear orderly sequence. They serve as a guide as to where people are in terms of their understanding and acceptance of the situation in which they find themselves.

PRACTICE KNOWLEDGE

This part will first of all consider the skills you need for breaking bad news before outlining in more detail the physical needs of the patient who is dying so that you can recognize these needs when assessing the patient for terminal care. Finally there is a discussion of the management of terminal care.

▶ BREAKING BAD NEWS

The breaking of bad news requires special skills, which can be learnt rather than being a natural feature of that person's interactions with patients. Buckman (1992) identifies the key stages as follows:

- ▶ get the physical environment right;
- ▶ find out what the patient already knows;
- ▶ find out what the patient wants to know;
- ▶ share the information;
- ▶ respond to the patient's feelings;
- ▶ plan any coping strategies and follow these up.

The fact is that bad news is bad news no matter how sensitively or carefully it is broken, but the long term outcome of breaking bad news in a sensitive and appropriate way will be apparent in the way in which the patient copes with the information. The practice of telling relatives before the patient or instead of the patient is one that often causes alarm among nursing students (Kiger, 1994; Saunders and Valente, 1994). There is a notion that deceiving people protects them and that the truth will harm them. Ian Ainsworth Smith, a hospital chaplain and author was interviewed on this theme and made the rejoinder that finally it is the truth that heals (Ainsworth Smith and Speck, 1982). Nurses need to be wary of colluding with relatives to deceive patients. When relatives say that the patient would not cope with the news, more often it is the relative saying 'I cannot cope with the news' (Buckman, 1992)

> Reflect on your practice experience and note when the relatives rather than the patient or client have been told 'bad news' first.
>
> - **Reflect on how this made you feel at the time.**
> - **Can you justify this activity, even with children? What are your justification arguments?**
> - **Discuss with your fellow students at what age (if age is a criteria) should a child be told 'bad news'.**

▶ RECOGNIZING THAT DEATH IS APPROACHING

Many experienced nurses may say that being able to recognize that death will occur soon is intuitive, a 'gut feeling'. However, it is a number of events that jointly suggest to the experienced nurse that this is the case. Lindley Davis (1991) discusses the physiological changes that occur using a systems based approach. In your assessment of the patient's needs around the time of death, the following knowledge will underpin your decision making about the most appropriate care to give your patients.

▶ *Cardiovascular System*

The heart rate initially increases, but as hypoxia increases then the heart rate and the blood pressure decrease. As peripheral perfusion fails, the patient becomes clammy due to failure of the insensible loss to evaporate from the skin. Because of a decrease in metabolic functioning, the heat lost from the body decreases, but the temperature of vital organs is maintained. The patient is cyanosed, cold and clammy when touched, and the skin appears mottled.

▶ Respiratory System

With failing cardiac output and greatly reduced lymphatic drainage, the lungs become congested, resulting in hypoxia. Breathing decreases and the rhythm can become irregular. As the levels of circulating carbon dioxide increase, so the brain becomes less sensitive and the periods of apnoea increase. The pattern of breathing is often referred to by experienced nurses as Cheyne Stokes respiration, even if at times this may not be strictly physiologically true.

▶ Musculoskeletal System

Severe muscle weakness can occur due to the failing circulation and the frequently reduced intake of nutrients by the dying person. The muscles of the tongue and tissues of the soft palate may fall back into the throat, resulting in a loud snoring sound commonly called the 'death rattle'.

The sphincters controlling the bladder and bowels relax leading to a loss of bowel and bladder function and subsequent soiling in the last hours before death. Walker (1973) discussed her observation that in the moments before death, patients became restless and appeared to struggle even when they had previously been moribund, and that this was followed by a period of calm.

▶ Special Senses

As the level of hypoxia increases, all the special senses are affected and their sensitivity is decreased, in particular the ability of the eyes to focus and distinguish in poor light. As the sensations of taste, smell, hearing and vision fail, the patient may experience changes in mental state. It has been believed that the sense of hearing is the last to fade and that nurses and relatives should continue to communicate verbally with the patient right up to the moment of death.

▶ Renal System

With the fall in cardiac output, there is a corresponding drop in kidney perfusion. This prevents the kidney from functioning efficiently and therefore the amount of urine produced decreases.

▶ Pain

Although pain is often associated in the mind of the public with dying, it is generally the case that pain, if present at all, is well controlled. We usually think of pain as a physical sensation, but if the patient is in mental anguish the perceptions of the family about the level of pain and distress the patient may have are enhanced because they are in the terminal stages of an illness and will soon die. One of the greatest wishes surrounding death is not to die alone or in pain. Many of the features of pain can be recognized through the verbal and non-verbal responses of the patient. Pain may manifest itself as a physical symptom, but may have psychological, spiritual or other roots when it may be unrelieved by analgesia – the concept of 'total pain' as outlined by Saunders (1990) (see also Chapter 2.3 for a fuller discussion on pain and its management).

RESEARCH BASED EVIDENCE

Yeager et al. (1995) have reported that family caregivers:
- *perceive that patients have significantly higher levels of pain compared to patient reports;*
- *perceive that patients experience significantly greater distress from their pain than the patients report themselves;*
- *experience significantly greater distress from the patient's pain than the patients themselves report.*

These results have replicated findings from previous research in this area over the past 30 years. The nurse needs to clarify what pain means to the individual and their carer if support is to be offered to ease the distress.

DECISION MAKING

Mrs Atheterton is terminally ill, having being diagnosed with an inoperable cancer. She wishes to go home to die and her relatives agree. However, she still has an intravenous infusion *in situ* and her son perceives that this is keeping her alive. He becomes quite aggressive towards the multidisciplinary team because if he agrees for the 'drip' to be removed he would be 'murdering his mother'. His mother is afraid to speak out as are the rest of the relatives.

- *Whose wishes should the multidisciplinary team consider as the most important in this situation?*
- *What stage of the grieving process is the son displaying?*
- *What strategies could be employed in order to resolve the situation and allow Mrs Atheterton to die at home*

CARING FOR THE DYING INDIVIDUAL

In order to manage the care of the patient, nurses need to develop their listening skills and be familiar with symptom relief methods. The management of care has been greatly influenced by the hospice movement (Parkes and Parkes, 1984) and by nursing development units such as that run by Dr Jessica Corner at the Royal Marsden Hospital. To promote good quality care, the approach taken by professionals should be empowering so that the patient's wishes matter until they die. To fulfil wishes there should be non-judgemental advocacy so that all requests are met and the team should work closely together to ensure that all understand and comply with the patient and the family's wishes. Caring for the dying child's symptom control follows the same pattern as that for adults with the need for a particular sensitivity to the child's wishes regardless of age or mental ability (Brady, 1994)

PHYSICAL CARE OF THE DYING PATIENT

Each of the symptoms outlined above in the systems assessment (Lindley Davis, 1991) will be dealt with in turn.

Breathing

The symptoms of breathlessness are distressing and unnecessary in many dying patients. Giving antibiotics to treat chest infections can ease the condition, but will not have any significant effect on the outcome for the patient. Regnard and Tempest (1992) suggest administering 100% oxygen if the patient is hypoxic and has no previous respiratory disease. This will help manage the patient's fear, which is very distressing and acute if he or she continues to fight for breath. Hyoscine hydrobromide can be introduced via the syringe driver to reduce the 'death rattle' as it will reduce secretions that the patient has not the energy to expectorate. Sedation should never be seen as an easy option, but is used if more appropriate and if the patient is less aware of the problem. Ideally, drugs are used with the patient's permission. Positioning is often significant while the patient remains conscious, but the patient should be encouraged to adopt the position he or she finds most helpful. Sitting in a well-padded chair may be more comfortable than being bedbound.

Nutrition

The notion of feeding dying people is controversial. As a general rule of thumb, if they want to eat, food is provided in a form that they can manage, including enteral feeding if the patient wishes. Anorexia is a fairly common problem and nausea and vomiting are experienced by 40% of dying people with cancer (Regnard and Tempest, 1992). In the final stages many individuals do not want to eat or drink, but controversy has arisen where discontinuing feeding has led to the death of the individual, for example in the Tony Bland case (Airedale National Health Service Trust v Bland (1993)). This whole area is discussed by writers in both the ethics and the medical field (Jennett, 1996).

More common in everyday nursing practice is the discontinuation of hydration. However, in such cases, the continuance of mouth care is vital to the patient's sense of wellbeing. According to Gallagher–Allred (1993) dehydration is a natural anaesthesia for terminally ill patients because it appears to decrease the patient's perception of suffering by reducing the level of consciousness. However, the nurse must be acutely sensitive to when a patient may be thirsty and wish to drink, especially if too weak to hold a glass and take the drink for him or herself (Hall, 1994).

▶ *Movement*

The use of corticosteroids to control the pressure symptoms of an encapsulated tumour coupled with poor nutritional status and limited mobility may lead to the development of pressure sores. Keeping the patient dry and clean can assist the person's sense of wellbeing. Where the client has advanced bronchitic or cardiac problems then the poor gaseous exchange rather than corticosteroids are a major contributory factor to pressure sore development. Within hospice units, patients are nursed on pressure-relieving beds to obviate the need for turning. Routines and rituals in turning should give way to patient comfort and the patient's wishes are paramount.

▶ *Constipation*

This is a major consideration with all terminally ill people because of their reduced mobility and reduced intake of food and fluids. It is even more of a problem for terminally ill individuals who are receiving opiates for pain management. The appropriate aperient must always be given with these drugs as the feeling of fullness and discomfort is a further cause of anorexia in the dying individual.

▶ *Weakness and Lethargy*

The combination of weakness and lethargy is possibly one of the most frustrating combinations of symptoms. The individual wants to do more, but is exhausted by minimal effort. Research is ongoing into this area and the issue of muscular weakness predominates (Regnard and Tempest, 1992). Physiotherapy and hydrotherapy can help keep the patient mobile, but weakness remains one of the most difficult symptoms to treat in the terminally ill patient.

PROFESSIONAL KNOWLEDGE

This part of the chapter primarily focuses on the ethical and legal issues related to the care of the dying individual. However, it is important to discuss the issue of where a patient should die first. This part will also briefly explore the personal reactions and beliefs of nurses and how these reactions can affect their professional role in caring for the dying. The 'emotional labour' of nursing in the field of hospice care needs to be recognized.

▶ THE LOCATION OF DEATH

We need to be mindful that whereas death at home is the preferred option of most patients (Woodhall, 1986), the family may not be able to cope with the level of care involved. Likewise hospice care is available to a limited number of people and often only for short respite periods to allow the family to have a rest. According to national statistics most patients still die in a hospital bed. While dying in hospital may not be the ideal, nurses need to try to bring some of what makes hospice care desirable into the general or psychiatric ward. Unlike other ailments where we can re-evaluate care and improve on our previous treatments, the client only dies once and a poorly managed death is like a pebble in a pond – it has effects far beyond the patient and his or her family. Table 3.5.5 lists some of the possible advantages and disadvantages of dying in each location. You may be able to add equally valid advantages and disadvantages to the list.

For each individual patient the resources available may limit the fulfillment of their wishes. Much has been done in recent years to bridge the gap between home, hospital and hospice care by developing many specialist nursing services. There are numerous groups who provide support within the community and hospital. The community nursing staff have a vital role to play not only in providing care, but also in their ability to support the family and coordinate the involvement of other care workers. They keep the primary health care team informed about the patient's progress and assess need. The development of the Macmillan Nursing Service has provided specialist support and guidance to assist those who are involved with the care of the patient. They do not deliver hands-on care themselves, but are a resource for those involved with the patient. This includes family members, general practitioners, and community staff. Some Macmillan nurses are

Location	Advantages	Disadvantages
Home	Familiar and family involved Atmosphere routine Freedom to have visitors More control for person Less feeling of helplessness for relatives	Relatives can become resentful or exhausted Disruption to family life Lack of facilities Care fragmented Isolation Difficulty in getting help quickly
Hospital	24-hour access to care Rapid response to changes Multidisciplinary approach Eases burden on relative Equipment readily available	Inflexible routine Alien environment Relatives can feel excluded Care can be very technical Lack of continuity
Hospice	Home from home Highly skilled and motivated staff Expertise in all aspects of care High staff/volunteer ratio to patient	Lack of availability Bias towards middle class christianity Limited available treatment services on site Possibility of overnursing the client

Table 3.5.5 The advantages and disadvantages of death at home, in the hospital, or in the hospice.

As many patients now choose to die at home, on your community placements you may have been involved with the primary health care team in supporting dying patients and their families.

- *Reflect on whether these patients and their families received all the services that they needed or requested.*

- *How did you feel as part of the team giving support in the palliative and terminal care of a dying individual?*

- *How might your community experiences inform your practice in an acute hospital unit?*

very specialist, for example specializing in breast care, lymphoedema, haematology or paediatrics, while others work on a locality basis or are hospital based. Services are also provided by the Marie Curie nurses, and they can also provide a sitter service to allow the primary carer to have a break. In some areas there is access to 'hospice at home', but this is at present still sporadic. Day hospices are often available for those who wish to attend on a daily basis only. All offer social support for the patient and the family, and some provide ongoing assessment of the patient and can provide emergency admission to sort out troublesome symptoms. Berenthal (1994) also discusses the role of the voluntary sector in helping to meet the needs of dying people and their families.

▶ PROFESSIONAL COPING

As professional nurses, we need to ensure that we look after our own psychological wellbeing as well as that of the client. Becoming dysfunctional in our grief at the death of a client is of little benefit to anyone. Thankfully the idea that the nurse who is upset at the death of a client is acting in an unprofessional manner has largely disappeared from professional practice. In order to care for an individual you naturally invest emotional energy. What we need to consider is the degree of involvement that we can reasonably give to meet the needs of the client without depleting our reserves for other patients.

RESEARCH BASED EVIDENCE

Through questionnaires and interviews, Spencer (1994) carried out research aimed at identifying how nurses manage their grief in an intensive care unit. The results showed that 41.2% felt guilty when a patient died. This was lower than expected and did not replicate the work of Iveson Iveson (1985) or Herrle (1987). The nurses found that informal discussion and peer support were very useful in coping, which replicates the studies by Little (1992) and Adey (1987).

Nurses have problems in admitting *that they have difficulties in coping with their feelings and found consulting outside agencies difficult. Spencer's study revealed that many nurses had received little training in how to deal with grief and this was similar to findings in Hockley's work (Hockley, 1989). When asked what form of support would be most helpful, 15.7% replied that a counsellor might be of use, but Adey's study (Adey, 1987) suggests that a counsellor is of only limited benefit. Most respondents favoured an informal discussion and one to one chats.*

Fisher (1991) states that we can turn grief into growth and suggests the use of structured bereavement counselling as a way in which it can be handled positively. She suggests that nurses come to palliative care settings because death has been managed badly where they have worked previously. She also sees early identification of those who need help as vital in promoting mental wellbeing. Similarly Kubler Ross (1975), Parkes (1972), and Morris (1986) are cited by Fisher (1991) as having identified the growth potential in grief. Saunders and Valente (1994) suggest that nurses who care for a terminally ill patient need to develop an 'emotional muscle'. This can be achieved by understanding theory, recognizing their own mortality and using whatever support is available. The most common source of distress to student nurses is how the patients die. Wilkes (1993) addresses the issues relating to how students perceive death, the so-called good or bad death – 'These nurses see a 'good' death as one where the patient is comfortable, alert and pain free and where the person is accepting of the situation and is surrounded by loved ones in a personally determined environment. On the other hand nurses descriptions of a 'bad' death include images of pain, loneliness, distress, unacceptance and unpreparedness'.

▶ LEGAL ISSUES – THE ROLE OF THE CORONER

The coroner is appointed by the local authority, but totally independent of them, to investigate sudden and unexplained deaths. Coroners are drawn from solicitors or medical doctors of five years or more experience. They are supported by coroner's officers, which are civilian posts, but the majority are former police officers. Their role is to investigate the circumstances surrounding the death and report back to the coroner. The coroner convenes an inquest, calls evidence, questions witnesses and brings in a verdict. The coroner can be supported by a jury or act alone. Coroners are appointed for life, there is no statutory retirement age and the decision of a coroner is final. Table 3.5.6 lists the circumstances under which a doctor must legally report a death to the coroner.

Any death where the patient is in hospital for less than 24 hours

Any death where the patient has not been treated by a doctor during the last illness or has not been seen by a doctor within the 14 days before death

Any death due to violent or unnatural circumstances

Any death occurring while undergoing a surgical procedure or before recovering from the effects of the anaesthetic

Death following a surgical procedure if the procedure could have a bearing on the cause of death

Death caused by an industrial disease

Death of a person in receipt of a war pension

Where the cause of death is uncertain

Any sudden or unexplained death

Table 3.5.6 Deaths reported to the coroner.

The coroner may ask for a postmortem and the request cannot be refused despite religious objections, but the issue is dealt with sensitively. The coroner's officer attends each postmortem. If the death of an organ donor has to be referred to the coroner, then the coroner must be asked to give consent to the removal of the organ, since the removal could affect some important evidence. Consent can usually be given quickly (Home Office).

If the death may be due to murder, manslaughter or infanticide, the coroner must send the papers to the Director of Public Prosecutions. The coroner sits with a jury for certain cases such as deaths in custody, industrial accidents or those caused by police officers in the course of their duties.

Coroners are empowered to rule on the cause of death as being as follows:

- ▶ natural causes;
- ▶ open verdict;
- ▶ accident;
- ▶ misadventure;
- ▶ suicide;
- ▶ unlawful killing.

Coroners' inquests are open to the public and if you wish to attend one it is best to contact the coroner's officer at your local police station.

▶ ETHICAL ISSUES – THE LIVING WILL

Living wills or advance directives were first developed in the USA and derive from the work of Kutner (1969). In 1976, the State of California passed the *Natural Death Act* (1977), which recognized the principle of living wills. The purpose of a living will is to allow autonomous individuals to make decisions while in good health about the care or withholding of care that they would wish to receive in the event of suffering from a prescribed list of illnesses within clearly defined boundaries. The will can include the appointment of a health care proxy, that is someone who is well acquainted with the patient's wishes and can apply them in situations where the advance directives are felt to be ambiguous.

If we remain competent to the end of our lives, then we can clearly state what we would wish or not wish to happen to us. However, progressive mental illness can make this impossible. Patient autonomy can cause ethical dilemmas for health care professionals. Jean Harlow, the famous blonde actress died of a treatable infection because she was a Christian Scientist who refused orthodox medical treatment. If we are to allow people to make their own choices, then we need to remember that they will not always choose as we would.

People with certain types of mental disorder who are subject to delusions can make 'a valid and legally binding (at common law) advance statement as long as they are clear about the consequences of the particular decision they wish to make' (Royal College of Nursing, 1994; British Medical Association and Royal College of Nursing, 1995).

DECISION MAKING

The British Medical Association and Royal College of Nursing 1995 report on *The Older Person: Consent and Care* cites the following case. 'In the 1993 case of 'C', a man in his 60s who was confined to Broadmoor, suffered from the delusion that he was medically qualified. C refused amputation of the foot and his anticipatory decision to continue to reject such an operation in the future was upheld at law. C suffered from a mental disorder, but was judged competent to make the particular decision in question'.

- *What is your immediate reaction to the above story – was the verdict the right one?*
- *Explore the legal and ethical literature on 'informed consent' and review the verdict again.*
- *Try to discuss the verdict with a group that includes members of the health care multidisciplinary team and note their individual reactions to the above decision.*
- *How would this debate relate to your particular field of nursing practice?*

At present, living wills are not legally binding in the UK and can be overruled by family members and clinicians. The Voluntary Euthanasia Society is currently lobbying parliament in the UK for the advance directives to carry the same weight as a last will and testament. The equivalent organization in South Australia is awaiting the enactment of *Consent to Treatment and Palliative Care Act*, which will make the living will legally binding in that particular state in Australia (Voluntary Euthanasia Society of South Australia).

▶ ETHICAL ISSUES – EUTHANASIA

Within the remit of a living will, the individual concerned cannot ask for assistance in dying. Euthanasia remains illegal throughout the world except in the Northern Territories in Australia where euthanasia legislation was enacted in 1995 (Voluntary Euthanasia Society – Northern Territories) although this has since been suspended by Australian law to prevent several other states taking similar action. In Holland, doctors carrying out euthanasia are not prosecuted only if they follow the clearly defined criteria and report the death to the coroner as euthanasia. Treatment used in modern palliative care may hasten a patient's death; however the intention is to treat the patient and not to bring about the death. This is the doctrine of double effect, and is most commonly seen in the administration of narcotic analgesia. The desired effect is to alleviate the pain, the unwanted effect is that it may cause respiratory depression. Even within Roman Catholic theology it is accepted as ethical to increase the dose of analgesia to alleviate the pain of the patient.

Euthanasia is illegal in Britain and yet it is practised, as demonstrated by the case of Dr Cox in the treatment of Lilian Boyes (Case of R v Cox (1992) 12 BMLR 38 Winchester CC). This elderly lady was crippled with both rheumatoid arthritis and osteoarthritis and begged her consultant whom she had known for many years to end her suffering. Having already tried very large doses of morphine, which sadly increased aspects of her pain, he resorted to intravenous potassium chloride, which has no therapeutic value and she swiftly died. This case is certainly not an isolated one – the physician attending King George VI later admitted euthanatizing him, while in a paper presented by McMichael and Barnett at the Fifth National Conference on Ethics in Medicine, 25% of those present acknowledged in confidence that they had accelerated the death of patients, 25% were totally opposed, and most accepted that doctors make life and death decisions concerning patients without consultation, for example 'do not resuscitate' orders. The legal system, while abhorring euthanasia, has obvious sympathy with medical practitioners who are involved with 'mercy killing'. A survey cited by the Voluntary Euthanasia Society in 1995 into doctors' attitudes towards euthanasia set the figure higher, with 30% of practitioners admitting to it. Nurses who are in the clinical area face a dilemma and may be perceived as trouble makers if they 'whistle blow'.

Euthanasia as a term was linked with the Nazi atrocities during the Second World War. Opponents of the concept cite this as the reason that no liberalization of the legislation should occur. The critical feature to be considered is the intention with which the act is carried out. In the literature, euthanasia (Greek: eu, good; thanatos, death) is categorized in four different ways:

- involuntary active;
- involuntary passive;
- voluntary active;
- voluntary passive.

We have already discussed Lilian Boyes, who was given active voluntary euthanasia by Dr Cox (Kennedy and Grubb, 1994). An example of involuntary active euthanasia would be where a doctor increases the narcotics given to a postoperative patient without the patient's consent and with the express purpose of killing the patient from respiratory depression. This is obviously totally unacceptable and is not supported by any campaigning body whatsoever. The case of Tony Bland (Jennett and Dyer, 1991) was involuntary passive euthanasia, involuntary in that he did not request it, and passive in that it involved withholding treatment rather than administering a noxious substance. Voluntary passive euthanasia would be the situation where a patient decides to refuse further treatment, for example refuses resuscitation in the case of a further cardiac arrest.

The most contentious issue for medical practitioners and nurses is voluntary euthanasia (Johnstone, 1994) (see Annotated Further Reading). The main argument for it centres on the right of the dying individual to choose and maintain control over his or her dying. By managing death, the individual may have choices about the location, manner and timing of the event. What is so noble about a painful lingering death? The pro-life campaign centres on the sanctity of life issues and the 'slippery slope' argument. The 'slippery slope' refers to the risks associated with any liberalization of the law. Pro-life campaigners fear that allowing euthanasia to be legalized would open the floodgates and that it would rapidly take on a life of its own like that resulting from liberalization of the *Abortion Act* (1967). The public would be at risk of devaluing the lives of disabled people and risk genocide.

▶ ORGAN DONATION

<table>
<tr><td colspan="2">DECISION MAKING</td></tr>
<tr>
<td>Francis is a 27-year-old married nurse with a two-year-old son. His wife Kate is a nurse teacher. One morning Kate wakes up with a very severe headache, which develops into a brain haemorrhage. She is in the intensive care unit and being ventilated. Within the next 24 hours the consultant asks to see Francis to discuss Kate's prognosis and he explains that there is nothing more that can be done. The transplant nurse who is a colleague of both Francis and Kate comes to see Francis to discuss donation of Kate's</td>
<td>organs. Kate did not carry a card and she and Francis had never discussed their views on it.
• From previous knowledge gained in this chapter decide what needs to be discussed more fully with Francis.
• What is the legal position in relation to the diagnosis of Kate's death?
• Decide whether Francis has sole responsibility for donating Kate's organs.</td>
</tr>
</table>

Organ donation and receipt remains the only hope for survival to many individuals in end stage organ failure. The problem of asking very distressed individuals if they will consent to their relative's organs being used is largely due to an absence of a clear expression of the individual's wishes. The living will and the new computerized register of donors can with adequate public information be much more user friendly than the previous card system and should provide the basis for discussion with the family (Dimond, 1993).

It is inevitable that in both your personal and professional life you will need to cope with death and dying. As stated at the beginning of this chapter, dying is a unique experience for each person. In your professional capacity as a nurse in whichever field you specialize you can make a difference to the experiences of dying patients and their families by providing informed and sensitive care. Through your knowledge of the contents of this chapter, your exploration of issues arising from the exercises, and your personal and reflective experiences in practice, you will be able to provide a high quality of care for the dying in whatever setting is appropriate for that person.

▶ PERSONAL REFLECTIONS

Having read the contents of this chapter, it is important for you to consider what death means to you personally.

> You may find it helpful to record on a piece of paper what words come to mind when considering death. Try and sort these into negative and positive notions.
>
> - *Is it really death you are writing about or the process of dying, which is quite separate?*
> - *Is death a good or a bad thing?*
> - *Can you identify why you feel as you do?*

It is often difficult to cope with negative attitudes towards dying. Personally, for me, it has sometimes been difficult to deal with my negative feelings about dying individuals. I had always assumed that caring for the dying would be rewarding and fulfilling, and in the majority of cases it is. Dying, however, does not make people saintlike, and we should not feel guilty that we are not drawn to every dying person, but what is vital is that we deliver a high standard of 'appropriate care' to our client. Nurses need to care for themselves and take their own good advice about coping with stress. Coping with the stress of caring is discussed in more depth in Chapter 4.1.

Think back to Worden's tasks of mourning (Worden, 1991) discussed in the Psychosocial part of Subject Knowledge. In your own life can you identify using these or do you tend to put problems that carry a high cost in terms of emotion out of sight? Some writers refer to this latter method of coping as 'shelving problems'. Sadly we can only do this for

> Can you remember Weisman's definition of an appropriate death in the Psychosocial part of Subject Knowledge (Weisman, 1988)? If not look back and refresh your memory. You may find it helpful to ask yourself the following questions.
>
> - *To what extent do patients in my area of nursing have an appropriate death?*
> - *What is the routine of my working area that helps or hinders an appropriate death?*
> - *What is the procedure for 'last offices' in my area? How much is it based on tradition? How much is it based on meeting the needs of relatives or undertakers?*
> - *How do I feel about carrying out the procedure for 'last offices'? What makes it better or worse?*
> - *What in my opinion is a good death?*

REFLECTIVE KNOWLEDGE

a time depending on our coping ability; eventually a significant loss will trigger memories of other losses and this can lead to severe depression and withdrawal, even breakdown.

Your answers in the above reflective exercise will be unique, but it may help to discuss and share them with a colleague. This is after all how we grow as human beings and develop the skills of nursing patients who are dying and who are receiving palliative care.

▶ CASE STUDIES

The following case studies are included so that you can consolidate the knowledge gained from reading this chapter and from the learning that has taken place through your experience in the practice of nursing.

▶ CASE STUDY: LEARNING DISABILITIES

A 50-year-old woman with Down's syndrome who was developing a dementing illness was admitted to a medical ward with increasing drowsiness and confusion. She lived in sheltered housing with her aged mother who was also in poor health. Physical examination was very difficult as she became very distressed when her abdomen was touched. She could not speak, other than by making grunting noises, and it was extremely difficult to assess her understanding. A very junior male student nurse spent time with her and she rapidly attached herself to him, and he to her. She was much calmer when he was around and allowed the nursing staff to care for her hygiene needs only if he was there. Sadly before she could have surgery she died. The student felt grateful that he had been able to help her to cope with her distress, and because he was junior, the staff had facilitated him spending time with her regularly during her hospitalization.

■ **Evaluate the benefits and the costs of getting involved with patients who are dying?**

■ **How might the ageing mother respond to her daughter's sudden death?**

▶ CASE STUDY: ADULT

Sarah Warner was a 41-year-old lady with two young children aged ten and six. Her husband Peter was a haemophiliac and contracted human immunodeficiency virus (HIV) from untreated factor VIII in 1990. Peter died in 1992 and Sarah died in 1994 after a short hospital stay from Pneumocystis carinii *pneumonia. The nurses caring for Sarah felt it was so unfair as neither Sarah nor her husband had done anything wrong and now the children were orphans.*

- How can we as nurses ensure that we do not blame people for their illnesses?

- How might our attitudes to the possible cause of death affect how we provide appropriate individualized care?

- Do children need special support to help them to grieve at their parent's death?

▶ CASE STUDY: MENTAL HEALTH

Mrs Groves was a 70-year-old lady who had been a long stay patient in a large psychiatric institution. She had schizophrenia as a young woman and this had become compounded by advanced dementia. She had had several falls over several months as she had become increasingly unsteady on her feet and she developed a persistent chest infection, which did not respond to antibiotics or chest physiotherapy. As it became apparent that she was dying, the nursing staff endeavoured to have a constant presence with her and she had a very peaceful and dignified death.

- What difficulties do you think you will have when dealing with patients who appear to have no insight into their condition?

- What is our role as nurses in such cases? (You might like to look at the *Code Of Professional Conduct* (UKCC, 1992) for this one.)

▶ CASE STUDY: CHILD

Sarah Lee was a six-year-old girl with meningitis. Sadly, despite a rapid diagnosis and rapid hospitalization, she died 48 hours later after initially showing some signs of improvement. Shortly afterwards her four-year-old brother developed the same symptoms, but he recovered with minimal damage and was soon allowed home.

- Using the tasks of mourning and the antecedents of death, can you give any view on the reason why Sarah's little brother may have suffered in the period following his sisters death?

- How far should doctors go to save the life of a child?

- Would you be happy to allow your child to have experimental therapy that offers a chance of recovery?

- When should we stop resuscitating? (The answers here may well be financial as well as moral.)

▶ ANNOTATED FURTHER READING

WRIGHT, B. (1996) *Sudden Death* (2nd edition). Edinburgh. Churchill Livingstone.
  Wright has written several books on sudden death from his perspective as

Clinical Nurse Specialist in Crisis Care based at Leeds Royal Infirmary and writes from extensive experience. I would particularly recommend this book for perusal and because it contains a clear commonsense approach based on work by Caplan (1964) and Worden (1991) (see also Chapter 2.1 on resuscitation).

HILL, L. (ed.) (1994) *Caring for Dying Children and their Families*. London. Chapman & Hall.

This is a comprehensive multi-authored book on care of the dying child and their families. Many chapters give research based evidence and Chapter 9 by Michael Brady gives a comprehensive outline of symptom control in the dying child.

KOHNER, N., HENLEY, A. (1991) *When a Baby Dies: The Experience Of Late Miscarriage, Stillbirth And Neonatal Death*. London. Pandora Press.

This current chapter has not dealt in any detail with issues surrounding perinatal deaths. However, this useful book is a valuable source if you need to learn more about families coping with the loss of a baby.

ROYAL COLLEGE OF NURSING (1996) *Verification of Death by Registered Nurses* (Leaflet N38 of Issues in Nursing and Health). London. Royal College of Nursing.

The above Royal College of Nursing guidelines are helpful in terms of the legal position of the nurse practitioner in verifying that a death has occurred.

ROYAL COLLEGE OF NURSING (1994) *Dealing with Living Wills* (Leaflet N4 of Issues in Nursing and Health). London. Royal College of Nursing.

The Royal College of Nursing has also published guidelines for nurses on how to deal with the issue of living wills. A copy of this leaflet can be obtained from the Royal College of Nursing on request.

JENNETT, B. (1996) Managing patients in a persistent vegetative state since Airedale NHS Trust vs Bland. In McLEAN, S. (ed.) Death, Dying and the Law. Part 1, Chapter 2. England. Dartmouth Press.

A good exposition of The Tony Bland Case can be found in this chapter by Brian Jennett. An interesting overview of this debate can also be found in Hall (1994), which the reader might care to peruse.

JOHNSTONE, M.J. (1994) *Bioethics – a nursing perspective* (2nd edition). Sydney. W.B. Saunders/Baillière Tindall.

Johnstone argues the case both for and against euthanasia in a systematic way, which will provide useful material for follow up reading.

▶ ANNOTATED VIDEOS

VOLUNTARY EUTHANASIA – THE FACTS. London. The Voluntary Euthanasia Society of England and Wales.

This video is available from The Voluntary Euthanasia Society of England and Wales, 13 Prince of Wales Terrace, London W8 5PG. The main arguments on both sides are well explored. The society is also willing to provide living wills and information about their campaigns and can be contacted by writing to the above address.

▶ THE MAIN ORGANIZATIONS TO CONTACT FOR PRO-LIFE VIEWS

HOPE (HEALTHCARE OPPOSED TO EUTHANASIA), 58 Hanover Gardens, London SE11 5TN

SOCIETY FOR THE PROTECTION OF THE UNBORN CHILD, 7 Tufton Street, Westminster, London SW1P 3QN, Tel: 0171 222 5845

◗ REFERENCES

ADEY, C. (1987) Stress: who cares? *Nursing Times* **83(4)**: 52–53.

AINSWORTH SMITH, I. and SPECK, P. (1982) *Letting Go*, 2nd edn. SPCK.

Airedale National Health Service Trust v Bland (1993) 2 WLR 316,343

ALEXY, W.D. (1991) Dimensions of psychological counseling that facilitate the grieving process of bereaved parents. In Worden, J.W. *Grief Counselling and Grief Therapy*, 2nd edition. London. Routledge.

BARNET COLLEGE (1992) *The Nature of Cancer*, 2nd edition. London. Manpower Services Commission.

BERENTHAL, J.A. (1994) A welcome break for the carers. *Professional Nurse* **9(4)**: 267–270.

BLACKMORE, S. (1988) Visions from the dying brain. *New Scientist* **118**: 1161.

BRADY, M. (1994) Symptom control in dying children. In Hill, L. (1994) (ed.) *Caring for Dying Children and their Families*. London. Chapman & Hall.

BRITISH MEDICAL ASSOCIATION AND ROYAL COLLEGE OF NURSING (1995) *The Older Person: Consent and Care*. London. British Medical Association.

BRITISH MEDICAL ASSOCIATION AND PHARMACEUTICAL SOCIETY (1997) *British National Formulary* (33rd edition).

BROOKBANK, J.W. (1990) *The Biology of Aging*. New York. Harper Row.

BUCKMAN R. (1992) *How to Break Bad News*. London. Papermac.

CANCER RESEARCH CAMPAIGN (1988) Fact sheet 6 (breast cancer) Fact sheet 7 (breast cancer screening) Fact sheet 8 (survival).

CAPLAN, G. (1964) Principles of preventive psychiatry. Cited in: WRIGHT, B. (1996) *Sudden Death Intervention Skills for the Caring Professions*, 2nd edition. London. Churchill Livingstone.

CASSELL, E. (1974) *Death inside out – Dying in a technological age*. In Steiners, P., Veatch, R.M. (eds) p. 43. New York. Harper and Row.

COLE, E.J. (1993) The near death experience. *Intensive and Critical Care Nursing* **9**: 157–161.

COPP, G. (1994) Palliative care nursing education: A review of research findings. *Journal of Advanced Nursing* **19**: 552–557.

COWLISHAW, S. (1993) *When My Little Sister Died*. Derby. Merlin Publications.

CUNNINGHAM, W.R., BROOKBANK, J.W. (1988) *Gerontology: The Biology, Psychology and Sociology of Aging*. New York. Harper Row.

DAY, L. (1995) Ethics and law. Practical limits to the uniform determination of death act. *Journal of Neuroscience Nursing* **27(5)**: 319–322.

DEPARTMENT OF HEALTH (1993) *Health of the Nation*. Key Area Handbook. London. HMSO.

DIMOND, B. (1993) Transplants and donor cards. *Accident and Emergency Nursing* **1**: 1.

DUNNE, E., MCINTOSH, J., DUNNE MAXIM, K. (1987) *Suicide and Its Aftermath*. New York. Norton.

EISENBERG, L. (1981) Foreword. In Koocher, G., O'Malley, J.E. (eds) The Damocles Syndrome. pp. XI–XV. New York. McGraw Hill.

ENGEL, G (1964) Grief and grieving. *American Journal of Nursing* **64**: 9.

FAULKNER, A., PEACE, G., O'KEEFFE, C. (1995) *When a Child Has Cancer*. London. Chapman & Hall.

FISHER, C. (1991) Brain death: A review of the concept. *Journal of Neuroscience Nursing* **23(5)**: 330–333.

FISHER, M. (1991) Can grief be turned into growth. *Professional Nurse* **7**: 3.

GALLAGHER–ALLRED, C. (1993) Nutrition and hydration in hospice care: needs, strategies, ethics. *Hospice Journal – Physical, Psychosocial and Pastoral Care of the Dying* **9**: 2–3.

GREEN, J. (1989) Death with dignity: meeting the needs of patients in a multi-ethnic society. *Nursing Times* **1**.

GREEN, J. (1993) Death with dignity. *Nursing Times* **2**.

HALL J.K. (1994) Caring for corpses or killing patients. *Nursing Management* **25(10)**: 81–82.

HENDERSON, V. (1966) *The Nature of Nursing*. London. Collier Macmillan.

HERRLE, S. (1987) Helping staff to cope with grief. *Nursing Management* **September** 33–34.

HILL, L. (ed.) (1994) *Caring for Dying Children and their Families*. London. Chapman & Hall.

HINDMARCH, C. (1993) *On the Death of a Child*. Oxford. Radcliffe Medical Press.

HINDS C.J., WATSON D. (1996) *Intensive Care: A Concise Textbook* (2nd edition). London. W.B. Saunders.

HOCKLEY, J. (1989) Caring for the dying in hospital. *Nursing Times* **85(39)**.

HOME OFFICE (1984) *The Work of the Coroner. Some Questions Answered*. London. Her Majesty's Stationery Office.

IVESON IVESON, J. (1985) Part of the spiral of life. Cited in SPENCER, L. (1994) How do nurses deal with their own grief? *Journal of Advanced Nursing* **19(6)**: 1141–1150.

JENNETT, B. (1982) Brain death. *Intensive Care Medicine* **8(1)**:1–3.

JENNETT, B. (1996) Managing patients in a persistent vegetative state since Airedale NHS Trust v Bland. In: McLean, S. *Death, Dying and the Law*. Aldershot. Dartmouth Press.

JENNETT, B., DYER, C. (1991) Persistent vegetative state and the right to die. *British Medical Journal* **302(6787)**: 1256–1258.

JOHNSTONE, M.J. (1994) *Bioethics – a nursing perspective* (2nd edition). Sydney. W.B. Saunders/Baillière Tindall.

KIGER, A. (1994) Student nurse involvement with death. **20(4)**: 679–686.

KUBLER ROSS, E. (1975) *Death: the Final Stage of Growth*. London. Prentice Hall.

KUHSE, H., SINGER, P. (1993) Voluntary euthanasia and the nurse. *International Journal of Nursing Studies* **30(4)**: 311–322.

KUTNER (1969) Due process of euthanasia. Cited in LUSH, D. (1993) Advance directives and living wills. *Journal of the Royal College of Physicians* **27(3)**: 276.

LINDLEY DAVIS, B. (1991) Process of dying. *Cancer Nursing* **14**: 6.

LITTLE, D. (1992) Informal trauma support urged. Cited in: SPENCER, L. (1994) How do nurses deal with their own grief? *Journal of Advanced Nursing* **19(6)**: 1141–1150.

LOUIS, P. *et al.* (1993) Barbiturates and hyperventilation during intracranial hypertension. *Critical Care Medicine* **21(8)**: 1200–1206.

MONTAGUE, S., KNIGHT, D. (1996) Cell structure and function, growth and development. In: Hinchliffe, S., Montague, S. and Watson, R. *Physiology for Nursing Practice*, 2nd edition. London. Baillière Tindall.

MORRIS, P. (1986) Loss and change. Cited in FISHER, M. (1991) Can grief be turned into growth? *Professional Nurse* **7(3)**: 178–182.

NARAYANASAMY, A. (1993) Nurses' awareness and educational preparation in meeting their patients' spiritual needs. *Nurse Education Today* **13**: 3.

NARAYANASAMY, A. (1995) Spiritual care of chronically ill patients. *Journal of Clinical Nursing* **4(6)**: 397–398.

NORTON, D.J. (1992) Clinical applications of brain stem death protocols. *Journal of Neuroscience Nursing* **24(6)**: 354–358.

OFFICE OF POPULATION CENSUSES AND SURVEYS (1991) *Mortality Statistics*. London. Her Majesty's Stationery Office.

OPEN UNIVERSITY (1992) *K 260 Death and Dying*. Open University.

OSIS, K., HARALDSSON, E. (1986) *At the Hour of Death*, 2nd edition. New York. Marmaroneck.

PALLIS, C. (1983) *ABC of Brain Stem Death (Articles from the BMJ, 1982–1983)*. London. BMJ Publications.

PALLIS, C., HARLEY, D.H. (1996) *ABC of Brain Stem Death* (2nd edition). London. BMJ Publications.

PARKES, C.M. (1972) Determinants of outcome following bereavement. *Omega 6.* Cited in FISHER, M. Can grief be turned into growth? *Professional Nurse* **7(3)**: 178–182.

PARKES, C.M. (1975) *Bereavement: Studies of Grief in Adult Life.* Penguin.

PARKES, C.M. (1987) Models of bereavement care. *Death Studies* **11(4)**: 257–261.

PARKES, C.M. (1991) Studies of grief in adult life. In Fisher, M. Can grief be turned into growth. *Professional Nurse* **7**: 3.

PARKES, C.M., PARKES, J. (1984) Hospice v hospital care: Reevaluation after 10 years as seen by the surviving spouse. *Postgraduate Medical Journal* **60**: 120–124.

PRAILL, D. (1995) Approaches to spiritual care. *Nursing Times* **91(34)**: 55–57.

PRIESTMAN, T. (1989) *Cancer Chemotherapy: An Introduction.* London. Pharmatalia Carlo Erba Ltd.

REGNARD C., TEMPEST, S. (1992) *A Guide to Symptom Relief in Advanced Cancer Care* (3rd edition). London. Haigh and Hockland.

RING, K. (1980) *Life at Death : A Scientific Investigation of the Near Death Experience.* New York. Coward, McGann and Geoghegan.

ROYAL COLLEGE OF NURSING (1994) *Dealing with Living Wills.* London. Royal College of Nursing.

SABOM, M. (1982) *Recollections of Death: a Medical Investigation.* New York. Harper and Row.

SAUNDERS, C. (1990) (ed.) *Hospice and Palliative Care: An Interdisciplinary Approach.* London. Edward Arnold.

SAUNDERS, J., VALENTE S. (1994) Nurses' grief. *Cancer Nursing* **17**: 4.

SCHOENBECK, S.B. (1993) Exploring the mystery of N.D.E. *American Journal of Nursing* **93(5)**: 42–46.

SINCLAIR, D. (1989) *Human Growth after Birth* (5th edition). Oxford. Oxford University Press.

SOURKES, B. (1987) Siblings of the child with a life-threatening illness. *Journal of Children in Contemporary Society* **19**: 159–184.

SPENCER, L. (1994) How do nurses deal with their own grief? *Journal of Advanced Nursing* **19(6)**: 1141–1150.

STONE H.W. (1995) Suicide and grief. In Smith, B., Mitchell, M., Constantino, R. *et al.* Exploring widows' feelings after the suicide of their spouse.

Journal of Psychosocial Nursing **33**: 5.

UKCC (1992) *Code of Professional Conduct.* London. UKCC.

VINEY, C. (1996) *Nursing the Critically Ill.* London. Baillière Tindall.

WALKER, M. (1973) The last hour before death. *American Journal of Nursing* **173**: 9.

WEISMAN, A.D. (1988) Appropriate death and the hospice program. *Hospice Journal – Physical, Psychological and Pastoral Care of the Dying* **4**: 1.

WILKES, L.M. (1993) Nurses' descriptions of death scenes. *Journal of Cancer Care* **93(2)**: 11–16.

WOODHALL, C. (1986) Care of the dying: a family concern. *Nursing Times* **82(43)**: 31–3.

WORDEN ,W.J. (1991) *Grief Counselling and Grief Therapy* (2nd edition). London. Routledge.

WRIGHT, B. (1996) *Sudden Death Intervention Skills for the Caring Professions*, 2nd edition. London. Churchill Livingstone.

YEAGER, K., MIASKOWSKI, C., DIBBLE, S.L., WALLHAGEN, M. (1995) Differences in pain knowledge and perception of the pain experience between outpatients with cancer and their family caregivers. *Oncology Nursing Forum* **22**: 8.

Supportive to restorative practice

4.1 Stress and Anxiety

D. Howard

▶ INTRODUCTION

Stress and anxiety are terms that are commonly used interchangeably. In this chapter the concepts of stress and anxiety are defined and the relationship between them explored. Stress affects nurses, clients and their relatives. Consequently, in this chapter, emphasis has been placed on developing awareness and management of your own stress as well as stress in others.

▶ OVERVIEW

▶ Subject Knowledge

The chapter is divided into four main parts. Part one, Subject Knowledge, addresses the nature of stress, its effects on individuals and the role stress plays in everyone's lives, together with the physiological, psychological and social changes that occur in response to stress. At the end of this part the consequences of exposure to very stressful events and prolonged exposure to stress are addressed in sections on burnout and post-traumatic stress syndrome.

▶ Practice Knowledge

In part two, Practice Knowledge, the nursing assessment of stress and strategies for planning stress management are explored. First stress in clients is addressed. The reasons why clients may suffer from stress and what should be assessed and why are examined. Nurses will also encounter clients' relatives who may be suffering from stress. Reasons why they may be stressed and the signs that may indicate this are explored.

The workplace is potentially a very stressful environment that nurses encounter. This is given attention in the final part of this section where signs of stress in colleagues and stress in the self are identified.

Following assessment, strategies for implementing stress management for yourself, in the workplace and for clients are addressed. Proactive and reactive strategies are identified and classified into cognitive and behavioural techniques.

▶ *Professional Knowledge*

Part three of the chapter, Professional Knowledge, examines the context in which stress arises. Emphasis is placed on the ability of the individual to control stress and the relationship between stress and employment.

▶ *Reflective Knowledge*

This chapter has been designed to enhance your learning through developing your self awareness. In the final part of the chapter, Reflective Knowledge, you are encouraged to consolidate this by reflecting on the main parts of the chapter and thinking about your responses to the exercises.

On pp. 507–509 there are four case studies, each one relating to one of the branch programmes. You may find it helpful to read one of them before you start the chapter and use it as a focus for your reflections while reading.

SUBJECT KNOWLEDGE

▶ THE CONCEPT OF ANXIETY

Anxiety is a term that is sometimes used to describe the feelings that are experienced in response to stress. It is also used as a diagnostic label and consequently its use can become blurred. To address this Sims and Owens (1993) distinguished between normal anxiety and abnormal anxiety. Normal anxiety is seen as essential for survival. It is the feeling that everyone experiences in response to a danger or threat. The intensity of the feeling is proportionate to the degree of threat; however, the significant criteria of normal anxiety are that it occurs to an appropriate degree for the level of threat and that it recedes when the threat is removed. Abnormal anxiety in contrast, is inappropriate to the threat and may continue long after the threat has been removed.

Sims and Owens (1993) suggest a clear differentiation between normal and abnormal anxiety. In reality, identifying the point at which normal anxiety becomes abnormal is not so simple though. Greene (1989) for example, viewed the relationship between normal and abnormal anxiety slightly differently. She suggested that normal and abnormal anxiety were end points on a continuous scale where anxiety developed through four categories of mild anxiety, moderate anxiety, severe anxiety and panic (Table 4.1.1).

▶ THE CONCEPT OF STRESS

Greene (1989) suggests that some level of anxiety is desirable for individuals to achieve their optimal performance. If this anxiety becomes too great, however, performance and ultimately health will deteriorate. This

Level of anxiety	Effect on thought process, verbal communication and non-verbal communication	
Mild anxiety	Thought process	Logical. Heightened cognitive functioning and perception.
	Verbal communication	Logical content. Normal rate and volume. Able to discuss one topic appropriately.
	Non-verbal communication	Appears alert, confident and secure.
Moderate anxiety	Thought process	Some blocking of thought. Frequent changes of topic. Loss of concentration. Hesitant. Diminished perception.
	Verbal communication	Accelerated rate and increased volume. Verbose. Attempted jocularity.
	Non-verbal communication	Restless. Excessive gesturing. Aggressive body postures frequently adopted.
Severe anxiety	Thought process	Distorted perception and cognitive processes.
	Verbal communication	Accelerated rate and volume. Express their anxiety by articulating how they feel, their helplessness or their desire to escape the stress invoking situation.
	Non-verbal communication	Fine and gross tremors. Restlessness usually observed in pacing, wringing of hands and picking clothes.
Panic	Thought process	Disjointed and irrational.
	Verbal communication	May scream. May plead or bargain.
	Non-verbal communication	May run about uncoordinated. May cling to objects of perceived security.

Table 4.1.1 Classification of levels of anxiety. (Adapted from Greene, 1989.)

reflects the arousal curve (Hebb, 1954). In the arousal curve the individual's performance increases in proportion to the level of arousal, but once the individual's maximum capacity for arousal is reached, the level of performance falls and negative effects on health begin to appear (Figure 4.1.1). This suggests that all individuals require a certain amount of stress to achieve optimal functioning, but once this is reached, any increase in the stress will result in negative effects.

People in high-paid, high-pressure jobs are consequently at risk of developing stress-related disease because of overstimulation. Think for example of the stereotypical business executive who develops a peptic ulcer.

If this singular explanation of the pathology of stress is true why do people who have low stimulating repetitive jobs also suffer from stress-related diseases? This question was asked by Sutherland and Cooper (1990). They agreed that overload caused stress, but additionally they argued that stress could be caused by underload. They developed the arousal curve into the inverted U hypothesis. This identified an optimal stress level in the centre of excessive stress levels characterized by underload and overload (Figure 4.1.2). This shows that boredom, apathy and poor morale are just as stressful as overload and the effects on individuals are just as damaging.

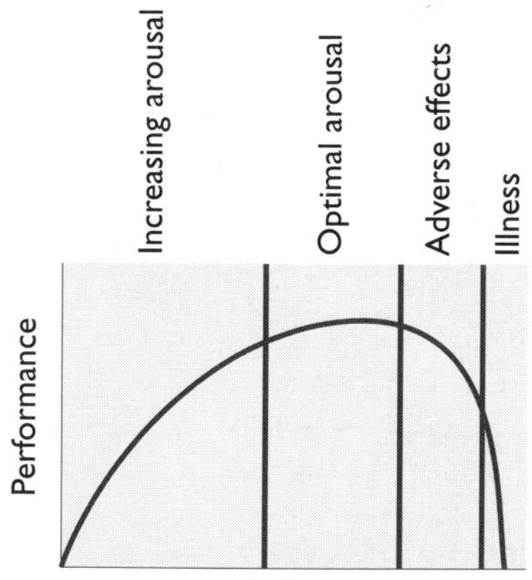

▶ THE NATURE OF STRESS

You may have noticed a similar pattern between the development of the stress response and that of the pattern of anxiety. This similarity has led

Figure 4.1.1: The arousal curve. (From Hebb, 1954.)

DECISION MAKING

- *What significance may the inverted U hypothesis hold for the nurse working in a health promotion clinic?*
- *How would the nurse use this knowledge to help a client manage a stress related health problem?*

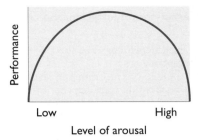

Figure 4.1.2: The inverted U hypothesis. (From Sutherland and Cooper, 1990, with permission.)

to a general interchangeability of the terms stress and anxiety. There is a difference, however, in that anxiety refers to how the individual feels in response to situations where they feel threatened. In contrast the stress response is a more generalized reaction, which may or may not encompass anxiety.

Seyle (1984, p. 74) defined stress as 'the non-specific response of the body to any demand', and argued that excessive stress results in detrimental effects to the individual, which ultimately manifests as illness. Seyle also found that some types of stress were pleasant whereas other types of stress are not so pleasant. He felt the single term stress was inadequate as it encompassed both positive and negative aspects of stress. Consequently he differentiated between the two types of stress. Positive stress he called eustress (Greek: *eu*, good), which was likened to excitement or euphoric feelings. Negative stress was called distress (Latin: *dis*, bad). Seyle found that the body underwent similar immediate physiological changes on exposure to both types of stress, however, the long-term effects of distress were seen to be far more damaging than those of eustress.

The eustress/distress hypothesis integrates with the inverted U hypothesis in that individuals require a certain amount of arousal to perform optimally. This occurs in eustress stimulation. If the arousal is too great or too little then eustress is replaced by distress.

You may have also noticed that whether stress is positive or negative can also be related to whether the individual has control of the stress or not. Stress that occurs where the individual retains control is positive and exhilarating. On the other hand where the individual has little control of the threat then the experience is negative and damaging.

DECISION MAKING

Following the advice from her occupational health nurse, Paula took up swimming once a week as a method of combating stress. She had always enjoyed swimming, and when she was younger had represented her school in swimming competitions. Paula felt refreshed from swimming and found it a positive way of relieving her stress. One day she met an old school friend at the pool who suggested that she joined her swimming club. Paula joined the club and was soon persuaded to enter competitions where she was successful in winning trophies. Paula needed to train intensively to maintain her competitiveness, however, and soon found herself training five evenings each week with competitions most weekends. In contrast to her initial intention to use swimming as a method of stress management, Paula now found that swimming was an additional stress in her life.

- *At which stage was Paula experiencing eustress from her swimming activities?*
- *At which stage was Paula experiencing distress?*
- *What advice should the nurse give clients who decide to use sport as a stress relieving activity?*

Biological ▶ BIOLOGICAL RESPONSES TO STRESS

▶ *The Immediate Physiological Response to Stress*

- *Think how you feel when you become anxious. What physically happens to you?*
- *Compare your responses with those listed in Tables 4.1.2 and 4.1.3.*

Imagine you are taking a pleasant stroll in the country one warm autumn evening when all of a sudden you are confronted by a very large, unaccompanied, angry, rottweiler dog. There are basically two courses of action for you to take. Either you can confront and fight the dog or run away from it at the utmost speed. This is the fight or flight response. The physiological responses are summarized in Figure 4.1.3.

The limbic system is stimulated by the stressor (in this case the dog) and sets in motion the physiological response. Initially the hypothalamus is stimulated and this responds in two ways. First it secretes corticotropin releasing hormone (CRH). CRH stimulates the anterior pituitary to secrete adrenocorticotropic hormone (ACTH). ACTH stimulates the adrenal cortex to increase the secretion of cortisol. The action of cortisol increases glycogenesis and also catabolism of body proteins. In turn this leads to hyperglycaemia.

Figure 4.1.3: Physiological stress response.

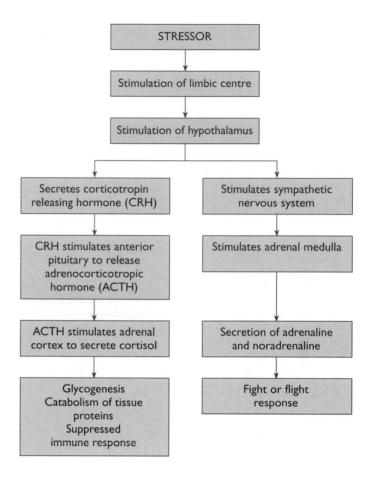

The hypothalamus also stimulates the sympathetic nervous system and the adrenal medulla. This leads to an increase in the secretion of adrenaline and noradrenaline and brings about the fight or flight syndrome. The physiological changes are summarized in Table 4.1.2. The specific signs that are associated with the fight or flight response are listed in Table 4.1.3.

The stress reaction occurs when individuals perceive themselves to be in danger. (A similar response is invoked each time you encounter a stressful event, for example, a job interview, taking an exam or going into hospital.) The physiological responses to stress prepare the body for intense physical action to either escape or fight the stressor.

The heart contractions increase in rate and volume. This is accompanied by constriction of peripheral blood vessels. The purpose of this is to concentrate the blood in the body core, increase the blood pressure and speed up the flow of the blood. In turn, this ensures an abundant blood supply to the large skeletal muscles, which will be used either in fighting or running away.

Respiration increases and the bronchi dilate to facilitate this. In turn this increases the oxygenation of the blood and provides the muscles with the copious amount of oxygen they will require in anticipation of the vast aerobic respiration involved in major exertion.

To enable respiration, muscles also require energy in the form of glucose. In the first instance the blood glucose level is increased by the

System	Effect
Circulatory system	Increased heart rate and force of contraction Peripheral vasoconstriction
Respiratory system	Increased respiratory rate Dilation of bronchi
Skin	Sweat gland stimulation Erection of body hair by pilomotor contraction Constriction of peripheral blood vessels
Eyes	Pupil dilation
Adrenal gland	Secretion of adrenaline and noradrenaline
Digestive system	Dry mouth Increased peristaltic activity
Skeletal muscles	Increased tension Fine tremor
Metabolism	Glycogenesis leading to hyperglycaemia Catabolism of protein Lipolysis

Table 4.1.2 Physiological changes associated with the flight or fight response.

Frequent urination
Diarrhoea
Restlessness
Poor concentration
Aggressive manner
Rapid speech
Feeling of impending doom
Feeling of nausea
Lump in the throat
Palpitations
Tightness of chest
Headache
Backache
Aching limbs

Table 4.1.3 List of symptoms of flight or fight reaction.

DECISION MAKING

When a patient is admitted to hospital the baseline observations of temperature, pulse, respirations and blood pressure are taken.

- *How may the anxiety associated with admission to hospital affect these readings?*
- *What strategies could be employed by the nurse to overcome these? Compare your response with your observations of clinical practice.*

process of glycogenesis. This releases the glucose stored as glycogen in the liver and muscles. A reserve of energy is also obtained by catabolism of body protein and lipolysis. (For a detailed explanation of this process see Chapter 3.2 on nutrition.)

In preparation for the fight or flight the body also needs to lighten itself. It does this in two ways:

- first it removes excess fluid by producing more urine, resulting in the frequent desire to urinate;
- second it removes, as much as possible, the contents of the alimentary tract. Peristaltic action is increased, which is often observed as diarrhoea. A full stomach entails extra weight, which would handicap fighting or running. Therefore the contents of the stomach may also be ejected. Additionally the feeling of a lump in the throat and a dry mouth dissuades the individual from eating, so preventing adding to the body weight.

Finally the skeletal muscles are put on alert and muscle tone increases. This prepares the body for immediate physical action. Skeletal muscles work in antagonistic pairs. Each joint has an extensor and a flexor muscle (Figure 4.1.4). If both these muscles contract then the joint will not move until one muscle relaxes. This allows a more rapid response than if both muscles were relaxed and one muscle had to contract.

Vast amounts of heat are generated by the aerobic respiration involved with the increased muscle activity. In anticipation, the body increases sweat production to begin cooling. Piloerection also occurs and at first this appears to be contradictory as piloerection is usually used to conserve heat. The function of piloerection in this instance is not thermoregulatory, however, but is a form of non-verbal communication. Man has little body hair and consequently this is not really observable. In animals with copious body hair the effect is dramatic. The piloerection causes the animal to appear much bigger than it is, therefore dissuading its foe to engage in combat with it.

Figure 4.1.4: An antagonistic pair of muscles – triceps and biceps.

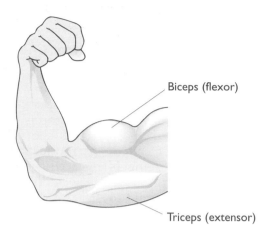

Biceps (flexor)

Triceps (extensor)

▍ *Long-term Physiological Changes in Stress*

Sometimes, although we experience the fight or flight reaction, we are unable to enact it because of adverse social pressures. For example, you may have an argument with your manager. Your immediate action, under the fight or flight response, would be to either hit your manager or run away. If you did either then it is unlikely that you would retain your employment for long. Instead you have to suppress your instinct. You 'bite your lip'. Social pressure therefore overrides the fight or flight reaction.

- *What do you think happens if this sort of reaction occurs frequently and you are unable to resolve it?*

The physical manifestations in response to long-term stress fall under the category of psychosomatic disorders. These used to be based on the premise that some physical disorders were exacerbated by psychological stress although contemporary theory focuses on the relationship between physiological and psychosocial factors contributing to the development of any organic disease (Doscher, 1989).

One of the most obvious effects of the fight or flight reaction is on the circulatory system. Heart rate increases and blood pressure rises. Continued exposure to stressful events can ultimately lead to damage as the circulatory system compensates for the maladjusted psychosocial responses and, in the event, becomes damaged itself.

In Figure 4.1.3 it was seen that the action of cortisol suppressed the immune response. A suppressed immune response leaves the individual less able to fight off disease. You may have noticed that if you are particularly tired, such as when you have not had a holiday for a while, you become more susceptible to colds and that they are more difficult to shake off. Many managers exploit this factor when monitoring stress in the workplace by using the incidence of sickness as an indicator of employee stress. The immune system also protects the body against more sinister disease, however.

We can use the holistic philosophy of health to explain these phenomena (Aggleton, 1990; Ewels and Simnett, 1992; Naidoo and Wills, 1994). This views individuals as comprised of interrelated systems such as the physiological, social, psychological and spiritual systems. In health there is a balance between the systems. In ill-health one system fails to function adequately and the equilibrium between the systems is disturbed. This imbalance is compensated by variation of the other systems. Therefore it follows that disturbance in one system leads to imbalance in the others. For example, you may be starting a cold. Although the cold is caused by a biological agent (a virus) and results in a physical illness you may feel psychologically tired or depressed.

RESEARCH BASED EVIDENCE

In the short-term physiological response to stress there is an increase in the heart rate and respiration. It has also been found that, in the long term, stress can lead to an increased incidence of heart and circulatory disease (Friedman and Rosenman, 1974; Patel et al., 1985; Totman, 1990; Legault et al., 1995).

RESEARCH BASED EVIDENCE

Following major life events it has been observed that people have an increased susceptibility to cancers (Totman, 1990). This effect has also been demonstrated by Fawzy et al. (1993), who evaluated the survival of individuals with malignant melanoma to find that those who had early psychological intervention to reduce stress had an improved survival rate.

Psychosocial

Take a few minutes to think back to periods when you have felt stressed.

- *How did you feel?*
- *How were you affected psychologically and socially?*

▶ PSYCHOSOCIAL RESPONSES TO STRESS

▶ *Psychological Changes in Stress*

Psychological responses to stress vary according to the level of threat. Greene (1989) asserts that mild anxiety is accompanied by a feeling of wellbeing. This was confirmed by Hebb's (1954) arousal curve and the inverted U hypothesis of Sutherland and Cooper (1990), which both state that cognitive functioning and alertness are increased with mild levels of stress. As the level of stress increases, however, the feeling of wellbeing is replaced by overwhelm. The individual's functioning ability decreases. The individual may be aware of what is happening, but be afraid to delegate or say 'no'. In consequence individuals find they have an ever-increasing workload that they are unable to complete, which in turn perpetuates their feelings of stress.

▶ Affective (emotional) changes

Initially the individual feels slight elation and competent to take on and achieve all tasks. As the level of stress increases this will be replaced by a feeling of unease and overwhelm. Individuals feel that they are struggling to keep their head above water. Interpersonal relationships may deteriorate as the individual becomes short tempered, aggressive and unapproachable.

▶ Behavioural changes

In mild levels of stress there is increased confidence, which is demonstrated by a confident posture. The individual also portrays a confident outlook. As the level of anxiety increases the confident behaviour is replaced by one of restlessness and urgency. Individuals appear to be competing against the clock and against others. The behaviour and posture they adopt are those associated with aggression. This may progress to panic where the behaviour either becomes uncontrolled or the individual clings to behaviours and objects of security. Eventually, in burnout, the behaviour is of resignation and compliance.

▶ Cognitive changes

Individuals may find that their concentration span decreases and find themselves moving from task to task, but never completing a task. Problem solving ability is severely curtailed and individuals drift between tasks. This worsens their plight and individuals find themselves locked into a stress cycle.

▶ Defence mechanisms

In response to stress the individual may attempt to cope by adopting defence mechanisms. These were identified by Freud (1934) who claimed they were used to defend the self against conflict, and have since been developed by many other writers.

Defence mechanisms are unconscious processes used to cope with negative emotions. In the short term they are used without any problem and they help the individual to survive the immediate period following exposure to the stress. Defence mechanisms do not alter the cause of the stress, however; they only alter the individual's interpretation of it. They

Mechanism	Definition	Example
Denial	When reality is too unpleasant or painful to face then individuals may deny that it really exists. In circumstances this is a healthy process as it allows the individual time to come to terms with the problem. Indeed it is the first stage of the grieving process (Kubler-Ross, 1969) (see Chapter 3.5 on death and dying). In other situations denial may be more serious (see example).	A woman may deny that she could have a serious illness and may delay seeking medical help for a lump she has recently found in her breast.
Displacement	When it is impossible to address the cause of stress then anger may be redirected on another, innocent, but reachable object.	You may have been given a hard time by your boss to whom you are unable to retaliate. When you return home you immediately have a blazing argument with your partner.
Intellectualization	To use intellectual powers of thinking, analysis and reasoning to detach oneself from emotional issues.	For people working in life or death situations, such as in high-dependency units, this defence mechanisms may be necessary for survival. If the emotional bluntness extends into other areas of the individuals' lives the mechanism becomes problematic.
Projection	Blaming someone else for how you feel.	The ward manager who is unable to manage the ward effectively may blame the situation on incompetent staff.
Rationalization	To find an acceptable explanation for an act that you find unacceptable.	'Its in the overall best interest'. 'You have to be cruel to be kind' 'I don't really care that I didn't get the interview. I didn't really want the job anyway'.
Reaction-formation	To conceal what you really feel by thinking and acting in the opposite way.	Some people who have an issue in their life they feel uncomfortable about and that may or may not be resolved, may campaign against the issue. For example, individuals who have led promiscuous lives may campaign strongly for the sanctity of family values.
Regression	Individuals engage in behaviours from an earlier, more secure, life stage.	Losing your temper and engaging in tantrums when things go wrong. Eating when feeling stressed.
Repression	Painful thoughts are forced into the unconscious. Although they are out of the conscious they may resurface in dreams.	An accident victim may use repression to have no recollection of the events surrounding the accident.
Sublimation	To redirect the energy from unacceptable sexual or aggressive drives into another socially acceptable activity.	Unacceptable aggressive energy focused into a sporting activity. This may not always be a positive mechanism. For example, a manager may use sublimation to secure promotions at the expense of family and social commitments.

Table 4.1.4 Defence mechanisms.

DECISION MAKING

- *Which defence mechanisms have you used?*
- *Which defence mechanisms have you seen other members of the health care team using?*
- *Have you seen clients or relatives using defence mechanisms?*
- *How will recognition of defence mechanisms influence decision making in nursing practice?*

create an illusion and consequently involve a degree of self-deception. Prolonged use of defence mechanisms is therefore unhealthy. The major defence mechanisms are outlined in Table 4.1.4.

Social Changes In Response To Stress

In the initial stages of stress, which are accompanied by a feeling of wellbeing, individuals feel confident and able to take on all tasks. As the level of stress increases, however, individuals may appear aggressive and their social interactions may reflect this increased hostility. They may have frequent arguments with others and become intolerant. As the level of stress increases they become overwhelmed and engrossed with the object causing their stress. They may reject all social contact, even with members of their family, and become isolated. Alternatively they may become hostile and react aggressively as discussed in Chapter 2.5.

Eventually, in burnout, individuals become emotionally blunted and cynical. Their relationships with others will have already deteriorated and they may struggle to maintain the relationships they still have.

▶ CAUSES OF STRESS

Think back to a period in your life that you found particularly stressful. Spend a few moments to jot down things that happened to you in the year preceding your stressful period.

(You will probably have written down a number of events that occurred. These are life events. One or more may be particularly significant such as getting married, moving house or getting a new job. Other events may be less significant such as going on holiday or buying a new car. On their own, life events may be manageable; however, their cumulative effect increases the overall level of stress that the individual experiences.)

DECISION MAKING

John is a student colleague who is having difficulty with his partner and, in consequence, moved out of their shared home into the nurses' home. This has caused him financial difficulties and he is having problems paying his credit card bills. John also has difficulty coping with the pressure of course work and the demands made upon him by clients in clinical placement.
- *What would you say to John, who feels that he is weak because he is unable to cope in situations that others appear to be able to manage?*

The cumulative effect of stress underpins the work of Holmes and Rahe (1967). They classified the significance of events in people's lives in the Social Readjustment Rating Scale (Table 4.1.5). This scale ascribes weightings to life events. The greater the stress invoked by the life event then the greater the weighting ascribed to it. As individuals go through life they are exposed to different stressors. In the Social Readjustment Rating Scale the rating of each new stressor is added to those that have occurred over the previous year. Individuals are then able to assess their level of stress using this scale by summating the ratings of all life events. Holmes and Rahe found that a rating of over 300 was associated with an increased occurrence of a stress related disease.

You may have noticed that some individuals appear to be able to cope with stress better than others. Using Hebb's model of arousal (Hebb, 1954) and the Social Readjustment Rating Scale (Holmes and Rahe, 1967) it is possible to see why one individual may be unaffected by an incident whereas to another individual the same incident may be catastrophic. The effect of stress is cumulative. If one individual has an accumulation of stressors and another has comparatively few then exposure to the same stressor will push the first individual into overload whereas the latter individual may have sufficient coping reserve.

A limitation of the Social Readjustment Rating Scale is that it only addresses long-term stressors. It does not take into account short-term stressors such as being late for work or sitting in a traffic jam, which may invoke a severe stress response, but only for a short period. It is also very difficult to quantify individuals' experiences of stress. Because of this the Social Readjustment Rating Scale should be seen as an indicator of an individual's underlying stress level. It should not be interpreted as providing an instant quantifiable snapshot of an individual's level of stress.

▶ INTERPRETATION OF STRESS

Up until this point we have assumed that the object of the stress is external to the individual and has more or less the same ability to cause stress to everyone. This is demonstrated in Figure 4.1.5 where the stimulus is seen identically by subject A and subject B.

The work of Lazarus (1966) and Cox (1978) suggest that stress should be explored from a different perspective. They take a phenomenological

Rank	Life event	Rating
1	Death of spouse	100
2	Divorce	73
3	Marital separation	65
4	Jail term	65
5	Death of close family member	63
6	Personal injury or illness	53
7	Marriage	50
8	Loss of job	47
9	Marital reconciliation	45
10	Retirement	45
11	Change in health of family member	44
12	Pregnancy	40
13	Sex difficulties	39
14	Gain of new family member	39
15	Business readjustment	39
16	Change in financial state	38
17	Death of close friend	37
18	Change to different line of work	36
19	Change in number of arguments with spouse	35
20	Mortgage over $10 000	31
21	Foreclosure of mortgage of loan	30
22	Change in responsibilities at work	29
23	Son or daughter leaving home	29
24	Trouble with in-laws	29
25	Outstanding personal achievement	28
26	Wife begins or stops work	26
27	Begin or end school	26
28	Change in living conditions	25
29	Revision of personal habits	24
30	Trouble with boss	23
31	Change in work hours or conditions	20
32	Change in residence	20
33	Change in school	20
34	Change in recreation	19
35	Change in church activities	19
36	Change in social activities	18
37	Mortgage or loan of less that $10 000	17
38	Change in sleeping habits	16
39	Change in the number of family get togethers	15
40	Change in eating habits	15
41	Holiday	13
42	Christmas	12
43	Minor violations of the law	11

Table 4.1.5 Social Readjustment Rating Scale. (From Holmes and Rahe, 1967.)

viewpoint. They agree that stressors can be external to the individual, but they say that how much the stress affects the individual depends upon how threatening the individual thinks the object is. Figure 4.1.6 represents this concept. Subjects A and B are exposed to the same stimulus as before, but the interpretation of threat is greater by subject B than by subject A.

The Social Readjustment Rating Scale attempts to generalize the severity of response to everyone; it does not allow for variability between individuals. Additionally, it only measures a restricted number of events. The ability of long-term stressors alone to predict an individual's stress response has been questioned and it is argued that a cumulation of minor day to day stresses or hassles is just as damaging as the long-term stresses identified by the Social Readjustment Rating Scale. Therefore an

Figure 4.1.5: Viewing the stimulus the same.

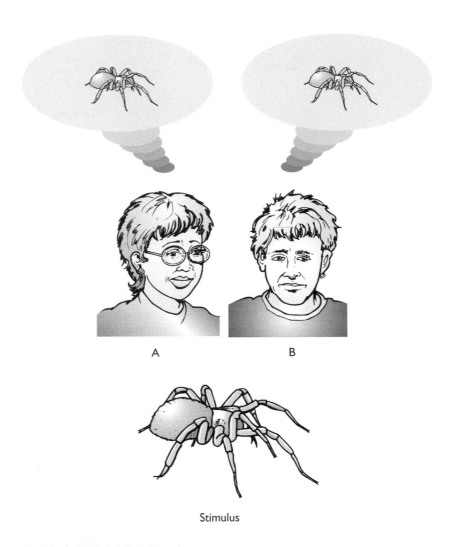

A

B

Stimulus

DECISION MAKING	
Jason, aged 15 years, is terrified of moths and will run out of a room if he thinks one is present. As a young child this behaviour was acceptable, but now it has become a focus of embarrassment. Jason has even begun declining invitations to go out with his friends at night in case he encounters a moth. • *Some people develop what appear to others to be 'irrational' fears of objects or of situations. These are called phobias. Using phenomenological stress theory explain how this*	*might occur.* • *How might this knowledge be used as a basis for a programme to help Jason overcome his fear.* (Most people have particular dislikes of certain objects or situations and will avoid exposure to them. This is normal behaviour. Phobias occur when the fear is grossly disproportionate to the amount of threat imposed by the object and the avoiding behaviour occurs to such an extent that it is impossible for the individual to continue with normal day to day life.)

assessment of an individual's stress should include a measure of an individual's hassles and an understanding of the individual's interpretation of stresses (Cox, 1978; Lazarus *et al.*, 1985; Reich *et al.*, 1988).

In a nursing assessment the use of the Social Readjustment Rating Scale to measure long-term stresses is useful in so much as it identifies a baseline of background stresses. From this baseline the effects of day to day stresses and the interpretation an individual attaches to the nature of stressful experiences must also be added.

▶ THE STRESSFUL PERSONALITY TYPE

Although individuals' responses to stressors vary according to their interpretations, some individuals have been observed to consistently respond

Figure 4.1.6: Interpretation of the stressor.

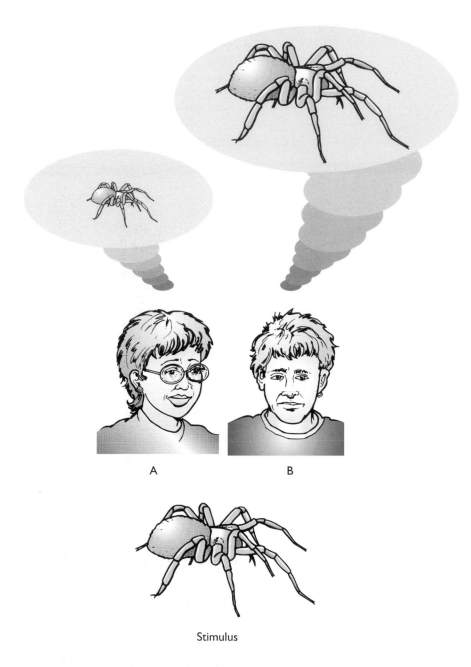

A   B

Stimulus

One form of stress management that is often suggested is taking up a sporting activity. Explain whether or not this strategy would be likely to be successful for Type A individuals?

to stress in similar ways. Friedman and Rosenman (1974) identified two dissimilar groups of individuals. The first group they classified as 'Type A' personality. These individuals are characterized by extreme competitiveness and an inability to place stress in perspective. They routinely work against the clock. They are unable to say no and they take on multiple commitments. The consequence of these factors is that they are unable to fit all tasks into the available time and they subsequently juggle tasks, switching from one to another, without completing any task. This is compounded by a lack of direction. Rather than taking a systematic approach to problem solving, Type A individuals will attempt to solve problems without first identifying the goals. They are also fiercely competitive. This leads them to appear aggressive and they often react to minor irritations in the form of temper tantrums.

In contrast, the characteristics of the second personality type, the Type B personality, are opposite to those of Type A. The Type B personality is totally relaxed almost to the point of unmotivation.

Type A and Type B personality types should really be viewed as the two extreme points of a scale. Most people have traits of both personality types and fit on a point somewhere along the scale (Figure 4.1.7).

Figure 4.1.7: From Type B personality to Type A.

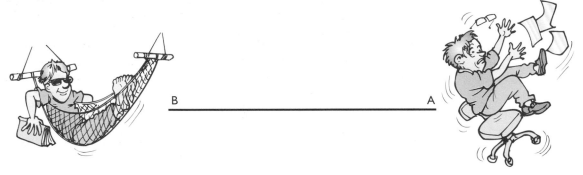

B ——————————————— A

RESEARCH BASED EVIDENCE

Type A individuals are more susceptible to stress related diseases. In particular Friedman and Rosenman (1974) found a relationship between Type A behaviour and coronary heart disease. They suggested a behaviour modification programme to replace Type A behaviour with that of Type B. This, in turn, reduced the stress related disease.

▶ CONTINUED EXPOSURE TO STRESSFUL EVENTS

▶ *Burnout*

Individuals who remain exposed to stressful events and who are unable to control them develop a response to the stress called burnout. Burnard (1991) asserts that due to the intense prolonged stressful nature of caring, members of the caring professions are particularly susceptible to the condition. Three main aspects of burnout were identified by Maslach (1982):

- ▶ emotional exhaustion – individuals feel that they are emotionally drained and unable to give more to individuals;
- ▶ depersonalization – individuals feel that they are becoming more isolated and hardened towards others;
- ▶ trivialization of personal accomplishments – individuals feel that they are becoming unable to deal with problems positively and may trivialize any achievements they make.

DECISION MAKING

Ken entered nursing at the age of 19. Throughout his career he had been very ambitious and developed himself academically and professionally and was now a ward manager. The NHS reforms, however, had led to many changes in the delivery and structure of health care in the UK, and Ken can no longer see a clear direction for his future career. He is even uncertain of the future of his present position and he resents the increasing amount of time that he has to spend away from patient care.

Although Ken feels insecure in his current position he also feels unable to move to another post. He feels trapped and under constant pressure to do more, but he is unclear what more the organization requires of him. He can see no real purpose in his life and is becoming very cynical. He suspects people of having hidden agendas and has become very confrontational, opposing any suggestions for change.

Ken has noticed that he is experiencing more arguments both at work and with his family. Because of this he has avoided events where he has to socialize with others as he tends to get into arguments. He is unable to relax and has found that he is increasing his use of alcohol in the evening to help him to sleep.

Ken was experiencing professional stress syndrome or burnout.

- ● *Using the list of symptoms of burnout, how do you think the quality of care offered by Ken is likely to be affected?*
- ● *How do you think Ken's leadership skills will be affected?*
- ● *What do you think will be the effects of Ken's condition on the rest of the ward staff and the consequences on the care that they give?*

Welch *et al.* (1982) categorized the symptoms of burnout into the areas of physical, intellectual, emotional, social and spiritual (Table 4.1.6).

There are two types of burnout (Welch *et al.*, 1982). In the first type, short-term burnout, individuals have mainly physical effects and feel run-down. It is relieved by a break from work, such as a holiday or a change to work such as a new project. This type of burnout is reversible and relatively short lived.

In contrast, the second type of burnout, long-term burnout, is signified by the profound psychological and social changes identified in Table 4.1.6. Individuals become emotionally blunted, their cognitive ability decreases and because they find it difficult to mix with others, they become isolated. The ramifications spill over from their work life and into their personal lives where they find relationships with their family and others deteriorating. The effects of long-term burnout are devastating and the recovery is long and difficult.

Physical	Lack of energy and persistent feeling of fatigue. Often accompanied by a lack of exercise and poor nutrition.
Intellectual	Loss of problem solving ability and cognitive ability. Lack of creativity. Often individuals have no distracting outlet such as hobbies.
Emotional	Feelings of helplessness and depression. Individuals severely at risk of burnout overinvest their energies in their job to the exclusion of other interests. When the job becomes difficult so do their lives. It was observed that people with interests outside work fared better than those without.
Social	Individuals with burnout do not share their problems with others. This may result from a fear of rejection or admission of weakness. It results in them withdrawing from others and becoming isolated. Conversely, if individuals feel threatened they may react aggressively towards others. In turn this will also make them isolated.
Spiritual	Individuals may have high expectations when entering their chosen career. In reality these expectations may be impossible to achieve, and as individuals experience burnout the achievement of these ideals becomes even more difficult. This leaves the individuals feeling unfulfilled, cynical and possibly cheated.

Table 4.1.6 Symptoms of burnout. (From Welch *et. al.*, 1982.)

▶ *Causes of Burnout in Nursing*

Burnout occurs as a response to continued stress. Individuals suffering from burnout may feel that it is a result of a weakness in their character, thus compounding their problem (Maslach, 1982). This is reinforced by the attitudes of others who may be less than sympathetic towards people admitting that they feel stressed. How many times have you heard phrases such as 'if you can't stand the heat get out of the kitchen'. Employers may encourage this attitude, blaming the individual who suffers the stress as being weak rather than addressing issues that may be causing the stress (COHSE, 1992). What must be remembered, however, is that burnout occurs as a result of external factors: 'no one burns out except in a climate that encourages burnout' (Welch *et al.*, 1982, p. 9).

Following the introduction of the health service internal market system in the UK, there is tremendous pressure on nurses to do more with less resources. Studies into burnout suggest that in this type of environment the incidence of burnout among nurses in the UK will probably increase unless individuals are aware of the signs of burnout and able to take action.

▶ *Post Traumatic Stress Disorder (PTSD)*

PTSD is a condition that occurs within six months following a traumatic life experience. It is defined in ICD-10 (World Health Organization, 1992, p. 147). as 'a delayed and/or protracted response to a stressful event or situation (either short or long-lasting) of an exceptionally threatening or catastrophic nature, which is likely to cause pervasive distress in almost anyone'.

PTSD occurs following exposure to a triggering event. Triggering events are any major psychological events outside the range of usual day to day experience. Examples are:

- ▶ natural disasters (e.g. earthquakes, floods, hurricanes);
- ▶ manmade disasters (e.g. major car, air or maritime accidents, industrial accidents);
- ▶ intentional manmade disasters (e.g. witnessing the violent death of others, being a victim of rape, torture or assault, prolonged combat).

Exposure to the trigger event leads to the onset of PTSD; however, there may be a latent period of up to six months before the symptoms develop.

The five major features of PTSD are:

- ▶ flashbacks, where individuals relive the experience during nightmares. Occasionally, when awake, they may also feel that the situation is about to recur;
- ▶ emotional numbing with emotional blunting and detachment from others;
- ▶ hypervigilance and an enhanced startle reaction;
- ▶ avoidance of anything reminiscent of the triggering event;
- ▶ confusion, anxiety and depression, which are common, and there may be suicidal attempts.

Other symptoms may include insomnia, somatic symptoms such as headaches, ulcers and circulatory problems, and an excessive use of alcohol or other drugs. Sometimes the individual may blame him or herself for the incident and, in addition, experience fear and guilt.

PTSD is usually diagnosed if it occurs within the six months following the triggering factor (World Health Organization, 1992). Sometimes an individual may experience PTSD-like symptoms months or years following the triggering event. In this case it may be referred to as a delayed PTSD (Greene, 1989; Charron, 1994).

It is argued that prompt intervention is the most effective strategy to restore normal health and prevent long-term psychological damage following exposure to trigger factors (Sims and Owens, 1993). You may have noticed that following major disasters teams of counsellors are deployed to provide this service to the victims. The crisis intervention strategies focus on the individuals' unique problems and assist them to make some sense out of their experience, adopt a problem solving strategy and to move through the crisis period.

PRACTICE KNOWLEDGE

We have discussed the nature of stress and how it affects individuals. Nurses are likely to experience stress from four main sources – clients, relatives, colleagues and themselves. This part of the chapter will assist you to make an assessment of stress in others and help you develop strategies to cope with stress you encounter.

▶ ASSESSMENT

▷ *In Clients*

Nurses may encounter clients in which stress is:

▶ a primary reason for referral;
▶ a cause of or a contributory factor to the client's condition
▶ occurring as a consequence of the client's illness.

The purpose of the nursing assessment is to gain understanding of the nature and meaning of both the causes and the individual's experiences of stress. Stress, as we have seen, is a phenomenon that cannot be generalized between individuals; everybody's experience of stress is unique. Similarly, individuals' responses to stress vary. Although the fight or flight syndrome classifies specific stress response behaviours, some clients may react by being very anxious and apprehensive, some may become very dependent upon the nurse to the point of compliance, whereas other clients may react with anger or violence.

If the nurse is to assist the client it is necessary to understand how that individual is experiencing stress and why he or she is reacting in that way. The pervasive nature of stress reinforces the need of an holistic assessment. This will enable the nurse to establish how the stress manifests and affects the individual's life and identify recurrent patterns of events that act as triggers.

Because stress results from interaction between the individual and the environment the nurse may use the Social Readjustment Rating Scale (see Table 4.1.5) to identify events that have led up to the stressful episode. This will give an estimate of the individual's underlying stress level, although as we saw previously, it is of limited value when trying to understand the way in which stress is perceived by the individual.

In completing the Social Readjustment Rating Scale the client will indicate some events that have occurred and contributed towards how they feel. This information can then be used by the nurse to provide a focus during the assessment interview where the client is able to expand on the areas they have indicated. In this way the nurse is able to gain an understanding of how the client feels about the stressful issues.

Clients may also be referred for a condition that is exacerbated by stress. This may take the form of a stress related mental or physical illness. The purposes of assessment in such an instance are to identify

---

DECISION MAKING

Kathleen has been admitted to the acute psychiatric ward from the outpatients department. She is 39 years of age and married with two daughters aged 16 and 14 years. This is her fifth in-patient admission in three years. Over the previous fortnight her family state that she has gradually become withdrawn and insular. She is neglecting her personal appearance and sleeping for prolonged irregular periods.

During the assessment the nurse uses the Social Readjustment Rating Scale to explore what issues have occurred in Kathleen's life over the previous year. It emerges that Kathleen's husband, who is employed as a fitter in the local car factory, has been told that the factory is to close and that he will be made redundant. The time that the factory closure was announced coincides with the onset of Kathleen's latest relapse.

Stress is often seen to precipitate a relapse of depression (Jacobson, 1980). The redundancy of her husband is seen as a major life event resulting in stress (Holmes and Rahe, 1967). This, in turn, has contributed to the recurrence of Kathleen's illness.

Using the Social Readjustment Rating Scale the nurse was able to quickly focus on the redundancy of Kathleen's husband and as Kathleen became able to enter into conversation, explore ways in which Kathleen and her family would cope.

- *Think of other reasons that may be contributing to Kathleen's level of stress (which may or may not be listed on the scale).*
- *Is the redundancy of Kathleen's husband eustress or distress?*
- *What are the disadvantages of the Social Readjustment Rating Scale?*

when stress occurs, why it occurs and how quickly it has led to the onset of the illness.

▌ Stress that accompanies other illness

The relationship between health and stress is established. A high stress level has negative ramifications on physical health (Totman, 1990; Fawzy *et al.*, 1993). A more immediate effect of the relationship between stress and physiological symptoms was noted by Hayward (1975). He found that an increase in anxiety was seen to increase the level of pain individual's experienced. Therefore, although the client's primary problem may be essentially physical the accompanying anxiety, if left unaddressed, will hinder recovery.

Clients may be concerned that they are going to die, that they are going to be in pain, that they may not wake up from an anaesthetic or that their prognosis may be poor. To the nurse working on a busy ward these may appear to be unfounded fears. To the client they are very real. It is very easy for the nurse to become desensitized to clients' fears in a busy environment.

Clients going into hospital may also worry about their continuing responsibilities. They may have dependent relatives and be uncertain about how they will be cared for. They may have a pet that requires care. They may worry about loss of income. They may be concerned that they will be unable to work again. The nurse, on identifying these problems, must spend time with the client and explore the issues from the client's perspective. It may sound obvious, but it is only when the client's problems have been identified that they can be addressed.

Where anxiety accompanies a physical illness the source of the anxiety must be identified. The nurse should identify the nature of the anxiety with the client, explore the nature of his or her problems and identify ways in which the problems may be resolved.

Many clients may not verbalize their concerns. For example, clients who adopt the closed position and do not make eye contact are displaying avoiding behaviour. This is the flight reaction. Conversely, clients may be hostile and aggressive. This is the non-verbal expression of the fight reaction. The nurse should therefore be aware of non-verbal expressions of anxiety and incorporate them into the assessment as discussed in Chapter 2.5.

▌ *Stress in Clients' Relatives*

In clients' relatives stress may result from concern at the client's illness, guilt that they are unable to cope and anger that the client is ill. Some relatives may avoid the client and neglect visiting the client. Although this may be interpreted as uncaring it may also be seen as the flight reaction. Other relatives may react with anger. The anger may be projected onto the nurse when the relative becomes hostile, or the relative may constantly find fault with the care given to the client. In this instance the relatives may be labelled as 'trouble makers' and in

---

> Imagine that you are to be admitted to hospital for an operation under general anaesthetic. What would you be worried about?

DECISION MAKING

Clients who are admitted to hospital for a physical illness will probably be anxious. This anxiety may be thought of as 'only natural' and not be deemed a significant problem by some nurses.

- *What would you say to a nurse who wrote the following care plan?*

Problem	Nursing Action
Anxiety	Give reassurance

DECISION MAKING

Lee is a lively seven-year-old boy who has enjoyed school and was a member of the school football team. His mother has recently noticed that Lee has developed frequent stomach aches. This has coincided with a change in his behaviour from being an enthusiastic boy who liked talking about school and football to a quiet boy who spends most of his time playing on his own with his handheld computer game.

His mother contacted the school, which had also noticed the change in Lee's behaviour and agrees to keep a close eye on him to determine whether there is a cause at school for the change. It emerges that Lee is being bullied by a group of older children. The school quickly addresses this and Lee begins to return to his usual self.

In Lee's case the non-verbal expression of stress manifested as symptoms of illness and a change of personality. Non-verbal expressions of stress can take many forms such as abrupt or aggressive interactions with others, avoidance behaviour or risk taking behaviour.

- *Think of the different client groups you work with. What non-verbal cues would suggest that they are feeling stressed?*
- *Think of your colleagues. What non-verbal cues would suggest that they are feeling stressed?*

DECISION MAKING

Jeanette is a junior staff nurse in a private nursing home for the elderly. She is primary nurse to George, a newly admitted man of 78 years of age. George's daughter visits regularly, but is always hostile towards Jeanette, constantly complaining about the care George is receiving.

- *Why do you think George's daughter could be reacting in this way towards Jeanette?*

Spend a few minutes thinking about your workplace. What indicators of excessive stress can you identify in yourself and in the environment you work?

turn be treated with hostility by the nurses. This perpetuates the situation. The nurse should recognize the stress felt by the relatives, acknowledge their concerns and pursue their complaints.

Relatives may also feel excluded from caring for their sick relative. This compounds their guilt and increases the hostility they may show to the nursing staff. Strategies such as flexible visiting arrangements and offering to involve them in the client's care (after obtaining the client's consent) may allow the relatives to take more control and collaborate rather than fight with the nursing staff. (For further information on managing hostility see Chapter 2.5 on aggression.)

▶ Stress in in the Nursing Workplace

Nursing is a stressful occupation. Nurses are expected to cope in traumatic life and death situations. They work unsocial hours and are expected to do more with less resources. Remuneration is minimal and many nurses no longer have job security, being placed on short-term contracts.

Stress is a reaction of the individual to a stressful environment. Individuals may incorrectly reason that if everybody else can cope then it is they who must be weak. This then leads the individual to have a poor self-esteem. It is therefore essential that nurses understand how stress affects them and others in the workplace. This is achieved by developing self-awareness.

Common indicators of excessive stress in the workplace are:

- bringing work home;
- not being able to switch off from work;
- feeling tense all of the time;
- poor self esteem;
- difficulty in mixing with others;
- deteriorating relationships;
- increase in arguments at work;
- talking malevolently about colleagues;
- feeling run down;
- increase in physical ailments.

These indicators signify the early stage of burnout. Monitoring is essential as individuals are often unaware of the signs and may progress rapidly into full burnout. Using feedback from others and self monitoring will enable individuals to detect early burnout and take stress limiting actions.

DECISION MAKING

Gail is manager of one of three care of the elderly wards in a hospital. The trust in which she works is in financial difficulty, however, and the level of services it offers is being reviewed. It is considering a rationalization of the elderly services, reducing the three care of the elderly wards to two.

Gail has vacancies for two staff nurses, but has been unable to fill the posts with permanent staff due to the uncertain future. The staff numbers are kept up by the use of bank staff for the busy periods although Gail is never certain which bank nurse will arrive and often it means that

she has to work over her hours to ensure that the bank nurse is familiar with the ward.

The ward staff are very unsettled. They often work more than their contracted hours. This is unpaid overtime and, due to the shortage of staff, they are unable to take their time back. Gail has noticed that there is a lot of 'backbiting' among the staff and that some staff are taking more sickness time. A number of the staff complain that their relationships with their partners are deteriorating; indeed one has recently divorced. Gail's partner is also fed up with her working

over and going into work on her day off.

Gail begins to feel that she is a poor manager as whenever she has asked for additional help her manager informs her that the other areas are managing and cannot see why she is unable to cope.

- *Referring to the indicators of stress in the nursing workplace, what would lead you to conclude that the staff are suffering a high level of stress?*
- *What factors could have led to this situation?*
- *What are the likely outcomes for Gail and her staff if this situation continues?*

▶ PLANNING

▶ *Drugs*

Both prescribed and non-prescribed drugs may be used by individuals to help manage the symptoms of stress. Examples of prescribed drugs are anxiolytics such as diazepam or lorazepam. Non-prescribed drugs you may encounter are alcohol, nicotine and some illegal substances.

Drugs provide immediate relief from the unpleasant feelings associated with stress. This is a very short-term effect, although in periods of crisis they may be used to reduce the level of anxiety to allow problem solving thinking to develop. If the underlying problems that have caused the anxiety are not addressed, however, the unpleasant feelings will return as the effects of the drugs wear off. This may encourage the individual to take the drug again. This then becomes a self-perpetuating cycle and may quickly lead to dependence upon the drug. For these reasons, the use of drugs is not advocated as part of long-term stress management and they have not been included in this chapter.

▶ STRESS MANAGEMENT

Stress management strategies fall into proactive and reactive methods. Reactive methods are used following a stressful event to help manage the problem. They therefore work on the assumption that there is stress to be managed in the first place. In contrast proactive strategies are taken to prevent or minimize the number of stressful events experienced. Most methods of stress management can be used either proactively or reactively; however, to effectively manage stress, the aim should be to use all strategies proactively.

The following methods of stress management have been classified into cognitive and behavioural methods.

▶ *Cognitive Methods*

Cognitive methods address the issues that underlie the stress. We have seen that stress is exacerbated when the individual lacks control. Cognitive methods aim to enable individuals take more control of stressors in their lives, so limiting their negative effects. The cognitive methods that will be addressed are:

- ▶ counselling;
- ▶ supervision;
- ▶ socialization;
- ▶ time management.

▶ Counselling

This focuses on assisting individuals to prioritize the importance of issues in their lives and to develop problem solving strategies for coping. Counselling aims to enable individuals to take control in stressful situations. Where this is not possible, for example, if the individual has become unemployed, then the individual is encouraged to take as much control of events associated with the stress as possible to limit the negative effects of the situation.

▶ Supervision

This is increasingly being used by nurses. It takes two forms:

- ▶ individual supervision;
- ▶ group supervision.

In individual supervision the supervisor is an experienced fellow professional whose role is to listen, evaluate and teach. The practitioner and supervisor meet weekly at pre-arranged sessions lasting for around one hour. In these sessions there is time for reflecting on issues that have occurred during the week and time for planning a strategy for implementation the following week. The value of supervision is that it provides an alternative perspective of events, it provides an outlet for the practitioner to discuss feelings held towards events and it facilitates learning via reflection, to enhance the practitioner's practice.

In group supervision 6–10 professionals working in similar areas meet weekly to reflect on their practice. The group is usually conducted by an experienced professional and the purposes, similar to those of individual supervision, are to provide a forum where practitioners can talk about their feelings and to provide an environment to learn and improve practice. The value of group supervision may be limited however, due to the number of people sharing the time and because individuals may not feel safe to disclose as much in a group as they would during individual supervision. Group supervision should therefore be used to support rather than to replace individual supervision.

▶ Socialization

Time should be made for all commitments in life. Under stress individuals may find that they have little time for anything other than work and work related issues. This is compounded should the individual work unsocial hours or shifts. It is essential that the individual continues with existing social contacts, for example friends and family, in order to retain an appropriate perspective on new stressors in life.

▶ Time management

One of the problems that occur when individuals become too stressed is that their organizational ability becomes curtailed. Individuals attempt to accommodate an ever increasing workload into an ever decreasing amount of available time. Life then loses structure and becomes overwhelming. Individuals may attempt to cope by multitasking – juggling between one task and another, but never completing a task. Because there is a finite amount of time individuals then prioritize which tasks are to be given most energy and may end up leaving little time for family and social commitments.

Effective time management is a fundamental part of proactive stress management. Essential equipment comprises:

- ▶ a diary;
- ▶ a year planner;
- ▶ a 'to do' list.

Make it a rule that you never make an appointment without your diary. When considering buying a diary it is important to select a format that will allow you to view at least one week at a time. Diaries that only allow you to view one or two days at a time are of limited use in personal time management as you are unable to appraise new appointments in the context of existing commitments. Personal organizers are very useful in this respect as they often contain yearly planners with monthly and yearly views so as to afford comprehensive views of commitments. The disadvantage is that information has to be entered two or three times. Many electronic organizers are becoming affordable, however, and these will update all sections automatically. Although this seems an ideal solution, before you rush out to buy one you should beware that many of the lower priced electronic organizers do not provide a facility to back up the data. This can be catastrophic should the batteries (or even the organizer) fail. Check before you buy!

The first items that should be entered into your diary and year planner are holidays and time for yourself. These are the most important entries you will make and should not be altered. All entries other than these will compete for the remaining space. Next enter dates and times that you know are committed into your diary. Work days for example.

This then concludes the initial entries in the diary.

The second stage of time management is to list all your objectives and construct a 'to do' list.

From the list identify end goals that will allow you to fulfil your objectives and the dates by which the goals must be achieved. Table 4.1.7 shows a competed list of goal statements.

Goal	To be completed by
Complete physiology essay	10th October
Complete sociology essay	21st October
Complete psychology essay	7th November
Decorate kitchen	14th November
Prune shrubs in garden	20th November

Table 4.1.7 Goal statements.

Take each goal statement and break it into smaller components. Set each component a target date for completion (Table 4.1.8).

Physiology essay	To be completed by
Literature search	10th September
Write plan	15th September
First draft	25th September
Second draft	30th September
Read second draft	5th October
Final draft	10th October

Table 4.1.8 Target dates for smaller goal components.

Transfer these goals onto your yearly planner. In your diary set aside time to achieve these goals. A completed diary page may then look like Figure 4.1.8.

This approach to time management is highly structured, but not inflexible. The structure is necessary as events can quickly get out of hand; however, once you are aware of what your commitments are, you are able to make adjustments to your schedule to accommodate alterations in demands on your time.

DECISION MAKING

The example of time management has addressed medium- to long-term management. Time management can also be used to help short-term management.

- *Look at your work objectives for a shift in clinical practice. Using the principles of time management organize how you will deliver your care.*

Figure 4.1.8: Completed diary page.

September	September
Monday 11th 7.30–14.30 Early shift 19.30–21.00 Write plan for biology	**Thursday 14th** Visit mum and dad for the day
Tuesday 12th 7.30–14.30 Early shift 19.30–21.00 Write plan for biology	**Friday 15th** 9.00–12.30 Finish plan for biology Afternoon – gardening 21.00 Go out to pub
Wednesday 13th 7.30–14.30 Early shift 19.30–21.00 Write plan for biology	**Saturday 16th** 12.30–21.30 Late shift
	Sunday 17th 7.30–14.30 Early shift

▶ *Behavioural Methods*

Behavioural methods only address the symptoms of stress and do not attempt to address the cause. This is rather like giving sedatives to manage stress – it is useful at the point of crisis; however, as the underlying causes of the stress are not addressed, there will probably be a recurrence of the individual's problems at a later date. The behavioural methods discussed are:

- ▶ progressive muscle relaxation;
- ▶ massage;
- ▶ meditation;
- ▶ biofeedback;
- ▶ assertiveness training;
- ▶ exercise;
- ▶ diet;
- ▶ cognitive behavioural therapy;
- ▶ desensitization.

▶ Progressive muscle relaxation

This is a behavioural technique used to help manage the effects of stress. We have observed that one effect of stress was an increase in muscle tone. This leads to a feeling of tension. Progressive muscle relaxation focuses the individual's attention on groups of muscles. The individual is asked to contract the muscle group and then to relax, to compare the difference and to remember the feeling of relaxation. This usually occurs when the individual is lying in a quiet room with relaxing background music. Each major muscle group is addressed in turn, leading to an overall reduction in muscle tone, and the individual feels relaxed.

▶ Massage

This is another form of muscle relaxation, but is combined with touch. It is a form of non-verbal communication and indicates that the person performing the massage cares about the individual receiving the massage. During massage individuals often feel sufficiently comfortable to discuss their main anxieties.

▶ Meditation

The individual sits in a relaxed and balanced posture. This is a position in which the body is balanced in such a way that it requires no muscle correction to maintain its position. The individual is asked to breathe slowly and deeply. This counters the increased shallow respiration that is experienced in anxiety. The individual is then asked to focus on a single object such as a lighted candle or to empty the mind of all thoughts. This aims to reduce the recurrent worrying thoughts that occur in anxiety.

▌ Biofeedback

This is a technique that uses operant conditioning to teach the client how to manage stress symptoms. It requires the use of a skin galvanometer to measure the electrical conductivity of the skin. We saw earlier, when discussing the physiological responses to stress (p. 482) that individuals perspire more readily when they are exposed to stress. This reduces the electrical resistance of the skin. Using a galvanometer designed for this therapy, a loudspeaker emits a tone that rises in pitch as the electrical conductivity (and stress level) increases. The individual is instructed in methods of stress management similar to those used in meditation and is asked to use these to reduce the pitch of the galvanometer and to maintain it at the low pitch. As the stress level decreases so does perspiration. This increases the electrical resistance of the skin, which is indicated by a lowering of the tone emitted by the galvanometer. This gives feedback to the user, who by this process learns to relax.

An adaptation of this technique can be used without the galvanometer. In this case the individual is asked to focus on respiration and the pulse and to attempt to reduce these in the same way as they would reduce the tone when using the galvanometer.

▌ Assertiveness training

Many individuals take on additional work or fail to stand up for themselves. This increases the individual's level of stress. By developing assertiveness skills individuals are better prepared to take more control of their life. In turn this allows better management of commitments and subsequently their stress.

▌ Exercise

Exercise can be used as part of a stress management programme. It provides an outlet for suppressed aggression. It also provides a diversion from stressful thoughts.

▌ Diet

Attention should be given to ensuring a well-balanced diet. A poor diet can worsen an individual's ability to cope with stress. Stress can result in changes to eating habits such as in over- or undereating. It can also lead to a reduction in the quality of food. In regression individuals may also use comfort foods such as those containing high sugar and fats. People may also increase their consumption of alcohol during stressful life periods.

▌ Cognitive behavioural therapy

This was developed by Beck (1979) and aims to stop negative destructive thoughts and replace them with positive constructive thoughts. Its original purpose was in the treatment of depression. Like people with depression, however, individuals who feel overwhelmed through excessive stress also experience a low self-esteem and often have negative thought processes. Cognitive therapy can therefore be successful for these individuals (Atkinson *et al.*, 1993; Sims and Owens, 1993)

▶ Desensitization

This is a behavioural method that helps individuals to overcome phobias. The phenomenological theory of stress, as we saw earlier, stated that individuals reacted to objects or situations according to their interpretation of the threat they imposed. It follows that to evaluate the object of stress as threatening the individual must have previously learned that it is threatening. Desensitization aims for individuals to unlearn that the object is threatening by learning that it poses no real threat. There are two variants:

▶ flooding;
▶ graded exposure.

Flooding exposes the individual to the object of stress with no means of escape. For example an individual who is phobic about spiders may be locked in a room with a spider. Initially this causes extreme anxiety and the individual may experience panic. This occurs only for a short period, however, as to sustain this reaction would become both physically and mentally exhausting. The normal coping mechanism of the individual when exposed to the object of stress would be avoidance and a hasty retreat. In flooding avoidance is prevented and when the object fails to harm, the phobic individual learns to re-examine his or her interpretation of the threat that the object poses. This reduces the phobic individual's level of stress and the phobic individual learns that the object no longer represents a threat to him or her.

In contrast to flooding, graded exposure works up slowly to confronting the object of stress by breaking the problem into smaller goals that must be systematically achieved. This process is shown in Figure 4.1.9.

DECISION MAKING

How might behavioural methods be applied in different areas of nursing? For example:

- *To help a 35-year-old woman develop a positive attitude towards newly diagnosed diabetes mellitus.*
- *To enable a child to overcome a fear of admission to hospital for minor surgery.*
- *To help a 25-year-old man with a moderate learning disability to develop the social skills to enable him to attend a local football match.*

Joan, a 63-year-old lady, was returning home from shopping one evening when she was attacked and robbed. Once she recovered from her immediate physical injuries she found it difficult to leave her house and eventually she refused to even go outside. Her general practitioner referred her to the Community Psychiatric Nurse (CPN) who commenced a programme of graded exposure.

Using biofeedback the CPN taught Joan how she could control her body and relax. Once Joan had learned these techniques the CPN then moved on to the graded exposure programme. Joan's ultimate goal was to return to her normal pattern of everyday life; however, at the start of the programme she could not imagine herself ever leaving the house again.

The CPN broke down the large goal into several smaller goals, which when worked through systematically would allow Joan to achieve the long-term goal as follows:

- *think about leaving the house;*
- *open the front door and look outside;*
- *step outside into the front porch;*
- *step into the front garden;*
- *walk to the end of the front garden path;*
- *walk into the street;*
- *walk to the end of the street;*
- *walk to the end of the street and catch the bus to the next stop;*
- *catch the bus into town and return home;*
- *catch the bus into town, go shopping and return home.*

First Joan was asked to think about leaving the house. Even thinking about this distressed Joan, but using the biofeedback method of relaxation control, Joan was able to control her anxiety. Joan practised this task between the CPN's visits and when she was able to think about leaving her house without feeling anxious the CPN moved on to the next stage of the plan, which was for Joan to open her front door and look outside. Again biofeedback techniques were used to control the anxiety Joan experienced and the stage was repeated until Joan again felt no anxiety.

The plan proceeded through each stage, with Joan practising anxiety control until no anxiety was experienced. At the end of the programme Joan's ultimate goal to return to her normal pattern of life was achieved and Joan felt freely able to leave her house once again without experiencing disabling anxiety.

Figure 4.1.9: An example of graded exposure.

PROFESSIONAL KNOWLEDGE

In this part the main emphasis is on the link between employment, stress and the effects on the profession of nursing. In particular the effects of employment changes in the NHS resulting mainly from the implementation of the Inquiry into NHS Management (Griffiths, 1983) and the *NHS and Community Care Act* 1990 (Department of Health, 1990) are explored.

▶ STRESS AND EMPLOYMENT

Consider the environment in which stress occurs. It is easy for employers to state that stress management is the responsibility of the individual as it is the individual who suffers the stress. It must be remembered that stress arises from the individual's reaction to the environment. Therefore, although the individual has some responsibility in managing stress, managing stress also requires some adaptation by the environment.

Employers claiming that individuals are responsible for their own stress are victim blaming. In times of high unemployment, when there is a ready supply of labour, employers may be unconcerned whether a workplace is stress inducing or not and may fail to provide appropriate support services. If employees become unable to work through stress then there are plenty more willing to take their place. Those in employment are also likely to tolerate stressful conditions for fear of losing their job as, in an environment of high unemployment, it is difficult to obtain alternative work. This is exploited by unscrupulous employers who increase workload and diminish resources, thereby maximizing their financial gains at the expense of the quality of their employees' lives.

The abolition of wage councils and removal of employment protection during the 1980s in the UK only served to increase employment related stress. Earnshaw and Cooper (1994) assert that because of the lack of employee protection, individuals are obliged to work overtime both in order to earn a decent living wage and because they feel obliged to do so under the threat of losing their jobs should they refuse. They cite the particular 'macho' culture that pervades workplaces where individuals feel compelled to take on additional tasks and work over their agreed hours to demonstrate their commitment to the organization.

In the UK, the change in workplace security for nurses coincided with the introduction of the radical changes to the National Health Service that took place during the 1980s and 1990s. Nurses are often given fixed or short-term contracts, ensuring that they remain compliant for their employers benefit. Those that complain about standards and workloads are disciplined or dismissed. Fatchett (1994) gives as examples the cases of Graham Pink who was dismissed for complaining of staff shortages in Stepping Hill Hospital, Stockport; Helen Zeitlin who was 'made redundant' after voicing her concern over nursing staff shortages at St Alexandra's Hospital, Redditch; and 20 Project 2000 students who were threatened with disciplinary action after complaining of poor standards of care in clinical placements at St Bartholomew's College of Nursing.

Some employers provide counselling services for employees. In many cases, however, the use of these services is limited to those who are desperate because of the stigma attached to them (Maslach, 1982). Maslach also noted that even when they provided support services, employers seemed to deliberately design work environments to discourage their use. Similar to Earnshaw and Cooper's (1994) observations, Maslach observed

---

DECISION MAKING

Nurses often have access to support systems to help them cope with stress. Find out the following:

- *Are stress support systems provided by your local Trusts?*
- *Are stress support systems provided by your school?*
- *Are stress support systems available through the professional organizations or unions?*
- *Are there any other stress support systems available to nurses working in your area?*

Once you have collected the information answer the following questions.

- *How well advertised was each support system?*
- *How accessible do you think each support system is?*
- *Which support systems would you feel confident using and why?*
- *Which support systems would you not feel confident using and why?*

One of the effects of short-term contracts in nursing is to encourage competition between nurses. This also happens in reorganizations where nurses may find themselves having to reapply for their jobs.

- **How likely is it that nurses will tolerate stressful working conditions in these circumstances?**
- **How likely are they to seek the help of supportive services and why?**
- **What effect do you think this will have on the care they give?**

RESEARCH BASED EVIDENCE

Matrunola (1996) identified that nurses' job satisfaction was related to the level of control they felt they had. In her study senior staff (ward managers) experienced more job satisfaction than the junior staff, indicating that a significant variable in job satisfaction is the role the individual has within the organization and the level of autonomy that accompanies it.

She went on to identify a relationship between burnout and job satisfaction where the less job satisfaction people experienced then the more burnout they experienced.

employers introducing competitiveness into the workplace. This discouraged the uptake of stress management services as those seeking support, even from peers, in this extremely competitive environment, were labelled lazy, incompetent or weak.

The competitive workplace strategy also affects the way in which line managers perform. Due to the competitive pressure, managers may be hesitant to refuse extra work on already hard pressed resources. In this situation the nursing staff subordinate to the manager find themselves pressurized and unable to control the situation. In the short term, productivity may appear to increase as the staff draw on their reserve strengths to cope. Neglecting individual employees and promoting a stressful work environment leads to an increase in burnout among nursing staff, however, (Duquette *et al.*, 1995). In the long-term this strategy consequently becomes counterproductive, as burned out staff result in decreased productivity.

A competitive work environment is stressful. We observed earlier that when under stress individuals begin to think negatively. In this situation it is easy for individual employees to become lost in the organization and for managers to concentrate only on the underachievement of the organization rather than to praise the good points. In her investigation of job satisfaction among nurse teachers, Harri (1996) found that although the main stressor was excessive workload, the negative effects were augmented by a lack of positive feedback from managers. The relationship between job satisfaction and employee behaviour was further explored by Matrunola (1996) who investigated whether nurses' poor job satisfaction led them to greater absenteeism. Although this was not upheld she found a relationship between job satisfaction and burnout. As burnout decreases the productivity of staff, it is important, she argued, that strategies should be developed to address this. Specifically she identified that managers should invest in the proactive use of stress awareness, seminars, counselling and support groups for staff.

The argument that employer attention to employee stress might be of mutual benefit was developed by Northcott (1996). He maintained that employers hold two contracts with employees. The first is the formal written contract detailing the terms and conditions of employment. The second is a hidden psychological contract. He argues that employers should focus on their responsibilities to employees in the hidden contract and he criticizes the 'macho management' culture that has developed following the implementation of the National Health Service reforms and setting up of hospital trusts in the UK. As a result of this policy he asserts that individuals' needs are often ignored, leading to poor morale. Although giving the managers power in the short term, it is eroded by low morale, difficult recruitment and consequently, poor staff performance. Addressing individuals' needs will accordingly provide mutual long-term benefit.

One of the reasons that the stressful workplace has evolved is that stress and stress induced disease are not yet classified as industrial diseases. Traditionally industrial injuries have gained compensation only where the employer's negligence has resulted in an employee's physical injury. Earnshaw and Cooper (1994) noted that where injuries are not directly measurable, such as in repetitive strain injury, the success of employees to seek redress from employers has been limited. Therefore individuals who find themselves unable to work through stress induced illness, even though it may have been invoked by their employer, find it difficult to obtain compensation.

Recently the way stress induced diseases are viewed by the legal establishment has altered. An increasing number of claims against employers have been successful in securing compensation for stress induced disease (*British Medical Journal*, 1994; Earnshaw and Cooper, 1994). Should this trend continue, and there is no evidence to suggest otherwise, then there are potentially enormous costs for employers and their insurers should they continue to ignore employee stress in the workplace. It is this financial penalty, rather that employee welfare that may influence the way in which employers treat stressful workplaces in the future.

This chapter has covered many theories on the causes of stress and how this affects individuals. To consolidate the knowledge gained from this chapter you should become more aware of your own response to stress and develop your individual stress management programme. If you have not already done so, work through the reflective exercises in this chapter and use the section on planning (p. 498) to develop your individual stress management package. Experiencing your own stress awareness and developing your own stress management programme will teach you many of the skills you will need to help others during your professional practice.

Four case studies now follow. Use the knowledge you have gained from this chapter to answer the questions at the end of each.

REFLECTIVE KNOWLEDGE

▶ CASE STUDY: LEARNING DISABILITIES

Robin is 32 years of age and has a moderate learning disability, which causes him difficulty in communicating. He lives with his elderly parents and attends a day centre each weekday. Over the past week, Robin's key worker has noticed that his behaviour has been deteriorating and he is starting to become aggressive towards other clients. The key worker can think of no obvious explanation for the change in behaviour and wonders whether the behaviour may be connected to changes in Robin's home.

The key worker discusses this change of behaviour with Robin's father when he arrives to collect him at the end of the day. He confirms that he has noticed the change in Robin's behaviour at home. During the interview Robin's father revealed that his wife had suffered a minor stroke the previous week and had been admitted to hospital. It was at this time that Robin's behaviour had changed.

■ **Why do you think Robin's behaviour changed following his mother's illness?**

■ **How could the key worker and Robin's father help to minimize any recurrence of the behaviour?**

▶ CASE STUDY: CHILD

Lucy is attending the health centre for examination of her 18-month-old baby. Lucy's partner was made redundant just before the baby's birth and has been unable to find work. This had caused the family severe financial problems. Lucy's partner had been unable to secure further employment and had begun to drink heavily. In consequence they had several major arguments and their relationship deteriorated to such an extent that three months ago Lucy's partner walked out.

Lucy complains to the nurse that the baby does not seem to feed properly and that he keeps waking up at night. This means that Lucy is not getting enough sleep at night and she feels that because of this she tends to become short tempered and ends up shouting at the baby. She feels unable to cope and finds looking after the baby, shopping, cooking and keeping the house tidy impossible to do on her own,

Weighing the baby at 12 months had shown that the baby's target of treble birth weight had not been achieved. Regular weighing since then had revealed a downward trend on the percentile scale. The baby is diagnosed as failing to thrive.

■ **Why do you think that the baby is failing to thrive?**

■ **How would you assess Lucy's level of stress?**

■ **What strategies would you use to help Lucy and her baby?**

▶ CASE STUDY: ADULT

Julian is 28 years of age and an ambitious sales executive with a double glazing company. He is admitted to your ward with a peptic ulcer. He has had the condition for some time, but has managed it, initially by using an unprescribed antacid medication and, latterly, Cimetidine. Julian enjoys his work and thrives on the pressure. He sets himself big targets and often works over 14 hours each day, using the weekends to catch up on his paperwork. Because of the hours he works he tends to live on take away food and often he will skip meals because he is so busy. He feels that he is fit though and he values the sales team's weekly squash evenings where he enjoys the competitiveness and, as he invariably wins, he concludes that this 'demonstrates [his] fitness in more than one way'. He has noticed that the indigestion becomes worse when he is under pressure, but up until now has suppressed the symptoms with the medication. He is worried that his stay in hospital will be seen as a weakness by his employers. He has beaten the sales of all the other members of the team for two years now and he is concerned that he will lose out on the promotion he hopes to achieve.

■ **How might Julian's lifestyle affect his mental and physical wellbeing?**

■ **What personality type would describe Julian?**

■ **What consequences could occur if Julian continues this lifestyle?**

■ **In what ways could Julian achieve his objectives yet lead a healthier lifestyle?**

▶ CASE STUDY: MENTAL HEALTH

Jo has been referred to the community mental health team for help with interview anxiety. She is 32 years of age and wishes to resume her career as a shop manageress. Jo has had a break *from work to have a family, but now that her children have started at school she wishes to resume her career. Jo states that she loses all confidence in herself and goes to pieces in the interviews to such an extent that she is on the verge of panic. She feels that she has little opportunity of securing an appointment as there are so many younger people around who do not have young families and are better qualified than her.*

- **What mental defence mechanism is Jo using?**

- **What behavioural techniques could the nurse use to help Jo in future interviews?**

- **How may the nurse increase Jo's self esteem?**

▶ ANNOTATED FURTHER READING

BUTTERWORTH, T., FAUGIER, J. (eds) (1992) *Clinical Supervision and Mentorship in Nursing*. London. Chapman and Hall.
This book is divided into three sections. The first section 'Theoretical Perspectives' examines the rationales underpinning the use of supervision in nursing and concludes with an examination of stress in health care workers and the role of support via clinical supervision. Part two 'Professional and Practice Perspectives' explores issues that may arise during clinical supervision in various areas of nursing. The final part 'Developmental Perspectives' suggests how clinical supervision may develop professional roles.

BURNARD, P. (1991) *Coping with Stress in the Health Professions: A Practical Guide*. London. Chapman and Hall.
A well written book that outlines the nature of stress and then concentrates on stress management. Many excellent exercises are included to raise self awareness and initiate behavioural management programmes. The book also contains mini case histories to illustrate the issues in the context of health care. This book concentrates on the practical rather than theoretical approach however, an extensive bibliography guides the reader towards further research should the reader require.

BACK, K., BACK, K., WITH BATES, T. (1991) *Assertiveness at Work: A Practical Guide to Handling Awkward Situations* (2nd edition). London. McGraw Hill.
This book contains many exercises to develop assertiveness skills using a cognitive behavioural approach to increase self-awareness and challenge self-defeating thoughts. This is useful; however, the limitation of the book is that you can only develop assertiveness skills by thought rehearsal. If you extend the exercises by bouncing them off a friend or in a supervised group session so much the better.

PAYNE, R.A. (1995) *Relaxation Techniques: A Practical Handbook for the Health Care Professional*. Edinburgh. Churchill Livingstone.
An overview of differing relaxation techniques. The intention of the book is to expose the reader to various methods of relaxation. This will allow the reader to appraise the appropriateness of methods in differing contexts. There is sufficient information to allow the reader to develop some of the techniques; however, further reading and instruction will be necessary for other methods the author includes. This is a good resource for relaxation exercises and with the information from this chapter you should be able to understand the rationale behind them.

▶ REFERENCES

AGGLETON, P. (1990) *Health*. London. Routledge.

ATKINSON, R.L., ATKINSON, R.G., SMITH, E.E., BEM, D.J. (1993) *Introduction to Psychology* (11th edition). Philadelphia, Harcourt Brace.

BECK, A.T. (1979) *Cognitive Theory of Depression*. New York. Guilford Press.

BRITISH MEDICAL JOURNAL (1994) Stress case paves way for damages claims (News). *British Medical Journal* **309**: 1391.

BURNARD, P. (1991) *Coping with Stress in the Health Professions*. London. Chapman and Hall.

CARSON, J., LEARY, J., DE VILLIERS, N., FAGIN, L., RADMALL, J. (1995) Stress in mental health nurses: comparison of ward and community staff. *British Journal of Nursing* **4(10)**: 579–582.

CHARRON, H.S. (1994) Anxiety disorders. In VARCAROLIS, E.M. (1994) *Foundations of Psychiatric Mental Health Nursing* (2nd edition). Philadelphia. W.B. Saunders.

COHSE (CONFEDERATION OF HEALTH SERVICE EMPLOYEES) (1992) *Tackling Stress from Health Care Work*. Banstead. COHSE.

COX, T. (1978) *Stress*. London. Macmillan.

DOSCHER, M.S. (1989) Psychophysiologic disorders. In SCHOEN JOHNSON, B. *Psychiatric–Mental Health Nursing* (2nd edition). Philadelphia. Lippincott.

DUNN, L.A., ROUT, U., CARSON, J., RITTER, S.A. (1994) Occupational stress amongst care staff working in nursing homes: an empirical investigation. *Journal of Clinical Nursing* **3**: 177–183.

DUQUETTE, A., KÉROUAC, S., BALBIR, K., SANDHU, R.N., DUCHARME, F., SAULNIER, P. (1995) Psychological determinants of burnout in geriatric nursing. *International Journal of Nursing Studies* **32(5)**: 443–456.

EARNSHAW, J., COOPER, C.L. (1994) Employee stress litigation: the UK experience. *Work and Stress* **8(4)**: 287–295.

EWELS, L., SIMNETT, I. (1992) *Promoting Health: A Practical Guide to Health Education*. London. Scutari Press.

FATCHETT, A. (1994) *Politics, Policy and Nursing*. London. Baillière Tindall.

FAWZY, F.I., FAWZY, N.W., HYUN, C.S., ELASHOFF, R., GUTHRIE, D., FAHEY, J.L., MORTON, D.L. (1993) Malignant melanoma. Effects of an early structured psychiatric intervention, coping, and affective state on recurrence and survival 6 years later. *Archives of General Psychiatry* **50(9)**: 681–689.

FREUD, A. (1934) *The Ego and the Mechanisms of Defence*. London. Chatto and Windus.

FRIEDMAN, M., ROSENMAN, R.H. (1974) *Type A Behaviour and Your Heart*. New York. Knopf.

GREENE, J.A. (1989) Anxiety and anxiety disorders. In SCHOEN JOHNSON, B. *Adaptation and Growth Psychiatric Mental Health Nursing* (2nd edition). Philadelphia. Lippincott.

GRIFFITHS, R. (1983) *NHS Management Inquiry*. London. Department of Health and Social Security.

HARRI, M. (1996) 'I love my work but…': the 'best' and the 'worst' in nurse educators' working lives in Finland. *Journal of Advance Nursing* **23**: 1098–1109.

HAYWARD, J. (1975) *Information: A Prescription Against Pain*. London. Royal College of Nursing.

HEBB, D.O. (1954) Drives and the conceptual nervous system. In BINDRA, D., STEWART, J. (eds) (1971) *Motivation*. Harmondsworth. Penguin.

HOLMES, T.H., RAHE, R.H. (1967) The Social Readjustment Rating Scale. *Journal of Psychosomatic Research* **11**: 213–218.

JACOBSON, A. (1980) Melancholy in the twentieth century: Causes and prevention. *Journal of Psychosocial Nursing and Mental Health Services* **18**: 18–21.

KUBLER–ROSS, E. (1969) *On Death and Dying*. London. Tavistock.

LAZARUS, R.S. (1966) *Psychological Stress and the Coping Process*. New York. McGraw Hill.

LAZARUS, R.S., DELONGIS, A., FOLKMAN, S., GRUEN, R. (1985) Stress and adaptational outcomes: the problem of confounded measures. *American Psychologist* **40**: 770–779.

LEGAULT, S.E., FREEMAN, M.R., LANGER, A., ARMSTRONG, P.W. (1995) Pathophysiology and time course of silent myocardial ischaemia during mental stress: clinical, anatomical, and physiological correlates. *British Heart Journal* **73(3)**: 242–249.

MASLACH, C. (1982) *Burnout: The Cost of Caring*. Englewood Cliffs. Prentice Hall.

MATRUNOLA, P. (1996) Is there a relationship between job satisfaction and absenteeism? *Journal of Advanced Nursing* **23**: 827–834.

NHS AND COMMUNITY CARE ACT (1990) London. Her Majesty's Stationery Office.

NAIDOO, J., WILLS, J. (1994) *Health Promotion Foundations for Practice*. London. Baillière Tindall.

NORTHCOTT, N. (1996) Contracts for good morale. *Nursing Management* **3(3)**: 23.

PATEL, C., MARMOT, M.G., TERRY, D.J., CARRUTHERS, M., HUNT, B., PATEL, P. (1985) Trial of relaxation in reducing coronary risk: four year follow up. *British Medical Journal* **290**: 1103–1106.

REICH, W.P., PARRELLA, D.P., FILSTEAD, W.J. (1988) Unconfounding the hassle's scale: external sources verses internal responses to stress. *Journal of Behavioral Medicine* **11**: 239–250.

RIDING, R.J., WHEELER, H. (1995) Occupational stress and cognitive style in nurses: 2. *British Journal of Nursing* **4(3)**: 160–168.

SEYLE, H. (1984) *The Stress Of Life*. New York. McGraw Hill.

SIMS, A., OWENS, D. (1993) *Psychiatry* (6th edition). London. Baillière Tindall.

SULLIVAN, P.J. (1993) Occupational stress in psychiatric nursing. *Journal of Advanced Nursing* **18**: 591–601.

SUTHERLAND, V.J., COOPER, C.L. (1990) *Understanding Stress. A Psychological Perspective for Health Professionals*. London. Chapman Hall.

THIBODEAU, G.A. (1987) *Anatomy and Physiology*. St Louis. Mosby.

TOTMAN, R. (1990) *Mind, Stress and Health*. London. Souvenir Press (Education and Academic).

WELCH, I.D., MEDEIROS, D.C., TATE, G.A. (1982) *Beyond Burnout: How to Enjoy Your Job Again When You've Just About Had Enough*. Englewood Cliffs, Prentice Hall.

WORLD HEALTH ORGANIZATION (1992) *The ICD-10 Classification of Mental and Behavioural Disorders*. Geneva. World Health Organization.

M. Gungaphul

▌ INTRODUCTION

Confusion is a negative characteristic of mental health. It is marked by poor attention and thinking, which lead to difficulties in comprehension, loss of short term memory and often, irritability alternating with drowsiness. It is also a word which, when used in everyday language, can mean different things to different people. For nurses especially, among other healthcare staff, the clinical meaning of confusion must be specific to prevent inappropriate care and support.

▌ OVERVIEW

This chapter explores how clients who are confused can be helped.

▌ *Subject Knowledge*

In Subject Knowledge the physiological factors that may lead to clients becoming confused are identified. This is followed by an exploration of the psychological and environmental factors that also may lead to or worsen confusion.

▌ *Practice Knowledge*

Practice Knowledge addresses the nursing assessment of confused clients and how nursing care may be planned. The specific therapies of reality orientation, reminiscence therapy and validation therapy are outlined and appraised.

▶ *Professional Knowledge*

In Professional Knowledge the common attitudes held towards people who are confused are considered. With the contemporary move to the delivery of more care in the community, the advantages and disadvantages of caring for confused clients in the community and the support of carers in the community are discussed. The focus is mainly on the elderly confused as it is this group who are likely to suffer long-term irreversible confusion.

▶ *Reflective Knowledge*

Finally, Reflective Knowledge summarizes the main points of the chapter to help consolidate your knowledge of confusion.

On pp. 527–529 there are four case studies, each one relating to one of the branch programmes. You may find it helpful to read one of them before you start the chapter and use it as a focus for your reflections while reading.

SUBJECT KNOWLEDGE

As a term used by nurses, confusion can be difficult to identify with. It is not easily distinguished from other terminology such as disorientation or delirium, with which it is sometimes used synonymously, and it is generally associated with negative mental health status.

Confusion is observed as behaviour. It results from adverse physiological, psychological or environmental factors, which in turn interfere with the functioning of the nervous system. Therefore confusion on its own is not a condition, but is a symptom of underlying pathology. Some of the factors that may lead to confusion are listed in Table 4.2.1. Although the physical, psychological and environmental precursors can cause confusion in individuals of all ages, confusion is, however, far more likely to be observed among elderly people. Some authors even contend that because of its prevalence, confusion is a feature in most aspects of medical care of the elderly (Brocklehurst and Hanley, 1976).

▶ CAUSES OF CONFUSION

There are two types of confusion – short term and long term. Short term or acute confusion is usually reversible and has a sudden onset. In the

Physical	Psychological	Environmental
Constipation	Anxiety states	Translocation
Diabetes mellitus	Depression	Stressful environment
Drugs or alcohol	Fear	Isolation or loneliness
Fatigue		External or internal stimuli
Hormonal disturbance		
Hypothermia		
Infection		
Neoplasm		
Vascular disorders		
Vitamin deficiencies		
Urinary retention		

Table 4.2.1 Factors that can lead to confusion.

older age group, almost any severe physical illness can cause an acute state of confusion (Liston, 1982; Lipowski, 1983). The younger age group can also develop acute confusion and factors that may lead to it include epilepsy (especially following a seizure), hyperpyrexia, post electroconvulsive therapy and poisoning. Generally, a confused episode that occurs during an acute physical condition is called delirium. Delirium is always secondary to an underlying medical condition, has a sudden onset, is usually reversible and involves no destruction of brain cells.

In contrast, long term or chronic confusion occurs following degenerative changes in the brain. This is called dementia. Dementia is slow in onset, is usually irreversible and involves substantial destruction of brain cells.

Biological ▶ PHYSIOLOGICAL CAUSES OF CONFUSION

The six major physiological factors that can lead to the development of confusion are:

▶ infections;
▶ endocrine disturbances;
▶ electrolyte imbalance;
▶ poisons;
▶ trauma;
▶ dementia.

▶ *Infections*

Infections causing fever can lead to confusion. Infections arise due to pathogens invading the body systems, commonly via the urinary or respiratory tracts. Additionally, a chest infection can lead to poor oxygenation of the blood. In turn this prevents adequate oxygenated blood reaching the brain, which also leads to confusion.

Pathogens can also be transported from the primary site of infection via the circulatory system to infect the nervous system. Angus (1989) noted over 50% of cases of meningitis in older people were due to bacteria that usually infect the lungs.

▶ *Endocrine Disorders*

Disorders of the endocrine system interfere with the operation of the nervous system and can subsequently cause confusion. In particular, malfunction of the thyroid gland can lead to the medical conditions of hyperthyroidism and hypothyroidism. Both these conditions affect the central nervous system and can cause behavioural disturbances, including confusion (Swanson *et al.*, 1981).

In diabetes mellitus, hypoglycaemia can also lead to confusion. When diabetes mellitus has not been stabilized or when food has not been taken after the administration of insulin, hypoglycaemia and the associated state of confusion can develop.

▶ *Electrolyte Imbalance*

Sodium is an important element of body tissues. In cases of chronic renal failure, congestive heart disease, cirrhosis of the liver, inappropriate intake of water or secretion of antidiuretic hormone, the resulting sodium

DECISION MAKING

On your next clinical placement find out the following:

- *What blood test is undertaken to determine whether an individual has an electrolyte imbalance?*
- *Why would individuals be prescribed diuretic medication over a prolonged period?*
- *How does the diuretic work?*
- *In people who are prescribed long-term diuretic medication such as frusemide how is the electrolyte balance maintained?*
- *Why is this information important to the nurse working in the community with elderly people who are confused?*

(You will need to be familiar with the physiology of the kidney before attempting this exercise. You may find your pharmacist and the *British National Formulary* (British Medical Association and the Royal Pharmaceutical Society of Great Britain, 1997) useful points of reference.)

deficiency leads to the electrolyte abnormality of hyponatraemia. This imbalance causes tiredness and confusion (Sheridan *et al.*, 1985).

Elderly people are often prescribed diuretics. These can also lead to an electrolyte disturbance, which may manifest as confusion. Furthermore, the habitual use of laxatives, a common practice by the elderly (Conn, 1992), can lead to problems of hydration and electrolyte imbalance and eventual confusion.

Electrolyte disturbance can also result from inadequate intake of food and drink, especially during febrile states. In addition to electrolyte disturbances this can also result in the body lacking essential vitamins such as vitamin B_{12}. The deficiency of this vitamin leads to changes in mental health observed by characteristics such as forgetfulness, depression, irritability and confusion (see Chapter 3.2 on nutrition). Butler and Lewis (1977) found that many older people were undernourished and had developed reversible brain syndromes associated with malnutrition and other metabolic disorders. In an institutional environment such as a hospital, nursing home or other such place managed by professional staff, this should not be difficult to remedy with appropriate changes to diet and dietary supplements. Increasingly, institutional care is becoming unavailable for the elderly, who following the implementation of the *NHS and Community Care Act* (1990) are being supported to live in their own homes (Knapp and Lawson, 1995). The elderly as a group are most likely to suffer poverty (Barr and Coulter, 1990) and be unable to obtain an adequate nutritious diet. Consequently difficulties occur when individuals remain in their home, as is increasingly common, and are unable to change their dietary regimen.

Poisons

Poisons include alcohol and drugs.

Alcohol

Intoxication with alcohol can lead to short-term confusion and sometimes memory lapses. Edwards (1982) found that alcohol-related brain damage of varying degree is common, leading to physical, psychological and social problems. In the long term, prolonged excessive consumption of alcohol can cause vitamin B_1 deficiency. In turn this leads to Korsakoff's syndrome and irreversible confusion is one of the characteristic features of this condition.

Drugs

Drug-related confusion may result from:

- an overdose;
- the drug's cumulative effect;
- an interaction between different drugs;
- the individual's reaction to the drug.

In particular, confusion can be induced by the use of certain neuroleptic drugs and compound analgesics. Additionally, some stimulants and sedatives can lead to disorientation and confusion if they are stopped suddenly. In people who have abused drugs or alcohol, for example, sudden withdrawal often produces a delirious state with associated confusion.

Elderly people over 60 years of age have two and a half times the

Wake (1995) found that contrary to popular belief the use of MDMA was not safe and noted a strong relationship between the use of the drug and a rise in MDMA-related hospital admissions and fatalities. Its adverse effects can lead to dehydration and a severe electrolyte imbalance. This alone causes confused behaviour and in a few cases has caused death.

The publicity surrounding the dehydrating effect of the drug has led users to compensate for the dehydration by drinking copious amounts of water. Again, this strategy is potentially dangerous as Day (1996) notes that some users of MDMA drink so much water that they severely disturb their electrolyte balance.

number of adverse drug reactions as people under 60 years of age (Hurwitz, 1969). This effect is compounded by the fact that the elderly are the age group most likely to make use of the health service because of longstanding illnesses (Blane, 1991) and therefore most likely to be prescribed medication.

Ghodse (1995) noted that a wide range of psychoactive drugs can impair an individual's general awareness and ability to concentrate. In particular, lysergic acid diethylamide (LSD or acid) results in altered perception and confusion. The illicit use of 3,4 methylene-dioxymeth-amphetamine (MDMA, better known as Ecstasy) has recently become a public concern. MDMA, banned in the UK since 1971 as a class A drug, has been popularized as a recreational drug among contemporary youth culture arising from the mistaken belief that it has relatively harmless properties (Henry, 1992). MDMA inhibits the uptake of serotonin leading to excessive amounts of this neurotransmitter. This in turn gives the euphoric feelings associated with taking the drug. Serotonin also has the effect of raising the body temperature, which in turn leads to dehydration, inappropriate blood clotting, convulsions and coma (Cook, 1995; Jones and Owens, 1996). In animal studies long-term exposure to MDMA damaged serotonin receptors in the neurones and reduced the natural secretion of the neurotransmitter. In humans, the deficit of serotonin is associated with depression. This is demonstrated by an observed long-term consequence of taking this drug where users have developed clinical depression (Cook, 1995; Day, 1996).

DECISION MAKING

On his eighteenth birthday, Jeremy Banjo visits a night club with a group of his peers. Later that evening he is admitted to the accident and emergency department after he collapses on the dance floor. He was reported to have taken Ecstasy tablets approximately 45 minutes earlier.

During the assessment the nurse notes that Jeremy is agitated and aggressive. Other physical characteristics of concern include hypotension, tachycardia, and pyrexia and he appears to be dehydrated.

- **What immediate nursing actions would be taken to stabilize Jeremy's physical condition?**
- **What medical interventions may**

be made to limit the damage of the drug?
- **How would the nursing and medical actions be affected by Jeremy's mental state?**
- **On your next clinical placement in accident and emergency or a medical ward find out how the National Poisons Centres may be used and how to contact them (you could also look in the British National Formulary).**
- **Following Jeremy's recovery, what would you include in a health promotion programme to help him avoid a recurrence of this problem?**

Trauma

Physical damage to the brain can result in confusion. The nature of the confusion will be governed by the part of the brain affected and the nature of the injury. If the injury is minor and reversible then the probability that the confusion will lessen is high. For example, the confusion that often accompanies concussion reduces as the concussion resolves. On the other hand, if the confusion arises from trauma that has caused permanent damage to the brain recovery from the confusion is less likely.

Dementia

Irreversible destruction of brain cells is the major feature of dementia. The most common type of dementia is Alzheimer's disease, which accounts for approximately 55% of all dementias. Multi-infarct dementia is also common and results from many 'mini strokes' over a period of time: the brain cells supplied by the damaged blood vessels are deprived of nutrients and oxygen and they subsequently die, leading to the onset of dementia and confusion.

In contrast to acute confusion, in dementia where there has been a severe irreversible destruction of brain cells, a permanent reduction in the level of confusion is unlikely.

Psychosocial ▶ **ENVIRONMENTAL INFLUENCES ON CONFUSION**

A variety of environmental factors can worsen the degree of confusion. They include:

▶ increased noise levels;
▶ lack of personal space;
▶ poor lighting;
▶ distortion of light and darkness;
▶ a lack of familiar faces.

DECISION MAKING

Joseph Black, aged 80 years, is a physically frail but mentally active man. He lives with his daughter and her family in the family home. His daughter is going on holiday, and as Mr Black requires constant care, he is admitted to a private nursing home for respite care.

Within one day of admission Mr Black becomes confused and refuses all help. He wants to 'get out of here' and warns the staff 'they will be in trouble if they insist on keeping me here'. However, he settles in gradually and is his usual self before his return to his family. On his return home his confusion relapses and continues for a short while, after which he becomes more familiar with his relatives and surroundings and the confusion once again disappears.

- *How would you explain to Mr Black's daughter why the changes in surroundings caused her father to be confused?*
- *Before Mr Black's admission, what nursing actions could have been taken to minimize the negative effects on his admission for respite care?*
- *Following his admission, what nursing actions could have been taken to minimize the negative effects?*
- *What do you think are the advantages and disadvantages of respite care?*

The environment is particularly important in the care of individuals suffering from chronic confusion, such as those with Alzheimer's disease, who are able to function in their usual environment, but will deteriorate rapidly if moved to a new unfamiliar environment. This is because the nature of the disease makes short-term memory ineffective. Long-term memory is preserved, however, Therefore the client is able to function when using information in long-term memory (e.g. about the familiar environment), but is unable to use short-term memory when required (e.g. for the new environment) and consequently becomes confused.

Attention to the immediate environment forms the basis of reality orientation therapy – a strategy that can be used to help clients who are confused.

▶ **PSYCHOLOGICAL CAUSES OF CONFUSION**

Confusion arising from psychological sources may be due to either an organic or a functional illness. With organic illnesses such as Alzheimer's

---

You will require a personal stereo and 2–5 colleagues to complete this exercise. It will take approximately 20 minutes to complete the task plus time for reflection on the questions at the end.

Obtain a pre-recorded cassette of someone speaking. I would advise you to obtain Alan Bennett narrating his diaries *Writing Home* (Bennett, 1994) if you can as he also gives his account of his mother's progression into Alzheimer's disease.

Put on the headphones and join your colleagues for a conversation on any topics that occur as the conversation develops. Aim for the conversation to last for around 20 minutes. Switch on the cassette player and set the volume level so that you can clearly hear the tape at a level just below ordinary conversation level. At the end of 20 minutes, switch off the personal stereo and discuss the following with your colleagues:

- *Could you participate in the conversation?*
- *Did your colleagues think you participated in the conversation?*

- *What difficulties (including difficulties with memory, nonverbal communication and verbal communication) did you encounter?*
- *What difficulties (including difficulties with memory, nonverbal communication and verbal communication) did your colleagues encounter?*
- *How might this experience help you when working with clients suffering from perceptual dysfunctions?*

disease, confusion has a slow insidious onset and during the early stage of the illness there may be lucid periods or 'flashbacks'. Confusion from organic illness is also accompanied by a deterioration of intellect, memory loss, sensory disturbances and disruption of the personality.

Confusion may also be experienced by a person with a functional illness. For example, an individual suffering a panic attack may also feel confused (Kaplan *et al.*, 1994). Functional disorders that give rise to perceptual dysfunctions such as delusions or hallucinations again can lead to confusion as the individual loses touch with reality.

▶ ASSESSMENT

PRACTICE KNOWLEDGE

It must be remembered that confusion is a symptom of an underlying pathological condition rather than a condition in its own right. The purpose of the assessment is to identify the condition causing the confusion as until this is addressed, strategies to help manage the confusion are of limited value. When assessing clients who are confused it is therefore important to consider them as a whole rather than dwelling only on the confusion. In addition to physiological assessment and recent history, a comprehensive biographical assessment should be made to record the client's 'life review'. This can facilitate the identification and interpretation of their needs or problems, lifestyle and circumstances (Butler, 1974). This life review can also be used as the basis of therapies such as reminiscence therapy to promote positive experiences in elderly people with confusion (Haight, 1992).

The individual who is confused will probably have difficulty in comprehending and communicating, so it is essential that the nurse possesses good interpersonal skills. This is facilitated by the active listening and observation outlined in Chapter 4.5, rehabilitation.

The three major areas that should form the basis of assessment are physiological, psychological and environmental.

▶ *Physiological Assessment*

This part of the assessment is to exclude underlying physiological factors that may be contributing to the confusion. This begins by recording the vital signs of temperature, pulse, respiration and blood pressure. Abnormal recordings may indicate physiological conditions that can lead to confusion. An overall visual impression of the client should also be made. In particular, observing the condition of the client's skin will indicate the level of hydration and nutritional state whereas cyanosis may indicate a poorly oxygenated blood supply to the brain.

The client's ability to communicate and comprehend should be determined. It may be that the client uses aids to communication such as spectacles or a hearing aid. If so it should be verified that these are worn correctly and are effective as sensory deficits may manifest as confused behaviour. Hearing deficits should always be investigated. Another stereotyped myth of old age is that old people become deaf. Often, when investigated, a build-up of ear wax is noted and once this is addressed the client's hearing is restored.

▶ *Psychological Assessment*

The term confusion is frequently used to describe a wide variety of other behaviours. Confusion may also be misdiagnosed for other mental health problems, especially in the elderly. Phillips (1973) noted several reports questioning the reliability of recognizing confusion.

▶ The Clifton Assessment

One particular instrument, the Clifton Assessment Procedures for the Elderly (CAPE) (Pattie and Gilleard, 1979) is commonly used in the assessment of elderly people who appear to be confused. It assesses:

- ▶ psychomotor activity;
- ▶ cognition;
- ▶ behaviour.

Psychomotor assessment is carried out using the Gibson Spiral Maze (Gibson, 1961) (Figure 4.2.1). It is used to assess the client's psychomotor ability. The client is required to trace a line from the centre of the spiral outwards, avoiding the obstruction and to complete this as quickly as possible. The time taken to complete the maze and the number of errors form the basis of the score – the lower the score the better.

For the cognitive assessment, the client answers 12 set questions relating to personal data, orientation and mental ability. These are scored out of the possible 12 items. Patients with depression are expected to score eight or more, while those with dementia are likely to score seven or less (Pattie and Gilleard, 1979).

Behavioural assessment is carried out using the Behaviour Rating Scale, which measures the level of dependence or independence based on 18 items, including bathing, dressing, mobility, eliminating and socializing. This scale, in contrast with that of the cognitive assessment, identifies dependency level with the highest scores. Therefore the less they can achieve in their activities, the higher their score. Blessed *et al.* (1991) in their study of 279 elderly people found that about 74% of the people studied rated as highly dependent and coined the term 'ceiling effect' with the Behaviour Rating Scale. In this context the term 'ceiling effect' means that the majority of the people studied achieved high scores for

Figure 4.2.1: The Gibson Spiral Maze. (From Gibson, 1961. Reproduced at about 45% of actual size, with permission from the publishers Hodder & Stoughton Educational.)

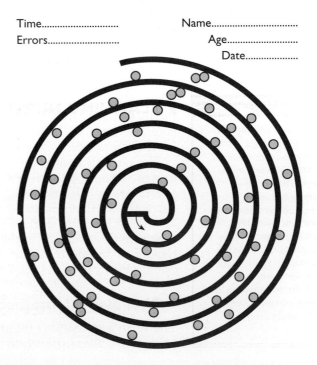

Time..........................
Errors........................

Name................................
Age..........................
Date..................

their levels of dependency. The remaining 26% with their low scores were fairly independent in comparison.

The CAPE score can be used immediately; however, it is usual to record the scores and repeat the test over a period of time to monitor the client's improvement or deterioration.

Nurses using CAPE are able to make reliable judgements about the client's confusion and mental impairment (Browne, 1984). If used appropriately this instrument facilitates the care and management of clients with confusion.

Although a helpful instrument, CAPE should be used with caution with some clients. Some people with mild confusion may be unable to carry out the activities or only partially achieve them. Others may have a different ethnic origin and a limited ability to understand the questions due to a limited knowledge of the language or cultural differences. Other clients may have sensory deficits or failings. Furthermore, considering the frail people involved, the assessment must not be rushed since inaccurate conclusions may result, as Goodwin (1991) noted.

▶ Environmental Assessment

It is important to include environmental factors in the nursing assessment. Confusion worsens in unfamiliar surroundings. For example, when clients are admitted to a new unit staffed with unfamiliar people their state of health may deteriorate with a consequent loss of sleep and increased distress. This is the 'translocation syndrome' (Smith, 1986). Therefore, when assessing clients in a new environment it must also be considered whether they can function to their fullest abilities in their usual surroundings.

▶ Risk Assessment

The nursing assessment should also consider whether the client should remain in their own environment or be admitted to an appropriate care facility. We saw earlier in the chapter that moving clients with a loss of short-term memory to a new unfamiliar environment will worsen their confusion. This must be balanced against the clients' risks to themselves and to others, their risks to and from carers, and the availability of adequate home support.

▶ PLANNING NURSING CARE

Whenever possible, the plan of care should be made with the cooperation of all involved in the care, for example informal carers, relatives and members of the multidisciplinary team. The care plan should also involve the client; however, with a severely confused client, this may sometimes be beyond the client's ability.

During the assessment the cause of confusion should be identified. In the planning stage strategies to address this should be put into place. Physiological causes of confusion should be addressed as a priority. In most instances this will lead to a rapid reduction in the level of confusion. If the confusion arises from a mental illness it is important that an accurate medical diagnosis is made as different pathways of treatment are required. In a functional mental illness such as depression with accompanying confusion, the symptoms become less severe and the confusion will improve as the underlying illness is treated. In contrast,

---

DECISION MAKING

In confusion, the operation of short-term memory is impaired. Long-term memory is often preserved.
- **Using this knowledge explain why clients may function adequately at home yet deteriorate rapidly if moved to a new unfamiliar environment.**
- **What strategies could a nurse working in a nursing home use to minimize this effect?**

RESEARCH BASED EVIDENCE

Achieving an accurate diagnosis is not straightforward. The symptoms of organic dementia and some functional conditions such as depression in the elderly are very similar. This may lead to an inaccurate diagnosis and treatment pathway. Homer et al. (1988) found that dementia was overdiagnosed in the elderly. A comprehensive and continuous assessment is therefore essential to exclude misdiagnosis and to ensure the appropriate care programme is enacted (Kozak-Campbell and Hughes, 1996).

if there is an organic cause of confusion, such as Alzheimer's disease, the pattern of care is likely to be progressively increasing care and support. An incorrect diagnosis will consequently lead to inappropriate care and perpetuate the client's confusion.

▶ *Long Term Confusion*

Treatment of an underlying cause of confusion usually leads to remission of the confusion. If the underlying cause cannot be treated, as in dementia, there are three main types of therapy the nurse can use to address the symptoms of confusion. These are:

- ▶ reality orientation;
- ▶ reminiscence therapy;
- ▶ validation therapy.

▶ Reality orientation

Confusion is accompanied by disorientation in which the concepts of time, place and person become disturbed. This causes difficulties for the individual regarding self, others, the environment and the relationship between them. Reality orientation helps the individual to refocus on the world about them (Birchenall and Streight, 1993). It uses a variety of cues, stimuli and tips to help the client remember time, place and names. Continued use of reality orientation decreases the need for the client to ask staff the time or the date or where the toilet is and decreases the chance that the client will be labelled confused or disorientated (Perko and Kreigh, 1988). It also helps to maintain a safe environment, promotes a sense of security, dignity, independence and self-esteem (Holden and Woods, 1982).

In practice, reality orientation requires the nurse to repeatedly confront the client with facts such as the day, date, names and news and wait for the client to respond correctly. For example, the nurse may say 'Hello Mr Smith. My name is Geoff. What is my name?' and repeat the greeting every time he meets the client throughout the day. Each correct response is given positive reinforcement, but it is important not to react negatively should the client give an incorrect response.

There are two modes of reality orientation:

- ▶ one occurs intensively during group sessions;
- ▶ the other is ongoing 24 hour reality orientation and relies on the use of cues, signs and colours placed at strategic points around the unit or in the client's house, for example, the client may have a colour coded bed area, the toilet may have an icon picture of a toilet on the door, and the living area may have a large clock, a calendar and weather description in a prominent area.

Criticisms of reality orientation are that it can distress both clients and carers if expectations have not been achieved, and for its repetitive nature. Distress to clients with perceptual difficulties is minimized by using remedial support such as spectacles or hearing aids, which should be given before the programme is started. Reality orientation is unlikely to help individuals suffering from severe dementia, but if the deterioration is not so advanced, it may slow the pace of deterioration and often improves the client's mental state.

▶ Reminiscence therapy

Reminiscence is an activity that everyone engages in. It is a common notion that older people live in the past and always talk about the 'good old days'. When considering Erikson's eighth stage of development 'ego integrity vs despair' (Erikson, 1980) it can be assumed that people in their later years look back over their life and accept its meaning. Older people, according to Klein *et al.* (1985), may hesitate to talk about their past, however, because they do not want to meet with rejection and may actually need help and encouragement to reminisce.

Reminiscence as a form of therapy has been promoted in elderly people with confusion (Norris and Eileh, 1982). It focuses on times when they were in full possession of their skills and abilities. Reminiscence therapy exploits the phenomenon that long-term memory remains relatively intact while short-term memory does not function. If short-term memory is not working it then becomes very difficult to engage in day to day social interactions. Reminiscence therapy therefore provides a means of using the functioning long-term memory to allow a conversation to develop. This, in turn, improves the client's self-esteem.

To enhance the process of reminiscing the nurse should formulate a comprehensive life review (Butler, 1974). Here, help from friends and relatives is invaluable. Norris (1986) uses the following criteria to select the material for the life review:

- ▶ it is relevant to the past experiences of the individual;
- ▶ it involves the stimulation of as many senses as possible;
- ▶ it is used sparingly so as not to overwhelm the client who is confused.

Care must be taken when selecting members of the reminiscence group that all members have similar life experiences. For example clients from different ethnic backgrounds may have totally different experiences of the war and this can lead to further confusion or even conflict.

People with confusion have the same feelings and needs as other people. Reminiscing can be a valuable form of therapy that brings the person with confusion into meaningful and enjoyable interaction. Reminiscing may also create feelings that are difficult to cope with, either by the client or the nurse or both and appropriate support strategies to enable these issues to be resolved must be arranged before the group begins.

▶ Validation therapy

It should be acknowledged that in some situations no effective treatment is available to prevent the progressive intellectual deterioration. Time spent promoting a reality orientation programme is then felt as frustrating with no progress in sight. Consequently, in this situation reality orientation provides little benefit and both the nurse and client become dissatisfied.

An alternative to reality orientation is provided by validation therapy (Feil, 1982). Like 24-hour reality orientation, it is an ongoing process; however, unlike reality orientation, it does not confront the behaviour, but seeks to find the underlying meanings. It involves not allowing any factual errors to interrupt the meaningful dialogue on topics of interest to the client. Therefore, when a client aged 80 years says something like 'My Father is waiting for me I must go home' the nurse does not confront the client with reality by replying 'Your father is dead and . . .'. In validation therapy, the nurse cultivates the statement to find the underlying meanings. Using this mode of therapy, interaction with the client who is confused should be on their ground, on their terms and on the subjects that they raise and choose to discuss (Morton and Bleathman, 1988). In validation therapy, communication and subject matter are matched to the stage of confusion. Clients who have a level of confusion that does not respond to reality orientation often show a significant improvement if validation therapy is used instead (Fine and Rouse-Bane, 1995).

PROFESSIONAL KNOWLEDGE

RESEARCH BASED EVIDENCE

In acute confusion, the client has some awareness of their forgetfulness and memory loss. It is therefore very important that a positive attitude is always maintained by the nurse. The statement that 'things would be different if more time was available' should be seriously considered. What would be done if only more time was available should be clearly identified. Amstrong-Esther et al. (1989) found in a study based in an acute care setting, 95% of the time elderly patients had no contact with nursing staff. In a more recent study, Amstrong-Esther et al. (1994) found that nurses had good intentions and when asked, responded that talking to patients was 'enjoyable, important and rewarding' and an 'objective' for themselves and the unit. However, in practice they did not talk to the patients.

▶ ATTITUDES TOWARDS PEOPLE WHO ARE CONFUSED

When working with clients who are confused nurses should be aware of their own feelings and behaviour. The passive acceptance of confusion and the notion that it is an inevitable characteristic of a particular condition or disorder promotes complacency in the nurse and adds to the burden of the client's low self-esteem, dependence and isolation. Nurses should look positively and objectively at the issues. They should promote a comprehensive assessment to help identify the cause(s) of the client's confusion and endeavour to promote a realistic programme of care or management.

Promoting relationships with a client with confusion is not easy, especially when exhibited behaviours are disturbing not only to the relatives, but also to the nurses themselves. In establishing a relationship, the nurse's attitudes should convey respect and the willingness to work with the client. The nurse should not give the impression that working with the client is only a job that has to be done or is part of his or her workload. The nurse's approach should be positive in outlook, promoting the potential of the client. Egan (1994) refers to concepts of attending and non-judgemental in promoting nurse–client relationship, attributes which are salient in any caring or nursing relationship, but particularly when working with a confused client.

▶ ATTITUDES TOWARDS THE ELDERLY

In the past, dependent clients have been treated very badly. Robb (1967) found the treatment of very dependent people distressing. She documented rudeness, rough handling and neglect of cleanliness. When these were brought to the attention of those with ultimate responsibility the matters were brushed aside. Even as late as 1982, Holden and Woods found that attitudes towards elderly people were discriminatory, rejecting and negative. If this was the view towards healthy elderly people, what would be the fate of those who had the added problem of confusion?

Elderly people, especially those with problems of cognition, are often discriminated against. This is reflected in the dilemma of whether or not to promote therapeutic activities. Were it a younger person with confusion, the same responses would not arise since they 'have a lot of life left'. This is ageism, a term coined by Butler (1969). Ageism is endemic in today's society and resides in everyone, including those who are old themselves (Scrutton, 1989).

A number of stereotypes exist about elderly people such as they are unproductive, they are asexual, they are senile and they are inflexible (Victor, 1987). These attitudes were reinforced by earlier studies such as that of Williamson *et al.* (1964), which represented the elderly in

---

RESEARCH BASED EVIDENCE

In contrast to the stereotyped views, the majority of elderly people are not dependent. Luker and Perkins (1987) in their study of 1400 individuals aged 65 years and over, found that more than 90% noted their health as being good. These findings are supported by the Office of Population Censuses and Surveys (1988, 1995), which revealed that the majority of older people are well and live reasonably happy lives.

Another continuing myth is that families no longer care for their dependent elderly members. Many studies have given evidence to the contrary, however, and shown that families do care. As far

back as 1966, Lowther and Williamson, in their study of 1115 elderly people discharged from hospital noted that in only 12 cases were the relatives unreasonable in providing little or no support. This was further supported by Isaacs (1971) who noted that in only one case among 200 admission referrals did the family want the client admitted so that they could enjoy their own social life rather than support their elderly dependent relative. Similar findings were made by Briggs and Oliver (1985) who also found that the majority of families with elderly dependent relatives cared for them in the community.

---

dependent roles, as people who were sick, or as people who were helpless. Stereotypes, myths and ageism are reinforced in a society that values the younger generation more than the old. With confusion more often observed in the debilitated older population, it is often the first impression of this age group. This may encourage the belief that all members of this group share this negative trait. It should be remembered, however, that elderly people are not a homogeneous group, but have differing abilities, skills and other positive attributes. Stereotyping them as all being confused is a cardinal mistake. There are endless positive characteristics among elderly people that enhance their status.

▶ ADVANTAGES AND DISADVANTAGES OF CARING FOR CONFUSED CLIENTS IN THE COMMUNITY

In the UK 94% of all elderly people live in their own homes (Skeet, 1989). According to Peace (1988), most old people prefer to live in their own homes. We have seen that because of the effects on short-term memory, moving a client from familiar surroundings to a new environment often results in a deterioration in their condition. It could therefore be argued that strategies to enable individuals to stay in the community are in the clients' best interests. Indeed, in the UK, there has been an increasing push towards community-based rather than institutional-based care. What then are the disadvantages to this policy?

The elderly are the largest users of the National Health Service and their numbers in proportion to the working population are growing (Central Statistics Office, 1994). The Conservative government elected into power in 1979 looked to the future of elderly care services. It saw community care as the way forward. This was a much cheaper option than providing institutional care. Underpinning this strategy was a re-definition of community care, first published in the report *Growing Older* (DHSS, 1981, para 1.9): 'the primary sources of support and care for elderly people are informal and voluntary. These spring from the personal ties of kinship, friendship and neighbourhood. They are irreplaceable. It is the role of public authorities to sustain, and, where necessary, develop – but never to displace – such support and care. Care in the community must increasingly mean care by the community'.

Caring by the community rather than providing care in the community was the view promoted throughout subsequent Conservative administrations to mark a return to 'family values' and taking responsibility for your own. Of course, if families care for their own dependent relatives instead of relying on the National Health Service, it would make for a cheaper (or more efficient) alternative. Therefore the government was able to reduce expenditure on services for the elderly, making for sounder, cost-effective, financial management while at the same time promoting their policy of sound family values.

The Griffiths Report (1988) further endorsed the government's position and formed the basis of the reforms to community care that were contained in the *NHS and Community Care Act* (1990). Griffiths argued that more care should be delivered in the community and that more use should be made of voluntary and commercial sectors to enhance the existing statutory services. He argued that this strategy would 'widen the individual's choice and increase flexibility and innovation'. Of course it paved the way for less investment in statutory services and made more demands upon voluntary and informal (unpaid) carers. Added emphasis was given to the strategy by the reduction of the National Health Service and local authority beds and the growth in the number of private nursing beds (Evandrou *et al.*, 1990). As private nursing beds were means tested it followed that elderly people with over £8000 of assets (assets includes the value of their house and contents) who required nursing or residential care were obliged to fund themselves, although elderly people with assets under this amount were funded by the Department of Social Security. This alone may have prevented some elderly people receiving the care they needed.

This initiative was compounded following the full implementation of the *NHS and Community Care Act* (1990) on 1st April 1993. On this date the responsibility for funding private nursing beds was transferred from the Department of Social Security to local authorities who received an increase in their central support grant to compensate. This money was not ringfenced however, and since then local authorities have chosen to invest more on domiciliary services to keep individuals who would previously have received residential or nursing home care in the community and to benefit from the associated financial savings (Knapp and Lawson, 1995).

▶ PROBLEMS EXPERIENCED BY INFORMAL CARERS

Informal carers comprise families, friends and neighbours (Hunter *et al.*, 1988). They perform an important part in the care of dependent people in the community. Before the 1980s there was patchy information available in the UK on informal carers. Green (1988), however, noted there were around six million informal carers in Great Britain providing regular service for someone who was sick or handicapped, either in their own household or elsewhere. Those caring in the same household comprised about 1.7 million, according to Richardson, Unall and Aston. (1989).

Family informal carers consequently play an important part in meeting the needs of their dependent relatives. Under the umbrella of community care, family informal carers are placed under great strain and often have to carry out their tasks without the resources, space and purpose-built environments that are available to formal carers. Unlike formal carers, they cannot remain detached from their role of caring. They are also

Imagine you have to look after your elderly dependent mother who is disorientated for time and place in your home. She is incontinent of urine and regularly gets up in the middle of the night, wanders outside, and if you do not catch her, quickly wanders off and gets lost. Recently she has also started to switch on the cooker, but forgets to light the gas.

Your mother is so dependent that you are unable to leave her for any length of time and you consequently have to give up your job. Your teenage children are too embarrassed to bring their friends home as they are ashamed of your mother's behaviour and complain that the furniture smells from where your mother has 'had accidents'.

- *What social problems are you likely to experience?*
- *What financial problems are you likely to experience?*
- *What psychological problems are you likely to experience?*
- *How will looking after your mother affect your health and wellbeing?*

unable to go home at the end of the day and have little opportunity to switch off. To make matters worse, some informal carers become ill themselves as a result of the stress of caring for their relative (Murphy, 1986). Wright (1986) identified medical and psychological health problems in carers, which included conditions such as arthritis, multiple sclerosis, stroke, alcoholism, back pain and obsessional neurosis. She also found that for some of the carers, their caring role was associated with sleep disturbance due to the dependent person waking up during the night. Braithwaite (1990) also demonstrated that increased levels of stress and emotional strain were experienced by informal carers when caring for their dependent relative, especially if the relative was suffering from dementia; according to Levin *et al.* (1989) this is the most stressful type of care. Levin and colleagues also found that carers' stress levels drop significantly when caring ceases.

In practical terms it is a matter of concern when carers experience high distress levels since they are less likely to continue caring or if they do the quality of care they give is likely to decline (Levin *et al.*, 1989). Unsupported, informal carers often battle on though. As Kirby and Kay (1987) noted, carers are the silent sufferers. Carers are, however, spared much of the overwhelming stress they experience if they are provided with adequate support. Therefore for informal carers to fulfil their roles, support is needed to reduce their stress levels.

Within the family the informal carer is likely to be the spouse or children. At first sight it would seem that advancing age suggests greater difficulty in managing as a carer. This was refuted by Fitting *et al.* (1984), however, who found that younger carers were more unhappy and resentful of their role than older carers. Mace *et al.* (1992) cited anger, helplessness, embarrassment, guilt and grief as the emotions frequently experienced by the carers. For those who give up paid employment to look after a dependent relative the reduced income may also result in financial hardship. Relationships can break down and the carer's health can begin to fail (Murphy, 1986). Unlike care professionals, informal carers cannot go home after their shift. Their responsibility for caring is for 24 hours every day.

DECISION MAKING

Elsie Graham, a 48-year-old spinster, shares a house with her 76-year-old mother. Elsie had to give up secretarial work five years ago to care for her mother who has become more and more dependent upon her. Left alone Elsie's mother cannot look after herself. She is at personal risk and has had many narrow escapes. Occasionally she has fallen and been unable to lift herself back to her feet. On other occasions she has left the gas cooker on or has turned on the gas and forgotten to light it. She wanders aimlessly during the day and often gets up in the middle of the night believing it is daytime.

Elsie feels obliged to look after her mother yet confides in the nurse that she is becoming a handful. Elsie is also worried that as the house in which she lives belongs to her mother, she will be evicted if her mother is admitted to a nursing home to pay the nursing home fees.

- *Are Elsie's fears of eviction valid?*
- *What support services are available to help Elsie care for her mother?*
- *How would you contact these services in your area?*

◗ SUPPORTING CARERS

Following the reforms in the *NHS and Community Care Act* (1990) and the greater reliance it placed on the contribution of informal carers, it is important that nurses include the carers as well as the client in the nursing assessment. Care and support to carers should be identified in response to the carers changing and complex needs.

With adequate support, informal carers can maintain a reasonable level of social activities, which may take the form of leisure, holidays and relationships with friends. Support in terms of family-based respite care

---

RESEARCH BASED EVIDENCE

In their study of caring for people with dementia in the community, Moriaty et al. (1995) identified that comprehensive, flexible, reliable and relevant local support systems must be available for carers if they are to successfully manage during the period of caring.

schemes such as befriending and home care are useful adjuncts to promoting care in the community. One scheme, organized by Age Concern, provides services such as respite in the helper's home, live-in respite in the home of the patient or carer, and day care (Thornton, 1989). Orlik *et al.* (1991) and Tyler (1987), however, found that like many schemes, these schemes were not widely known about by potential users and also had to overcome problems related to public acceptability, confidence and carers' guilt.

Support for informal carers may also take the form of practical help such as taking the client out, helping with dressing, bathing and toileting, and simply keeping an eye on the client to check that they are alright. Twigg and Atkin (1993) found that informal carers of individuals with dementia valued day care both for the relief it can bring and for the opportunities it gave them to go out and pursue tasks at home. They also identified that significant social and recreational facilities were of benefit to informal carers.

Support groups run by social workers and psychiatric nurses have been less well evaluated. Not all carers enjoy group activities according to Twigg (1992). She found that some informal carers were not interested in hearing about other people's problems and felt that they had enough problems of their own. Other problems that informal carers face when attending support groups are transport difficulties, particularly in rural areas, and arranging care for the dependent relative, especially if the meeting times are inflexible.

With the finite resources, reduction of services and the strong emphasis on community care, it is likely that unless in dire need dependent elderly people will be cared for in their own homes by informal carers, with the help and support of the statutory, voluntary and private sector services. The nurse's role has consequently evolved from providing care to facilitating care, in partnership with other carers, and to ensuring that informal carers have sufficient support.

This chapter has explored how physiological, psychological and environmental factors can lead to the development of confusion. Confusion is symptomatic of an underlying pathology and the focus of the initial nursing assessment must be to identify and exclude this. Nursing strategies to help manage confusion in different contexts were then explored and the indicative criteria for each identified.

The elderly are the group most likely to suffer long-term confusion. There are many stereotyped views on confusion and the elderly and the nurse needs to be aware of these in order to give appropriate assistance to clients and their carers.

The pattern of caring for the elderly is increasingly falling to informal carers in the community. The advantages and disadvantages of this policy have been debated and the nurse's role in the support of carers in the community discussed.

▶ CASE STUDIES

Four case studies now follow, one from each branch of nursing. You should work through each and answer the questions to consolidate the knowledge you have learned from this chapter.

▶ CASE STUDY: MENTAL HEALTH

Nancy Frederick, a 68-year-old widow, has been referred to the community psychiatric nurse at her daughter's request. Nancy has Alzheimer's disease and until three years ago she was a sociable independent person, well known in her village. Since that time, however, she has gradually caused increasing concern. She has had to be brought back from different parts of the village where she has been found wandering for no apparent reason and at very odd times. She is also finding it difficult to remember familiar objects and faces and is not looking after herself. Her daughter finds it difficult to cope with her mother.

- ■ **Why have Nancy's problems occurred?**

- ■ **What actions should the community psychiatric nurse take to promote a therapeutic relationship with Nancy?**

- ■ **What support services are available in the community to facilitate Nancy remaining at home for as long as possible?**

- ■ **At what stage would Nancy require admission to a hospital or nursing home?**

▶ CASE STUDY: ADULT

Tom Jennings is a 58-year-old retired coal miner who has lived on his own since his wife left him five years ago. He is admitted to hospital with a severe chest infection following a home visit from his general practitioner. He has not been eating

REFLECTIVE KNOWLEDGE

properly and his skin is dry, loose and putty-like. He is pyrexial and has difficulty in breathing. His extremities are cyanosed. On admission Tom is very agitated and restless. On interview he is disorientated of time, date and place. He thinks you are one of his children and keeps asking you why you are not at school.

■ **Explain why Tom's confusion has arisen.**

■ **What immediate actions should be taken to help reduce Tom's level of confusion?**

■ **How long would you expect to wait before the remedial action started to take effect and Tom became less confused?**

▶ CASE STUDY: CHILD

Helen Rhodes, aged nine years, was playing in the local park on the swings. She was working the swing vigorously and fell off, hitting her head on the ground as she landed. She is reported to have lost consciousness briefly and was brought into the accident and emergency department. A skull radiograph does not demonstrate a fracture, but she is to be kept in hospital overnight for observation.

Helen's parents were both at work when the accident happened and the babysitter is unable to stay with Helen in hospital as she has other children to look after. Helen is frightened and does not appear to know where she is or why she is there. She has no recollection of the fall.

■ **Why has Helen's confusion arisen?**

■ **What immediate actions should be taken to help reduce Helen's confusion?**

■ **How long would you expect Helen's confusion to last?**

▶ CASE STUDY: LEARNING DISABILITIES

Pravin Dutt is a 34-year-old man who suffered brain damage at birth. Since the death of his mother, nine years ago, he has been cared for in a group bungalow. Using the continued support from his carers Pravin has coped well with day to day activities of living. Along with three other residents he has also benefited from an active behaviour modification programme.

Recent changes in management and organization have resulted in Pravin becoming much more dependent upon others, in particular with elimination, and he has developed faecal incontinence. This has been followed by changes in his mental state manifesting as disorientation of time, date and place, restlessness and challenging behaviour.

- Identify the most probable cause for Pravin's change in behaviour.

- What actions should the carers take to relieve Pravin's distress?

- What actions could be taken to minimize Pravin's faecal incontinence?

- What are the likely outcomes of the actions taken and when would you expect them to be achieved by?

▶ ANNOTATED FURTHER READING

GLYNN, J.J., PERKINS, D.A. (1995) *Managing Health Care: Challenges for the 90s.* London. Saunders.
A useful book that evaluates the effects of recent legislation on the availability and delivery of health care. It contains pertinent chapters on community care and useful data on social trends in health.

HILLS, J. (ed.) (1990) *The State of Welfare: The Welfare State in Britain since 1974.* Oxford. Clarendon.
A useful resource of data underlying policy formation. This makes a critical appraisal of health and social policy between 1974 and 1990. This is particularly relevant to help locate contemporary health policy in the UK.

MACE, N.L., RABINS, P.V., CASTLETON, B.A., McEWEN, E., MEREDITH, M. (1992) *The 36 Hour Day.* London. Hodder and Stoughton.
This is identified as a 'family guide' to caring for people at home with Alzheimer's disease and other confusional illnesses. This is a useful text with comprehensive information on caring issues. It is suitable for both formal and informal carers.

▶ ANNOTATED VIDEO

BBC Video (1983) *Where's the Key?* Wood Lane, London. BBC Enterprises.
An excellent film lasting around one hour that looks at the effect of Alzheimer's disease on the individual and her informal carer. Although the setting of the film is the early 1970s most of the issues raised remain unresolved at the end of the 1990s.

▶ REFERENCES

ARMSTRONG-ESTHER, C.A., SANDILANDS, M.L., MILLER, D. (1989) Attitudes and behaviours of nurses towards the elderly in an acute care setting. *Journal of Advanced Nursing* 14(1): 34–41.

ARMSTRONG-ESTHER, C.A., BROWNE, K.D., MCAFEE, J.G. (1994) Elderly patients: still clean and sitting quietly. *Journal of Advanced Nursing* 19(2): 264–271.

ANGUS, R. (1989) Infectious diseases of the nervous system. In: TALLIS, R. *The Clinical Neurology of Old Age.* Oxford. John Wiley.

BARR, N., COULTER, F. (1990) Social security: solution or problem? In HILLS, J. (ed.) *The State of Welfare in Britain: The Welfare State in Britain since 1974.* Oxford. Clarendon.

BENNETT, A. (1994) *Alan Bennett Diaries 1980–1990.* London. BBC Radio Collection.

BIRCHENALL, J.M., STREIGHT, M.E. (1993) *Care of the Older Adult.* Philadelphia. Lippincott.

BLANE, D. (1991) Elderly people and health. In SCAMBLER, G. (ed.) (1991) *Sociology as Applied to Medicine.* London. Baillière Tindall.

BLESSED, G., BLACK, S.E., BUTLER, T., KAY, D.W.K. (1991) The diagnosis of dementia in the elderly. *British Journal of Psychiatry* 159: 193–198.

BRAITHWAITE, V.A. (1990) *Bound to Care*, Sydney. Allen and Unwin.

BRITISH MEDICAL ASSOCIATION AND THE ROYAL PHARMACEUTICAL SOCIETY OF GREAT BRITAIN (1997) *British National Formulary*, No. 33. London. BMA and RPS of Great Britain.

BRIGGS, A., OLIVER, J. (1985) *Experience of Looking After Disabled Relatives.* London. Routledge and Kegan Paul.

BROCKLEHURST, J.C., HANLEY, T. (1976.) *Geriatric Medicine for Students.* Edinburgh. Churchill Livingstone.

BROWNE, K. (1984) Confusion in the elderly. *Nursing* 12(24): 698–705.

BUTLER, R.N. (1969) Ageism: another form of bigotry. *Gerontologist* 9(4): 243–246.

BUTLER, R.N. (1974) Successful ageing and the role of the life review. *Journal of American Geriatrics Society* 22(12): 529–537.

BUTLER, R.N., LEWIS, M.I. (1977) *Ageing and Mental Health: Positive Psychological Approaches.* St Louis. Mosby.

CENTRAL STATISTICS OFFICE (1994) *Social Trends* 24. London. Her Majesty's Stationery Office.

CONN, V.S. (1992) Self-management of over the counter medicines by older adults. *Public Health Nursing* **9(1)**: 29–36.

COOK, A. (1995) Ecstasy (MDMA): alerting users to the dangers. *Nursing Times* **91(16)**: 32–33.

DAY, M. (1996) The bitterest pill – the drug ecstasy. *Nursing Times* **92(7)**: 14–20.

DEPARTMENT OF HEALTH AND SOCIAL SECURITY (1981) *Growing Older*. London. Her Majesty's Stationery Office.

EDWARDS, G. (1982) *The Treatment of Drinking Problems – A Guide For The Helping Professions*. Oxford. Blackwell Scientific Publications.

EGAN, G. (1994) *The Skilled Helper – A Problem–Management Approach To Helping* (5th edition). Pacific Grove, California. Brooks/Cole.

ERIKSON, E.H. (1980) *Identity and the Life Cycle*. New York. Norton.

EVANDROU, M., FALKINGHAM, J., GLENNERSTER, H. (1990) The personal social services: everyone's poor relation but nobody's baby. In HILLS, J (ed.) *The State of Welfare in Britain: The Welfare State in Britain since 1974*. Oxford. Clarendon.

FEIL, N. (1982) *Validation – The Feil Method*. Ohio. Edward Feil Productions.

FINE, J.I., ROUSE–BANE, S. (1995) Using validation techniques to improve communication with cognitively impaired older adults. *Journal of Gerontological Nursing* **21(6)**: 39–45.

FITTING, M.D., RABBINS, P.V., LUCAS, M.J. (1984) Care-givers for dementia patients: A comparison of men and women. In BARUCH, A.S., WANDA, M.S (eds) Gender Differences In Care Giving: Why Do Wives Report Greater Burden? *The Gerontologist* **25(5)**: 667–677.

GHODSE, H. (1995) *Drugs and Addictive Behaviour – A Guide To Treatment*. London. Blackwell Science.

GIBSON, H.B. (1961) *The Gibson Spiral Maze*. Sevenoaks, Kent. Hodder and Stoughton.

GOODWIN, S.E. (1991) Planning care: from admission onwards. In BENSON, S., CARR, P. (eds) *The Care Assistant's Guide to Working with Elderly Mentally Infirm*. London. Hawker.

GREEN, H. (1988) *Informal carers*. Office of Population Censuses and Surveys, Social Survey Division, Series GH5 No 15 Supplement A. London. Her Majesty's Stationery Office.

GRIFFITHS, R. (1988) *Community Care: Agenda for action – A Report to the Secretary of State for Social Services*. London. Her Majesty's Stationery Office.

HAIGHT, B. (1992) The structured life-review process: community approach to the ageing client. In JONES, G.,

MIESEN B.M.L. (eds) *Care-Giving In Dementia – Research and Applications*. London. Routledge.

HENRY, J. (1992) Ecstasy and the dance of death. *British Medical Journal* **305(6844)**: 5–6.

HOLDEN, U.P., WOODS, R.T. (1982) *Reality Orientation – Psychological Approaches To The 'Confused' Elderly*. Edinburgh. Churchill Livingstone.

HOMER, A.C., HONAVAR, M., LANTOS, P.L., HASTIE, I.R., KELLETT, J.M., MILLARD, P.H. (1988) Diagnosing dementia: Do we get it right? *British Medical Journal* **297(6653)**: 894–896.

HUNTER, D.J., MCKEGANEY, N.P., MACPHERSON, I.A. (1988) *Care of the Elderly*. Aberdeen. Aberdeen University Press.

HURWITZ, N. (1969) Predisposing factors in adverse reactions to drugs. *British Medical Journal* **1(643)**: 536–539.

ISAACS, B. (1971) Geriatric patients: Do their families care? *British Medical Journal* **4(5782)**: 282–286.

JONES, C., OWENS, D. (1996) The recreational drug user in the intensive care unit: a review. *Intensive and Critical Care Nursing* **12(3)**: 126–130.

KAPLAN, H.I., SADOCK, B.J., GREBB, J.A. (1994) *Kaplan's and Sadock's Synopsis of Psychiatry, Behavioural Sciences and Clinical Psychiatry*. New York. Williams and Wilkins.

KIRBY, D., KAY, P. (1987) Support for the silent sufferers. *Nursing Times* **83(19)**: 43–44.

KLEIN, W.H., LeSHAN, E.J., FURMAN, S.S. (1985) *Promoting Mental Health of Older People through Group Methods*. New York. Manhattan Society for Mental Health.

KNAPP, M., LAWSON, R. (1995) Community care and the health service. In GLYNN, J.J., PERKINS, D.A. *Managing Health Care: Challenges for the 90s*. London. Saunders.

KOZAK-CAMPBELL, C., HUGHES, A.M. (1996) The use of functional consequences theory in acutely confused hospitalized elderly. *Journal of Gerontological Nursing* **22(1)**: 27–36.

LEVIN, E., SINCLAIR, I., GORBACH, P. (1989) *Families, Services And Confusion In Old Age*. Aldershot. Gower.

LIPOWSKI, Z.J. (1983) Transient cognitive disorders: delirium and acute confusional states in the elderly. *American Journal of Psychiatry* **140(11)**: 1426–1436.

LISTON, E.H. (1982) Delirium in the aged. In JARVIK, L.F., SMALL, G.W. (eds) *The Psychiatric Clinic of North America*. Philadelphia. Saunders.

LOWTHER, C.P., WILLIAMSON, J. (1966) Old people and their relatives. *Lancet* **ii(7479)**: 1459–1460.

LUKER, K., PERKINS, E. (1987) The

elderly at home: service needs and provisions. *Journal of the Royal College of General Practitioners* **137**: 299.

MACE, N.L., RABINS, P.V., CASTLETON, B.A., McEWEN, E., MEREDITH, B. (1992) *The 36 Hour Day: A Family Guide to Caring at Home for People with Alzheimer's Disease and Other Confusional Illnesses*. London. Age Concern.

MORTON, I., BLEATHMAN, C. (1988) Does it matter whether it's Thursday or Friday? *Nursing Times* **84(6)**: 27.

MORIATY, J., LEVIN, E., PAHL, J., WEBB, S. (1995) *An Evaluation Of Community Care Arrangements for Older People with Dementia*. London. National Institute for Social Work.

MURPHY, E. (1986) *Dementia and Mental Illness in Old Age*. London. Papermac.

NHS AND COMMUNITY CARE ACT (1990) London. Her Majesty's Stationery Office.

NORRIS, A.D., EILEH, A.E. (1982) Reminiscence groups. *Nursing Times* **78(32)**: 68–69.

NORRIS, A. (1986) *Reminiscence with Elderly People*. London. Winslow Press.

OFFICE OF POPULATION CENSUSES AND SURVEYS (1988) *Disabilities in Great Britain. The Prevalence of Disability among Adults*. London. Her Majesty's Stationery Office.

OFFICE OF POPULATION CENSUSES AND SURVEYS (1995) *Morbidity Statistics from General Practice. Fourth National Study 1991–1992. A Study Carried Out By The Royal College Of Practitioners, The Office Of Population Censuses And Surveys, and The Department Of Health*. London. Her Majesty's Stationery Office.

ORLIK, C., ROBINSON, C., RUSSELL, O. (1991) *A survey of family-based respite care scheme in the United Kingdom*, Bristol. National Association For Family-Based Respite Care.

PATTIE, A.H., GILLEARD, C.J. (1979) *Manual of the Clifton Assessment Procedures for the Elderly (CAPE)*. London. Hodder and Stoughton.

PEACE, S. (1988) Living environment for the elderly – promoting the 'right' living institutional environment. In WELLS, N., FREER, C. *The Ageing Population – Burden or Challenge?* London. M Stockton Press.

PERKO, J.E., KREIGH, H.Z. (1988) *Psychiatric and Mental Health Nursing: A Commitment to Care and Concern*. New York. Prentice Hall.

PHILLIPS, L.R.F. (1973) A word about confusion. Cited in: WOLANIN, M.O., PHILLIPS, L.R.F. (1981) *Confusion–Prevention and Care*. St Louis, MI, CV Mosby.

RICHARDSON, A., UNELL, J., ASTON, B. (1989) *A New Deal For Carers*. London. King Edward's Hospital Fund.

ROBB, B. (1967) *Sans Everything*. Surrey. Nelson.

SCRUTTON, S. (1989) *Counselling Older People – A Creative Response To Ageing*. London. Arnold.

SHERIDAN, E., PATTERSON, H.R., GUSTAFSON, E.A. (1985) *The Drug, The Nurse, The Patient*. Philadelphia. W.B. Saunders.

SKEET, M. (1989) *Small Area Planning For The Elderly*. Regional Office for Europe. World Health Organization

SMITH, B.A. (1986) When is confusion translocation syndrome. *American Journal of Nursing* **86(11)**: 1280–1281.

SWANSON, J.W., KELLY, J.J., McCONAHEY, W.M. (1981) Neurologic aspects of thyroid dysfunction. *Mayo Clinic Proceedings* **56(8)**: 504–512.

TAYLOR, D. (1989) *Hospital-at-Home – The Coming Revolution*. London. Kings Fund.

THORNTON, P. (1989) *Creating a Break: A Home Care Relief Scheme for Elderly People and Their Supporters*. Mitcham. Age Concern England.

TWIGG, J. (1992) Carers in the service system. In TWIGG, J. (ed.) (1992) *Carers – Research and Practice*. London. Her Majesty's Stationery Office.

TWIGG, J., ATKIN, K. (1993) *Policy and Practice in Informal Care*. Milton Keynes. OU Press.

TYLER, J. (1987) Give us a break. *Nursing Times* **83(5)**: 32–35.

VICTOR, C.R. (1987) *Old Age in Modern Society – A Textbook of Social Gerontology*. London. Chapman and Hall.

WAKE, D. (1995) Ecstasy overdose: a case study. *Intensive and Critical Care Nursing* **11(1)**: 6–9.

WILLIAMS, M., HOLLOWAY, J., WINN, M. (1979) Nursing activities and acute confusional states in elderly hip-fractured patients. *Nursing Research* **28(1)**: 25–35.

WILLIAMSON, J., STOKOE, I.H., GRAY, S., FISHER, M., SMITH, A. (1964) Old people at home: their unreported needs. *Lancet* **i(7342)**: 1117–1120.

WRIGHT, F.D. (1986) *Left To Care Alone*. London. Gower Publishing.

S. Eastburn

KEY ISSUES

■ SUBJECT KNOWLEDGE
▷ defining sexuality
▷ sexuality: the historical context
▷ masculinity and femininity
▷ sexual development
▷ the sexual response
▷ sexual behaviour

■ PRACTICE KNOWLEDGE
▷ sexuality and nursing models
▷ assessment and sexuality
▷ discussing sexuality with clients

▷ problems related to clients' sexuality
▷ nursing actions

■ PROFESSIONAL KNOWLEDGE
▷ nursing as a female profession
▷ key issues in the four branches of nursing
▷ the law and sexuality

■ REFLECTIVE KNOWLEDGE
▷ self awareness
▷ case studies

▶ INTRODUCTION

The concept of sexuality is important for nursing practice because it is an essential element of people's lives and people's health. This chapter explores the nature of sexuality and suggests how nurses can incorporate it into their day to day work with clients. Nursing theory has acknowledged the significance of human sexuality, but it is an aspect of practice that nurses have great difficulty with. This is probably due to two factors:

▶ first, sexuality is not easy to define;
▶ secondly, it includes aspects of people's lives that usually remain private.

Sexuality is a delicate subject surrounded by mystery and misunderstandings. Consequently it can be easily avoided by nurses and clients. The aim of this chapter is to explore the meaning of sexuality and identify the relevance of the concept for nurses in practice.

▶ OVERVIEW

▶ *Subject Knowledge*

The chapter begins with an exploration of definitions and meanings of sexuality. It includes an overview of the historical context, and identifies some of the problems associated with our understanding and images of sexuality in the past. Masculinity, femininity and gender roles are then addressed, leading into an outline of the processes involved in the development of an individual's sexuality. This section includes information on the male and female reproductive systems and the biological control of human sexual development and the human sexual response. It also includes psychosocial theory related to the development of sexual identity and gender roles.

Following this is an overview of sexual norms and a summary of key research on sexual behaviour in Britain. This ends with a consideration of the relationship between emotions and sexual behaviour.

❯ *Practice Knowledge*

This section begins with an outline of sexuality as an aspect of nursing models and moves on to discuss the assessment of an individual's sexual health and sexuality-related problems. It includes guidance on how to discuss sensitive issues with clients. Following this is a section on types of sexuality-related problems, and the roles and actions nurses take in caring for people with such problems.

❯ *Professional Knowledge*

This section discusses the importance of nursing as a mainly female profession and identifies issues specific to the four branches of nursing. It ends with a list of legal issues related to sexuality and patient care.

❯ *Reflective Knowledge*

The final section considers self-awareness as an aspect of nursing expertise. It includes an exercise to assess your own sexual health and sexual fulfilment.

On pp. 566–569 there are four case studies, each one relating to one of the branch programmes. You may find it helpful to read one of them before you start the chapter and use it as a focus for your reflections while reading.

SUBJECT KNOWLEDGE

❯ DEFINING SEXUALITY

Defining sexuality is not an easy task. Sexual activity, including feelings, thoughts and actions, is central to such a definition, and the concepts of masculinity and femininity are also significant. Writers who have grappled with the nature of sexuality have often included these ideas, but the need to take a broad view has been emphasized. These views are perhaps best summarized by Byers (1989, p. 312) who states that 'Sexuality is the expression and experience of the self as a sexual being. It is, therefore, a state of both the body and mind and a crucial part of the personality. Sexuality is not limited to overt sexual activity, such as sexual intercourse, but includes solitary activities like studying, walking and relaxing. Sexuality is part of every relationship, whether it is primarily a sexual relationship or not; it is the rapport that is established between the self and body'.

Although this definition emphasizes the broad nature of sexuality as a component of people's lives, its generality may still leave you asking '. . . but what does it really involve?' There is no simple answer, but in the literature there are the following common elements:

- ❯ sex;
- ❯ sexual orientation;
- ❯ gender and associated roles;
- ❯ relationships;
- ❯ self-image;
- ❯ self-esteem;
- ❯ human attraction;
- ❯ love.

This list attempts to expand on the concept of sexuality, but it is not definitive. Because sexuality is a social construct and is open to change and interpretation, complete and accurate definitions cannot exist. You will see from the above list that the elements in themselves are complex and difficult to define. Also they are surrounded by notions of normality, what is right and what is wrong. In coming to an understanding of sexuality we must take into account its changing nature and the social and historical forces that shape it.

▶ SEXUALITY: THE HISTORICAL CONTEXT

Studies on the history of sexuality emphasize how people's attitudes and behaviour have changed (Foucault, 1979). These changes are difficult to appreciate because the language and concepts used to compare sexuality through the ages are based on our understanding of sexuality today. For example, promiscuity is defined by a society's behavioural norms and expectations. What might be seen as promiscuous now could have been accepted behaviour in the past. For this reason any historical view of sexuality must be treated with caution.

Van Ooijen and Charnock (1994) summarize a history of sexuality by focusing on a range of issues, for example common sexual practices, forbidden sexual activities, the relationships between men and women, religious influence on social norms and the portrayal of sexual symbols in art and language. You will see from this range of issues that understanding the historical context of sexuality is a complex business.

You may have beliefs about the nature of sexuality during historical periods. For example the popular image of Roman times is one in which sexual activity had a high public profile. Behaviours that would not be accepted today were seen as normal practice. Victorian times on the other hand have been characterized by repressive attitudes towards sex. These attitudes manifested themselves in the language of the day, and the delicate subject of sex was surrounded by taboos and managed through strict social etiquette. The 1960s are famous for 'free love' and the liberated youth. Although there may be some truth in these pictures they are nevertheless generalizations and tend to concentrate on sexual activity rather than a broader understanding of sexuality.

These stereotypical views of sexuality during previous generations have their inherent dangers. A nurse working with an older person may make assumptions about his or her sexuality based upon a view of the era in which the person was born and raised. For example the 1930s and 1940s may conjure up images of marriage for life, sexual faithfulness in the nuclear family setting, and sex as a taboo subject in day to day conversation. These images are arguably more myth than reality, but they can influence the way a nurse views an older person in the 1990s. It is easy to see how the subject of safe sex may not be considered appropriate by a nurse working with a 75-year-old person if the nurse believes that people from that generation think and behave according to the popular images.

Using your views of sexuality in history as a way of making judgements about people can therefore create problems. First these views may be inaccurate. Second there is an assumption that a person's sexuality develops during his or her 'formative' years and then remains stable.

An important development in the recent history of sexuality is the increasing acceptance of sexual activity as a valid topic for scientific

- *What are your views on the nature of sexuality during the era of your parents' youth?*

- *When your grandparents were teenagers, what do you think sexuality was like then?*

- *How do you think your parents or grandparents views on sexuality have changed during their lifetimes?*

- *How might these views influence your work with older people?*

study. This has perhaps resulted from more openness in society and also from the need to focus attention on human immunodeficiency virus (HIV) and acquired immunodeficiency syndrome (AIDS). Sexual problems and the impact of ill health on sexuality are recognized as issues that may require professional help. Also nursing and other professions are incorporating a holistic model of health into their practice that views sexuality as an important dimension of human life.

▶ MASCULINITY AND FEMININITY

> Being masculine or feminine probably brings to mind lists of commonly understood personal characteristics. These characteristics may include an individual's looks and the way he or she acts, thinks and feels.
>
> Spend five minutes writing down the words you associate with masculinity. Repeat the exercise for femininity.
>
> - *How easy did you find this?*
> - *How did it make you feel?*
> - *Are the characteristics positive, negative or neutral?*
> - *Does masculinity include more or less socially valued characteristics than femininity?*
> - *Are these characteristics relevant for the day to day lives of children and adults?*
> - *What is society's attitude towards men with feminine characteristics and women with masculine characteristics?*
> - *Use this exercise as a basis of group discussion with your colleagues.*

Sexuality is a broad term referring to an essential part of people's lives. It is reflected in a range of things we do, say and feel, and especially in the way we interact with others. A traditional way of interpreting sexuality is through our understandings of masculinity and femininity and the roles associated with being a man or woman. Although these understandings may be blurred in today's society, gender-specific roles are still influential in many aspects of people's lives. In starting to explore sexuality the ideas of masculinity and femininity are important.

You may feel that your descriptions of masculinity and femininity do not represent any sort of reality and are more easily associated with the stereotypical images of men and women. These images can be seen in films, cartoons and popular magazines and although these images can be the butt of jokes, they can also be ideals or sources of aspiration. It could be argued that these images are outdated and that to be masculine today the characteristics of the so-called 'new man' have to be taken into account. Some disagree, suggesting that the emergence of the new man is a myth and that many traditional gender differences and inequalities still exist (Hudson and Williams, 1995). Others suggest that the experience of being a woman has changed as many more women take on paid employment and the nature of family life has altered (Giddens, 1993). Whatever the case, the images we hold of masculinity or manhood and femininity or womanhood influence our day to day lives through our choice of jobs, the clothes we wear and the types of interests we develop.

> - *Do you think the popular images of masculinity and femininity have affected your thoughts and behaviour in any way?*
> - *Have they motivated you to do things in certain ways?*
> - *Do aspects of your life demonstrate both feminine and masculine characteristics?*

▶ Gender Roles

In society there is a distinction between men's and women's roles. This can clearly be seen by the sorts of jobs men and women take, and the social pressures influencing the decisions around job selection. From an early age children often have ideas about what they would like to be when they 'grow up'. With responses like 'I want to be a train driver' or 'I want to be a nurse' you can guess with some confidence the sex of the child. Although children's aspirations differ from one society to the next and from one generation to the next, boys' views of their future will clearly contrast with those of girls. Of course these childhood wishes

Through the processes of socialization, we learn to behave, think and feel in ways that express our gender. Some of these aspects of our lives are obvious, but others are more subtle. Consider the following – walking, holding a cigarette, waving, talking to a neighbour over the fence, dancing, driving – and answer the questions below.

- *How would you expect men and women to differ in the above activities?*
- *How do you explain these differences ?*
- *Do these differences have any particular significance?*
- *Discuss your answers with your colleagues.*

are not likely to come true for many, but nevertheless adult roles are largely gender-specific and comply with general expectations. There are exceptions, but being exceptions, they tend to reinforce the rule. For example, a female brick layer and a male office cleaner will probably be seen as unusual and may acquire local celebrity status.

It has been argued that with the changing employment market and the disappearance of traditional heavy jobs through automation and computer technology, men's and women's roles are less distinct (Beechey, 1987). This could be the case, but gender role differences are not the sole province of paid employment. They are also evident in leisure interests, household tasks and the relationships and interactions within a family. Some of these differences are inequalities. Men living in family settings often have access to a greater proportion of those activities generally viewed as rewarding or stimulating, for example, leisure time, careers, peer group interaction. There is evidence that marriage may affect men's and women's health differently. In simplified terms married men are healthier than single men whereas married women are less healthy than single women. Although this does not demonstrate cause and effect, the associations between family life and a number of indicators of health for men and women consistently point towards the conclusion that marriage is 'healthy' for men and 'unhealthy' for women (Gove and Tudor, 1972).

DECISION MAKING

Mary is 26 years old and married and has three children under six years of age. Her husband John is a long-distance lorry driver and works on average 60 hours per week, spending two or three nights away from home every week. Mary is devoted to the children and is proud that she can manage and maintain the home on the family's limited income. Mary also has a few friends, mostly other mothers from the playgroup and local primary school. During a routine visit to the practice nurse Mary admits to being very tired and having difficulty motivating herself. She has become irritable with the children recently and as a way of calming herself down, she has a few glasses of sherry in the afternoon.

- *How might Mary's conflicting roles contribute to her present state of health?*
- *How might the practice nurse enable Mary to manage her conflicting roles in a healthier way?*
- *What are the difficulties faced by Mary's practice nurse in helping her manage this situation?*

The roles we have in society, particularly those in paid employment and those within a family, express something about us as individuals. They express our sexuality to those around us and enable us to develop a positive image of ourselves. Sometimes these roles are associated with pressures. Role strain occurs when the duties or expectations associated with a person's roles become a burden. The individual finds it difficult to wear many hats. Role conflict occurs when a person's roles show signs of incompatibility. For example, a woman can be a mother and be expected to make decisions regarding her children. She can also be a daughter and be expected to take advice from and listen to the wisdom of her parents. Such pressures can make the fulfilment of these roles difficult or impossible at times.

The roles we have in society express our sexuality. Similarly our everyday behaviour says something about our gender identity.

▶ THE DEVELOPMENT OF AN INDIVIDUAL'S SEXUALITY

Sexuality is an important part of our lives and it influences much of our behaviour, especially the way we interact with others. How can we explain our sexuality, how does it develop and what are the forces that shape it? Answers to these questions are considered below. First the development of an individual's sexuality is described. It includes biological sciences, with an overview of the male and female reproductive systems and an outline of the significant changes associated with puberty, menopause and old age. Then in the section on behavioural sciences there is an outline of key psychological and sociological theories that attempt to explain the development of sexual identity.

Biological ▶ **DEVELOPMENT OF THE REPRODUCTIVE SYSTEM**

▶ *Embryo*

For the first few weeks after fertilization the embryonic internal and external genitalia for males and females are the same. At about the seventh week hormonal changes lead to sex differentiation and the male reproductive system develops under the influence of increased androgen levels.

▶ *Childhood*

In childhood, the greatest time of physical change related to sexuality occurs during puberty. These changes are hormonally controlled and the process begins at around 11–12 years of age for girls and 12–13 years of age for boys. It involves the development of fully functioning reproductive systems and the body changes that result in the characteristic adult male and female physiques (Figure 4.3.1).

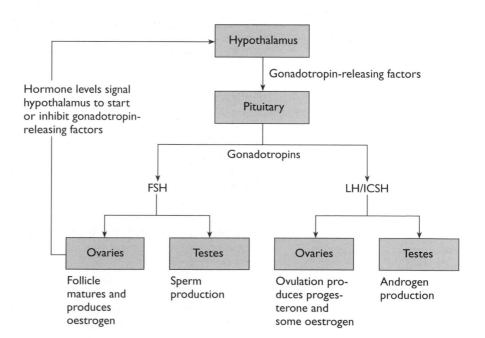

Figure 4.3.1: Hormonal control of sexual development (after Offir, 1982).

▶ *Adult Male Reproductive System* (Figure 4.3.2)

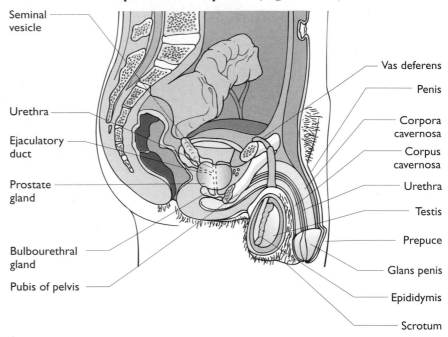

Seminal vesicle

Urethra

Ejaculatory duct

Prostate gland

Bulbourethral gland

Pubis of pelvis

Vas deferens

Penis

Corpora cavernosa

Corpus cavernosa

Urethra

Testis

Prepuce

Glans penis

Epididymis

Scrotum

Figure 4.3.2: Anatomy of the male reproductive system. (Redrawn from Hinchliff *et al.*, 1996.)

▶ Testes

Testes have two functions:

- ▶ production of sperm;
- ▶ secretion of testosterone.

The testes are made up of a fine network of convoluted seminiferous tubules. Under the influence of hormones, stem cells in the convoluted seminiferous tubules undergo a series of changes. These result in the production of spermatozoa, which pass into the epididymis to mature before ejaculation. During ejaculation the sperm pass out of the tail of the epididymis and into the vas deferens. As the sperm pass along the vas deferens and ejaculatory duct, the seminal vesicle, prostate gland and bulbourethral gland secrete fluid containing chemicals and nutrients. This mixture is called semen and its purpose is to allow the sperm to survive and move along the female reproductive tract.

Testosterone is a hormone needed for spermatogenesis and the sex drive. It is also responsible for the development of the following male secondary sex characteristics:

- ▶ enlargement of the penis and testes;
- ▶ enlargement of the larynx producing a deeper voice;
- ▶ growth of facial hair and pubic hair;
- ▶ increased sebaceous gland activity;
- ▶ muscle development.

▶ Penis

The penis contains three cylindrical masses of erectile tissue: two corpora cavernosa running along the top and sides, and a smaller corpus cavernosa on the underside, which contains the urethra. The glans penis at the end of the shaft of the penis is normally covered by a fold of skin, the prepuce or foreskin. This is sometimes surgically removed (circumcision). During sexual arousal the erectile tissue fills with blood and the penis enlarges and becomes firm.

▶ Adult Female Reproductive System

▶ Internal genitalia (Figure 4.3.3)

The ovaries have two functions:

- ▶ production of ova;
- ▶ secretion of progesterone and oestrogen.

The ovary contains many oocytes. These are the cells that undergo a series of changes to develop into mature Graafian follicles. Ovulation occurs when a follicle ruptures and releases an oocyte into the fallopian tube. This happens once a month during the menstrual cycle.

Progesterone 'prepares' the woman's body for pregnancy. It increases the growth of the endometrium and breasts and influences cervical mucus production and uterine muscle activity. Oestrogen influences oogenesis and follicle maturation, the onset of puberty and the development of female secondary sex characteristics, and the growth and maintenance of reproductive organs. Female secondary sex characteristics include:

- ▶ growth and development of breasts;
- ▶ body hair, e.g. pubic hair;
- ▶ changes in fat distribution to produce the female physique;
- ▶ vaginal secretions.

Fallopian tubes extend from the uterus towards the ovaries. They open into the peritoneal cavity with funnel-like projections. The oocyte moves into the first part of the fallopian tube and is fertilized in the ampulla partway along its length. Peristalsis and ciliated cells help the oocyte move to the uterus, which is a hollow, thick-walled muscular structure that assists in the implantation of the embryo, nurtures the developing fetus and moves the baby out through the vagina at birth. The epithelial layer is the endometrium and this changes in thickness and structure under hormonal control during the menstrual cycle. The cervix is at the lower end of the uterus.

The vagina is a canal connecting the cervix to the external genitalia. It expands during childbirth and intercourse and has an acidic environment to protect it from pathogenic organisms. It becomes lubricated

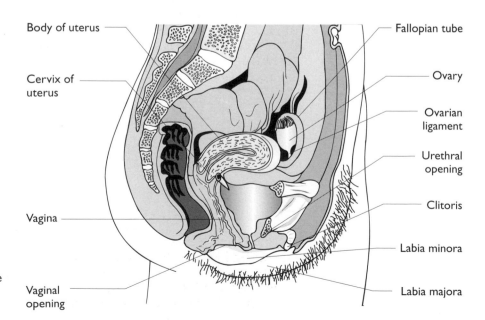

Figure 4.3.3: Anatomy of the female reproductive system. (Redrawn from Hinchliff *et al.*, 1996.)

during sexual arousal with secretions from the vestibular glands and with some fluid leakage from the vaginal walls. The distal end of the vaginal orifice is partially occluded by the hymen. This usually ruptures during first intercourse, but it can also be ruptured by tampons or exercise.

▌ External genitalia (Figure 4.3.4)

The mons pubis is a fatty pad over the pubic bone. The labia majora are covered in skin and have many sebaceous glands and the labia minora meet at the anterior end at the clitoris. The clitoris is rich in nerve endings and plays an important part in the sexual response. The vestibular glands secrete a fluid which lubricates the vagina during sexual arousal.

▌ The menstrual cycle

This is controlled by circulating hormones, but can be influenced by emotional factors. It has the following three phases:

▌ the proliferative phase (oestrogen causes cell proliferation in the uterus, the endometrium thickens and the cervical mucus becomes thinner and more profuse), which ends with ovulation;

▌ the secretory phase (vascularity of the endometrium increases under the influence of progesterone and cervical mucus thickens to block the cervical canal; hormonal secretion from the corpus luteum declines if fertilization does not take place and the endometrium begins to degenerate);

▌ the menstrual phase (the flow of blood and endometrial tissue, which lasts 3–6 days); prostaglandins stimulate the uterus to contract and this causes the characteristic pain (dysmenorrhoea).

Figure 4.3.4: The female external genitalia. (Redrawn from Hinchliff *et al.*, 1996.)

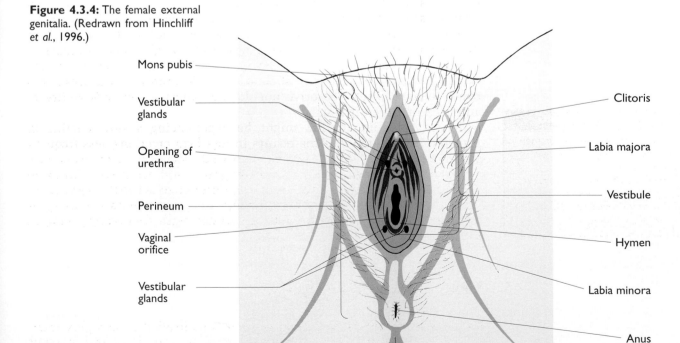

Mons pubis

Vestibular glands

Opening of urethra

Perineum

Vaginal orifice

Vestibular glands

Clitoris

Labia majora

Vestibule

Hymen

Labia minora

Anus

DECISION MAKING

How could a detailed understanding of the anatomy and physiology of the reproductive systems and the phases of the menstrual cycle help nurses in the following settings?
- *A school nurse working with primary schoolchildren.*
- *A nurse working with women with learning disabilities.*
- *A practice nurse running a 'well man' clinic*

▶ PREMENSTRUAL SYNDROME

Before the menstrual phase some women experience a range of symptoms. Pelvic congestion and overall body water retention can give a feeling of distension. Also tiredness, irritability, depression and loss of concentration are not uncommon. The increase in body weight alongside these symptoms can lead to body image changes and feelings of low self-esteem. The reasons for these symptoms are unclear. Some theories suggest fluid retention is the cause, others that a vitamin deficiency (vitamin B_6) resulting from hormonal variations affects the functioning of the brain leading to mood changes.

The intensity of the premenstrual syndrome varies from individual to individual, but these variations do not seem to be linked to the degree of hormonal change. Also the significance and character of premenstrual changes have varied throughout history. This suggests that the premenstrual syndrome is influenced by social and psychological as well as biological factors (Webb, 1985).

▶ MENOPAUSE

Some of the changes in sexual response for women are associated with the menopause. This usually happens between the ages of 45 and 55. It is the time when the ovaries cease to function and a woman's reproductive life ends. The hormonal changes are sometimes associated with a range of symptoms, and the pattern of symptoms can vary. Sweating, hot flushes, insomnia, depression, fatigue and headaches are sometimes experienced at this time of life. Webb (1985) believes that the evidence to link these symptoms with hormonal changes is far from conclusive. Coming to terms with the end of a reproductive life plus other stressful life events commonly experienced at this age might be the causes of such symptoms. She cites the variations between women from different social classes and women from different societies as evidence to suggest that the menopause has significant social and psychological determinants.

It is important to stress that the hormonal changes occurring during the menopause do not directly affect a women's interest in sex. Oestrogen levels do not control sex drive nor do they affect a woman's ability to enjoy sex or have orgasms.

Men at this time of life might be experiencing a slow decline in testosterone production. This results in less firm erections, less frequent ejaculations and a longer refractory period. Men can also experience social and psychological pressures leading to a 'mid-life crisis'. (Atkinson *et al.*, 1990). In the same way that it is difficult to attribute menopause purely to biological factors, any changes in a man's sexual activity at this time of life cannot always be associated with decreasing androgen levels.

DECISION MAKING

List common life events for men and women between the ages of 45 and 55.
- *How might these events affect their intimate relationships with those close to them?*

▶ THE SEXUAL RESPONSE

The sexual response in men and women is controlled by complex interactions between the central nervous system, the peripheral nervous system, neurotransmitters, hormones and the circulatory system (Boone, 1995). It has four stages:

- arousal, which in men results in penile erection, testicular elevation and flattening of the scrotal skin, and in women results in vaginal lubrication, clitoral enlargement, upper vaginal dilation, vaginal constriction of the lower third, uterine elevation and breast and nipple enlargement;
- plateau, which in men is associated with an increase in secretions from the urethral Cowper's glands and an increase in blood pressure, heart rate, respiratory rate and muscle tone, and in women is associated with retraction of the clitoris against the pubic bone and increases in blood pressure, heart rate, respiratory rate and muscle tone;
- orgasm, which in men is characterized by a rhythmical contraction of the perineal muscles, closure of the bladder neck and ejaculation, while in women may be single or multiple and involves contractions of the perineal muscles, uterus and fallopian tubes, although not all women experience orgasm;
- resolution, when the physiological changes are reversed. There is also a refractory period, which is the resting time that must elapse before the next sexual response can be initiated, and this may be shorter for women (Masters and Johnson, 1966).

▶ *Physiological Changes due to Age and the Male Sexual Response*

These are as follows:

- arousal – erections may occur less frequently and more and longer direct stimulation of the penis is required to establish and maintain an erection;
- plateau – may be prolonged and ejaculation more easily controlled;
- orgasm – the number and force of contractions decrease, but the sensation may be equally satisfying;
- resolution – the length of time between orgasm and the next possible erection increases.

▶ *Physiological Changes due to Age and the Female Sexual Response*

Reduced oestrogen levels result in thinning of the vaginal mucosa, replacement of breast tissue by fat and shrinking of the uterus. These may affect the sexual response in older women as follows:

- arousal – longer direct clitoral stimulation may be required, the vaginal opening expands less and vaginal lubrication may be reduced;
- plateau – sensation may alter due to a decrease in vasocongestion and a reduced tenting of the vagina;
- orgasm – contractions may be fewer;
- resolution – the clitoris loses its erection more rapidly, but the refractory period after orgasm does not seem to lengthen for women as it does for men.

DECISION MAKING

From the information on the effects of ageing on the sexual response:

- *Can you see any physiological reasons why sexual activity might have to stop for older people?*
- *Can you see any physiological reasons why older people might not enjoy sexual activity?*
- *What implications do your answers have for nurses working with older people?*

Psychosocial   A number of sociologists and psychologists have attempted to explain how people develop a sexual identity. There is agreement among many that relationships and interactions with those close to us play an important part. Others emphasize the biological factors and believe that our genetic makeup determines our sexual identity. The key theories are outlined below.

▶ FREUD'S PSYCHO-ANALYTICAL THEORY

Freud's pscho-analytical theory (1923) offered an explanation of why boys and girls grow up differently, and has since been developed by many psychologists. Freud focused on five stages of development. At each stage he identified the way in which individuals learned to balance the satisfaction of the 'libidinal' or pleasure drive of Id against Ego and Superego. The effectiveness of resolution at each stage, Freud contended, had lasting ramifications on the subsequent personality development.

▶ *Oral Stage: 0–18 Months of Age*

Newborn infants are unable to do little more than suck and drink and the libidinal drive finds its outlet in this activity. The infant derives its gratification orally, both for food and for pleasure. In early life sucking is passive to gain nourishment, although as the infant develops this occasionally turns to aggressive biting. During this stage of life only Id is present in the personality. Superego and Ego have not yet developed. Consequently the infant becomes frustrated if his demands are not met immediately.

▶ *Anal Stage: 18 Months–3 Years of Age*

During this period restrictions are placed upon the child's life for the first time. Initially the child discovers that the breast is no longer available immediately when it is wanted. Then potty training begins, restricting bowel evacuation and urination to specific times. These constraints frustrate Id and result in temper tantrums. Eventually, with the development of Ego, the child learns to exert some control over Id and uses the potty. It is at this time that the libidinal drive passes to the anus and the child finds the control of bowel movements to be pleasurable, both from expelling the bowel contents and by retaining them.

During these first two stages of development the infant is unaware of gender differences. All children are seen as 'little males'.

▶ *Phallic stage: 3–5 Years of Age*

The child becomes aware of its gender and discovers that pleasure can be derived from the penis or clitoris. The libidinal drive then centres on this body area and the child derives satisfaction from playing with its sexual organ. This continues until the behaviour is shamed into cessation by the child's parents. During this phase the child forms an incestuous desire for the parent of the opposite sex. In the male child this is called the Oedipus complex. The boy's love for his mother becomes very intense and this leads him to become very jealous of anyone who competes for his mother's attention. Consequently conflict arises with his father. The child wishes to replace his father as the object of his mother's attention; however, he fears that if he does so then he will be punished. He has noticed that girls and his mother do not have a penis. This, he suspects, is because they were castrated as a punishment when they were younger. He fears that if he continues with the feelings he has for his mother then his father will also castrate him. To protect his penis he represses the feelings he holds for his mother and identifies with his father. This way he both retains his penis and by identifying with his father he also fulfils his desire for his mother.

In the female child a different process, the Electra complex, occurs. Initially the female child is drawn towards her mother. She discovers, however, that unlike her father and boys, she does not possess a penis. She assumes that she has been castrated, for which she blames her mother and feels inferior. Freud called this phenomenon 'penis envy'. The girl realizes that she will not get a replacement penis and consequently sublimates the desire for a penis with the desire for a baby. She looks to her father to provide her with this and transfers her affections to him. This also brings problems though. If the girl looks to her father to provide affection then she will be in direct competition with her mother. In consequence she fears that her mother may withdraw her love for her. To prevent this she internalizes the images of her mother as carer, so that her mother will continue to love her. This final part of the Electra complex, where the girl identifies again with her mother, is called anaclytic identification.

This is a very ambivalent period for a child of either gender and parental attitudes during this stage have profound ramifications on the child's development.

▶ Latency Stage: 5 Years of Age–Puberty

Following the traumas of the phallic stage, this period is relatively quiet. The child's sexual interests are replaced by interests at school, playtimes, sports and a range of new activities. Possibly for the first time the child meets people from outside the family and with whom new relationships are formed. Children who were unsuccessful in passing through the earlier stages can find the world outside the family confusing and threatening and they often have difficulty forming new relationships in this period.

▶ Genital Stage: Puberty–Adulthood

With the onset of puberty the individual experiences a jolt from the sexual dormancy of the latency stage. The individual has an intense libidinal drive to engage in full sexual activity. The capacity for full physiological sexual responses have also developed by this stage and for the first time the individual experiences themself as a complete sexual being.

At this stage boys lose sexual attachment for their mother. Similarly girls lose their attachment for their father. This allows them to make sexual attachment to members of the opposite sex; however, during this stage, the individual has to learn to express sexual energy in socially acceptable ways.

Despite the criticisms, Freud's theory highlighted the importance of relationships and interactions between children and the adults around them. It also identified the importance of sexuality in many aspects of life, and stimulated a wealth of research in this area.

The nature and quality of relationships during these formative years seem to be significant in the development of an individual's sexuality. The difficulties people have in forming relationships with others result in part from early childhood experiences with parents. In certain settings nurses will work with people who have problems with their identity. Crises with an individual's identity, in particular their sense of sexuality, are likely to have their origins in childhood development, and advanced

There are a number of assumptions in Freud's theory: the penis is somehow superior to the clitoris or vagina; man is naturally active and woman naturally passive; women have a natural 'maternal' instinct; children become aware of their gender identity at about five years of age; and homosexuality represents a fault in childhood development.

- *Do you think these assumptions are valid?*
- *What might the repercussions for nursing be if we believe that these assumptions are always true?*

(For critiques of Freud's theory of psychosexual development see Webb, 1985; Giddens, 1990; and Gross, 1992.)

nursing practice may involve the exploration of patients' relationships with their parents.

▶ NEOANALYTICAL THEORY

Some writers have modified Freud's ideas, basing their explanations of gender identity on other experiences in early childhood. Chodorow (1978) emphasizes the importance of the early maternal bond that exists apparently in all societies. Girls never completely break this bond and their consequent identity incorporates a significant relational element. Boys on the other hand have to break this bond in order to develop a masculine identity. This masculine identity is characterized by independence, individuality and a rejection of the feminine. Girls grow up being able to relate closely to others whereas boys take a more analytical view of the world and value achievement rather than caring or compassion. As a result, women require a close relationship in order to maintain their self-esteem, but men feel threatened by such close emotional attachments.

This theory is based on the primary role of the woman as the main carer of children, especially in the early years. It has been criticized for assuming a straightforward female psychological makeup that fails to take into account other feelings, for example aggression and assertiveness (Sayers, 1986). On the other hand it may help us make sense of some men's apparent inability to express their emotions.

DECISION MAKING

- *What groups in society are stigmatized because of the ways in which they express their sexuality?*
- *How might this knowledge be useful for nurses?*

▶ SOCIOBIOLOGY

Sociobiologists use ideas from evolutionary biology to explain human behaviour and sexual identity. Symons (1979) argues that sexual behaviour is influenced by our biological need to reproduce. People strive to be successful in reproduction so that genetic information can be passed on to the next generation. Sexuality concerns those activities that help achieve this success.

Men have many sperm and it makes sense for men to seek to use as many as they can. This has been given as an explanation for men being more promiscuous than women. Women have relatively few ova, and these being precious, their owners need to make sure that they are used carefully. It is in the interests of women therefore to be selective in whom they chose as a mate. They need to make sure that their genes are amalgamated with others of a high quality. This theory has implications for the development of attitudes. Men should approve of casual sex and have many partners, whereas women should be less approving of casual sex and should seek long-term commitment from a small number of partners. Related to this is the explanation of men's jealousy and desire to control women's sexuality. Because a man provides for the mother and child he needs to make sure that his work is being used to rear his own offspring and not anyone else's. For this reason men would be disapproving of their wives engaging in extramarital sex.

This sociobiological theory has its critics. Travis and Yeager (1991) argue that society is more complex than the picture painted here and sexual behaviour has meanings other than the purely reproductive. For example, the theory does not take into account the developing nature of sex and sexuality throughout an individual's lifespan. Also it attempts to legitimize inequalities between men and women by suggesting that they are natural and normal. This fails to explore the importance of socialization and the use of power in establishing and maintaining gender inequalities.

▶ SOCIAL LEARNING THEORY

This is concerned with the processes through which boys and girls learn their gender-related roles (Mischel, 1966). It does not see biology as particularly important in determining behaviour, but emphasizes the association and interactions between children and others. This is, in the first place, the communication that takes place with parents. Behaviour consistent with gender is reinforced through rewards. So when parents and others react in a positive way towards a girl in a pretty dress playing with dolls and an urchin of a boy climbing trees, this behaviour is likely to be repeated. Initially children look to others for models of behaviour and these can include parents, siblings, teachers and people in the media. This means that learning how to behave as a woman or a man is partly influenced by parental upbringing, but the influence of people and images outside the family explain why children can differ from their parents. This theory is dynamic in that it takes account of an individual's changing nature and incorporates such things as trends and fashions. However, it tends to see people as initially shapeless, waiting to be moulded by the environment and those around them. In this sense, self-will, motivation, and the ability to manipulate the environment and other people, are ignored.

Social learning theory attempts to explain how we learn our culture, that is how we acquire certain patterns of beliefs, values, attitudes and norms. Our culture has a strong impact on sexuality. Different cultures assign different meanings to sexuality. Some emphasize equality between partners, including goals of mutual pleasure and psychological disclosure. Others believe that the exchange of pleasure or communication of affection through sexual touching plays no major role in the expression of sexuality (Monga and Lefebvre, 1995). Some cultures permit premarital sex, while others condemn it. Formal rituals can play an important part in the development of a sexual identity, for example the circumcision of Jewish boys and the practice of female circumcision in some African countries. Nurses need an understanding of these cultural differences so that they can give 'culture-specific' care (Lavee, 1991)

> • Do the theories that attempt to explain the development of an individual's sexual identity have implications for our understanding of the situation where children are raised by a homosexual couple or by single parents?
>
> • How can a nurse ensure that patients receive care that is culture-specific?

▶ NORMS AND SEXUAL BEHAVIOUR

The things we learn from others as well as the forces and pressures that exist in society help us acquire an understanding of what is 'normal', 'right' and 'good' You could argue that we need some clues to help us know what we 'ought' to be doing and thinking in our relationships with others. We pick up these clues during our observations and interactions with others and this socialization process is useful in teaching us social rules. Unfortunately the same process may help us acquire prejudicial attitudes towards individuals or groups.

Norms are the standards of behaviour seen as socially acceptable and may help us define what is morally right. As discovered by Kinsey *et al.* (1948) and Kinsey and Gebhard (1953), the so-called norms of sexual

What is your attitude towards the following?

- *Sex before marriage.*
- *Men having many female sexual partners.*
- *Women having many male sexual partners.*
- *Men having many male sexual partners.*
- *Women having many female sexual partners.*
- *People wearing clothes normally associated with the opposite sex.*
- *Masturbation.*

- *People of the same sex kissing passionately in public.*
- *Anal sex between a man and a woman.*
- *Anal sex between two men.*
- *How does your attitude compare with public attitudes or norms?*
- *How does your attitude compare with those of your colleagues?*
- *How do you think present day attitudes compare with those from the past?*

DECISION MAKING

Michelle is 15 years old. She sees the practice nurse at her general practitioner's surgery for some advice. She has been sexually active for two years and has had a number of partners, most of them being 'one night stands'. Her present partner has been seeing Michelle for two months and they are both wondering about safe sex and contraceptives. They do not like condoms and Michelle wants to discuss alternatives. She asks the practice nurse about oral and anal sex because she knows that these will at least prevent her from becoming pregnant. Michelle is also concerned because she had unprotected sex with a previous partner when she was drunk at a party last weekend.

- *How might the nurse react to Michelle and her situation?*
- *Do you think that there could be some conflict between the nurse and Michelle?*
- *If so, why?*
- *How do you think the practice nurse should handle the situation?*

- *How does society view infidelity or promiscuous behaviour for men?*
- *How does society view infidelity or promiscuous behaviour for women?*
- *How does society view child rearing in a stable heterosexual relationship?*
- *How does society view child rearing in a stable homosexual relationship?*

- *What might society's attitude be towards a 25-year-old man with a sexually transmitted disease?*
- *What might society's attitude be towards an 80-year-old man with the same condition?*
- *Use this exercise as a basis of a group discussion.*

behaviour do not closely match the lived experience of a large proportion of the population. This might be a case of people not acting according to their public beliefs. Turned the other way round it may mean that people feel unable to display attitudes that are faithful to their private and innermost thoughts. Because people have feelings and beliefs that may run contrary to the popular social norms, the discovery of sexual behaviour and the private world of individuals is fraught with difficulties.

There may be differences between expressed social attitudes and private behaviour. Also these public attitudes can include considerable variations, so that groups in society have their own associated norms and appropriate forms of behaviour. Here we have potential for conflict. For example the norms of sexual behaviour held by the youth culture could be very different from those held by parents or by professionals. There is a possibility that people such as parents, teachers, doctors, and nurses will see their own 'standards' as right and impose them on those they feel they have a responsibility for.

There may be inequalities in the way norms are applied to groups within society. For example certain behaviours may be viewed as acceptable for men, but not for women. Similarly the public attitude towards a stable heterosexual couple is likely to differ from that towards a stable homosexual couple.

The differences between norms and actual behaviour are beginning to be uncovered as we find out more about the sexual behaviour and practices people are involved in. There are difficulties with this type of research, for example the range of terms used to describe sexual activity, and the potential unwillingness of respondents to tell the truth, but it might be argued that with sophisticated research methods and with the increasing social acceptance of the subject, people are more open to discuss sexual behaviour. Nevertheless it is worth bearing in mind that the accuracy of research in this area is always open to question because of people's unwillingness or inability to discuss such issues.

▶ *Homosexuality*

The idea of a homosexual identity, in which people attracted to others of the same gender have their own culture and their own lifestyle is a relatively new phenomenon. Gay bars and clubs, newspapers, associations, and holidays have not existed in an organized and overt way for very long. In past centuries individuals were not clearly labelled with a sexual identity that described them as either heterosexual or homosexual. Homosexual activity has always existed, but it was not necessarily seen as exclusive to a specific group of people. In Roman times, for example, it formed part of a range of experiences for some people. Bancroft (1989) describes the development of a gay culture through history, noting varying periods of acceptance and repression of homosexual activity.

In the recent history of developed countries homosexuality has been characterized by its rejection. This has been seen in public attitudes and the prejudice and institutionalized inequalities within the legal frameworks of many countries.

Minority groups are used as scapegoats for things going wrong in society. 'Homosexuals' have been perceived as the minority group responsible for the downfall of the Greek Empire and for the spread of the AIDS virus.

The high incidence of homosexual activity in single-sex restrictive institutions such as prisons, monastic orders and boarding schools and the numbers of people reporting homosexual experiences are viewed as examples of the flexibility of our sexual nature or the fact that we cannot be pigeonholed into clearly definable orientations. The hostility towards homosexuality may be a denial of the 'naturalness' of a mixed sexual identity. Similarly the laws of 'nature' have been used to support hostility towards homosexuality. 'Our bodies are not made for it' is the sort of argument put forward. This relates sexual activity to procreation, and homosexuality therefore has no function. A further explanation for the non-acceptance of homosexuality is its association in history with other types of antisocial behaviour, for example witchcraft and heresy.

The medical profession in the nineteenth century gave a different interpretation of homosexuality from that of the church. Rather than it being a sin, it was seen as a sickness that individuals were either born with or acquired. Treatments were developed to 'cure' homosexuality. The twentieth century saw some ambivalence in medicine's attitude towards homosexuality, but the idea that it was something to treat predominated. It was not until 1974 that the American Psychiatric Association removed homosexuality from its list of pathological diagnoses.

Female homosexuality is written about less frequently and has had a lower profile throughout history. This may not mean that women have been less likely than men to be involved in homosexual activity, but could be a reflection of the domination of women by men across a range of social institutions.

Biological and behavioural sciences tell us something about the development of a sexual identity. Our sexuality seems to be a complex mix of biological, psychological and social factors. After exploring the nature of sexuality and how it develops we need to know how it manifests itself. One of the obvious ways in which we express our sexuality is through sexual relationships and sexual activities. How do people do this and what activities do they participate in? The next section looks at research in this area.

DECISION MAKING

You witness a group of nurses making jokes about a client's homosexuality.

- *How can you explain the nurses behaviour?*
- *How might the client's care be influenced by these nurses' attitudes?*
- *How would you handle this situation?*

❱ *Sexual Behaviour*

Compared with other aspects of people's lives sexual behaviour has received little academic attention. *The National Survey on Sexual Behaviour in Britain* (Wellings *et al.*, 1994) had a difficult start because the Department of Health withdrew its backing at the last minute and the researchers had to find alternative support. The impetus for the work came from the need to find out more about the relationships between sexual practices and the spread of HIV and AIDS, but the social and political sensitivity of the subject meant that the researchers had problems in starting. Similarly Kinsey in the 1940s in the USA (Kinsey *et al.*, 1948) and Lanval (1950) at about the same time in Belgium suffered in their attempts to discover more about sexual behaviour. This type of research was seen as pornographic and not worthy of academic attention. Despite these problems Kinsey persisted, and his findings have been seen as highly significant in developing our understanding of sexual behaviour. Essentially he tried to discover through interviewing over 10 000 people what sexual practices were common, for example how many people masturbated and how many had experienced homosexual activities. It was apparent from the findings that individual's experiences were very different from the official social norms at the time. The reported incidence of homosexuality, masturbation and premarital intercourse, and the active role of women in sexuality differed from what might have been expected and caused some social and political disquiet (Gagnon, 1988).

DECISION MAKING

One of the major findings from Kinsey's research on sexual activity was the difference between the social norms and the actual behaviour of individuals.

- *If this is still true today, what might the implications be for nurses working with problems related to a patient's sexual activity*

❱ *Findings of The National Survey on Sexual Behaviour in Britain (Wellings et al., 1994)*

Wellings *et al.* (1994) is the most extensive study on sexual behaviour in Britain. It was initiated to discover how the spread of AIDS and HIV might be related to certain sexual practices and it therefore concentrates on things like unprotected sex, number of partners and activities involving risks. Because of its broad quantitative nature it tells us little about the meaning of sexual experiences to individuals. It does give details of who does what with whom, at what age and how often, and relates these sorts of things to class and educational level. One of its major drawbacks is its failure to include people over 60 years of age. This perhaps reflects the commonly held view that 'old people don't do that sort of thing'.

Some of the findings are given below.

❱ Heterosexual behaviour (Wellings *et al.*, 1994)

- ❱ Over the last 40 years the median age of first heterosexual intercourse has fallen from 21 to 17 years of age for women and from 20 to 17 years of age for men.
- ❱ Less than 1% of women who were 55 years of age in 1991 reported that it happened before they were 16, compared with nearly 20% of women in their late teens.
- ❱ Early sexual intercourse is associated with lower social class and educational attainment, but this is much weaker than it used to be.
- ❱ First intercourse is now more likely to involve contraceptive equipment (usually the condom) than for previous generations, but the younger first timers are less likely to use contraception than those in their late teens.

▶ First heterosexual intercourse tends to be associated with more planning and less spontaneity than previously, and for the majority this is within an established relationship.

▶ Women tend to have older partners for this experience whereas men have age peers. It rarely occurs for the first time during marriage and it is very rare for a man's first intercourse to be with a prostitute.

Heterosexual partnerships (Wellings *et al.*, 1994)

▶ There are extreme variations in the numbers of partners reported. Young people, divorced people and single people reported the highest numbers and there was a significant trend towards increasing partner change with higher social class.

▶ In general, people appear to be having more partners these days, but this may be clouded by older people's memory difficulties, and their unwillingness to report the facts.

▶ Men tend to have partners younger than themselves, but more than 50% of men were found to have partners within two years of their age.

Heterosexual practices (Wellings *et al.*, 1994)

▶ The frequency of heterosexual sex (oral, anal and vaginal intercourse) varies considerably, with the peak activity occurring in the mid-twenties and then a gradual decline, which is more marked for women.

▶ People in longer relationships reported a lower frequency of heterosexual sex and the decline in activity with age seemed to be associated with this factor rather than other age-related changes.

▶ Vaginal intercourse was the most frequently practised activity.

▶ 70% of people had experienced oral sex (cunnilingus or fellatio) and the evidence suggests an increasing popularity of orogenital contact especially in the younger age group.

▶ An experience of anal intercourse was reported by 13.9% of men and 12.9% of women, and those reporting recent experience tended to be in the younger age groups.

▶ Manual classes were more likely to report anal sex and non-manual classes were more likely to report oral and non-penetrative sex, although these associations are weak.

Homosexual behaviour (Wellings *et al.*, 1994)

▶ 6.1% of men and 3.4% of women reported a homosexual experience in their lifetime and 1.1% of men and 0.4% of women reported having had a homosexual partner that year.

▶ It appeared that homosexual experience was transitory for many and was reported across a wide cross-section of society.

▶ A minority of men reported larger numbers of male partners than those reporting female partners. Also men regularly participating in homosexual anal intercourse did so both as a receptive partner and as a penetrative partner. There was no evidence to suggest that men exclusively adopted one or other role in homosexual practices.

▶ An important finding supported by other studies is the high prevalence of bisexual behaviour. This means that the popular image of being either heterosexual or homosexual is inappropriate and that the classification of people's sexuality is complex.

▶ EMOTIONS AND THE SEXUAL RESPONSE

Webb (1985) believes that many studies on sexual behaviour emphasize the physical aspects and do not tell us much about the social and psychological factors involved. For example what is it that makes things sexually arousing to some people and not to others and how do we explain the desires and attractions between people?

The human sexual response is a complex process and sexual attraction towards others is not easily explained. Emotions are central to these experiences and they can influence and be influenced by the physical aspects of sexual activity. Bancroft (1989) describes the psychosomatic circle of sex, which emphasizes the importance of social and psychological factors in sexual activity and their ability to influence the physiological processes involved.

The evidence on how anxiety may influence the sexual response is not clear, perhaps because of the difficulty in defining anxiety. Also it may be important to distinguish between anxiety generated by the sexual activity itself and anxiety resulting from other sources. Anxiety might be seen to influence sexual responses through a number of mechanisms as follows:

▶ anxiety excites the peripheral autonomic nervous system, which controls important physiological changes associated with sex – as a result the neurological control of vasocongestion of the genitals and of orgasm for example may be affected and this may prevent these changes from occurring, slow them down or speed them up;

▶ anxiety may disrupt thought processes so that erotic stimuli are not perceived – this is equivalent to having something on your mind, making it difficult to concentrate on anything else.

▶ anxiety and the sexual response become associated through past experiences and the individual may subconsciously inhibit sexual responses in order to avoid anxiety, thereby reinforcing the initial anxiety;

▶ anxiety occurs as a reaction to a failure of sexual response.

Bancroft (1989) also discusses the role of anger and mood in influencing the sexual response. Anger may stimulate the sexual response or impair it and this seems to be difficult to explain. Some people are able to be sexually aroused and angry at the same time, but others are not. Sexual response may facilitate anger, but on the other hand a sexual interaction may have a calming affect. Also a failure to respond sexually could generate an angry reaction and an individual's avoidance of sex may be a way of expressing anger.

The relationship between mood and sexual response appears to be less complex, but it has received relatively little investigation. It is easy to appreciate how feeling low or depressed could influence a person's sexual desire or interest in sexual activity. Feeling low leads to more negative thoughts, particularly about oneself, and this generates a low self-esteem. What is not easy to determine is the role sexual dysfunction has in creating the depression in the first place. Also sexual problems and depression may be related to other underlying causes, for example biochemical or hormonal changes.

Spend a few moments thinking about someone you find sexually attractive.

- *What are their characteristics that make you feel this way about them?*
- *Do you know anyone who has the same characteristics, but is not sexually attractive to you?*
- *Are there particular situations or experiences that you find sexually arousing?*
- *Do they always have this effect on you or does sexual arousal depend upon other factors?*

DECISION MAKING

- *What might you need to explore with a client who expresses a fear of intimate sexual contact with his or her partner?*
- *How might your understanding of the relationship between anxiety and the sexual response assist you in helping this client?*

PRACTICE KNOWLEDGE

This section focuses on the inclusion of sexuality in nursing models, communication issues as part of the assessment process, the types of sexuality problems and frameworks for nursing actions.

▶ MODELS OF NURSING

Some models of nursing include explicit definitions of health, and identify the nature of the problems people experience that require nursing assistance. For example Roper *et al.* (1996) focus on the activities of living and the difficulties people may have in carrying them out. Within this model 'expressing sexuality' is seen as an important activity and one that ought to be considered by nurses in all settings with all patients. The activity is very broad and includes sexual activity, gender identity and relationship issues. The model describes the nurse's role in helping people express their sexuality and there is an emphasis on the impact of health conditions and illnesses on this part of people's lives.

Orem's model (1995) has 'self-care' as a central concept and nursing is a helping activity introduced when individuals are having difficulty managing their own 'self-care'. Life is seen as the meeting of a range of needs. Health conditions and illnesses have a direct impact on the types of needs and the skills and knowledge an individual requires to meet them. One of the 'universal needs' relates to 'being normal'. This is obviously a broad concept and it includes ideas on 'reaching one's potential' and living according to social norms and values. Although being less specific than the Roper *et al.* (1996) model, Orem (1995) sees sexual activity and gender identity as important areas of concern for nurses because they are part of 'being normal'.

Other models of nursing tend to be more process orientated. This means that they do not try and define the nature of human problems requiring help. They concentrate on the nature of the activity of nursing and what nurses have to do to help people. Peplau (1988) focuses on the relationship between the nurse and the patient and how this is 'used' to help the patient develop. This relationship moves through a number of stages. Together the patient and nurse identify and explore the patient's problems. They move on to discuss methods for coping with the problems, and end by evaluating what they have both learned, and how they have both developed. The nurse relies on the patient's perceptions, experiences and feelings to identify the nature of the problems to be 'managed'. This model therefore does not explicitly include sexuality as a relevant area of nursing concern. Implicit though is the importance of this aspect of people's lives and how there may be particular problems for some individuals

During your clinical placements, make a point of looking at the assessments of clients.

- *Is sexuality included?*
- *What issues do nurses identify in this part of the assessment?*
- *How well do you think this is carried out?*
- *Ask your colleagues to complete this exercise and compare your results.*

▶ ASSESSING SEXUALITY AND SEXUAL HEALTH

The World Health Organization (1975, p. 6) defines sexual health as '. . . the integration of the somatic, emotional, intellectual, and social aspects of sexual being, in ways that are positively enriching and that enhance personality, communication and love'. This is a positive definition, but being very broad it helps little in our direct work with patients. The Department of Health (1992) in *The Health of the Nation* literature focuses on specific diseases and behaviours as indicators of sexual health, for example the incidence of sexually transmitted diseases including gonorrhoea and HIV, and the number of teenage pregnancies. This is a negative way of viewing sexual health because it emphasizes the 'bad things'. The hidden assumption here is that if we are free from disease and successfully delay pregnancies until late teens or early twenties then we will be sexually healthy. This is a dangerously limited view and like the World Health Organization (1975) definition gives nurses little guide to their work for promoting sexual health in clients. A similar emphasis on prevention rather than promotion has been evident in a number of sections within the health service in the UK, for example family planning clinics and genitourinary medicine clinics. Although providing very important services it could be argued that these departments are unable to have much impact on the broader view of sexual health for individuals. This broader view includes feelings about one's sexual self and the maintenance and development of enriching relationships.

Discussing Sensitive Issues

Sexuality is a sensitive subject and it may be for this reason that nurses regularly fail to address it with patients (Webb, 1988; Smook, 1992; Matocha and Waterhouse, 1993; Gamel *et al.*, 1993; Lewis and Bor, 1994).

Like many aspects of human interpersonal activity there is no easy guide to instruct nurses on how to manage conversations about sexuality. It has been argued that nurses face serious ethical issues by even considering that such conversations are theirs to be managed (Batcup and Thomas, 1994). Take for example a client who has a health problem that the nurse feels could be seriously affecting his or her sexuality. If the client says nothing about the way he or she feels about him or herself or does not 'admit' to any such sexuality problem does the nurse have a duty to 'dig deeper' on the understanding that it may be the client's embarrassment that prevents him or her from telling the truth? If the nurse does this is the nurse in danger of setting the agenda and putting ideas into the client's mind? By asking specific questions the nurse can demonstrate to the client that it is legitimate to talk about issues related to sexuality or sexual activity. On the other hand, the questions could lead the client to consider aspects of their lives in detail, and begin to see 'new' problems. For example 'Does the pain affect your sex life?' implies that the client ought to have a sex life and suggests that a sex life might normally be affected by such pain. This type of question could lead the client along a line of discussion they had not previously considered. Sociologists have described this management of the conversation as a form of professional control, with the nurse exerting power over the patient (Foucault, 1973).

Language

One of the difficulties in conversations on delicate or sensitive subjects is deciphering the true meaning. The nurse will sometimes need to take the lead and make sure that there is a mutual understanding. This will involve exploration and clarification.

RESEARCH BASED EVIDENCE

There is a danger with the type of questions asked and the way in which they are asked during conversations with patients on sex and sexuality. Weijts et al. *(1993)* investigated such conversations between doctors and patients during gynaecological outpatient appointments. They uncovered tactics used by both the patient and the doctor to avoid and delay discussions on sex. The research highlighted three common themes during these conversations: delaying, avoiding and 'tuning in'.

Delaying

Concerns and worries about sex tended to creep into conversations at the last minute, either as a result of the doctor or patient raising the issue. This left very little time to discuss matters thoroughly. On occasions the doctors blocked discussions when patients attempted to talk about sex. A short-term delaying tactic during the conversations was the tendency to hesitate immediately before a delicate word or topic. This hesitation announces to the listener that the item to be introduced is delicate and embarrassing. For example 'Are you having any problems with .....errrr.......intercourse' may send a hidden message to the patient that intercourse is a delicate subject and one that the patient must also handle with some

tact and 'delicacy'. There was also a tendency for doctors to be aware of the patient's hesitations and on occasions to finish off the patient's sentence. Sometimes the patient's hesitations resulted from an uncertainty about the words to use to describe their specific worries.

Avoidance

The doctors used a number of ways of avoiding sensitive or delicate subjects:

- first, there was the use of vague terms such as 'down below' and 'marital relations';
- second, delicate terms were simply omitted, for example 'the pain that you get is it during or afterwards'?
- third, there was a tendency to use pronouns and adverbs once terms had been introduced and understood early in the conversation and this could become quite difficult as the doctor might use 'it' several times in one sentence to refer to more than one thing – here is an excerpt from one conversation with a patient discussing painful intercourse: 'You should think over with your husband whether its a technical problem. Maybe it's a little too narrow or very tough or may be the

problem is that you just don't feel like having it';
- fourth, the conversations were frequently depersonalized by the doctor as the subjects and terms used were made abstract and distant, giving the impression that although they were discussing sensitive and delicate issues, the conversations were not really about the patient sitting in front of him or her, but about hypothetical cases and the problems of the 'generalized other', for example 'How is the penis?' 'How do the breasts feel now? and 'Do the tablets have any effect on the sex life?'

Tuning

The researchers described the doctors attempts at being on the patient's wavelength as a process of 'tuning', and this involved adopting the patient's language and style of speech during conversations on sexual issues. A doctor would use a patient's terminology as a way of encouraging a deeper exploration of the issues. Similarly if the patient avoided certain explicit terminology the doctor would mirror this as a way of showing a sensitive respect for the patient's difficulty with these words or phrases.

Using the client's language and terminology may help the nurse and client feel at ease with some of these delicate subjects. However, there is still a danger that, despite using the same words, there is not a mutual understanding. The use of 'proper' or medical terms can also be misunderstood and can act as a barrier in the conversation. Using slang or colloquial terms may be at odds with the client's perception of a professional nurse and can present as patronizing or condescending. The way to proceed is to be open with the client about the difficulties with terminology and to agree to use words you are comfortable with and ones that you both understand.

DECISION MAKING

Look at the statements below. For each identify the range of possible meanings, would you assume one particular meaning? and how could you check with a client exactly what is meant?

- '**We no longer sleep together**'.
- '**I can't stand her anywhere near me now**'.
- '**I haven't had a relationship since it happened**'.
- '**Since the operation I can't stand him to see my bits and pieces**'.
- '**I'm not the man I used to be**'.
- '**I got around a bit in my younger days**'.
- '**The tablets have stopped me from getting it up**'.

▶ Essential communication skills in assessing problems related to client's sexuality

These include:

- using silence to allow the client to talk;
- listening to what the client says and does not say, being aware of and sensitive to the way he or she expresses ideas, picking up clues and hints;
- reflecting the client's ideas by repeating and paraphrasing their words;
- clarifying the meaning behind statements, making sure that you both understand things in the same way;

- interpreting the client's words to uncover the significance of events and explore the hidden feelings and meanings in the conversation;
- focusing on certain topics as a way of encouraging and guiding patients to discuss areas of their concern.

> Specific suggestions for initiating conversations on sexuality with clients

These include:

- 'Has 'anything' (e.g. a recent experience, illness, operation) affected your relationships with people close to you?'
- 'Tell me about your partnership/relationship/marriage.'
- 'How do you feel about yourself as a woman/man/wife/husband/partner/mother/father?'
- 'Has your illness/operation/being in hospital changed the way you feel about yourself?'
- 'Has your illness/operation/being in hospital affected your sex life?'
- 'How are things between you and your partner?'
- 'Some of the tablets you are taking can affect aspects of your sex life. Have you noticed anything?'

Potential Problems Related to Clients' Sexuality

Nurses will need to consider clients' sexuality across the spectrum of health care settings. This means that the way sexuality becomes part of an assessment will depend upon the nature of the client's presenting health conditions.

Sexuality can be an issue as:

- the client's primary reason for referral;
- a problem secondary to another health condition;
- a problem arising from difficulties coping with normal developmental changes.

> Sexuality as a primary problem

Primary problems with sexuality include:

- difficulties with sexual activities or relationships;
- unfulfilling sexual activity;
- antisocial or inappropriate sexual behaviour;
- fertility problems;
- contraceptive difficulties.

These kinds of problems usually require the input of a specialist nurse. In some cases clients will raise these problems with 'generic' nurses, for example practice nurses, health visitors or community psychiatric nurses. It is important for these staff to be aware of the specialist services available, for example sex therapists, psychosexual counsellors, fertility clinics and family planning clinics.

▶ Sexuality problems secondary to other health conditions

Most nurses will be concerned with these types of sexuality problems. Since there are many diseases, illnesses and health conditions that can affect an individual's sexuality, the potential for nurses in this area is massive. Sexuality is a complex blend of physical, psychological and social factors. It is not always possible to identify the cause and effect relationship between illness and sexuality problems. For example a client with diabetes mellitus might have a low self-esteem. He might also have difficulties obtaining and maintaining an erection. It would be difficult to judge just how the diabetes mellitus, the low self-esteem and the erectile dysfunction interrelate in terms of cause and effect. Physiological changes could cause the erectile dysfunction, which in turn could cause a low self-esteem. On the other hand the diagnosis of diabetes mellitus could induce feelings of poor self-worth, which in turn could generate

Type of health condition	Sexuality-related problems
Musculoskeletal conditions	Sexual activity Body image Work and leisure activities Dressing and hygiene
Cardiovascular and respiratory conditions	Energy levels Breathing Body image Emotional state Male and female sexual response
Neurological conditions	Sensations Movement and coordination Male and female sexual response Libido
Endocrine and hormonal conditions	Libido Male and female sexual response Body image Growth and development The onset of puberty
Skin conditions	Body image Sensations Emotional state
Genitourinary conditions	Male and female sexual response Body image Libido Choice of clothing
Mental health problems	Self-concept Body image Libido Male and female sexual response Work and leisure activities Interpersonal relationships
Learning disabilities	Relationship skills The development of socially acceptable sexual behaviour Emotional state Work and leisure activities Vulnerability to sexual abuse Self-concept

Table 4.3.1 Sexuality-related problems sometimes associated with certain types of health conditions.

erectile dysfunction. Sexuality problems that coexist alongside physical ill-health can therefore be difficult to understand.

Table 4.3.1 lists the sexuality-related problems that are sometimes associated with types of health conditions. The list is not exhaustive, but gives an indication of some of the problems to consider when working with clients.

▌ Medications and sexual function

A number of medications have potential side effects on sexual activity and some of these are listed in Table 4.3.2. Nurses assessing clients' problems need to be aware of these side effects and will need to give advice on them when helping clients develop regimens for managing their medications. This advice will enable clients to make fully informed decisions about the benefits and disadvantages of medications (Holzapfel, 1994; Burns-Cox and Gingell, 1995).

The list given in Table 4.3.2 is not exhaustive. It is possible that many clients taking prescribed medications experience side effects that affect their sexuality and sexual activity. As well as this, alcohol and nicotine are known to contribute to impotence. It is therefore important to find out about clients' medications and their use of leisure drugs.

Type of medication	Drug	Side effects on sexual activity
Diuretics (e.g. used for patients with heart failure)	Thiazides	Erectile dysfunction Decreased libido
	Spironolactone	Erectile dysfunction Decreased libido Gynaecomastia (enlargement of male breast)
Beta-blockers (e.g. used for patients with high blood pressure and patients with anxiety)		Erectile dysfunction
Sympatholytics (e.g. used for patients with high blood pressure)	Methyldopa	Erectile dysfunction Ejaculatory failure
	Prazosin	Erectile dysfunction Retrograde ejaculation in patients with benign prostatic enlargement
Antidepressants	Tricyclics and monoamine oxidase inhibitors	Erectile dysfunction Ejaculatory failure
Antipsychotics	Phenothiazines	Erectile dysfunction
Anxiolytics	Benzodiazepines	Erectile dysfunction
Cytotoxics		Amenorrhoea Decreased sperm count
Antihistamines		Decreased vaginal lubrication Erectile dysfunction
Glucocorticosteroids		Weight gain Changed fat distribution

Table 4.3.2 Potential side effects of medications on sexual activity.

▷ Sexuality and normal developmental changes

People can experience difficulties in managing and coming to terms with normal developmental changes. Nurses have an important role in helping individuals understand these changes and also in offering support and practical advice on how these changes can be managed. For example, school nurses are in an ideal position to help children understand the changes experienced during puberty and adolescence. These changes are physical, psychological and social, and nurses can explore issues such as menstruation, nocturnal emissions ('wet dreams'), masturbation, sexual relationships, safe sex, contraception, social roles and becoming an adult. Because these subjects are still surrounded by myth and taboo, there is a risk that children can grow up misinformed. This misinformation can result in a lack of awareness in the practical management of some of these changes. Also it can lead to the acquisition of uncomfortable and unhealthy attitudes and behaviours such as guilt and repression, and these can affect individuals for the rest of their lives.

Other developmental changes require individuals to adapt and readjust. In many cases these changes have an impact on sexual identity and sexual activity. For example menopause can be associated with dryness of the vagina. Women can experience problems coping with this physical change. Also around this time, children leave home and middle-aged adults might be involved in caring for ageing parents. As a result of decreasing androgen production in the late forties or early fifties, men experience less firm erections and an increased refractory period. At the same time men and women can be involved in important career decisions and planning retirement. These physical and social changes require psychological and behavioural adjustment. People having difficulties making the necessary adjustments can develop a low self-esteem and a negative body image. These can have a direct impact on the quality of relationships, sexual identity and sexual activity.

▷ NURSING ACTIONS

Clients present with a wide range of problems related to sexuality. Also, clients are individuals and their experience of these problems will be unique. Consequently, it is impossible to describe appropriate nursing actions in detail here since a full assessment is required in order to plan care. Nevertheless there are guidelines to help nurses plan appropriate care. Annon (1974) describes levels of intervention using the P-LI-SS-IT model:

- P, permission;
- LI, limited information;
- SS, specific suggestions;
- IT, intensive therapy.

Permission

This is when the nurse openly acknowledges to the client that sexuality is a legitimate issue for discussion. This means that the nurse must be seen to be willing to discuss sexuality, either by asking specific questions or by allowing and encouraging clients to raise the issue themselves. This says to the client that it is within the nurse's role to discuss sexuality and also that it is 'normal', usual and OK for clients to have concerns or problems related to their sexuality.

Limited Information

This next stage requires the nurse to give explanations, facts or reasons about why the client might be having the sexuality problem. Obviously the nurse must have sufficient knowledge and experience to understand and interpret sexuality problems. Also this demands communication and teaching skills so that explanations can be understood and remembered. This level of intervention enables the client to make sense of the problems, and gives him or her the opportunity to consider ways of resolving or improving the situation. This stage might involve the nurse helping the client to correct any misconceptions or dispel any myths surrounding sexuality.

Specific Suggestions

A client having difficulty resolving his or her own problems is likely to need specific guidance or advice. This means that the nurse must draw on research and previous experience to make practical, acceptable and realistic suggestions. The nurse must assess the client's abilities, knowledge and attitudes so that appropriate suggestions are made. Some suggestions could involve referral to other agencies. The nurse must be aware of the range of specialist services available, the nature of the services provided and the appropriate reasons for referral so that the client can decide how to proceed.

Intensive Therapy

This level is usually beyond the skills of the 'generic' nurse. Clients and partners can be involved in a programme of sessions to instruct, coach and demonstrate ways of overcoming the particular sexual problem. This could focus for example on relationship and communication difficulties between partners on alternative ways of 'pleasuring' or sexual expression between partners or on medical and surgical interventions to treat or improve the sexual response.

Like Annon's model (Annon, 1974), Webb (1985) outlines a number of roles for nurses in their work with clients' sexuality problems. These are as:

- facilitator – the nurse encourages the client to open up and discuss sexuality using a non-judgmental approach;

DECISION MAKING

Think about a client you have worked with recently who had a sexuality problem.
- *Using Annon's (1974) and Webb's (1985) ideas above, identify the levels of intervention and the roles adopted by the nurses in caring for this patient.*
- *Could the nurses have worked at other levels or adopted other roles as ways of improving the care to this patient?*

- validator – the nurse helps to dispel misunderstandings about sexual activity and perceptions of 'normality' and it is emphasized that acceptable sexual practices are those that participants enjoy and freely consent to;
- teacher – the nurse uses a range of teaching skills to pass on information;
- counsellor – the nurse uses listening and counselling skills to enable the client to explore his or her own sexuality;
- advocate – the nurse supports and encourages clients to make their own fully informed decisions about treatment and care;
- referral agent – the nurse gives advice on other services available and discusses appropriate referrals with the client.
- specialist sex therapist – the specialist nurse is experienced in assessing complex sexual problems and can provide a range of specific interventions to solve these problems.

PROFESSIONAL KNOWLEDGE

This section has three parts:

- nursing as a female profession;
- information specific to the four branches of nursing;
- an outline of key legal issues related to nursing and clients' sexuality.

NURSING AS A FEMALE PROFESSION

The concepts of masculinity and femininity are especially important for nursing because the profession itself is associated very strongly with being feminine. This has implications for men in nursing, and also for women in nursing wanting to move into areas traditionally associated with masculine characteristics, for example management and positions of leadership. In a broader context the feminine characteristics have been used to explain the subservient role of nursing in the political hierarchy of health care professions (Versluysen, 1980). Because nursing is viewed by many as a female profession and women are often seen as subservient, nurses as a group command little political power (Salvage, 1995). What is beginning to be touched upon here is the political nature of gender and sexuality. The descriptions of femininity and masculinity indicate the traditional views of the differences between men and women. These views are arguably not 'neutral' because some characteristics are seen as more important for society and consequently attract higher social prestige and status. This is evident in the health service where medicine maintains power and prestige and is still seen as a male profession. Male nurses and female doctors as exceptions to these stereotypical images might be viewed with suspicion in some clinical areas. Also the day to day working relationships between doctors and nurses can be influenced by these gender politics (Stein, 1976).

DECISION MAKING

- *How could the working relationship between a male doctor and a female nurse be affected by their genders?*
- *How could this relationship influence patient care?*
- *Taking into account male and female nurses and male and female patients, identify specific situations in which sexuality and gender might adversely affect the nurse/patient interaction and the care given?*
- *Identify potential situations in which gender relationships could lead to an abuse of power by a nurse over a patient.*
- *What would you do if a patient refused to be seen by you because of your gender?*

Nurses must also be aware of the potential effects of their own gender on patients. Nursing often involves intimate activities. Patients are required to expose their bodies and to be touched in sensitive, sometimes erogenous zones. Many of these activities are normally only associated with sexual encounters. This can result in embarrassing situations for the patient and the nurse, and both can use a range of strategies to diffuse or cope with this embarrassment (Lawler, 1991). These situations can be compounded by the gender mix between the patient and the nurse. For example, a male nurse washing the genitals of a male patient could generate a range of thoughts and feelings for both parties, some of which might be uncomfortable and difficult to deal with.

▶ INFORMATION SPECIFIC TO THE FOUR BRANCHES OF NURSING

▶ *Adult Nursing*

Staff working in this branch need to be aware of the relationship between sexuality and ageing. The degenerative changes associated with ageing can affect sexual desire and response. For example a decrease in circulating androgens will lower libido, and changes in neurological and vascular systems can affect sensation and response. These changes may not be important for some people, but many of these potential problems can be overcome by practical advice and medical intervention. These physiological changes do not in themselves prevent older people from having an active and pleasurable sex life and research suggests that sexual activity plays an important part in people's lives well into old age (Bretschneider and McCoy, 1988).

Decline in sexual activity in older people is perhaps more to do with demographic and social factors than a decrease in ability or desire. (Diokno *et al.*, 1990). Many older people are widows or widowers. They have fewer social contacts and their chances of meeting a new partner are reduced. Also the attitudes that youth is beautiful and that older people should not be sexually active may force older people to believe that they are no longer sexually attractive and that it is not right for them to have sexual desires. Comfort and Dial (1991) suggest that 'most of our aged stop having sex for reasons similar to those why they stop riding a bicycle; general infirmity, fear that it would expose them to ridicule, and for most, lack of a bicycle'.

▶ *Learning Disabilities Nursing*

A key concept to consider in caring for clients with learning disabilities is consent. If there are doubts about an individual's knowledge or level of understanding, then any sexual activities he or she is involved in could constitute abuse. This judgement of the ability to consent is difficult, but rests on a consideration of the individual's cognitive functioning and ability to assert his or her wishes in pressured situations (Gunn, 1991). This will have implications for nurses, in particular how such a judgement is reached and how clients can be helped to gain the appropriate knowledge and skills (Sundram and Stavis, 1994).

A central issue here is deciding what we mean by appropriate knowledge and skills. If a client expresses a desire to wear clothes normally worn by the opposite sex should nurses discourage this or should nurses help the client to understand, promote and actively enjoy his or her chosen cross-dressing identity? On the one hand nurses might aim to encourage client decision making and choice, but on the other hand aim to help clients develop attitudes and behaviour that allows for a degree of integration in the 'community'. The difficulty in this case is that such an expression of sexuality may prevent what is usually understood as social integration. There may, however, be a 'cross-dressing community' into which the client can integrate, but this may prove difficult because of the client's level of social skills or the stigma associated with learning disabilities. With regards to consent and choice nurses may have to consider whether it is appropriate for clients to make decisions about some aspects of their lives, but not others. Like many other aspects of learning disabilities nursing there is a danger that nurses might impose their norms of sexuality, overtly or covertly, and restrict the client's potential.

McCarthy and Thompson (1995) identify how staff's norms and attitudes have led to restrictive practices in relation to the sexuality of people with learning disabilities, to the extent that help and guidance has failed to take into account recent changes in attitudes towards sexuality in the community at large. For example same-sex relationships are 'pathologized' and discouraged, women are seen to have a passive role in sexual activity, and cross-dressing can be prevented by promoting heterosexual relationships. Carr (1995) suggests the following important points for nurses dealing with the sexuality of adults with learning disabilities:

▶ sociosexual education is vital because of people's vulnerability in the community;

▶ a sociosexual educator needs to liaise closely with parents and other professionals as a way of sharing knowledge and reducing unnecessary anxiety;

▶ a sociosexual educator needs to understand the legal implications of carrying out this role to protect all individuals concerned – this relates in particular to the teaching methods used to help people develop appropriate skills and how practical demonstrations and client participation for subjects like masturbation and the management of menstruation might be interpreted as assault.

▶ *Children's Nursing*

Illness can intrude in the development of a child's sexuality. A variety of endocrine conditions as well as some chronic illnesses can directly affect growth and physiological development to the extent that puberty is delayed or absent. Similarly chronic illness in childhood can influence exposure to the social and psychological experiences that seem to be important in the development of sexual identity. Smith (1993) and Hakalkse and Mian (1993) identify a number of factors influencing normal sexual development in children as follows:

▶ the involvement of an adult same-sex role model in the child's immediate environment;

▶ witnessing displays of affection between others (touch and language);

▶ receiving comforting touch and praise that result in feelings of trust and security;

▶ exploring one's own body and being allowed to gain pleasure from it (e.g. through masturbation);

▶ learning that your body is your property and that others need your permission to touch it;

▶ learning appropriate levels of privacy related to the body, in a way that prevents a feeling of guilt;

▶ learning about other's needs for privacy;

▶ encouraging a child's curiosity about gender and sexuality, giving open and honest answers appropriate to the child's level of understanding;

▶ having opportunities for play with peers of the same and of the opposite sex;

- being free to participate in gender-based play;
- being free to participate in mutually agreed private sexual play with peers;
- learning about physical changes during puberty;
- learning that sex is 'good, natural and healthy'.

Adolescence is characterized by experimentation, rebellion and risk-taking behaviour. There are obvious risks in relation to unwanted pregnancies, sexually transmitted diseases and emotional trauma during this stage of development. A healthy sexual development should include an understanding of rights, responsibilities and relationships as well as the mechanics of sexual activity. This has implications for nurses in many areas, particularly those in primary health care, school nursing, and health education and promotion.

Mental Health Nursing

The interrelationship between sexuality and mental health is complex. There is a two-way relationship in which problems in expressing sexuality can seriously affect an individual's self-concept. Also, low self-esteem and anxiety can intrude into personal relationships affecting libido and sexual function. This relationship can become a vicious circle, with low self-esteem limiting sexual expression, which further reduces self-esteem. In this situation the client can feel out of control.

Ferguson (1994) discusses the relationship between sexuality and mental health and stresses the significance of social, political and financial forces as determinants of this relationship. Sexuality incorporates the idea of social roles and social norms, and in order to express 'masculinity' or 'femininity' within our society there is an expectation of people to adopt gender-specific attitudes and behaviour. This is where the nurse can be caught in a trap because he or she might see it as valuable to help the client fit back into these social roles as a way of regaining self-esteem and control. On the other hand it could be argued that the roles in themselves are 'pathological' because of the associated stresses and inequalities. Does the nurse in these types of cases strive to help the client conform or challenge these social roles to help the client adopt a new perspective? There is a problem when the origins of mental ill-health are located not so much in the individual, but in the organization and structure of society. As an example, Ferguson (1994) outlines how differences in the patterns and types of mental illness experienced by men and women are more a product of social forces than genetic makeup. This has implications for the role of the nurse and suggests that as well as having an individual focus, nursing should be involved in social and community action as a way of addressing social forces and social inequalities.

Other important issues in this relationship between sexuality and mental health are:

- the function of assertiveness and communication within personal relationships and how inability in these areas may lead to feelings of low self-esteem;
- the impact mental illness can have on personal relationships, in particular on the expression of intimacy within relationships;
- the function of the psychiatric services in defining, monitoring and treating sexual deviance, and their social role in maintaining the stigmas surrounding certain sexual practices.

DECISION MAKING

How do you think each of the following key areas in law might relate to the care of clients with sexuality problems and what is the relevance of each of these areas for the four branches of nursing?
- *Employment and equal opportunities.*
- *Sex discrimination.*
- *Family.*
- *Child care.*
- *Reproduction.*
- *Abortion.*
- *Sexual deviance.*
- *Sexual abuse.*
- *Assault and rape.*
- *Gross indecency.*
- *Consent.*
- *Confidentiality.*
- *Privacy.*

◗ the potential for therapeutic relationships between clients and professionals to develop into relationships involving inappropriate sexual expression – this can create difficulties for clients and staff and needs to be handled openly and sensitively;

◗ the balance required between the client's right to sexual expression and the need to protect vulnerable clients from exploitation – this will be an important issue for nursing and care staff working in homes for people with long-term serious mental health problems.

◗ LAW AND SEXUALITY

Sexuality is central to an individual's life. It influences a wide range of thoughts, feelings and behaviours. Because of this, the relationship between the law and sexuality is wide ranging. It is beyond the scope of this chapter to cover the legal aspects of sexuality in any detail. It is, however, important for you at this stage to be aware of the areas of law that might need to be considered by nurses across a range of settings. For a more detailed introduction to these areas see Dimond (1995).

▶ SELF-AWARENESS

This chapter has explored the meaning of sexuality and has identified its relevance for nursing practice. The reflective exercises throughout the chapter will help you consolidate your knowledge of sexuality and in particular will help you consider your own attitudes to this important aspect of human life. Self-awareness is essential if nurses are to address sexuality with patients.

Brash (1990) believes that in order for nurses to be able to work with patients and sexuality they need to have an understanding about themselves and their own sexual health. This includes an awareness of our feelings about our sexual self and knowledge of the ways in which we can develop our sexuality. There is an implication here that nurses need to be role models for sexual health. Although there are obvious problems with this idea, Brash's suggestion that nurses need to have self-awareness seems to make sense. She describes a model of sexual health that nurses could use to enhance this self-awareness as well as a framework for understanding patients and their sexuality (Table 4.3.3).

> Set aside 30 minutes. Using Brash's framework (Brash, 1990) shown in Table 4.3.3 consider your own sexual health.

Brash has a particular interest in sex, marital and relationship therapy and her emphasis is on sexual activity and ways of improving people's sex lives. She gives detailed suggestions for becoming more sexually fulfilled as follows:

▶ give yourself and your partner regular time and attention and set time aside for planning enjoyable experiences;
▶ look after your body physically and make sure you obtain adequate rest and nourishment;
▶ be sexually creative and encourage experimentation;
▶ tune in to your own and your partner's likes and dislikes;
▶ enjoy your mind and imagination through sexual fantasy – it may not be necessary to act out this fantasy, but sharing your thoughts with your partner can increase pleasure.

Brash's ideas emphasize sexual activity and its contribution to health in general. They can be used as a basis for assessing the impact of a health problem on a patient's sexuality.

DECISION MAKING

How could Brash's ideas (see Table 4.3.3; Brash, 1990) assist in your assessment of the following people?
- *A man with impotence resulting from diabetes mellitus.*
- *A woman who had a mastectomy six weeks ago.*
- *A man being treated for alcohol dependency in an inpatient unit.*
- *A woman with learning disabilities in the early stages of her first sexual relationship.*

REFLECTIVE KNOWLEDGE

Statement of sexual health	Questions to ask yourself
I know and accept my sexual self and my body as OK	Do I like my body? Does it give me pleasure? Am I attractive? Do I know what happens to my body during sexual stimulation? Do I know how aspects of my life have or are likely to affect my sexual self, for example puberty, adolescence, middle age, pregnancy, menopause, old age? What have been my most and least satisfying sexual experiences? What are my sexual needs? Am I able to articulate and communicate these needs?
I have chosen a sexual lifestyle that fits and satisfies me	Am I happy with the lifestyle I have chosen? Is it compatible with my needs and desires? Are there pressures that make me choose certain things? Am I happy with these pressures?
I am sexually assertive	Can I ask for what I want? Can I say no if I am not ready or do not want sexual activity? Can I negotiate with my partner on sexual issues?
I am free to express both my masculine and feminine sides	Can I be active and passive? Am I able to give and receive pleasure? Are my sexual relationships flexible and not confined by traditional stereotypical behaviour?
I am sexually competent and sexually responsible	Can I combine the above skills to achieve a satisfying lifestyle? Am I able to recognize and face sexual difficulties? Do I know the sorts of things that can cause sexual difficulties, for example unresolved anger between couples, depression, medications, stress, repressed feelings from childhood? Is my behaviour safe for me and my partners? Do I show respect for my partners? Is my judgement on sexual issues affected by drugs or alcohol? Do I encourage open and honest discussion with my partners? Do I respect my partner's confidentiality?

Table 4.3.3 Brash's model of sexual health. From Brash, K.C. (1990) Toward a model of sexual health for nurses. *Holistic Nursing Practice* **4**(4): 62–69. © 1990, Aspen Publishers, Inc.

▶ CASE STUDIES

Four case studies follow, one for each branch of nursing. Use the information in the chapter to help you answer the questions.

▶ CASE STUDY: ADULT

Mrs Ellis is a resident in a private nursing home. She is 75 years old and has been a widow for ten years. Despite having severe osteoarthritis in her knees and hips she sees herself as relatively fit. She is mentally alert and enjoys mixing with other residents, especially during meal times and organized social events. She has early signs of heart failure, which prevents her from having surgery for her arthritis and also makes her feel tired and 'out of sorts' at times. She requires assistance with dressing, personal hygiene and going to the toilet, but is able to move around the home independently in her wheelchair. She has made a close association with a man in the home and they spend time together most afternoons.

■ **How might Mrs Ellis' age and disability affect the way she sees herself as a woman?**

■ **What would your reaction be if you were Mrs Ellis' primary nurse and she said she would like to develop the relationship with her friend into a sexual one?**

■ **What are the potential problems with confidentiality and what should Mrs Ellis' primary nurse do to maintain confidentiality?**

▶ CASE STUDY: LEARNING DISABILITIES

John Brown is 26 years of age and has moderate learning disabilities. He lives at home with his parents and visits a day centre every day where he participates in a social skills training programme, which is partly organized by a community nurse. The nurse discovers from the day centre staff that John regularly visits a local public toilet to participate in homosexual activities. This emerged at a day centre group meeting when another of the service users, who openly admits to visiting the same toilets, said he had seen John there.

John is usually withdrawn and initiates little conversation or interaction with people at the day centre. He has a close relationship with the nurse, but is reluctant to talk about his sexual activities with anyone. John is not used to making decisions in his life and has everything organized for him by his parents. Generally the staff see John as an inoffensive young man who creates no fuss in the day centre because on the whole he does as he is told.

■ **Supposing the claim about John's sexual behaviour is true, Is this behaviour 'normal' in society?**

■ **Should the nurse be concerned about this behaviour? Why or why not?**

■ **Do you think the nurse should do anything and if so, what?**

■ **How do you think John's parents might react if they discovered what he was doing?**

■ **Do you think John's parents have a right to know?**

▶ CASE STUDY: CHILD

Susan Jones is 15 years old and has cystic fibrosis. This is a hereditary condition affecting a number of body systems. The respiratory system produces large amounts of thick, sticky sputum, breathlessness can be particularly disabling, and the illness is likely to lead to a premature death. Susan needs oxygen therapy much of the time and requires regular physiotherapy to keep her chest clear. Like other children with this condition, Susan's physical development has been retarded and she is short for her age and underweight.

Susan lives at home with her parents and 12-year-old sister. She has missed a lot of school over the last year and although a couple of friends visit on occasions she has lost touch with her peer group. Her parents are very caring and worry about her repeated chest infections. They believe that the infections flare up after Susan has had friends around and as a result they discourage too many visitors.

■ **How might Susan's ill-health have affected her self-concept?**

■ **Adolescence is a crucial time for the development of a sexual identity. What important aspects of adolescence might Susan have missed out on?**

■ **How could a community nurse promote the development of Susan's sexual identity?**

▶ CASE STUDY: MENTAL HEALTH

David Anderson is a 35-year-old single man who lives alone in his new four-bedroom detached house on the outskirts of a large city. He has been admitted to an acute admission ward in a psychiatric hospital suffering from severe depression. He has recently split up from his partner of six months and the advertising business he owns is struggling, to the extent that he is considering laying off staff. His career has been all-consuming and David has never been one for 'getting married and settling down'. He has had a number of short-term relationships over the last ten years and he explains the breakdown of his recent relationship as mainly his fault. He has not been interested in sex and 'found it difficult to perform these days'.

■ **How might recent events be contributing to the way David feels about himself?**

■ **Describe the possible relationship between David's lifestyle and his sexual difficulties.**

■ **As David's primary nurse what could you do to help him regain his ability to express his sexuality?**

▶ FINALLY

- ■ Have you been surprised by anything in this chapter?

- ■ Has anything in the chapter challenged your attitudes in any way?

- ■ How do you feel about incorporating sexuality into your practice with patients?

- ■ Are there any aspects of sexuality you feel uncomfortable with?

▶ ANNOTATED FURTHER READING

AGGLETON. P. (1996) *A Compendium of Family Planning Service Provision for Young People*. London. Health Education Authority.

This short text provides a regional breakdown of services for young people. It is a useful resource for discovering what is available in your area (in the UK). The services included are advice and counselling on contraception, termination of pregnancy, sexually transmitted diseases and a full range of sexual issues likely to affect young people.

ENGLISH NATIONAL BOARD FOR NURSING AND MIDWIFERY (1996) *Caring for People with Sexually Transmitted Diseases Including HIV Disease*. London. The Board.

This open learning pack is designed to help nurses, midwives and health visitors involved in the care, management and education of people with sexually transmitted disease. The first four sections are general in approach and are useful for all nurses caring for clients with sexuality-related problems. These sections include discussions of sexuality and health and ways of working with clients.

TALLMER, M. (1996) *Questions and Answers about Sex in Later Life*. Philadelphia. Charles Press.

A short but readable text that attempts to dispel some of the myths surrounding sexuality and older people. It is based on the author's counselling experience and uses case histories and research to illustrate the importance of sexuality in later life. Its question and answer format gives the text a practical and matter of fact approach. It would be useful for anyone working with older people.

WATERHOUSE, J. (1996) Nursing practice related to sexuality. *Nursing Times Research* **1(6)**: 412–418.

A comprehensive review of mainly American literature on sexuality and nursing practice. It confirms the view that sexuality as an aspect of people's lives receives little attention from nurses. The article is a useful source of research ideas and it makes suggestions for future practice and education.

▶ REFERENCES

ANNON, J.S. (1974) *The Behavioural Treatment of Sexual Problems*. Honolulu. Enabling Systems.

ATKINSON, R.L., ATKINSON, R.C., SMITH, E.E., BEM, D.J., HILGARD, E.R. (1990) *Introduction to Psychology* (10th edition). Orlando. Harcourt Brace Jovanovich.

BANCROFT, J. (1989) *Human Sexuality and Its Problems*. Edinburgh. Churchill Livingstone.

BATCUP, D., THOMAS, B. (1994) Mixing the genders, an ethical dilemma; how nursing theory has dealt with sexuality and gender. *Nursing Ethics* **1(1)**: 43–52.

BEECHEY, V. (1987) *Unequal Work*. London. Verso.

BOONE, T.B. (1995) The physiology of sexual function in normal adults. *Physical Medicine and Rehabilitation: State of the Art Reviews* **9(2)**: 313–322.

BRASH, K.C. (1990) Toward a model of sexual health for nurses. *Holistic Nursing Practice* **4(4)**: 62–69.

BRETSCHNEIDER, J., McCOY, N. (1988) Sexual interest and behaviour in healthy 80- to 102-year-olds. *Archives of Sexual Behaviour* **17**: 109–129.

BURNS-COX, N., GINGELL, C. (1995) Drugs and sexual dysfunction. *Practice Nursing* **6(19)**: 32–34.

BYERS, S. (1989) Sexuality and sexual concerns. In SHOEN JOHNSON, B. (ed.) *Psychiatric–Mental Health Nursing: Adaptaion and Growth* (2nd edition). Philadelphia. Lippincott.

CARR, L. (1995) Sexuality and people with learning disabilities. *British Journal of Nursing* **4(19)**: 1135–1141.

CHODOROW, N. (1978) *The Reproduction of Mothering*. Berkeley. University of California Press.

COMFORT, A., DIAL, L. (1991) Sexuality and aging: An overview. *Clinical Geriatric Medicine* **7(1)**: 1–7.

DEPARTMENT OF HEALTH (1992) *The Health of the Nation*. London. Her Majesty's Stationery Office.

DIMOND, B. (1995) *Legal Aspects of Nursing*, 2nd edition. London. Prentice Hall.

DIOKNO, A., BROWN, M., HERZOG, R. (1990) Sexual function in the elderly. *Archives of International Medicine* **150**: 197–200.

FERGUSON, K. (1994) Mental health and sexuality. In WEBB, C. (ed.) *Living Sexuality. Issues for Nursing and Health*. London. Scutari.

FOUCAULT, M. (1973) *The Birth of the Clinic*. London. Tavistock.

FOUCAULT, M. (1979) *The History of Sexuality, Volume 1; An Introduction*. London. Allen Lane.

FREUD, S. (1923) *The Ego and the Id*. London. Hogarth.

GAGNON, J.H. (1988) Sex research and sexual conduct in the era of AIDS. *Journal of AIDS* **1**: 593–601.

GAMEL, C., DAVIS, B.D., HENGEVELD, M. (1993) Nurses' provision of teaching and counselling on sexuality; a review of the literature. *Journal of Advanced Nursing* **18**: 1219–1227.

GARRETT, G. (1994) Sexuality in later life. *Elderly Care* **6(4)**: 23–28.

GIDDENS, A. (1993) *Sociology*. Oxford. Blackwell.

GOVE W.R., TUDOR, J.F. (1972) Adult sex roles and mental illness. *American Journal of Sociology* **78**: 812–835.

GROSS, R.D. (1992) *Psychology. The Science of Mind and Behaviour*. London. Hodder and Stoughton.

GUNN, M. (1991) *Sex and the Law: A Brief Guide for Staff Working with People with Learning Difficulties*. London. Family Planning Association.

HAKA-IKSE, K., MIAN, M. (1993) Sexuality in children. *Pediatrics in Review* **14(10)**: 401–407.

HINCHLIFF, S., MONTAGUE, S., WATSON, R. (1996) *Physiology for Nursing Practice*, 2nd edn. London. Baillière Tindall.

HOLZAPFEL, S. (1994) Aging and sexuality. *Canadian Family Physician* **40**: 748–766.

HUDSON, R., WILLIAMS, A.M. (1995) *Divided Britain*. Chichester. Wiley.

KAUTZ, D.D., DICKEY, C.A., STEVENS, M.N. (1990) Using research to identify why nurses do not meet established sexuality nursing care standards. *Journal of Nursing Quality Assurance* **4(3)**: 69–78.

KINSEY, A.C., POMEROY, W.B., MARTIN, C.E. (1948) *Sexual Behaviour in the Human Male*. Philadelphia. Saunders.

KINSEY, A.C., GEBHARD, P.H. (1953) *Sexual Behaviour in the Human Female*. Philadelphia. Saunders.

LANVAL, M. (1950) *An Inquiry into the Intimate Lives of Women*. New York. Cadillac.

LAVEE, Y. (1991) Western and non-western sexuality: implications for clinical practice. *Journal of Sex and Marital Therapy* **17(3)**: 203–213.

LAWLER, J. (1991) *Behind the Screens. Nursing: Somology and the Problem of the Body*. London. Churchill Livingstone.

LEWIS, S., BOR, R. (1994) Nurses' knowledge of and attitudes towards sexuality and the relationship of these with nursing practice. *Journal of Advanced Nursing* **20**: 251–259.

McCARTHY, M., THOMPSON, D. (1995) No more double standards: Sexuality and people with learning difficulties. In PHILPOT, T., WARD, L. (eds) *Values and Visions. Changing Ideas in Services for People with Learning Difficulties*. Oxford. Butterworth Heinemann.

MASTERS, W., JOHNSON, V. (1966) *Human Sexual Response*. London. Churchill.

MATOCHA, L.K., WATERHOUSE, J.K. (1993) Current nursing practice related to sexuality. *Research in Nursing and Health* **16**: 371–378.

MISCHEL, W. (1966) A social-learning view of sex differences in behaviour. In MACCOBY, E.E. (ed.) 1966 *The Development Of Sex Differences*. Stanford. Stanford University Press.

MONGA, T.N., LEFEBVRE, K.A. (1995) Sexuality: an overview. *Physical Medicine and Rehabilitation: State of the Art Reviews* **9(2)**: 299–311.

OFFIR, C. (1982) *Human Sexuality*. San Diego. Harcourt Brace.

OREM, D. (1995) *Nursing; Concepts of Practice*. London. Mosby.

PEPLAU, H. (1988) *Interpersonal Relations in Nursing*. London. Macmillan.

ROPER, N., LOGAN, W., TIERNEY, A. (1996) *The Elements of Nursing*. Edinburgh. Churchill Livingstone.

SALVAGE, J. (1995) *The Politics of Nursing*. London. Heinemann.

SAYERS, J. (1986) *Sexual Contradiction; Psychology, Psychoanalysis and Feminism*. London. Tavistock.

SMITH, M. (1993) Pediatric sexuality: promoting normal sexual development in children. *Nurse Practitioner* **18(8)**: 37–44.

SMOOK, K. (1992) Nurses' attitudes towards the sexuality of older people; an investigative study. *Nursing Practice* **6(1)**: 15–17.

STEIN, L. (1976) The doctor–nurse game. *Archives of General Psychiatry* **16**: 699–703.

SUNDRAM, C.J., STAVIS P.F. (1994) Sexuality and retardation: unmet challenges. *Mental Retardation* **32(4)**: 255–264.

SYMONS, D. (1979) *The Evolution of Human Sexuality*. New York. Oxford University Press.

TRAVIS, R., YEAGER, C. (1991) Sexual selection, parental investment and sexism. *Journal of Social Issues* **47(3)**: 117–130.

UKCC (1992) *Code of Professional Conduct*. London. UKCC.

VERSLUYSEN, M.C. (1980) Old wives' tales? Women healers in English history. In Davies, C. *Rewriting Nursing History*. London. Croom Helm.

VAN OOIJEN, E., CHARNOCK, A. (1994) *Sexuality and Patient Care: A Guide for Nurses and Teachers*. London. Chapman and Hall.

WEBB, C. (1985) *Sexuality, Nursing and Health*. Chichester. Wiley.

WEBB, C. (1988) A study of nurses' knowledge and attitudes about sexuality in health care. *International Journal of Nursing Studies* **25(3)**: 235–244.

WEIJTS, W., HOUTKOOP, H., MULLEN, P. (1993) Talking delicacy; speaking about sexuality during gynaecological consultations. *Sociology of Health and Illness* **15(3)**: 295–314.

WELLINGS, K., FIELD, J., JOHNSON, A.M., WADSWORTH, J. (1994) *Sexual Behaviour in Britain; The National Survey of Sexual Attitudes and Lifestyles*. London. Penguin.

WORLD HEALTH ORGANIZATION (1975) *Education and Treatment in Human Sexuality; the Training of Health Professionals. Report of a WHO Meeting*. Geneva. World Health Organization.

4.4 Sleep and Rest

M. Reet

▷ INTRODUCTION

Sleep, relaxation and rest are essential requirements to human wellbeing and yet they are concepts that are not yet fully understood by scientists and researchers. It is, however, evident that there are patterns of sleep that are similar between individuals and this has led to the generation of theory around which nursing care may be based.

The need for sleep varies through life according to an individual's age, and quality and quantity of sleep may be affected by an individual's state of health. Conversely, the amount of sleep an individual is able to enjoy may affect his or her health and wellbeing. It is essential that clients are facilitated in ensuring that they are able to relax effectively and gain an optimum amount of sleep. The context of care is also an essential consideration for nursing since much care takes place out of the clients usual setting for sleep, and, away from a home environment.

Individuals may have anxieties and concerns, which must be addressed in order to enable effective rest and relaxation. Even at home a client with a newly diagnosed illness may suffer anxieties that affect their ability to relax, rest or sleep.

Skill is required in understanding individual client's needs for sleep and in ensuring the best possible circumstances for relaxation, rest and sleep to take place.

Professionally, although it is important to recognize the importance of sleep, relaxation and rest for clients, sleep is also important in order to ensure fitness for personal practice. This is especially important within nursing, for shift work that includes late evening finishes and early morning starts as well as night duty, and stresses at work such as an increased number of critically ill clients or limitations of resources may result in a reduction in an individual's capacity for relaxation and rest.

In this chapter, the concepts of sleep, relaxation and rest are explored, appraising existent theory and research and applying this integrally in offering strategies for the facilitation of nursing care of clients. Additionally, these concepts will be considered at a personal and professional level, offering you the opportunity to reflect on your effectiveness in ensuring adequate sleep and rest.

The chapter aims to help you to understand how you can enable patients and clients in your care to achieve optimum sleep, relaxation and rest using a decision making approach. All branch areas are considered in terms of the specific problems they may have, and case studies reflecting all branch areas are used as illustrations in the Reflective Knowledge part of the chapter.

▶ OVERVIEW

▶ *Subject Knowledge*

In the biological part of Subject Knowledge the physiology of sleep is explored and sleep patterns seen over 24-hour periods are examined. The effects of ageing on sleep pattern and duration of sleep are presented and discussed.

In the psychosocial part the effects of culture and social factors on sleep are explored, and the value of bedtime routines are considered. Finally the influences of circadian rhythms on routines are identified. The physical effects of relaxation and rest on an individual require acknowledgement, as well as the consideration of psychosocial influences. These concepts are therefore explored in detail here. Definitions of rest and relaxation are considered and also potential problems associated with enforced rest.

▶ *Nursing Knowledge*

This focuses on the assessment of patients' needs for sleep, relaxation and rest. Discussion of non-pharmacological approaches to sleep is followed by a short consideration of pharmacological aids to sleep. The four nursing branch areas are presented in turn to establish particular client needs.

▶ *Professional Knowledge*

The application of knowledge about sleep and rest is applied to the profession of nursing. In caring for others it is our professional duty to be alert and able to carry out our job safely, and ensuring adequate personal sleep and rest is essential. The role of the night nurse is briefly discussed.

▶ *Reflective Knowledge*

Five case studies are offered as illustrations to aid reflection of the knowledge acquired in this chapter to inform decision making.

On pp. 591–594 there are five case studies, each one relating to one of the branch programmes. You may find it helpful to read one of them before you start the chapter and use it as a focus while reading.

SUBJECT KNOWLEDGE

Nurses have the opportunity to influence the quantity and quality of sleep and rest received by clients. This is achieved in a variety of ways, which we will explore throughout this chapter. In this section, the biological bases to sleep, rest and relaxation are addressed, and psychosocial influences are explored.

Biological

▶ SLEEP

There are many similar attempts to define sleep within the existing literature. Taking all factors into consideration it may be described as 'a recurrent natural condition where consciousness is temporarily lost and bodily functions are partly suspended. It is reversible, either by natural return of consciousness or by external stimulation, for example by an alarm clock'.

▶ *Physical Aspects of Sleep*

Most people when asleep have their eyes closed and make occasional movements, but are generally still. The face and neck muscles relax, the jaw tends to sag and the mouth falls open. Breathing becomes slower and deeper. There is little or no response to gentle stimulation.

▶ *Development of Sleep Research*

- **What can you identify from your previous experience as the physical manifestations of sleep?**
- **How would you decide that someone was asleep?**

Sleep is essentially a mystery to science. The objective measurement of someone else's subjective experience is difficult to achieve in practice, but even more so when the experience is not shared. When we sleep what occurs in our minds and our bodies remains unknown. Scientists have attempted to understand what happens when we sleep, but it must be recognized that they are far from being able to describe exactly what happens and the exact reasons for sleep.

Originally, objective observations of pulse, blood pressure, temperature and muscle movements were used to describe sleep until the discovery of the electroencephalogram (EEG) in the 1920s (Borbely, 1987). It was then discovered that the electrical activity of the brain could be monitored, not only while the subject was awake, but also while asleep. Using the traces obtained theories began to emerge about the physiology of sleep.

Today, much of the scientific knowledge about sleep is achieved in sleep laboratories. Borbely (1987) describes this process in some detail. The subject is monitored using a polysomograph, which uses electrodes to record the EEG, electro-oculogram (EOG) and the electromyogram (EMG), which records the electrical activity in the chin muscles. Other external observations may also be recorded, for example temperature, pulse, blood pressure, pulse oximetry and external movements. This external monitoring obviously has disadvantages as its use may in fact interrupt normal sleep patterns. The usual method for investigations of this nature do attempt to take this into consideration and subjects spend a night in the laboratory being monitored before the experiment begins. The room used for the subject is comfortably furnished and soundproofed and there is ample length to the monitoring wires for the subject to move comfortably in bed when asleep.

▶ *Stages of Sleep*

As suggested above, theories have developed about the stages of sleep identified from EEG tracings. Four main stages were identified and are now commonly referred to as orthodox sleep (Horne, 1988).

▶ Stage 1

The subject is in the process of falling asleep and becomes drowsy and barely conscious, although any slight sound would arouse him or her. The EEG demonstrates alpha waves, which are associated with the wakeful state.

▶ Stage 2

The subject is now asleep. There is greater relaxation of muscles and joints and movements are still; however, the subject remains easily roused. The EEG shows the appearance of slow waves called K-complexes, as well as bursts of rapid waves known as sleep spindles (Borbely, 1987). Stage 2 accounts for more than half the total time spent asleep.

▶ Stage 3

The subject is now completely relaxed and is not aroused by familiar noises. EEG waves become slower and larger and are known as delta waves (Borbely, 1987).

▶ Stage 4

The subject rarely moves and is difficult to awaken. An increase in the percentage of delta waves is noted on the EEG recording. Sleep walking or enuresis occurs during this stage of sleep.

▶ REM (paradoxical) sleep

Further studies revealed a further stage of sleep characterized by rapid eye movements (REMs). This fifth stage of sleep became known as REM (or paradoxical sleep), while the previously identified Stages 1–4 became known as non-REM sleep (Horne, 1988).

REM sleep is characterized by a period of light sleep during which dreaming is thought to mainly occur. During this stage of sleep REMs are recorded using an EOG.

▶ *The Sleep Cycle*

The five stages of sleep follow an organized ultradian cycle (Brugne, 1994a). Initially individuals move through Stages 1 to 4. From Stage 4 the subject may change position in bed, usually indicating a move back into Stage 2. A period of REM sleep then occurs and the individual returns to Stage 2. The cycle progresses to Stage 4 and again repeats until the individual awakes. Each ultradian cycle is thought to last 90–100 minutes in an adult, but the length of time spent in each stage alters during the night. During the early part of the night the percentage spent in Stages 3 and 4 is larger in comparison with REM sleep, while in the later hours of sleep the percentage of REM sleep increases and the percentage of Stage 3 and 4 sleep decreases (Figure 4.4.1).

The sleep cycle is characterized by sudden changes from deep to light

Figure 4.4.1: Sleep pattern in a young adult illustrating sleep stage changes. (Developed using data from Horne, 1988.)

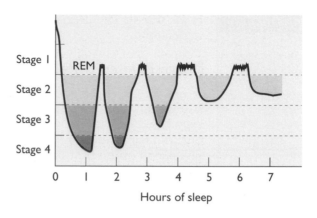

> • *How can knowledge of the sleep cycle inform nursing practice?*
>
> • *Identify three ways in which such knowledge may aid the nurse in caring for clients.*

sleep, which are often indicated by positional changes, while light to deep sleep occurs more gradually.

Physiological Changes During Sleep

Borbely (1987) describes other physiological patterns noted in sleep. When subjects are in non-REM sleep:

- body temperature falls by a few tenths of a degree;
- breathing becomes slower;
- pulse rate decreases;
- blood pressure falls;
- blood cortisol concentration decreases;
- in deep sleep blood growth hormone concentration increases (Brugne, 1994a).

The release of growth hormone is thought to promote growth in children. It is also responsible for body maintenance, speeding up the production of new cells, strengthening bone, building muscle and supporting tissues. However, this is disputed by Horne (1988), who suggests that this may reflect the need for nutrients in response to the fasting state of the body during sleep.

When subjects are in REM sleep:

- bodily function activities increase – there is increased blood flow to the brain, freeing waste products and increasing efficiency, leading to the belief that REM sleep is important for restoring brain function;
- breathing becomes irregular;
- pulse and blood pressure recordings fluctuate;
- erections are common in males of all ages (Borbely, 1987).

Larger quantities of REM sleep coincide with active growth in the brain. Babies are noted to spend proportionally more time in REM sleep than adults (Borbely, 1987). This has led to the belief that REM sleep is the most important for restoring brain function.

Towards the end of a period of sleep:

- body temperature rises;
- blood cortisol concentration rises;
- the sleeper changes position more frequently.

> As a nurse working at night, what changes in critical observations might you observe when your clients are asleep?

The precise control over sleep remains a mystery. It is now thought that a region of the brain known as the reticular formation regulates sleep physiologically (Green, 1987; Tortora and Anagnostakos, 1987; Nie *et al.,* 1988). The precise information about how it works is not yet fully understood.

Age-Related Differences in Sleep

It has already been mentioned that babies enjoy more REM sleep than adults, but the whole pattern of sleep varies with age. Newborn babies spend much of their time asleep, although they sleep for shorter periods of time. Babies have a shorter sleep cycle than adults. Their cycle usually last 45–50 minutes at one year, increasing to 60–70 minutes at 5–10 years and thereafter increasing to the 90–100 minute average in adults (Borbely, 1987). The pattern of sleep also changes with age as shown in Table 4.4.1.

Age	Two months	Three years	25 years	75 years
Amount of sleep in 24 hours	18 hours	13 hours	8 hours	5 hours
Pattern of sleep	Asleep between feeds	Night sleep and daytime nap	Night sleep	Night sleep and day nap(s)

Table 4.4.1 Pattern of sleep changes according to age.

It is important to note that individuals' needs for sleep differ and it is therefore impossible to generalize absolutely from the above.

Effects of Ageing on Sleep

Morgan (1987) in his book on sleep and ageing offers many suggestions for the changes observed in the sleep patterns of the elderly including:

• changes in bladder function;
• disordered breathing – sleep apnoea, snoring;
• increased limb movements during sleep;
• pain and physical discomfort;
• depression;
• dementia, where sleep becomes short, shallow, broken and desynchronized;
• bereavement;
• living alone due to a lack of security, reassurance and comfort;
• financial hardship due to inadequate diet and cold;
• institutionalization due to noise (auditory awakening thresholds decrease with age).

Some of the above may be responsible for the altered or disturbed sleep patterns of the elderly and these can be addressed during assessment.

In contrast, Kearnes (1989) found that bedtime routine, the prevention of anxiety and the promotion of relaxation were the key considerations in promoting sleep in the elderly.

Sleep in Pregnancy

Pregnancy also causes a change in sleep pattern. There may be an increased need to void urine, causing a disturbed night. Movements of the baby and achieving a comfortable position in bed as the woman's shape changes may contribute to disturbed sleep. Increasing tiredness during the pregnancy also means that it is common to take daytime naps.

Biofeedback training has been used to help pregnant mothers relax and therefore keep their blood pressure low, although it has to be said this has been most effective when used with middle class and older mothers rather than with young mothers from working class backgrounds (Little *et al.*, 1984).

▶ *Dreams*

Scientists have been interested in the various stages of sleep and what occurs during them. Subjects may be awoken at various stages to find out for instance whether they have been dreaming and what they can remember of their dreams. It has been found that sleepers woken during REM sleep report that they were dreaming, but when woken from non-REM sleep only 25% report dreaming (Atkinson *et al.*, 1993).

Dreams have provided much interest to scientists and many psychologists have spent a great deal of time trying to identify the causes for certain types of dream. It is known that we all dream when asleep even if we do not remember our dreams. We are able to recall dreams when we awakened while dreaming, but the memory fades quickly unless a conscious effort is made to remember the dream.

Psychosocial   ## ▶ PSYCHOSOCIAL ASPECTS OF SLEEP

▶ *Sleep Pattern*

Many areas of our lives occur as a pattern of culture and it is evident that one type of sleep pattern is not relevant for all cultures (Brugne, 1994a).

The habit of sleeping once at night by adults in North European countries for instance is not reflected in some of the Mediterranean cultures. Here a siesta taken in the hottest part of the day is more culturally acceptable, with retiring for night-time sleep being much later than is common in North Europe. In China workers are expected to have a sleep in the middle of the day as part of the lunchtime break and employers are expected to provide for this time (Borbely, 1987).

▶ *Sleep Environment*

Many people choose to sleep in a bed in a room that is designed for sleeping. There are many differences in this, however. Children in large families may be used to sharing a bed with a brother or sister and many children are at least used to sharing their bedroom. In other families all the family members sleep in a room alone. The increasing number of families forced to live in bed and breakfast accommodation as a result of being without a house or flat of their own means that many families become used to living and sleeping in the same room (National Children's Home, 1992). The numbers of homeless people who sleep under bridges and underpasses must not to be forgotten when considering where sleep occurs. This has to be remembered when as nurses we are assessing the patients and clients and enabling them to sleep and rest. For instance it may be that an elderly man finds sleeping more comfortable in a chair as he does not sleep in bed at home. Or it may be that an elderly lady finds it hard to sleep after the death of her husband because she has not slept alone for 40 or 50 years. Others may find sleep difficult as they have always slept alone and sleeping in a

---

DECISION MAKING

Sita aged four years lives with her parents who are unemployed, and her two brothers aged 18 months and three years. They are living in one room.

- **What kind of problems may be related to sleep for this family?**
- **Sita is admitted to hospital with infectious diarrhoea. She is nursed alone in a cubicle. What considerations would you need to take into account in helping Sita to sleep while in hospital.**

shared ward may prove disturbing in itself. Sleeping with a partner can cause problems with sleep patterns, particularly if the partner snores or has a disturbed night.

Psychosocial knowledge about sleep is perhaps best explored by considering what enables us to sleep ourselves.

▶ Sleep Hygiene

Borbely (1987) suggests sleep hygiene to promote sleep and this includes the following items:

▶ establish a regular bedtime;
▶ reserve the evening hours for leisure activities and relaxation;
▶ avoid naps;
▶ avoid caffeine, alcohol and nicotine especially in the hours before sleep;
▶ create favourable conditions for sleep.

He suggests that when unable to sleep the individual should get up and do something relaxing rather than lie worrying about the lack of sleep.

▶ Circadian Rhythm

Circadian rhythm is the term used to describe the daily pattern of life for organisms including humans. It has been found that the human body when deprived of light or other sources of time-keeping adopts a sleep–wake routine that resembles a 24-hour clock. In experiments it has been found that the average circadian rhythm for humans is around 25 hours, although the range of circadian rhythms for different subjects varied from 16–48 hours. This rhythm is thought to be biologically controlled, as the experiments removed the sociological time-setters for sleep (Folkard, 1991; Brugne, 1994a). These time-setters are called zeitgebers, which are defined by Borbely (1987, p. 181) as an 'external signal that synchronizes the circadian rhythm of an organism'. Examples of zeitgebers are:

▶ the light/dark cycle;
▶ knowledge of clock time;
▶ behaviour of others in society;
▶ meal times.

In experiments the most powerful zeitgebers for humans appeared to be those of an essentially informative or social nature (Folkard 1991; Hodgson, 1991).

The individual circadian rhythm can be blamed for the emergence of two personality types:

▶ 'Morning types' who rise early and do much of their best work in the hours before noon, but become tired by early evening and do not then function as efficiently;
▶ 'Evening types' who have difficulty rising in the morning, often have difficulty facing breakfast and do not really perform at their best until the afternoon – many are at their peak of alertness in the late evening and often settle late (Folkard, 1991; Duxbury, 1994a).

▶ *Sleep Deprivation*

One of the ways scientists have tried to understand our need for sleep has been to undertake trials on volunteers who agree to go without sleep to monitor the effects of sleep deprivation on the body. Some understanding has been achieved as a result of such studies.

You have probably thought of several symptoms of a poor night's sleep. For example:

- ▶ sore heavy eyes, which often feel 'gritty';
- ▶ difficulty carrying out monotonous jobs;
- ▶ difficulty concentrating;
- ▶ difficulty remaining alert;
- ▶ being irritable;
- ▶ headache;
- ▶ feeling tense;
- ▶ feeling cold;
- ▶ visual misperceptions (Irwin, 1992).

In tests of severe sleep deprivation (longer than 72 hours without sleep) the main complaints were related to the effect on the senses and included:

- ▶ hallucinations;
- ▶ poor cooperation;
- ▶ paranoia;
- ▶ doing and saying strange things;
- ▶ falling asleep when undisturbed, even when doing something (Oswald and Adam, 1983).

In the remaining part of this section it is intended to explore the concepts of relaxation and rest and how physical needs for these may be influenced by psychosocial issues. The potential effects on clients of failing to relax and rest effectively are examined.

▶ RELAXATION

Relaxation is defined as 'a lessening of tension'. This can imply a lessening of either muscular tension or a lessening of stress, which is often referred to as tension. A more detailed consideration of stress and anxiety is provided in Chapter 4.1.

▶ REST

In *Baillière's Encyclopaedic Dictionary of Nursing and Health Care* (Weller, 1989) rest is defined as 'repose after exertion'. This fits well when we consider cell life, for instance that of the myocardium. These muscle cells are responsible for the continued beating of the heart from just after conception to death. As part of their cycle they have an active phase followed by a resting phase when they prepare for the next impulse. It could be reasonable to apply this to the human organism and think of the human need for rest after exertion. Exercise cannot usually be sustained for long periods without an opportunity for rest.

Think of the last time you felt deprived of sleep.

- *How did it make you feel?*
- *What was the worst part about it?*

DECISION MAKING

- *During an admission assessment, what signs might lead you to suspect that a client was deprived of sleep?*
- *What kinds of questions might you ask in order to verify (or annul) your suspicions?*

- *What do you think to relax means?*
- *How do you relax?*
- *Compare your thoughts with the definition of relaxation below.*

DECISION MAKING

If you were told to rest what would you do? Ask two or three other adults the same question and compare their replies with yours.

- *What does this tell you about the lay understanding of the concept of 'rest'?*
- *How might a broad and varied understanding of the concept of 'rest' cause problems in the health education of clients?*

- *How do you feel after a period of rest?*
- *Think about how you felt before you rested. What change has occurred?*

To rest can mean different things to different people. For some resting means to be doing something different from work or normal pursuits. In resting then they can be active, for example cycling or gardening as they find this a restful pursuit. To others resting means sitting down and doing little, for others it may mean lying in bed, and for still others it may be interpreted as sleep.

In the application of terms it appears that resting can be interpreted as relaxing. As professionals working in society we work with members of the public and it is as well to remember the kind of language they use to describe certain activities and to attempt to use culturally relevant language when talking with them.

It is evident that people will interpret the term 'to rest' in a variety of ways. If a specific need for rest is identified then there must be a specification of what we mean by the term so that clients understand what they must do. It can mean little to clients to say that they should get more rest, if to them that means digging the garden when we mean sitting or lying down.

▌ Defining Rest for Patients

The increasing use of day surgery for patients can provide unrealistic expectations that because they are treated as a day case that they will rapidly be able to resume normal activities. They need to be prepared for the lassitude they are likely to feel postoperatively, the length of time they should allow for recuperation, and the activities they will be able to do (Raper, 1992; Reid, 1992; Smith, 1992).

▌ Bed rest

DECISION MAKING

The use of bed rest for antenatal care of mothers can raise difficulties that are not always of a physical nature (Taylor, 1985). Bed rest may be recommended for individuals at any point in the life span and can have both physical and psychological implications as well as offering the benefits of treatment.

- *Imagine that you have to rest in bed at home for a month. Jot down the problems you may face.*
- *What if you had a toddler at home with you? Amend your list in the light of this.*
- *Identify the potentially damaging effects of prolonged bed rest for an elderly client.*

We use the term bed rest in nursing to describe the immobilization of a patient within the confines of a bed. This can refer to resting on the bed, but allowing the patient to walk to the toilet with support or supervision. Conversely it may refer to a client who is forbidden to weight-bear and must remain in bed at all times. It is important that this is clarified in the nursing records to ensure that all members of staff are aware of the appropriate care for the client and its rationale. It is important that the nurse pays attention to the positioning of patients who are likely to spend long periods of time confined to bed. This is in order to prevent deformities and breaches of skin integrity. You should refer to Chapter 3.4 for a more detailed description of the care of the immobile patient and Chapter 2.4 for a consideration of skin integrity.

▌ Problems of enforced bed rest

There are many physical and psychologial problems associated with enforcing bed rest and the physical aspects are addressed in more detail in relation to mobility in Chapter 3.4.

Some of the main psychological problems of enforced bed rest are boredom and frustration that accompanies it. Visitors can help alleviate this, although at times they can prove tiring and a reminder that life is going on without the patient. Suggesting pastimes is part of the nurse's role in providing holistic care for his or her patients and clients.

What kind of pastimes could you think of if you were on enforced bedrest?

▶ PSYCHOSOCIAL INFLUENCES THAT MAY AFFECT OPTIMUM RELAXATION AND REST

It is important to remember that rest is not limited to a physical position, but is more complex. Psychosocial aspects can be important in the promotion of rest. For instance, a client may appear agitated and unable to settle and there may be a physical reason for this, for example he or she may need to micturate. However, this agitation could equally be a symptom of psychological distress, such as anxiety about a situation at home. Identification of such worries and anxieties can enable the nurse to involve other professionals to assist the client or members of his or her family to reduce the anxiety.

> **DECISION MAKING**
>
> Decide what signs may lead you to suspect that a patient or client is anxious. (Refer to Chapter 4.1 of this book to supplement your answer and to explore means of alleviating anxiety.)

▶ *Pastimes and Play*

To play means to 'occupy or amuse oneself pleasantly'. For children, play is an important part of their daily lives. It is the medium through which all aspects of their development progress. For example children who are not exposed to play are unable to manipulate simple toys and will not attempt to explore their environment. This demonstrates the importance of play to the normal development of children. However, play or pastimes are discussed here in this chapter more in terms of people who have to relax as part of their care. Pastimes are an option to enable clients to relax. The ability to 'amuse oneself pleasantly' is not necessarily natural and some will require help to explore how they can achieve this. In particular those patients and clients who have been stressed or depressed may find this aspect a difficult area to resolve.

> **DECISION MAKING**
>
> Peter Swift is a 55-year-old business executive. He is admitted to hospital after a suspected mycardial infarction and has been advised by the doctors to relax. However, Peter appears agitated and stressed.
> - **What physical and psychological factors may prevent clients like Peter relaxing in an institutional setting?**
>
> - *How could Peter be helped to relax?*
> - *Imagine you are working in a health care of the elderly setting where there is a large dayroom in which the majority of the residents spend a large part of their day. What kind of amusement might you suggest to enhance their relaxation?*

As part of their care clients should receive strategies to enable them to amuse themselves and these may improve their ability to rest and relax. In a busy institutional setting this can be difficult to organize or encourage, but it is still important. The provision of items to assist this can be a simple way to promote this aspect of care. For instance, (complete) jigsaw puzzles, books, magazines, packs of cards and games suitable for the client group can offer some choices. In some health care of the elderly settings where the elderly are 'at home' this must be an important planned part of their week. Otherwise there is a danger that the majority of their contact with others is through staff meeting their physical needs. Some may need encouragement to undertake these pastime activities. However, respect for the patients or clients right to refuse to take part must be maintained.

PRACTICE KNOWLEDGE

When caring for patients and clients whether in the community or at home the nurse is in an ideal position to offer support and advice about sleep.

Some of the main problems encountered by people when ill are sleep and rest disturbances although there has been relatively little research into this area of care (Southwell and Wistow, 1995). Here is a list of reasons given by a group of individuals for poor sleep.

▶ REASONS FOR POOR SLEEP

These include:

- ▶ anxiety or worry;
- ▶ fear (e.g. of burglars, death in sleep);
- ▶ depression;
- ▶ bereavement;
- ▶ change in routine (shift work, long distance air travel, institutionalization);
- ▶ too much or too little exercise;
- ▶ pain or discomfort (e.g. due to an unsettled stomach or coughing or breathing problems);
- ▶ stimulants (e.g. caffeine, alcohol, nicotine);
- ▶ hunger or overeating;
- ▶ temperature of the room (too hot or too cold);
- ▶ unfamiliar place/bed/room/pillows/covers;
- ▶ light;
- ▶ noise;
- ▶ gender (men tend to be more disturbed, although women complain more);
- ▶ genetics (hyperactivity);
- ▶ alcohol or drug withdrawal;
- ▶ long period of bedrest (can affect circadian rhythm);
- ▶ excitement.

> Who is responsible for ensuring adequate rest and sleep of patients and clients?

Although the nurse in an institutional setting may identify more problems that can potentially affect the patients and clients, all nurses should be aware of the potential problems of poor sleep.

▶ ASSESSMENT

In order to assist clients in promoting healthy sleep, it is important to perform an assessment of their sleep habits and routines. It is only by asking the right questions and applying them that a full picture will emerge that can inform individualized care planning (Wilkie, 1990). Hodgson (1991) suggests that the nursing assessment should consider the following aspects:

- ▶ age;
- ▶ normal pattern of sleep during health;
- ▶ current pattern of sleep;
- ▶ nutritional status;
- ▶ emotional status;
- ▶ daytime and night-time symptoms;
- ▶ sleeping environment;
- ▶ sleep-related rituals;
- ▶ presence of dreams or nightmares;
- ▶ present medication;
- ▶ wake-time behaviour.

It is to be remembered that assessments will be subjective as they will be based on individuals' perceptions. Knowledge gained from initial assessments can be used to promote sleep in the therapeutic environment.

Finally, it is also important to remember that illness itself may contribute changes to sleep habits and it is possible to develop a vicious

RESEARCH BASED EVIDENCE

The following studies have been carried out to investigate sleeping in hospital. Closs (1988) found that the majority of patients in her sample described sleep in hospital as worse than at home. Sleep was shorter with an earlier awakening. Patients were often disturbed during the sleeping period. The main reasons given for disturbed sleep were pain or discomfort, noise, the environmental temperature and dissatisfaction with the beds. It can be seen that nurses can contribute to at least the two main problems and to some extent the others.

Southwell and Wistow (1995) looked at patients' experiences of sleep in hospital and demonstrated differences between the perceptions of the staff and those of the patients about the quality of sleep.

Finally, a small study by Hill (1989) challenged routine practice, which did not necessarily consider patient or client needs. For example, waking everyone at 6 a.m. for medication, tea or observations of temperature, pulse and respiration.

circle. Ryan (1995) describes a cycle of sleep disturbance in patients with fibromyalgia where fatigue and pain leads to sleep disturbance, which in turn reduces the quantity of deep restorative sleep, which increases fatigue and therefore pain.

▶ AIDING RESTFUL SLEEP

Nurses need to be aware of the available research in this area in order to be able to promote sleep and rest for their clients (Duxbury, 1994b).

In Chapter 2.3 the nurse's role in pain management is described and should be considered when promoting sleep and rest.

▶ *Noise*

The noise levels in ward environments can be controlled to some extent by nursing staff. Simple measures like using soft-soled shoes that do not squeak (squeaking can be almost as bad as clicking heels!), making sure that trolleys are well maintained so that their wheels run smoothly without clattering, ensuring that any talking as far as possible takes place away from the patient areas and having call lights instead of buzzers at night, can all aid sleep for the patients and clients.

▶ *Comfort*

The control of ward temperature can be a difficult but essential component to aiding clients' sleep. The use of more or less blankets and of fans to aid air flow can be helpful. Nurses are also involved in purchasing equipment including beds. Consideration of client comfort is as important as the maintenance of a safe environment.

Management of the ward environment to allow for individuals differences in sleep patterns should enable many patients and clients to follow as near normal a pattern of sleep as possible. For instance, being aware that some patients will be ready for sleep at 9 p.m. while others will not feel tired until after midnight should as far as possible fit in with the patients' care. The process of working in partnership with patients and clients if they are able to participate or with their carers should enable the planning of care that will promote sleep and rest and will be individually appropriate and therefore potentially achievable (Department of Health and Social Security (DHSS) and the Welsh Office, 1976).

DECISION MAKING

- *Find a copy of the DHSS and Welsh Office report 'The Organisation of the In-patients Day' (1976) in your local library.*
- *On reflection, how much does your care planning in practice address the promotion of sleep and rest for individuals?*
- *Have the criteria set by the DHSS report been acheived over 20 years on?*

▶ ANXIETY AND ITS EFFECT ON SLEEP

One area of concern not mentioned yet is that of anxiety, which can create a great deal of disturbance for the individual patient or client. The opportunity to discuss the patient's anxiety and fears may provide adequate relief to aid sleep. Talking to patients can be an important part of the nurse's role, as already discussed in earlier chapters and its potency should not be minimized when aiding rest and sleep.

▶ AIDS TO SLEEP

The measures described so far relate mostly to environmental methods that the nurse can use to assist patients or clients to sleep. It is now appropriate to consider some of the potential aids to sleep that can be used to promote sleep if difficulties are encountered. These fall into two categories: the non-pharmacological and the pharmacological.

▶ *Non-Pharmacological Aids to Sleep*

The nurse has the opportunity to choose many of these as alternatives to aid the rest and sleep of patients and clients rather than choosing pharmacological aids as a first resort. They include:

- darkness – often difficult to achieve in hospital as dim light is needed in many areas to promote safety, but if this is a problem, blindfolds could be suggested, if patient safety will not be compromised;
- silence – as mentioned before noise at night is a common problem for patients and clients attempting to sleep, and earplugs could be suggested if noise is a serious problem;
- relaxation and a comfortable position – in order to sleep the patient or client should be in a position that is comfortable and in which he or she is able to rest. For the immobile patients this will have to be achieved by the carer, but many partially mobile clients may need assistance with this;
- feeling tired – many patients who are used to being physically active when well, may find that they are not as tired and this can affect the time they take to settle to sleep;
- food and drink – many people settle after a light supper or snack and many are in the habit of taking a night-time drink, which aids sleep, so the provision of a suitable drink or snack at an appropriate time can be important for the promotion of sleep and rest and should be considered in the nursing assessment;
- warmth – this can be ensured by the provision of extra blankets or the use of warm bedwear;
- security – the confidence of patients or clients in their carers can contribute to this, including their belief that they are 'safe' in hospital and this may be undermined by media coverage of criminal investigations;
- familiarity – the use of familiar bedtime routines can promote this, or having familiar objects from home, for instance photographs and cuddly toys for children;
- reading – bed lights that do not disturb other patients can be used and selection of books in the day room can help;
- hot bath with aromatic bath salts or foam;
- pillows – using comfortable pillows, perhaps even shaped pillows

can help some patients and clients;

▶ avoiding daytime naps if this is not a usual pattern of sleep – often if there is little stimulation during the day it can be easy for patients and clients to nap, which can mean that they are less tired at bedtime;

▶ complementary therapies – several therapies can be used to promote rest and sleep including acupuncture, massage, aromatherapy, magnetic pillows and herb pillows, although for some of these the efficacy is not proven; Mantle (1996) provides a useful summary of some of these alternatives to drug therapy.

RESEARCH BASED EVIDENCE

Massage and aromatherapy are sometimes used to aid relaxation, rest and sleep. Deakin (1995) describes the use of relaxation techniques with patients and clients with disruptive behaviour. Using a programme to manage disruptive behaviour using individual relaxation sessions enabled other clients to benefit from group relaxation sessions. Eventually disruptive clients were able to participate in the group.

Dunn et al. (1995) looked at the effectiveness of massage, rest and aromatherapy in an intensive care unit. One of their findings was that periods of undisturbed rest were as important to the patients as the use of aromatherapy or massage. They highlighted that these techniques and their use needs to be

considered on an individual basis and with careful consideration regarding the client's beliefs, values and understanding of the use of therapeutic touch. This should ensure that as far as possible no offence is caused and cultural taboos are not broken. To this end patients or clients should have the opportunity to express their informed consent or if unable to do so this should be obtained from their next of kin. Dunn et al. (1995) found that aromatherapy and massage did prove beneficial to most patients.

Cannard (1995) reports on a small study at a nursing development unit in Ireland looking at the use of aromatherapy with older people to promote sleep and rest, which met with some success.

Relaxation training may help some

patients and clients, but others may be helped by a technique researched by Childs-Clarke (1990) called stimulus control. This method seeks to strengthen the association of behaviour with sleep, which is the reward for falling asleep. Instruction for those in the study were: only go to bed when feeling tired; if not asleep in 10–15 minutes get up and return to bed when sleepy; do not read, listen to the radio, watch television, eat, drink or smoke in bed; get up at a regular time every morning; do not catnap during the day (Childs-Clarke, 1990, p. 53). The results described appear to be encouraging as the sleep quality of the subjects was increased with little nursing input.

RESEARCH BASED EVIDENCE

Studies investigating the use of sleep medication include that of Halfens et al. (1994) which raised some important concerns. These researchers provided evidence to suggest that dependence on sleep medication can begin as a result of a hospital admission where drugs tend to be offered as a routine to aid sleep. Our responsibilities as nurses are to be aware of this and to use non-pharmacological aids where possible.

A small study by Duxbury (1994c) found that primary nurses (who take responsibility for coordinating the care of specified patients) used less night sedation than those nurses who worked in teams. This could imply that effective assessment and planning for sleep may serve to reduce the amount of required night sedation.

▶ *Pharmacological aids to sleep*

If non-pharmacological suggestions are ineffective, the use of drugs to aid sleep can be considered. Some of the disadvantages of medication to aid sleep can be that the sleep it promotes is qualitatively different from natural sleep. It has been shown to contain a reduced amount of REM sleep. In addition, many preparations have a hangover effect, leaving the patient with a 'muzzy head' (Burton, 1992), and some can contribute to difficulty with concentrating and balance. In the long term they can create dependency. Following withdrawal the patient is likely to have an increased amount of REM sleep, which often leads to increased reports of dreaming (Borbely, 1987).

The main sleeping pills prescribed belong to two groups: hypnotics and anxiolytics. A few barbiturates are, however, still used. The hypnotic drugs act on the central nervous system to induce sleep. These include nitrazepam and temazepam, chloral hydrate and chlormethiazole. Anxiolytics are tranquillizers that can be given to calm the anxious patient. Their use can be appropriate for the highly anxious patient, particularly before surgery (Burton, 1992).

▶ SETTLING CHILDREN TO SLEEP

Previously discussion has concentrated on the experiences of adults. Children can pose particular problems with sleep patterns. The disturbances are not necessarily only related to hospitalization. Many parents

DECISION MAKING

- *Thinking about your reading into the effects of sleep deprivation, what effects are likely to be experienced by parents after a period of disturbed sleep.*
- *How might this affect judgement and temperament.*
- *What strategies could you suggest to parents in order to enable them to get the best possible sleep during this difficult period in their lives?*

may express their concerns about their child's sleep pattern when their children attend hospital or at routine health visitor appointment. In fact in some areas sleep clinics have been set up to address the problems that parents experience (Fardell, 1989; Boomer and Deakin, 1991; Galbraith *et al.*, 1993). If you talk to many parents they will express the problems they have experienced in settling their children into a socially acceptable routine of sleep. Parents accept as a rule that a newborn baby will awaken during the night for feeds or changing, but can become dissatisfied when nights remain disturbed later and other parents report that their child sleeps through. Parents are not just considering how to enable their child to adopt a sleep routine, but they are also struggling themselves with chronic sleep deprivation.

▶ Developing Good Sleep Habits

There have been various suggestions for parents to achieve a good sleep habit in their child. In the past, parents were advised that a child awakening in the night should be left to cry so that the behaviour was not rewarded by being comforted or fed. Indeed some parents have tried this method with some success. However, thought now revolves around the adoption of a positive sleep routine before settling the child so that particular events will be associated with preparation for sleep (Crawford *et al.*, 1989; Roberts, 1993). The use of quiet activities – bath or wash and dressing ready for bed, drink or snack, and perhaps the reading of a story or a cuddle with a parent – before being laid to sleep in a darkened room after cleaning teeth as an example can train the child that it is now bedtime and sleep will follow. This is not to say this method is always effective, however, and not all children will respond to this type of training. Disturbances to routines can cause sleep problems, which can be persistent. These disturbances can have a variety of causes including illness, holidays (or sleeping away from home), admission to hospital, disturbances by siblings, visitors to the family home or essentially any activity that affects the child's routine.

Many authors have tackled this topic within the popular press (Douglas and Richman, 1984; Weissbluth, 1987; Haslam, 1992). Weissbluth (1987) offers some useful practical advice for parents. His book is useful as an informed resource for health care professionals. He highlights the four elements of a healthy child's sleep as:

- ▶ the duration of sleep – the length of sleep in a day varies between individual babies, but it is thought that babies' needs for sleep are essentially governed by biological functions when they are under 3–4 months of age, but after 3–4 months of age the parents can influence sleep duration;
- ▶ naps – daytime sleeps that restore the baby or toddler and are necessary to ensure that the correct amount of daily sleep is achieved (children can show signs of sleep deprivation if they miss their nap);
- ▶ consolidation of sleep – the settling of children for a period of time without interruptions as allowing babies to sleep and not to awaken them unnecessarily is important, though this can be difficult for parents to judge as excessive sleeping can be a sign that a baby is ill;
- ▶ a sleep schedule – the establishment of a routine for sleep where parents interpret cues for sleep as well as establish a regular pattern for sleep and naps for their child.

◗ *The nurse's role*

When children are admitted to a hospital environment, during assessment, attention must be paid to their normal sleep routine at home, including nap routines. Where possible these should be respected in hospital so that as little disruption as possible occurs to the child. Optimally children should be continued to be cared for by their parents in hospital with the support of children's nurses. In the event of parents not being able to stay with their children the attention to sleep routines is a vital part of the assessment information needed to enhance their care. Actions of parents when their child awakens in the night are an important element of the assessment of the child's normal sleep routine. Nurses may cuddle a crying baby for long periods of time at night, but this may not be what parents would normally do at home. Parents may offer a dummy, drink of water or merely pat the child as a reassuring gesture that they are present rather than picking the child up. The child can quickly develop 'bad' habits. These may include waking up crying and becoming inconsolable unless they are picked up and cuddled. This can have a deleterious effect on the parents in particular on their own sleep habits when their child returns home again. It can take some time to re-establish routines.

◗ LEARNING DISABILITIES

Clients with learning disabilities can have many problems in terms of their sleep patterns. Their carers often require respite support to enable them to manage to continue caring in the home environment because of the demands placed on their own sleeping patterns. Many children with learning disabilities have to be trained to sleep in order to promote sleep as adults. Work by Quine *et al.* (1991) looked at specific behavioural techniques that parents could use to improve bedtime behaviour. The solution lay in enabling parents to understand the following three aspects of the behaviour:

◗ the antecedent conditions;
◗ the behaviour itself;
◗ the consequences of the behaviour.

Following this parents were given options of a behavioural approach to change the behaviour. The four approaches were:

◗ to set a bedtime routine as many of these children have not established a bedtime routine, but this approach is hampered as it is thought that such children may lack biological sleep control mechanisms;
◗ to remove incentives for sleep disturbance (i.e. do not reward undesired behaviour by attending the child if they cry), but this can be hard to achieve in practice, requires the commitment of both parents and should not be used when the child is ill;
◗ to use a phased-in version of removing incentives for sleep disturbance by attending the child, but not cuddling, and gradually on successive occasions reducing contact until none is offered, by which time the habit may be broken;
◗ positive reinforcement, which rewards the child for desired behaviour and should be used so that it is achievable for the child – the main reward should be the praise of the parent although star charts

and using a small reward for a certain number of stars can provide some success.

▶ MENTAL HEALTH

Many mental health problems interfere with the normal sleep pattern. Depression and anxiety are common mental health problems that can disturb sleep patterns. Clients or patients with predominantly physical problems can also suffer anxiety and depression and may require extra support to promote sleep and rest.

Dunwell (1995) talks of the problems of insomnia in mental health. The strategies to assist patients and clients include those we have already mentioned, but include some other suggestions, which may also prove useful, such as thought jamming. Thought jamming involves using a neutral word to interrupt unwanted thoughts. It is important to use alternative methods of sleep induction in preference to drugs.

Many people with mental health problems exhibit sleeping problems such as sleepwalking (somnambulism) or night terrors and the level of consciousness during these episodes can be debated. However, Crisp *et al.* (1990) felt that this behaviour could be evidence of a client's ability to dissociate when awake and found that people with these types of disorders tended to have difficulty controlling anxiety and were prone to hysteria.

In caring for all patients and clients it must be remembered that disturbances to their sleep may affect other members of the household. The needs of the carers should be considered and it may be necessary as a nurse to encourage carers to take a break or make opportunities to enhance their own sleep and rest. Carers often feel obliged to continue to care, unwilling to say that they cannot cope. Nurses should remain alert to the needs of carers and observe for signs that the carers are not getting adequate rest themselves.

PROFESSIONAL KNOWLEDGE

It is important that the nurse retains a high degree of self-awareness as this can enhance the care that patients receive. If nurses' sleep is disturbed and they are not able to function correctly the lives of those for whom they provide care can be placed in jeopardy. The most obvious area for consideration appears to be the night shift, which has received a great deal of attention in the nursing press, but the sleep patterns of nurses on day shifts can be equally important. Lack of sleep for a variety of reasons (many of which have already been mentioned) can affect nurses as well as any member of the public. Nurses and other health care professionals are not immune to the effects of sleep deprivation.

As a professional nurse, the welfare of clients must come first and the *Code of Professional Conduct* governs professional behaviour (UKCC, 1992). This means that attention must be paid to personal health in order to look after the needs and requirements of clients. In some respects it is important that health care professionals are able to rest and sleep in order to offer constructive advice to clients. If nurses are unable to rest or sleep, it not only potentially affects their judgement, but it also calls into question the validity of the advice that they offer. The nurse's role should be to educate clients about sleep and rest (Brugne, 1994a).

Clients who require 24-hour care rely on nurses to provide that care. Shiftwork can affect health. Northcott and Facey (1995) considered the

Reflect on your present pattern of lifestyle.
• **Are there any changes you will need to make to accommodate shift working?**

use of 12-hour shifts used in many areas and preferred by some, but concluded that tiredness at the end of the shift predisposed to mistakes. This is the conclusion also reached by Totterdell *et al.* (1992). Barton (1995, p. 32) suggests that problems for some nurses on shift systems include 'chronic fatigue, anxiety, digestive complaints, disturbed sleep and disruptions to social and domestic life'. However, Skipper *et al.* (1990) challenge this view. In their study they found that shift work was not necessarily associated with poorer physical or mental health, although they did recognize that shiftwork was an issue for some workers. Managers need to consider the most appropriate form of rostering to ensure that the needs of staff are considered. In addition nursing professionals need to consider their personal need for rest and relaxation. Patterson (1991) highlights the need for staff to ensure an appropriate level of rest and play in order to ensure continued excellence of practice.

▶ NURSING AT NIGHT

There are two main issues to consider regarding night nursing: first, the effect of the disturbance of the circadian rhythm on the individual nurse; second, the issue of the role of the nurse at night to enhance patients' and clients' sleeping patterns.

▶ *Circadian Rhythm and the Night Nurse*

Earlier in the chapter there was some discussion about circadian rhythms and their effect on the individual. Nurses on night duty effectively reverse their daily working and sleeping pattern. Research into the biological rhythms suggest that for short periods of time the body does not significantly alter its biological routines (Folkard, 1991). Therefore daytime sleep is often disturbed by the need for the nurse to get up to pass urine for example. Folkard (1991) discusses the problems associated with circadian rhythms and shift work and offers some evidence to suggest that rapid shift changes are more beneficial in the long term to the shift worker.

Brugne (1994b) describes the poor attention span between 2–4 a.m. He suggests the use of flash sleep – short periods of sleep which refresh the nurse – to prevent them falling asleep while on duty. He suggests that managers should consider implementing breaks for this to prevent nurses falling asleep at night.

The long-term sociological implications of working permanent nights are mentioned by Folkard (1991). In particular the difficulty in being involved with social committees and groups can affect individuals and their role in their own community, and their ability to rest and relax, unless they ensure that this remains a priority to maintain their own mental health.

The importance of sleep and rest to clients for improving health has been neglected in many textbooks on nursing. To some extent sleep is a subjective experience of the patients and it can be difficult for nurses to realize the potential implications of sleep promotion because if successful the patient will not complain of sleep disturbances.

The night nurse can sometimes be regarded as a less important member of the ward team; however, the ability to plan and implement strategies to promote sleep should prove a vital contribution to client health within the actions of the multidisciplinary team. Hewitt-Sayer and Mayfield

(1992) and Hicks (1992) describe how night nurses were involved in the establishment of standards for the care of patients and clients during the night. The increasing number of institutions that have internal rotation onto night duty can go some way towards reducing the existing 'second class' image, but for some nurses home circumstances can make permanent night duty a more practical option. It is important that the night nurses' contributions to patient care are recognized and encouraged to promote their personal professional development (Duxbury, 1994d).

In conclusion, the promotion of relaxation, rest and sleep is an area that has not always received the attention it deserves. It is pertinent to consider that this is an essential part of the role of all nurses and midwives and should not be minimized. As professional nurses constant monitoring must take place to review current practice to ensure that good practice is maintained.

An awareness of the effect of poor sleep and rest on our own health as health care professionals should ensure that we recognize potential health risks in ourselves.

The consideration of promoting sleep and rest is vitally important in all areas of nursing and midwifery. Patients and clients may have difficulty in asking for help as they may feel, especially in institutional settings, that poor sleep is inevitable. As nurses it is therefore important for us to remain vigilant to patient and client needs in this area of their care. We need to observe and ask our patients and clients specifically about their rest and sleep to identify potential problems. It must be remembered that our objective observations do not always match the subjective experiences of patients and clients.

It is important that a clear and full assessment of sleep is undertaken in order to ensure appropriate planning of care.

Apart from the benefits to patients and clients directly from our increased understanding and awareness of relaxation, rest and sleep, they will also benefit indirectly from our consideration of our own needs in this aspect of care. As professional carers it is important that we monitor our own health in order to be able to care for our patients and clients to the best of our ability.

REFLECTIVE KNOWLEDGE

▶ CASE STUDIES

Using the information previously examined consider the following case studies representative of the different branches and use the questions posed to guide your reflections.

▶ CASE STUDY: ADULT

Mr Frederick Jacobs is 72 years old and lives with his wife, Amy, in a new bungalow. They moved six weeks ago from their lifetime family home because Amy was finding it increasingly difficult to manage the stairs. The bungalow has one bedroom and is part of a warden-controlled complex for the elderly.

Mr Jacobs has always been active and worked on the railway for 45 years before retiring seven years ago. Since retirement he had been gardening for themselves and for their two neighbours in their previous home. The bungalow has a small garden, but it is still very rough and will need some work to make it usable.

Yesterday Mr Jacobs had a bout of angina while digging the garden. The general practitioner was called and advised him to rest for a few days and not to overexert himself. The district nurse has now called to dress an ulcer on Mrs Jacobs' leg and Mrs Jacobs tells her that she is worried about Fred because he is finding it hard to rest.

■ **What do you think could be some of the factors affecting Mr Jacobs' ability to rest?**

■ **What kind of advice could the nurse offer to Mrs Jacobs to enable Mr Jacobs to rest?**

■ **While talking to Mrs Jacobs she tells the nurse that Fred has had difficulty sleeping since they moved. What are the likely reasons for Mr Jacobs' difficulties in settling?**

■ What are some strategies the nurse could suggest to promote Mr Jacobs' sleep?

▶ CASE STUDY: CHILD

Joel is an 18-month-old toddler. He has an older brother Joshua, who is seven years old and a sister Naomi, who is four years old. They live with their parents in a two-bedroomed terraced house. The children share a bedroom. Joshua and Naomi have a bunk bed and Joel is still in a cot. Their parents, Samuel and Clarissa Jones are happily married. Samuel works shift work at a local factory and Clarissa is a full-time housewife.

Since being a baby Joel has been a poor sleeper at night. He wakes two or three times and is difficult to settle. He was initially breastfed until nine months of age, but is now fully weaned. He occasionally wants a drink when he awakens.

Clarissa is becoming increasingly tired. Samuel has been working nights for the last two weeks and she has found herself becoming irritable with both him and the children. Joel has been waking every night and the longest period of unbroken sleep that she has had over the past fortnight is four hours.

Samuel's family live some miles away and can provide little support. Clarissa's father is terminally ill and is being cared for at home by her mother. They live locally and it tends to be Clarissa supporting them rather than them supporting her. There are no other family members locally, and though they do have some friends, their friends all have families of their own.

The health visitor pops in to see Clarissa to do a developmental assessment on Joel and notices how tired Clarissa is looking. Clarissa pours out the story to her and asks for advice.

■ What are likely to be some of the reasons for Clarissa's poor sleep pattern?

■ What could be some of the reasons for Joel's poor sleep pattern?

■ What kind of strategies could the health visitor suggest to promote sleep and rest for Joel . . . . . . and Clarissa?

▶ CASE STUDY: LEARNING DISABILITIES

Francis Milligan is 18 years old. He had a birth injury, which has left him with a cerbral palsy. This has resulted in a spastic quadriplegia and he needs constant help with all activities of daily living. He is unable to use verbal communication, but his non-verbal behaviour indicates that he is able to understand what is said to him. He is normally cared for in a residential school, going home to his parents and six brothers for weekends and during the school holidays. He spends some time at a short-term respite centre funded by charity. He usually sleeps throughout the night, although he has to be moved three or four times a night to prevent the disruption to his skin integrity. Francis has now been admitted to hospital with a severe chest infection, which is compromising his airway. His spine has a severe scoliosis and he has a pigeon chest. He is difficult to position due to his disability, but this is exaggerated by his chest infection.

■ **What information would the nurse need to enable her to meet Francis' needs for rest and sleep?**

■ **How might the nurse assess the quality of Francis' rest and sleep?**

▶ CASE STUDY: MENTAL HEALTH

Marlene Meadows is a 32-year-old executive working in a large city firm. She works long hours every day and frequently takes paperwork home to complete in the evenings. She is married to Roger who is a chartered surveyor and they are buying a large Victorian house, which requires renovation. They have decided not to have children and to pursue their careers. However, Marlene is having some regrets about this decision and is feeling the lack of children quite acutely. She has been referred to the community psychiatric nurse (CPN) with anxiety and depression. One of her most upsetting symptoms is disturbed sleep, which has made it difficult for her to function during her working day. She has refused to take time off work at the present and finds it hard to describe how she relaxes in the evenings. The CPN suspects that she does not rest at all before attempting to settle to sleep. Marlene says that as soon as her head hits the pillow she wakes up and is no longer tired and she constantly thinks of the days events and prepares for the following day. She does settle eventually, but then wakes early in the morning and is unable to settle again.

■ **How would a detailed analysis of Marlene's sleep routine assist the planning of strategies to aid sleep?**

■ **What suggestions could be made about lifestyle that could enable Marlene to rest and relax?**

■ **What kind of sleep plan could be drawn up in partnership with Marlene to promote sleep?**

▶ CASE STUDY: STUDENT NURSE

Jennifer Stephens is a 20-year-old student nurse. She is at the end of the first year of the Common Foundation Programme. She has two assignments to be submitted in three weeks time and has barely managed to have a very rough draft of one and has not yet started the other. She knows that time is running out and she must work hard over the next few weeks to have them ready in time.

However, she is about to spend one week in practice placement at a nursery school. She did work experience at a junior school before joining the course and she remembers how tired she was at the end of each day. She is becoming quite worried about how she will cope with both her placement and her work.

She is living in the nurses' home at present and goes home most weekends. She finds it hard to settle to sleep in the nurses' home as it is often noisy in the late evenings. As a consequence she is often tired when she goes home and spends time 'catching up', particularly on a Sunday morning. In order to supplement her money she works at a local chip shop on a Saturday from 11 a.m. to 11 p.m. Sitting in the social club one evening she is talking to you about her situation and asks for your advice.

■ **What is the importance of resting and relaxing for Jennifer?**

■ **What suggestions would you make for her to promote rest and relaxation?**

■ **Think of your own situation. Is there a need for you to review your methods of resting and relaxing? What can you learn from this chapter that will inform your lifestyle and enable you to remain healthy?**

▶ ANNOTATED FURTHER READING

Within this chapter it has not been possible to fully explore all issues relating to sleep and rest. The literature on rest is limited; however there are some useful texts on sleep, which you may find it useful to extend your knowledge.

BORBELY, A. (1987) *Secrets of Sleep*. Harlow. Longman Scientific and Technical. (Translated by Schneider.)
This book provides an excellent overview of the science of sleep. The author has long experience in the study of sleep. The book is written in an easy to understand style and provides some insight into sleep problems.
DOUGLAS, J., RICHMAN, N. (1984) *My Child Won't Sleep*. Harmondsworth. Penguin Books.
This book is written for parents of children who are experiencing difficulties with sleep. The book offers an overview of common sleep problems in childhood and offers some practical solutions.
HODGSON, L.A. (1991) Why do we need sleep? Relating theory to nursing practice. *Journal of Advanced Nursing* **16**: 1503–1510.
This article offers a comprehensive insight into the physiology of sleep and its relevance to nursing practice.
MCMAHON, R. (ed.) (1992) *Nursing at Night: A Professional Approach*. Harrow. Scutari Press.
This edited book offers useful and practical insights into nursing at night. It has very useful chapters on promoting sleep and considers a wide range of quality and policy issues from a management perspective.
OSWALD, I., ADAM, K. (1983) *Get a Better Night's Sleep*. London. Martin Dunitz.
This book written for the lay public offers some useful insights for the health care professional. The authors of this book have some experience in the investigation of sleep and have some good advice for promoting a better night's sleep, as the title of the book suggests.

▶ REFERENCES

ATKINSON, R.L., ATKINSON, R.C., SMITH, E.E., BEM, D.J. (1993) *Introduction to Psychology* (11th edition). Orlando. Harcourt Brace and Company.

BARTON, J. (1995) Is flexible rostering helpful? *Nursing Times* **91(7)**: 32–33.

BOOMER, H., DEAKIN, A. (1991) Getting children to sleep. *Nursing Times* **87(12):** 40–43.

BORBELY, A. (1987) *Secrets of Sleep.* Harlow. Longman Scientific and Technical. (Translated by Schneider.)

BRUGNE, J.. (1994a) Sleep, Wakefulness and the Nurse. *British Journal of Nursing* **3(2)**: 68–71.

BRUGNE, J.F. (1994b) Effects of night work on circadian rhythms and sleep. *Professional Nurse* **10(1)**: 25–28.

BURTON, E. (1992) Something to help you sleep? *Nursing Times* **88(8)**: 52–54.

CANNARD, G. (1995) On the scent of a good night's sleep. *Nursing Standard* **9(34)**: 21.

CHILDS-CLARKE, A. (1990) Stimulus control techniques for sleep onset insomnia. *Nursing Times* **86(35)**: 52–53.

CLOSS, S.J. (1988) *A Nursing Study of Sleep on Surgical Wards.* Report prepared for the Scottish Home and Health Department Nursing Research Unit, Department of Nursing Studies. Edinburgh.

CRAWFORD, W., BENNETT, R., HEWITT, K. (1989) Sleep problems in pre-school children. *Health Visitor* **62(3)**: 77–81.

CRISP, A.H., MATTHEWS, B.M., OAKEY, M., CRUTCHFIELD, M. (1990) Sleepwalking, night terrors and consciousness. *British Medical Journal* **300**: 360–362.

DEAKIN, M. (1995) Using relaxation techniques to manage disruptive behaviour. *Nursing Times* **91(17)**: 40–41.

DEPARTMENT OF HEALTH AND SOCIAL SECURITY AND THE WELSH OFFICE (1976) *The Organisation of the In-patient's Day*: Report of a Committee of the Central Health Services Council. London. Her Majesty's Stationery Office.

DOUGLAS, J., RICHMAN, N. (1984) *My Child Won't Sleep.* Harmondsworth. Penguin Books.

DUNN, C., SLEEP, J., COLLETT, D. (1995) Sensing an improvement: an experimental study to evaluate the use of aromatherapy, massage and periods of rest in an intensive care unit. *Journal of Advanced Nursing* **21**: 34–40.

DUNWELL, F. (1995) Insomnia and mental health. *Nursing Times* **91(37)**: 31–32.

DUXBURY, J. (1994a) Understanding the nature of sleep. *Nursing Standard* **9(9)**: 25–28.

DUXBURY, J. (1994b) Avoiding disturbed sleep in hospitals. *Nursing Standard* **9(10)**: 31–34.

DUXBURY, J. (1994c) An investigation into primary nursing and its effect upon the nursing attitudes about, and administration of, prn night sedation. *Journal of Advanced Nursing* **19(5)**: 923–931.

DUXBURY, J. (1994d) Night nurses are they undervalued? *Nursing Standard* **9(11)**: 33–35.

FARDELL, J. (1989) Children who don't sleep. *Nursing Times* **85(17)**: 39–41.

FOLKARD, S. Circadian rhythms and hours of work. In WARR P. (ed.) *Psychology of Work* (3rd edition). Chapter 2, pp. 30–52. Harmondsworth. Penguin Books.

GALBRAITH, L., HEWITT, K.E., PRITCHARD, L. (1993) Behavioural treatment for sleep disturbance. *Health Visitor* **66(3)**: 169–171.

GARFINKEL, D., LAUDON, M., NOF D., ZISAPEL, N. (1995) Improvement of sleep quality in elderly people by controlled-release melatonin. *The Lancet* **346** 541–544.

GREEN, S. (1987) *Physiological Psychology: An Introduction.* London. Routledge and Kegan Paul.

HAIMOV, I., LAUDON, M., ZISAPEL, N., SOUROUJON, M., NOF D., SHLITNER, A., HERER, P., TZISCHINSKY, O., LAVIE, P. (1994) Sleep disorders and melatonin rhythms in elderly people. *British Medical Journal* **309**: 67.

HALFENS, R., COX, K., KUPPER-VAN MERWIJK, A. (1994) Effect of the use of sleep medication in Dutch hospitals on the use of sleep medication at home. *Journal of Advanced Nursing* **19(1)**: 66–70.

HASLAM, D. (1992) *Sleepless Children: A Handbook for Parents.* London. Piatkus.

HEWITT-SAYER, W., MAYFIELD, S. (1992) Night-Watch. *Nursing Times* **88(16)**: 32–35.

HILL, J. (1989) A good night's sleep. *Senior Nurse* **9(5)**: 17–19.

HICKS, F.M. A quality assurance programme for night nurses. In McMAHON, R. (ed.) (1992) *Nursing At Night: A Professional Approach.* Chapter 9, pp. 127–148. Harrow. Scutari Press.

HODGSON, L.A. (1991) Why do we need sleep? Relating theory to nursing practice. *Journal of Advanced Nursing* **16**: 1503–1510.

HORNE, J.A. (1988) *Why We Sleep: The Functions of Sleep in Human and Other Mammals.* Oxford. Oxford University Press.

IRWIN, P. The physiology of sleep. In

McMAHON, R. (ed.) (1992) *Nursing At Night: A Professional Approach.* Chapter 2, pp. 30–52. Harrow. Scutari Press.

KEARNES, S. (1989) Insomnia in the elderly. *Nursing Times* **35(47)**: 32–33.

LAURENT, C. (1991) Perchance to dream. *Nursing Times* **87(24)**: 16–17.

LITTLE, B.C., HAYWORTH, J., BENSON, P., HALL, F., BEARD, R.W., DEWHURST, J., PRIEST, R.G. (1984) Treatment of hypertension in pregnancy by relaxation and biofeedback *The Lancet* **i**: 865–867.

MANTLE, F. (1996) Sleepless and unsettled. *Nursing Times* **92(23)**: 46–47.

MORGAN, K. (1987) *Sleep and Ageing.* London. Croom Helm.

MUSSEN, P.H., CONGER, J.J., KAGEN, J., HUSTON, A.C. (1990) *Child Development and Personality* (7th edition). New York. Harper Collins.

NATIONAL CHILDREN'S HOME (1992) *The NCH Factfile: Children in Britain 1992.* London. National Children's Home.

NIE, V.M., HUNTER, M., ALLAN, D. (1988) The Central Nervous System. In HINCHLIFF, S., MONTAGUE, S. (eds) *Physiology for Nursing Practice.* pp. 88–139. London. Baillière Tindall.

NORTHCOTT, N., FACEY, S. (1995) Twelve hour shifts: helpful or hazardous to patients? *Nursing Times* **91(7)**: 29–31.

OSWALD, I., ADAM, K. (1983) *Get a Better Night's Sleep.* London. Martin Dunitz.

PATTERSON, D.L. (1991) Achieving excellence in nursing. *Journal of Pediatric Nursing* **6(6)**: 391–395.

QUINE, L., WADE, K., HARGREAVES, R. (1991) Learning to sleep. *Nursing Times* **87(48)**: 41–43.

RAPER, J. (1992) Practised advice. *Nursing Times* **88(36)**: 26–27.

REID, S. (1992) After the big sleep. *Nursing Times* **88(36)**: 28.

ROBERTS, S. (1993) Tackling sleep problems through a clinic based approach. *Health Visitor* **66(5)**: 173–174.

RYAN, S. (1995) Fibromyalgia: what help can nurses give? *Nursing Standard* **9(37)**: 25–28.

SANDERSON, H., CARTER, A. (1994) Healing hands. *Nursing Times* **90(11)**: 46–48.

SKIPPER, J.K., JUNG, F.D., COFFEY, L.C. (1990) Nurses and shiftwork: effects on physical health and mental depression. *Journal of Advanced Nursing* **15(7)**: 835–842.

SMITH, S. (1992) Tiresome healing. *Nursing Times* **88(36)**: 24–25.

SOUTHWELL, M.T., WISTOW, G. (1995) Sleep in hospital: Are patients needs being met? *Journal of Advanced Nursing*

21(6): 1101–1109.
TAYLOR, A. (1985) In for a rest? *Nursing Times* **81(36)**: 29–31.
TORTORA, G.J., ANAGNOSTAKOS, N.P. (1987) *Principles of Anatomy and Physiology* (5th edition). New York. Harper and Row.
TOTTERDELL, P., SMITH, L., FOLKARD,

S. Nurses as night workers. In McMAHON, R. (ed.) (1992) *Nursing at Night: A Professional Approach.* Chapter 8, pp. 109–126. Harrow. Scutari Press.
UKCC (1992) *Code of Professional Conduct* (3rd edition). London. UKCC.
WEISSBLUTH, M. (1987) *Sleep Well:*

Peaceful Nights for You and Your Child. London. Unwin Paperbacks.
WELLER, B.F. (ed.) (1989) *Bailliere's Encyclopaedic Dictionary of Nursing and Health Care.* London. Baillière Tindall.
WILKIE (1990) Golden slumbers. *Nursing Times* **86(51)**: 36–38.

4.5 Rehabilitation

J. Barker

KEY ISSUES

■ SUBJECT KNOWLEDGE
▶ social and political context of rehabilitation
▶ body image, social roles and self-esteem
▶ stigma and labelling
▶ altered body image, loss and grieving
▶ motivation and change
▶ teams and leadership

■ PRACTICE KNOWLEDGE
▶ nursing assessment for beginning a rehabilitation programme
▶ risk assessment
▶ goal setting and prioritizing
▶ communication skills
▶ the nurse as an educator

▶ health beliefs and change

■ PROFESSIONAL KNOWLEDGE
▶ the implications of the NHS and Community Care Act 1990 for rehabilitation
▶ the ethics of rehabilitation and who benefits most
▶ health rationing
▶ the role of the nurse in the multidisciplinary rehabilitation team

■ REFLECTIVE KNOWLEDGE
▶ the nurse's role in rehabilitation
▶ the wide scope of rehabilitation
▶ rehabilitation in professional practice

▶ INTRODUCTION

There has been a shift from custodial care to rehabilitation in a variety of contexts ranging from care of the elderly to children's disorders and physical disorders to enduring mental illness. Indeed legislation in the form of *The Health of The Nation* (Department of Health, 1991) identifies rehabilitation as a key area in the strategy for health. This would seem to suggest that rehabilitation is becoming an area of increasing importance.

Various definitions of rehabilitation are available, but Waters' definition (1994, p. 239) is the most comprehensive suggesting the term relates to 'the whole process of enabling and facilitating the restoration of a disabled person to regain optimum functioning (physically, socially and psychologically) to the level they are able or motivated to achieve.'

The word 'process' in the above definition suggests an activity that moves forward through a series of actions aimed at achieving an identified result. Williams (1993, p. 67) asserts that 'rehabilitation is a process not an end in itself, where the greatest steps are usually the smallest, sometimes literally, and every day gives the opportunity to see someone win a major victory over his or her own body or mind'.

Rehabilitation is seen by Doughty (1991) as not only the province of the old, immobile or physically disabled, but for all who experience health problems, both acute and chronic. She suggests that whenever it is necessary for choices to be made relating to the achieving of a full, active, healthy lifestyle following illness, a rehabilitation process is necessary. If this is so, rehabilitation is an aspect of every nurse's practice and as such warrants close consideration.

▶ OVERVIEW

This chapter addresses the various factors that may have a bearing on the process of rehabilitation. It is divided into four main parts.

▶ *Subject Knowledge*

Part one, Subject Knowledge, develops the scope of rehabilitation. Rehabilitation is undertaken in a wide range of settings and as such it would be impossible to address physical aspects here. However, the social, psychological and social policy aspects are common and have great relevance to all forms of rehabilitation and for this reason form a large section of this part. Interpersonal aspects of care provision are also discussed in relation to communication between nurses and clients and interprofessionally. The development of such skills is central to professional practice in the rehabilitation setting.

▶ *Practice Knowledge*

Part two of the chapter, Practice Knowledge, looks at the nurse's role in the process of rehabilitation through assessment, goal setting and health education. The use of decision-making exercises and reflective exercises help to promote consideration and development of knowledge essential to the provision of nursing care.

▶ *Professional Knowledge*

Part three of the chapter, Professional Knowledge, focuses on three main issues: the impact of the *NHS and Community Care Act* (Department of Health, 1990a), the nurse's membership within a multidisciplinary team and ethical issues in rehabilitation.

▶ *Reflective Knowledge*

Finally, in Reflective Knowledge the main points of the chapter are revisited.

On pp. 620–622 there are four case studies, each one relating to one of the branch programmes. You may find it helpful to read one of them before you start the chapter and use it as a focus for your reflections while reading.

RESEARCH BASED EVIDENCE
Gibbon and Thompson (1992) found that nurses had difficulty in defining their role in the process of rehabilitation. Although they thought they made a contribution this was usually in collaboration with other members of the care team such as occupational therapists and physiotherapists. They concluded from this that nurses should recognize their own role in rehabilitation and develop the confidence to implement their own rehabilitation programmes rather than taking their lead from other disciplines.

SUBJECT KNOWLEDGE
Psychosocial

▶ THE SOCIAL AND POLITICAL CONTEXT OF REHABILITATION

Rehabilitation appears to be an area of increasing interest in health care. With the growing number of individuals suffering from chronic disorders and the advent of the *NHS and Community Care Act* (Department of Health, 1990a) rehabilitation is seen as an effective way of returning people to or maintaining people in the community. This is reflected in the social policies of various governments. An understanding of social policy and its impact on the health care of individuals is therefore important.

Social policy relates to central and local government activities associated with the provision of services related to health, education, housing and social services, including social security and income support. It addresses questions concerning how much welfare the state should provide and how this is to be funded.

Developed countries are viewed as having a mixed economy of welfare made up of:

‣ state sector;
‣ private sector;
‣ voluntary sector;
‣ informal carers.

The term welfare state is used to describe the type of society that developed in the UK after 1945. Successive governments intervened positively in the economic and social interests of the general public with a view to achieving a minimum standard of living for all. This approach grew out of a distinct set of social ideas – ideology – known as collectivism where all individuals have certain social, economic and political rights. Before this the ideology had been that of *laissez faire* associated with minimal state interference in social and economic affairs.

The growth of the welfare state continued from 1940s until the late 1970s due to what is known as consensus politics. Here political parties have a basic agreement about the desirability of a welfare state. This consensus broke down in the late 1970s due to a growing dissatisfaction with the welfare state as it became seen as ineffective and expensive to maintain. Criticisms of the welfare state were offered by the New Right (Table 4.5.1)

Inequalities in society are inevitable
The welfare state has not delivered equity of welfare
The welfare state undermines enterprise and initiative
The welfare state is incompatible with wealth creation
The welfare state keeps people in the poverty trap
State involvement is wrong and dangerous
A need to move towards thrift, self-reliance and self-help

Table 4.5.1 The New Right views on the welfare state.

Look at Table 4.5.1.

• *Do you think the criticisms of the welfare state offered by the New Right are valid?*

• *Why have you arrived at your decision?*

Since the 1970s there have been four major developments in the provision of welfare:

‣ the growth of the private sector;
‣ restriction on public expenditure;
‣ a focus on efficiency and selectivity;
‣ the introduction of an internal market.

Although community care has been a major feature of health policy since the 1950s (Table 4.5.2) only gradual progress had been made. The *NHS and Community Care Act* (Department of Health, 1990a) intended to address this and provided plans for the move towards community care from the 1990s and beyond.

The *NHS and Community Care Act* (1990) proposed to provide services and support for the disabled and elderly individuals to enabe them to live independently in their own homes or in homely surroundings (Table 4.5.3).

1959	*Mental Health Act* aimed at providing a 'comprehensive' community care service
1961	*Hospital Plan* begun to run down large mental hospitals
1963	White paper *Health and Welfare, the Development of Community Care*
1971	White paper *Better Services for the Mentally Handicapped*
1974	Statutory requirement for *Joint Planning* between health and local authorities.
1975	White paper *Better Services for the Mentally Ill*
1976	*Joint Finance Initiative* to allow health services' moneys to be used to develop community services run by local authorities
1978	Discussion document *Happier Old Age*
1983	*Community Care Initiative* promoting the transfer of clients to community-based resources from long-stay hospitals
1984	Voluntary sector formally involved in planning initiatives
1985	*Commons' Social Services Committee Report* recommends that hospital closures should be slowed down
1986	Audit Commission report *Making a Reality of Community Care* identifies a fragmentation of services and perverse incentives encouraging residential care
1988	*Griffiths' Report* identifies the need to provide services geared to individuals' needs in the form of care packages
1989	White paper *Caring for People*
1990	*NHS and Community Care Act*

Table 4.5.2 A chronology of community care.

To promote the development of domiciliary day and respite services to enable people to live in their own homes wherever feasible and sensible

To ensure that the service providers make practical support for carers a high priority

To make proper assessment of need and good care the cornerstone of high quality care

To promote the development of a flourishing independent sector alongside good quality public services

To clarify the responsibilities of agencies and so to make it easier to hold them to account for their performance

To secure better value for tax payers' money by introducing a new funding structure for social care

Table 4.5.3 Policy objectives for community care (Department of Health, 1990b).

▶ SOCIAL ROLES

The social and political context explains how a society views rehabilitation. To explore what it actually means for individuals requires an understanding of how individuals interact within society.

Individuals and society interact through taking various social roles. This provides a sense of purpose and belonging for all individuals within society and allows the individual to develop a concept of self. A loss of social role can occur following illness or disability or as a result of the often prolonged process of rehabilitation. In enabling an individual to achieve their optimum level of functioning, Smith and Clark (1995) suggest that within the rehabilitation process an individual's ability to resume his or her normal social role is of great importance. This is supported by McGrath and Davis (1992), who also propose that a major aim of rehabilitation is to enable individuals to resume valued social roles. An understanding of social roles is therefore central to planning rehabilitation programmes.

Social roles are associated with the individual's status within his or her society. Status relates to things such as:

▶ gender (e.g. male or female);
▶ occupation (e.g. nurse, farmworker, tailor);
▶ family relationships (e.g. daughter, brother, parent).

> • Consider your role as a nurse. Is this role fixed or negotiated?
>
> • How might this affect your interaction with clients?

Status is culturally defined and may be either:

▶ fixed or ascribed (e.g. gender or caste);
▶ achieved (e.g. marital status or class).

For each status there are identifiable expected and acceptable ways of behaving. These are known as 'norms'. The group of norms attached to a particular status is a 'role'. Therefore each status is accompanied by a role, which shapes and directs social behaviour. Individuals then perform this role in relation to one another (Table 4.5.4). This enables individuals to interact with one another, predict how each other will behave and have a clear idea of what is expected in terms of their own and related roles. For example, in the interaction between nurse and client, each knows what is expected of them and how the other should respond. Both nurse and client can then concentrate on the situation they are in without being inhibited by other aspects of their lives.

When someone becomes ill they may not be able to fulfil their normal roles and this affects their perceived status and self-esteem. For example, if a woman experiences a stroke that affects her ability to do domestic chores, she may feel that this affects her role as a provider of care for her husband. This may have an impact on the way the husband and wife interact and their expectations of each other.

So far it seems that social roles and obligations are clearly identified and explicit. Such a view of role is adopted by a particular perspective in sociology known as 'functionalism'. An alternative theoretical stance is that of 'interactionism'.

From an interactionist perspective the idea of role is less defined. Although roles are viewed as a part of the social system, role is seen as a set of general guidelines, which allows negotiation between two individuals. A role is not fixed, but fluid and changeable. Therefore there is no script as to how a student nurse should behave; rather this is negotiated between students and their teachers, ward supervisor and clients. This negotiation occurs in relation to an individual's understanding of the role and their beliefs.

▶ Sick Role

From all sociological perspectives individuals have a variety of roles, which are culturally defined and carry obligations. When people become ill, they are unable to continue their normal roles. In a definitive analysis on the impact of illness on social status, Parsons (1951) suggested that this inability of sick people to perform their usual social roles is viewed as deviant behaviour and requires some form of regulation. Normally within a society any behaviour that is viewed as deviant and is preventable is regulated through sanctions such as the imprisonment imposed on those who commit crimes. As illness cannot be prevented, Parsons suggested regulation is achieved through a socially prescribed role to control the behaviour of the sick person (i.e. a defined sick role). This sick role contains four expectations, consisting of two rights and two obligations (Table 4.5.5).

The granting of the rights of the sick role is dependent upon the individual fulfilling the obligations. If a person fails to meet the obligations the rights may be suspended and the individual is seen as responsible for his or her illness. The sick role is viewed as a temporary role with the main function of minimizing the disruptive effect of illness on society and ensuring that individuals return to a healthy state as soon as possible. This is very limiting and various criticisms are therefore levelled at Parson's (1951) proposed sick role (Table 4.5.6).

Status	Nurse
Norms	Knowledge of illness
	Cares for people
	Gentle and kind
Role	Wears a uniform
	Practical
	Busy

Table 4.5.4 Role of the nurse

DECISION MAKING

Think of a client in whose care you have recently been involved during a clinical placement.

- *Identify the various roles that individual may have.*
- *How might their illness or disability affect these roles?*
- *How could the nurse help the client adjust to the new role demands in the short term?*
- *What long-term role adjustments might this client be required to make?*

- **On your last practice placement, did the clients meet Parson's (1951) criteria for the sick role (see Table 4.5.5)?**
- **If they did, how?**
- **Have you ever taken the sick role?**
- **Did you fulfil the demands and obligations?**
- **What problems are there in applying the sick role to individuals with mental health problems who do not comply with medical advice?**

Right or obligation	Provisos
Two Rights	
The sick person is exempt from performing his or her usual social role	This exemption is relative to the severity of the illness It must be legitimized by others – often the doctor is the legitimizing agent
The sick person is not responsible for his or her illness	The person is not expected to 'pull themselves together' As he or she is exempt from responsibility there is an expectation of 'being taken care of'
Two Obligations	
The sick person must get better as soon as possible	Being ill is unacceptable and the person must be motivated to get well
The sick person must seek medical advice and comply with the treatment prescribed	Help must be sought from a competent and acceptable source in relation to the severity of the illness

Table 4.5.5 The sick role (Parsons, 1951).

People with minor illnesses are not expected to adopt the sick role
The sick role usually applies only to acute physical illnesses
People with mental illness are often reluctant to adopt the sick role
The sick role is seen as non-applicable to chronic illnesses as these are not temporary and the individual may not be able to return to previous roles

Table 4.5.6 The limitations of the sick role.

▌ LABELLING AND STIGMAS

Becoming ill can be viewed as deviant and the sick role offers a way of describing how behaviour is regulated. An alternative way of viewing this is through labelling theory. This offers an interactionist view of society and an explanation as to how a client's role is negotiated and maintained.

Lemert (1951) suggested two forms of deviation: primary and secondary. Primary deviation relates to acts that an individual may engage in before being publicly labelled as deviant. These acts are seen as relatively unimportant as they have little impact on an individual's self-concept. What is important is society's response to the individual. Public recognition and labelling of deviant behaviour coupled with the consequences of such identification produces a response from the individual. This response is the secondary deviation. Society's reaction to the individual assigns a new role and status, which has an impact on the individual's self-concept and future actions. The transformation from primary deviance to secondary deviance occurs when an individual labelled deviant accepts the 'new' social status and role.

Williams (1987) discusses primary deviance in relation to a medical diagnosis. Secondary deviation occurs where the diagnosis is accepted and associated with a negative social status. As a result of illness or surgery, labels such as diabetic, schizophrenic or amputee may be applied. Therefore the labelled individual is marked as different from the rest of society and may invoke negative social reactions. 'Stigma' is the term applied to such responses.

The classic work on stigma was produced by Goffman (1963), who identified various sources and attributes in relation to this phenomenon (Table 4.5.7). The negative social responses to conditions that attract stigmas are related to feelings such as fear or disgust associated with certain labels and the attributing of stereotypical traits to individuals. Therefore people in wheel chairs are often viewed as both mentally and physically disabled, while someone with a mental illness is considered to be potentially violent.

Sources	Abominations of the body	Physical disabilities
	Blemishes of character	Mental illness, sexual deviance
	Tribal stigmas	Race, nation, religion
Attributes	Discreditable	Those that are not visible or known and are therefore only potentially stigmatizing such as epilepsy, acquired immuno-deficiency syndrome (AIDS), diabetes mellitus
	Discrediting	Known, visible and provoking a reaction in others, for example facial disablement or deformities, symptoms of mental illness

Table 4.5.7 Sources and attributes of stigma (Goffman, 1963).

Stigmatized ideas are culturally determined, that is they are based on the society's norms and values, which are learned early in life and reinforced through every day conversations and the media. Individuals with stigmatizing illnesses may be viewed as socially inferior and may also be subject to discrimination and socially disadvantaged. The imposing of such social disfavour may result in poor self-concept and identity. Goffman (1963) suggests that the stigmatized individual may adopt various responses when interacting with a non-stigmatized individual (Table 4.5.8.)

Passing	Tries to conceal attribute and 'pass' as normal (e.g. an individual not disclosing a history of mental illness to an employer)
Covering	Tries to reduce the significance of the condition (e.g. attempts to resume 'normal behaviour')
Withdrawal	Opts out of social interaction with 'normal' people (e.g. all social activities involve others with a similar disorder)

Table 4.5.8 Responses to stigma (Goffman, 1963).

▶ BODY IMAGE

Many stigmatizing illnesses have an impact on the way an individual perceives his or her body and therefore his or her body image. Body image is a much used term that has wide applications in holistic care. Body image affects the social, spiritual, physical and psychological aspects of wellbeing, and as such, an understanding of this subject is vital to the provision of care. Price (1990) suggests that a client's body image has an impact on the process of rehabilitation, having consequences for and affecting the client's wellbeing. He identifies three components to body image:

- ▶ how individuals perceive and feel about their bodies (body reality);
- ▶ how the body responds to commands (body presentation);

▶ how the first two components compare with an internal standard (body ideal) (Table 4.5.9).

Reality	As it really is: tall/short, fat/thin, dark/fair Norm for race and relative to wider social group Not a constant state, dependent upon age and physical changes
Presentation	Dress and fashion Control of functions, movement and pose How others receive us
Ideal	How a body should look and act (culturally determined and includes contours, size, proportion, odours and smells) Personal norm for personal space Body reliability, which may be unrealistic Applied not only to self, but to those around us

Table 4.5.9 Components of body image (Price, 1990).

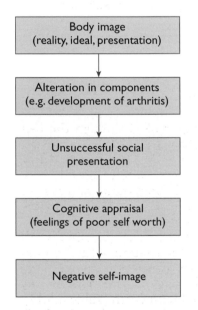

Figure 4.5.1: Impact of body image on self-image.

Throughout life there is an attempt to achieve and maintain a balance between the three elements.

Body image depends not only upon the individual's response to his or her own body, but also upon the appearance, attitude and responses of others. This is important for nurses to remember when delivering care, as their own responses may have a great impact on how clients perceive themselves.

Body image and self-image are interconnected, self-image being central to an individual's confidence, motivation and sense of achievement. It is a product of an individual's personality, being moulded by socialization and represents an assessment of self-worth (Price, 1990). There is a high valuing of attractiveness within developed countries, with an associated stereotyping of beautiful as good (Bercheid and Walster, 1974). When the three elements of body image are in a state of equilibrium, meeting both personal and social expectations and therefore enabling a successful presentation of self, there is a corresponding positive self-image. If, however, changes occur that result in an alteration of one or more of the body image components, a negative self-image may follow (Figure 4.5.1).

Altered body images can arise from two sources

▶ open (i.e. visible) as with arthritis;
▶ hidden (i.e. not readily observable) such as a colostomy.

Personal responses to altered body image will arise from the interaction of a variety of factors, including:

▶ visibility;
▶ associated shame or guilt;
▶ significance for the future – work, social life, personal;
▶ support during transition;
▶ personal coping strategies;
▶ stage of the grieving process.

In discussing the types of problems that an individual with spinal injuries may encounter in relation to altered body image, Brennan (1994) identifies three main areas of concern as physical, psychological and social (Table 4.5.10).

Physical	Arise from altered body reality related to reduced ability to care for self and presence of inhibiting factors such as catheter, sutures, drains
Psychological	The extent to which the body reality deviates from the body ideal will have a psychological impact on the individual
	These problems may arise from a sense of loss related to appearance, ability and function, resulting in the person experiencing the grieving process
	Self-esteem may be lowered
Social	Body presentation is altered through the use of equipment (e.g. wheel chair, cervical collar, walking frame)
	This may cause anxiety relating to how the person thinks he or she will be viewed by others and in turn this has an impact on self-image and confidence
	Social isolation can result

Table 4.5.10 Problems related to altered body image in people with spinal injuries following surgery (Brennan, 1994).

▶ LOSS AND GRIEVING

The concept of grief is usually associated with death and dying, but it can also be examined in terms of loss in more general ways. Costello (1995) suggests that grief relates to the feelings evoked through the loss of something valued, and as proposed by Sheppard (1994), individuals requiring rehabilitation have to come to terms with many losses. These losses relate to things such as lifestyle changes, altered physical or psychological functioning and loss of body parts. This can give rise to the grieving process.

In her work with terminally ill people and their families Kubler-Ross (1970) identified a number of emotional stages experienced by people faced with death (Table 4.5.11). She suggests that not all individuals will go through all these stages, that some may never reach acceptance, and that individuals may move to and fro between the stages. Although this process is viewed in terms of the individual's impending 'loss' through their own death, it can also have relevance to losses experienced from illness and disability.

DECISION MAKING

Gareth Pearce, aged 23, is developing his career as a professional footballer. He played for a third division team when he was spotted by a scout for a premier league team, who subsequently signed him on. He appears to have a promising career ahead of him. However, in his fourth match in the first team as a result of a bad tackle, Gareth finds himself in the accident and emergency department with a fractured left tibia and fibula. He is accompanied by his wife and young son. The orthopaedic surgeon informs Gareth that he will not be playing football again for the rest of the season and that the fracture is so severe that at this stage he is uncertain whether Gareth will be able to play football again.

- *What losses might Gareth and his family experience as a result of the accident and during his hospitalization?*
- *What responses or behaviour could this evoke?*
- *How might a knowledge of the grief reaction help the nurse to support Gareth and his family over the immediate crisis?*

(For further information on the grief reaction see Chapter 3.5 on Death and Dying.)

Stage of grief	Features
Denial	Feeling that 'this can't be true', emotions are not expressed and the person tries to continue as if nothing has happened.
Anger	Following acknowledgement of the reality an individual may express anger. This may be directed at themselves, friends, family, carers, God, everyone or everything in general.
Bargaining	The person seeks to avoid the inevitable by proposing 'bargains' such as becoming a good person or going to church regularly if only they are allowed to live longer or have less pain. These 'bargains' are made privately or silently.
Anger, depression, acceptance	As the individual begins to feel that bargaining is futile they may lapse into depression or revert to their anger, questioning 'why me'? For the person to feel this way there has to be a certain element of acceptance
True acceptance	

Table 4.5.11 Stages of grief (Kubler-Ross, 1970).

▶ MOTIVATION

One of the most important factors in the process of rehabilitation is that of the client's motivation. Where a client's physical ability is present, but motivation is lacking, Squires and Wardle (1988) propose that rehabilitation becomes a most frustrating experience for those providing care. There is a need to understand what motivates people and why some individuals appear more motivated than others.

Atkinson *et al.* (1993) suggest three different types of motives drive behaviour and are:

- ▶ survival needs – related to those activities necessary to ensure the individual's survival such as eating and drinking, and have a biological basis;
- ▶ social needs – may have a biological basis, but require interaction with others, for example sexual drives where the need to reproduce the species has a biological basis, but the behaviour is culturally determined in terms of what is acceptable or not;
- ▶ the need to satisfy curiosity.

Various theories of motivation have been put forward and Sternberg (1995) suggests that the concept has captured the imagination of psychologists from varying academic backgrounds. The theories are classified into three general approaches:

- ▶ physiological approaches, which address the relationship between the central nervous system and behavioural aspects of motivation;
- ▶ clinical approaches, which consider the relationship between personality and motivation;
- ▶ cognitive approaches, which are viewed as examining the thought process underlying behaviour.

Examples of these various approaches are given in Table 4.5.12. As Sternberg (1995) identifies, an individual's physiology, personality and cognitive processes cannot be examined in isolation as each interacts with the others. Therefore it may be necessary to adopt an integrated approach to the understanding of motivation.

Approach and example	Features
Physiological approach e.g. Arousal theory (cited in Sternberg, 1995)	Activity in the central nervous system dictates level of arousal Each person has their optimum level of arousal Individuals perform most efficiently at the optimum arousal level Low levels of arousal result in boredom, inactivity and poor motivation High levels of arousal result in anxiety and tension
Clinical approach e.g. Maslow's hierarchy of needs (Maslow, 1970)	Needs are hierarchical in nature, having the following seven levels: 1. Food, water, air 2. Safety, shelter 3. Belonging, love, companionship 4. Self-esteem 5. Cognitive needs – knowledge 6. Aesthetic needs – goodness, beauty 7. Self-actualization Each level of need (beginning with physiological) must be satisfied before moving onto the next Having achieved or satisfied one level individuals are motivated to satisfy the next level of need
Cognitive approach e.g. Intrinsic and extrinsic motivators (cited in Sternberg, 1995)	Intrinsic motivators come from within – doing things because they are interesting and important to the individual Extrinsic motivators come from outside the individual in the form of perceived rewards or punishments Motivation results from either one or a combination of both intrinsic or extrinsic factors

Table 4.5.12 Examples of different approaches to motivation.

▌ MANAGEMENT OF CHANGE

The alteration of an individual's health status may necessitate lifestyle changes to reduce risk factors associated with particular disorders. The rehabilitation process therefore involves the developing of skills, attitudes and norms in individuals to enable the achievement of optimum wellbeing. For example, someone with hypertension may be asked to stop smoking, lose weight, take up an exercise routine and reduce their stress. Such a regimen involves major lifestyle changes, an increased knowledge relating to diet and exercise and the development of alternative coping skills.

Change is described by Keyser (1986, p. 103) as 'an attempt to alter or replace existing knowledge or skills, attitudes, norms, and styles of individuals or groups'.

To facilitate change the nurse must adopt the role of 'change agent'. A change agent is someone who creates an environment conducive to change, overcomes resistance to change, understands how to encourage acceptance of the need for change, generates ideas and implements and evaluates the process. Lancaster and Lancaster (1982) identified specific skills that are required to successfully facilitate change (Table 4.5.13).

People prefer the familiar and often show resistance to change, seeing it as a threat. This may relate to the nature of the change or beliefs (real or imagined) about what the change will mean. The anxiety invoked by change may be related to:

Communication
Group process
Self-awareness
Interpersonal
Assertiveness
Assessment
Planning
Implementation
Evaluation
Prioritizing

Table 4.5.13 Skills needed to be a change agent (Lancaster and Lancaster, 1982).

⬗ fear of the unknown;
⬗ uncertainty;
⬗ lack of knowledge or skills to achieve change;
⬗ low confidence;
⬗ feelings of powerlessness;
⬗ resentment to need for changes.

Resistance to change manifests itself in a variety of ways as the experience is a personal one, but there are some common responses (Table 4.5.14).

Lip service	Individuals listen to suggestions, agree while change agent is present, but do not undertake proposed action or behaviour in their absence
Aggression	Person displays aggressive behaviour, which results in them not having to face or undertake the change
Destruction	In an attempt to reduce feelings of anxiety individuals may demonstrate destructive behaviour (e.g. a family member may encourage the client not to adhere to a diet when trying to lose weight or to have a cigarette when attempting to give up smoking)
Lack of continuity	Individuals may find excuses not to do certain things – 'I'm too busy today to do my exercises'; the excuses increase until the proposed change is shelved completely

Table 4.5.14 Common resistance to change behaviours (Vaughan and Pillmoor, 1989).

The process of change also provokes an emotional response in those involved, which has been described as 'the emotional cycle of change' (Kelley and Connor, 1979; Table 4.5.15). Here individuals experience a variety of highs and lows as change occurs, the process ends in 'the glow' of satisfaction (Vaughan and Pillmoor, 1989).

Stage	Features	Individual experiences
Uninformed optimism (certainty)	Ideas look good Obstacles are trivial Morale at its peak	Highs
Informed pessimism (doubt)	Problems occur Energy wanes Solutions difficult to identify Why did I ever start this?'	Lows
Hopeful realism (hope)	Deals with emotions and doubts Modifies goals	
Informed optimism (confidence)	Individual gains confidence in abilities to succeed Encouragement, recognition and support are needed	
Rewarding completion (satisfaction)	Successful implementation of change	Glows

Table 4.5.15 Stages of the emotional cycle of change (Kelley and Connor, 1979).

To summarize so far then, to reduce resistance to change and to help individuals through the cycle of change, a change agent must:

RESEARCH BASED EVIDENCE

Davis et al. (1992) implemented changes to working practice in a rehabilitation centre where they moved from a multidisciplinary to an interdisciplinary approach. This led to the adoption of a more client-centred method of care, which was directed by a specific 'care coordinator'. They described the process of change and highlighted the problems that occurred. From the experience they identified that:

- **The terminology used by all involved on the process of change must be clearly defined and understood.**
- **Aims and objectives must be clearly stated.**
- **Sufficient time must be given for the change to occur.**
- **Records should be kept throughout the process and should include all successes and failures.**
- **Evaluation must occur.**

- communicate effectively – this includes listening;
- develop trust among all participants;
- clearly identify goals, plans, priorities and problems;
- ensure necessary resources are available;
- define responsibilities of others, allowing individuals freedom to do their part;
- evaluate at regular intervals to review provide feedback on progress (Lancaster and Lancaster, 1982).

In selecting the appropriate strategy to facilitate change, two criteria are essential (Haffer, 1986). First, it is necessary to focus on an appropriate goal. Second, the individual should be both willing and able to make the change. For example if implementing a fitness regimen the goal of walking ten miles every day may not be appropriate for an 80-year-old woman. She may be neither willing nor physically able to undertake such a proposal. To implement change successfully then, a variety of factors must be considered and used effectively (Table 4.5.16). Without these elements in place change is unlikely to occur.

Element	Features
Involvement	Of all individuals who will be affected, professionals and carers
Motivation	Valuing of everyone's contribution Listening to and respect for all involved
Planning	Must be flexible
Legitimization	Sanctioned or owned by those involved
Education	Individuals have the necessary skills or knowledge
Management	Aimed at developing the necessary skills
Expectations	To expect the unexpected To respect other's experiences
Nurturance	Recognition of individuals' needs Support
Trust	

Table 4.5.16 Implementing change requires the following elements (Lancaster and Lancaster, 1982).

Promoting Effective Communication

To communicate is generally taken to mean to 'impart', 'transmit' or 'share'. Thurgood (1990) states that communication is central to the rehabilitation programme as without good communication the client ultimately suffers. From Thurgood's perspective, effective communication is essential to the rehabilitation process, ensuring that all involved – nurse, client, family, friends and members of the multidisciplinary team – are fully aware of and can participate in the process. Therefore a general understanding of the factors that promote and hinder the process of effective communication is essential.

To communicate effectively various skills need to be developed. These include:

- active listening;
- use of appropriate questioning;
- awareness of non-verbal communication.

▶ Active listening

Active listening or attending is more than hearing what an individual says. It involves showing people that you are interested in them and that you value what they have to say and encouraging the disclosure of information and expression of feelings. This is achieved through the use of both verbal and non-verbal strategies and observing individual behaviour to pinpoint meanings behind words.

The listener must be aware of his or her own body language. People believe what they say is most important, but up to 80% of communication is via body language. If verbal and non-verbal communications are not synchronized, non-verbal communication will take priority. It is easy to convey lack of interest through simple gestures. The listener may say verbally 'I'm interested', but if their body language is saying 'I haven't got time for this' (e.g. looking at the time, wringing hands, glancing towards paperwork), the 'talker' will pay more attention to the body language and communication will stop.

The use of non-verbal prompts such as nods and smiles and paralinguistics such as 'mmms' and 'uh huhs' can also encourage an individual to continue talking.

To convey interest and promote active listening you might consider the use of Egan's (1986) acronym SOLER (Table 4.5.17). Responding in this manner conveys interest and suggests active listening.

	Sit squarely
(Adopt an)	**O**pen posture
	Lean forward as appropriate
(Maintain good)	**E**ye contact
	Relax

Table 4.5.17 SOLER to convey interest and promote active listening (Egan, 1986).

Observing the talker's non-verbal and paralinguistic behaviours can provide the nurse with important cues about the talker's feelings. For instance in response to 'How are you?' the client may say 'I'm fine' while his or her facial expression suggests distress and hunched shoulders, a bowed head and a low and anguished tone of voice suggest that all is not well. Recognizing these cues enables the listener to adopt appropriate interventions.

▶ Questioning

Skilled questioning is essential in communication. Questioning can serve many functions, for example:

▶ to encourage conversation;
▶ to promote information gathering;
▶ to clarify issues, feelings or beliefs;
▶ to identify problems;
▶ to check the listener's understanding of issues;
▶ to focus the discussion on specific issues.

There are two main types of questions: open and closed. Closed questions restrict the possible responses to either yes or no or the giving of direct information. Such questions are useful in obtaining specific information or facts, but do not allow for the expression of feelings, thoughts or opinions. Open questions encourage the expression of thoughts and

DECISION MAKING

Your client, George Rowe, appears to be distressed. Following a road traffic accident in which he sustained a severe head injury George has become dysphasic. You think that his distress may be related to his concern about his wife's ability to care for herself in his absence.

* *How would you encourage George to discuss his feelings?*
* *What questions would it be appropriate to ask?*
* *What aids to communication would you consider using?*

feelings, place no restrictions on the responder and usually begin with 'how', 'what', 'where', 'when', and 'why'. Table 4.5.18 gives examples of open and closed questions. Both types of questions have their uses, but open questions promote the disclosure of issues most relevant to an individual and offer the individual some control over his or her response.

Type of question	Example
Open	How well did you sleep?
	Tell me how you feel?
	What would you like to have for your dinner today?
Closed	What is your name?
	Are you feeling OK?
	Did you sleep well?

Table 4.5.18 Examples of open and closed questions.

▶ BARRIERS TO COMMUNICATION

Communication between client, family and care team sometimes goes wrong. Reasons for poor communication are wide ranging, but some of the factors involved are examined here.

▶ *Physiological Factors*

A variety of physical problems can act as barriers to communication. A visual or hearing impairment can reduce an individual's ability to communicate with others unless appropriate strategies are used. Touching a person who is blind to make them aware of your presence allows the person to orientate towards communication. Similarly someone with hearing difficulties may have problems if the communicator does not face them or is unable to use sign language or if hearing aids are appropriate, but are not used.

Neurological damage following stroke or head injury can give rise to dysphasia, poor concentration, confusion or memory impairment, all of which can serve as barriers to communication.

▶ *Cognitive Factors*

Cognitive barriers relate to those factors that affect processes such as attention, perception, thinking, problem solving, reasoning, memory and language. Neurological damage can give rise to problems in some of these areas, as can some mental health problems and learning disabilities. For example, someone with schizophrenia may have a poor attention span resulting from altered perceptions and thought disorder.

Stress and anxiety can have an impact on all cognitive processes. Individuals who are only just beginning to come to terms with an illness or new situation may have high levels of stress and anxiety. In such situations the individual's perception of information being given and interpretation of things said can be affected (see Chapter 4.1 on stress and anxiety).

In health care medical jargon is common, but can appear as a foreign language to someone receiving care. Use of words that are not within the client's own vocabulary generally results in misunderstandings and poor communication.

▶ Environmental Factors

Trying to talk to someone in a noisy environment where there are continual interruptions leads to frustration, lack of understanding and poor concentration. Similarly individuals are often disinclined to discuss personal information or the expression of strong emotions if they can be overheard or seen.

Other environmental factors may relate to time available to talk. Nurses often feel under pressure to 'get the job done' and their workloads may either inhibit clients 'I don't want to bother the nurses they're so busy' or result in the nurse communicating poorly because of pressure of work.

▶ Personal Factors

Individual nurses may lack the knowledge, experience and skills to promote effective communication. There is a belief that communication is just about talking, but effective communication requires the learning of skills, practice and confidence.

> Some people are perceived by others as 'easy' to talk to. What particular communication skills do you think these people possess?

▶ TEAMS AND LEADERSHIP

A rehabilitation programme requires the involvement of a variety of health care professionals in the bid to return the client to their optimum level of functioning. Multidisciplinary involvement necessitates a coordinated approach to ensure that the needs of the client are addressed. This is best achieved through teamwork.

A team is a group of people working together; it is more than an aggregate of individuals, but rather what Huczynski and Buchanan (1985) describe as a 'psychological group' where individuals have a sense of collective identity and interact in a significant way. A multidisciplinary team is also a 'formal group'. It is created by an organization to achieve specific goals related to identified tasks.

Groups do not come into being fully formed and functional; they grow and develop over time. Groups form by passing through sequential steps – forming, storming, norming, performing (Table 4.5.19).

Forming	Feelings of uncertainty, anxiety and looking for leadership
Storming	People try to find a role within the group and conflict and competition arise as bids for dominance are made
Norming	Group identity emerges – there is an acceptance of common rules and a sense of belonging
Performing	Solidarity, commitment to group goals, individual responsibility for work, agreed objectives

Table 4.5.19 Group formation and stages of group development (Tuckman, 1965).

Argyle (1969) suggests that in all groups a hierarchy appears with a leader at the top. In formal groups, such as teams, this leader is either formally appointed or becomes the person with the highest status. Leadership is concerned with the guiding, directing and influencing of others towards an identified goal or result. In a formally appointed leader, control is based upon power and the leader is able to exert power to influence the group. This is not the same for all leaders, however, and styles of leadership can vary (Table 4.5.20).

Autocratic	Defensive, restrictive, fearing, obedience, punishment, reward, threat, constant surveillance
Democratic	Open, accepting, trusting, recognition, satisfaction, self-discipline, challenge
Laissez faire	Permissive, abdicating, indifferent, self-direction, differences, ultraliberal, equality

Table 4.5.20 Leadership styles and their characteristics.

The ability of the leader to influence others in the group relates to the power structure within the group, which may stem from a variety of sources. The way in which communication occurs within a group will vary according to the group structure and the style of leadership. With autocratic leadership communication tends to go in one direction – from the leader to the other members. The democratic style encourages multi-directional communication that flows between group members and the leader. Communication within a group with *laissez faire* leadership only occurs when the leader is asked to provide information. The different styles of leadership and communication structures are appropriate to use in particular situations.

> Identify in which care situations the three different styles of leadership (see Table 4.5.20) and communication would be most appropriate?

PRACTICE KNOWLEDGE

▶ ASSESSMENT IN REHABILITATION

Assessment is often described as the first stage of the nursing process. This suggests that it is a one-off activity that only occurs within the nursing domain. Such assumptions are inappropriate in the sphere of rehabilitation where the emphasis is placed on continuous multi-disciplinary assessment. The process of rehabilitation requires an assessment of multiple factors in an effort to ensure an individual's needs and abilities are fully identified. This allows for rehabilitation to be ability-led and therefore reflect the needs of the individual. Wing (1983, p. 55) suggests that 'the value of assessment is to determine the severity and the chronicity of disablement and its main causes, to discover what talents might be developed, to lay down a plan of rehabilitation, to allocate the appropriate professional help to the client and relatives, and to monitor progress and update the plan as necessary'.

Although Wing (1983) is referring to the assessment of individuals with schizophrenia, this statement applies to all aspects of rehabilitation. It is only through rigorous assessment that an appropriate rehabilitation programme can be developed. Within such a programme reassessment to monitor progress is essential. One-off assessment only tells how an individual functions at a particular time. On-going assessment allows identification of changes in the client's status.

Assessment is also essential to provide a baseline from which to measure improvement and rehabilitation success. This should include identification of an individual's capabilities before the illness episode to provide a true picture of what is achievable. Often the client's family and friends will be involved in the assessment if this does not compromise confidentiality. This information is helpful to identify the client's previous level of social, cognitive and practical skills.

Assessment requires the collection of data based on:

▶ direct observation;
▶ interviews;
▶ assessment tools.

RESEARCH BASED EVIDENCE

Lewinter and Mikkelsen (1995) emphasized that the nursing assessment should encompass an holistic approach to care and not focus on what appears to the nurse to be the primary problem. They interviewed individuals who had undergone rehabilitation following a stroke. Generally, the physical retraining aspects of the rehabilitation programmes were evaluated well. It was found that the care programmes were inadequate in that they failed to address psychological and social needs, in particular counselling and group support. Individuals were also critical of the lack of sexual counselling (a topic that staff evaded) and cognitive training.

DECISION MAKING

Think of a client you have recently been involved in caring for.
- *What data would you need to collect to develop a rehabilitation programme?*
- *How could these data be collected?*
- *Identify specific assessment tools to aid this process.*

The focus of observations and interviews and the types of assessment tools used will be dictated by the individual's illness or disorder. For example, Appleton (1994) suggests that in the rehabilitation of children with head injuries a strong emphasis should be placed on emotional, intellectual and cognitive needs as well as physical requirements. In the

Assessment tool	Description	Use
Clifton assessment procedures for the elderly (CAPE)	Two parts: the cognitive assessment scale measures cognitive impairment; the behaviour rating scale measures various areas of disability.	Discriminates between dementia and functional psychiatric disorders, predicts likelihood of discharge from hospital.
London Psychogeriatric Rating Scale (LPRS)	Four subscales: mental disorganization or confusion; physical disability; social irritating behaviour; disengagement. Rated on a three-point scale by someone who knows the person well.	Orientated towards hospital patients, but can be adapted for community. Shown to predict patient outcome.
Echelle Comportment et Adaptation (ECA)	32 items covering physical independence, social integration, occupation and orientation, mobility, and language. Each item gives a choice of several levels of function.	Filled in by someone in close contact with the individual
Structured Assessment of Independent Living Skills (SAILS)	50 items covering expressive language, receptive skills, time and orientation, money-related skills, instrumental activities, social activities. Gives a combined motor score, cognitive score and total score.	Involves direct observation of performance in a testing situation.

Table 4.5.21 Assessment tools for individuals with dementia (Form, 1994).

Skill	Associated activities
Self-awareness	Own values, attitudes, prejudices and their management; motives and needs; competence and limitations; non-verbal communication; effect on others
Observing	Verbal and non-verbal communication; group and family dynamics; interaction with others
Data collection	Recognize sources; identify factors that may affect data collection; acknowledge range of observations available in relation to activities of living; ability to identify relevance or validity of data; awareness of policies and procedures; present data in a logical manner
Interviewing	Formulate strategies in relation to individual differences; consider environment, time, individual needs; communication skills – for example listening and attending, questioning, paraphrasing; being non-judgmental
Identifying needs	Identify factors influencing need; classify need; prioritize need
Diagnosis problems	Independence or dependence level; consider motivation, level of cooperation and possible constraints; base judgements on available data; identify problems; identify areas for nursing intervention and those requiring interventions from other agencies
Recording and disseminating information	Assemble, document, process and organize data accurately; comply with legal requirements; formulate a nursing history; maintain confidentiality; disseminate information quickly

Table 4.5.22 Assessment skills (Department of Health, 1994).

elderly, however, assessment should address physical, mental and social functioning (Williams, 1993). Various assessment tools are available and the most appropriate for the situation should be chosen. Table 4.5.21 lists examples of assessments available to measure disability in individuals with dementia.

Although particular illnesses or disorders may require specific assessment criteria, the basic principles of data collection and assessment skills remain the same. When considering the role of mental health nurses, the Department of Health (1994) identified skills of assessment (Table 4.5.22). These are relevant to all areas of rehabilitation and cannot be emphasized too strongly.

The development of a trusting relationship is also central to assessment. Without such a relationship with both the clients and their families the gathering of relevant information becomes difficult, if not impossible. To facilitate this, good communication skills are essential, and as identified earlier, those factors that promote and act as barriers to communication must be considered.

▶ GOAL SETTING

Goals are viewed as facilitating communication interprofessionally and between health professionals, clients and informal carers. Goals also have a motivational aspect, giving a sense of direction, and when achieved, increasing self-esteem and feelings of satisfaction. Scut and Stam (1994) identify that goal setting in rehabilitation is an essential prerequisite to effective teamwork, and promote a problem solving approach to care.

There are two different types of goals, long-term and short-term. The overall goal of a rehabilitation programme may be to restore an individual to a certain level of functioning. This is a long-term goal. Rehabilitation is often a lengthy undertaking and the daily grind of working towards a too distant goal is demoralizing and demotivating. To maintain a sense of progress there is a need to identify smaller goals that are attainable in a shorter space of time. Short-term goals provide the means of evaluating the rehabilitation programme. This is essential both from the clients' perspective – to enable clients to see their own improvement – and from the formal and informal carers' view to determine whether the care they are giving is appropriate.

Goals are an expression of desired outcomes or objectives that identify the direction of care. The rehabilitation process can be said to stand or fall on the quality and relevance of the goals set, and the importance of this aspect of rehabilitation cannot be emphasized too strongly.

Goal setting is not without its problems (Table 4.5.23). When identifying goals it must be remembered that what is important to the nurse or carer may not be so to the client, therefore mutual goal setting is essential. If a goal is viewed by anyone involved in the rehabilitation process as irrelevant, the motivation to achieve the goal will be lacking and difficulties will arise (see Table 4.5.14 for those behaviours associated with resistance to change), whereas goals that are too complex will act as a disincentive if they are beyond the client's ability. There is a need for discussion, negotiation, and at times, compromise between all involved.

Goals also need to be set in order of priority. In addition, different members of the multidisciplinary team may have conflicting views about what is essential for the rehabilitation of an individual and the priority each goal takes. Additionally, what is a priority to the team may not be so for the client. If the priorities of goal setting are not universally agreed,

Incompatibility of goals (within a discipline, between disciplines, between patient and professionals, between patient and family or friends)

Setting appropriate time scales

Setting at an appropriate level

Table 4.5.23 Problems with goal selection (McGrath and Davis, 1992).

there may be a resistance to change and the rehabilitation plan may well be undermined. It is essential therefore that all individuals communicate effectively and openly in the setting and prioritizing of goals.

The goal should express what is to be accomplished rather than describing what is to be done to or by the individual. Goals should also be phrased in a positive manner, proposing the outcome to be achieved, for example 'be able to make a cup of tea unaided' as opposed to 'reduce dependency upon others'. This approach puts the process in a positive framework and clearly states what is expected as opposed to identifying what is not wanted. If this is coupled with the writing of goals in behavioural terms, for example stating what is to be observed if the goal is achieved and when it is expected to be achieved by (Table 4.5.24), goals become well defined, unambiguous and easy to evaluate (Binnie *et al.*, 1984).

Behavioural goal	Evelyn is becoming mobile following a hip replacement and will walk for 30 m using a walking frame without sitting down twice daily for five days
1) Who will demonstrate behaviour	Evelyn?
2) What he or she will do?	Walk 30 m
3) Under what conditions?	Using her walking frame
4) To what standard?	Without sitting down
5) Expected time or interval by which the behaviour will occur	Twice a day for five days

Table 4.5.24 All behavioural goals must contain the five elements listed here with examples.

▌ THE NURSE AS AN EDUCATOR OR FACILITATOR OF CHANGE

An integral part of rehabilitation is the education of individuals in terms of health promotion and self-care. This includes the identification of risk factors associated with certain illnesses or disorders and the facilitating of changes to reduce such risk factors and adopt healthier lifestyles. This aspect of rehabilitation helps to reduce the dependency of an individual on others and encourages the client to take responsibility for his or her own wellbeing. Individuals must accept such responsibilities if they are to become more than passive consumers of care. Successful rehabilitation programmes require active client participation.

Health care professionals have a responsibility to promote health through increasing awareness of risk factors and facilitating appropriate changes in lifestyles. This is enabled by the acquisition of skills identified by Priest and Speller (1991) in Table 4.5.25.

Goeppinger (1982, p. 373) identified that 'Life-style factors are amenable to change only by individuals who understand the rationale to change and are sustained in their efforts by strong family ties, assistance of friends, community support systems, and relevant social policy'. This is echoed by Sheppard (1994) who suggests it is imperative that nurses educate clients about the meaning of rehabilitation and what it entails. This is not only to enable the individual to take part more fully in the process, but also to allow a full understanding of the various responsibilities of those involved. The nurse must, however, beware of prescribing lifestyles; informed choice is the most appropriate intervention. An example of the aims of a health education programme is given in Table 4.5.26.

Knowledge relating to risk factors

Awareness and understanding of an individual's attitudes to the identified health problem

Ability to apply knowledge and skills to facilitate change

Table 4.5.25 Skills of effective practitioners undertaking risk assessment (Priest and Speller, 1991).

An understanding of their physical capabilities and the knowledge to maintain a reasonable level of fitness

An awareness of the adverse effects of smoking, obesity, poor diet, lack of exercise and stress

An appreciation of the benefits of a healthier way of life

An ability to identify individual risk factors and take measures to modify them.

Table 4.5.26 Example of aims for participants in a cardiac rehabilitation programme (Doughty, 1991).

Priest and Spiller (1991) suggest the use of the Health Belief Model (Table 4.5.27) and the Stages of Change Model (Table 4.5.28) to structure nurse interventions with the individuals when identifying lifestyles, risk factors and areas for change. This enables the identification of beliefs related to risk factors and the individual's readiness to change.

Health related behaviour is related to
How much the health goal is valued by individual
The strength of belief.that a change will result in avoidance of ill health

The ramifications of these are
The client's perceived susceptibility 'Will it happen to me?'
The client's perceived severity 'How badly will it affect me?'
Perceived benefits for the client 'What do I get out of changing?'
Perceived barriers for the client 'Is it worth the discomfort?'

Table 4.5.27 Health Belief Model (Mainman and Becker, 1974).

Stage	Description
Precontemplation	'There is no problem for me, why change?'
Contemplation	'OK so its a problem but I'm not sure if I'm ready to do anything about it'.
Action	'I'm ready to do something now'.
Maintenance	'I'll keep going even though its difficult'
Relapse	'I didn't really want to change I'll go back to the old behaviour'

Table 4.5.28 Stages of Change Model (Priest and Speller, 1991).

PROFESSIONAL KNOWLEDGE

▶ IMPACT OF *NHS AND COMMUNITY CARE ACT* (1990) ON THE PROVISION OF CARE

The implementation of the *NHS and Community Care Act* (Department of Health, 1990a) led to a massive reorganization of the health and social services available in the UK. The thrust behind these changes was the desire to provide a flexible service tailored to meet individuals' needs. Added to this was a need to contain the spiralling cost of health care. Although the principles embodied in community care were generally widely supported and welcomed, the ability of health and local authorities to meet their commitments in relation to the act is questioned. The initial result of the act was a massive closure of 'long-term' NHS beds and an expansion in the number of private residential and nursing homes. Following full implementation of the Act on 1st April 1993 when the funding for nursing and residential care was transferred from the Department of Social Security to local authorities, residential care has increasingly been rejected in favour of (cheaper) domiciliary services (Knapp and Lawson, 1995).

Bakheit and McLellan (1995) suggested that the act failed to meet its promise of targeting resources more appropriately. The matching of services to need did not materialize and the majority of care was provided by (unpaid) relatives. Very dependent clients remained in hospital as local authorities were unable to meet their community care requirements. Often this was related to the lack of funds to provide equipment or suitable residential care.

The success of a rehabilitation programme depends upon the availability of support and resources in the individual's own home. Where resources are limited it is essential that needs are prioritized to ensure that the individual receives the optimum level of care available. Williams (1993) suggests that the future of rehabilitation rests on the ability to maintain and support individuals in the community.

▶ THE NURSE AS A MEMBER OF THE MULTIDISCIPLINARY TEAM

Most literature relating to the nurse's role within the rehabilitation team suggests that the nurse has a vital part to play. The Royal College of Nursing (1991) sees the 24-hour presence of nurses during the individual's stay in hospital as a significant aspect of the nurse's role in rehabilitation. This is echoed by Williams (1993), who identifies that no other health professional has such close and continuous contact.

Key aspects of the nurse's role in rehabilitation of the elderly identified by the Royal College of Nursing (1991) are:

▶ intimate care;
▶ prevention of complications;
▶ skin care and wound care;
▶ personal hygiene;
▶ bowel and bladder functions;
▶ provision of adequate nutrition;
▶ promotion of self-medication.

Added to these is the assertion that the nurse's role is dynamic and changes in relation to the client's needs. A broader view of the nurse's role is offered by Williams (1993) who suggests the nurse's role encompasses:

▶ observation;
▶ assessment;
▶ coordination of care and treatment;
▶ client advocacy;
▶ social, therapeutic and recreational activities;
▶ delivery of essential care;
▶ health promotion and education;
▶ family support.

The key role of ensuring effective communication between members of the multidisciplinary team, health professionals and clients and their families is viewed as falling within the domain of nurses.

The relationship between the nurse and client is proposed by O'Connor (1990) as central to a therapeutic programme. It is suggested that the nurse should match interventions with the physical, psychological and emotional needs of the individual. This ensures that the rehabilitation process keeps pace with the client's needs and progress. This aspect of the nurse's role is essential to ensure the rehabilitation process takes account of the client's current and changing needs.

The process of rehabilitation often begins in hospital, but as Appleton

- *Should people with cardiac problems be admitted to a rehabilitation programme if they continue to smoke?*
- *Should scarce resources be allocated only to those who show a willingness to adapt their behaviour or does everyone have a right to treatment regardless of their lifestyle?*

(1994) proposes, it is continued in the community taking days or months depending upon the severity of problem. Although Appleton referred to children with head injuries, this principle is true of most aspects of rehabilitation. In mental health, for example, rehabilitation is often conducted over a number of years with a gradual reintroduction of the individual into the community. This blend of hospital and community care underlines the need for nurses in both settings to develop skills and knowledge related to the process of rehabilitation.

▶ ETHICAL CONSIDERATIONS

Ethics is said to be about the 'rights and wrongs' of a situation, the value judgements and decisions made relating to how people should and should not act. The promoting of individual responsibility for health is central to rehabilitation, but as Goeppinger (1982) suggested, such an approach may give rise to dilemmas, which grow out of differing political ideologies. On one side the responsibility of individuals for their own health is seen as paramount. Therefore if individuals do not reduce identified risk factors in their lifestyles they are viewed as responsible for their own ill health. The opposing argument suggests that there are extraneous factors that make it difficult for individuals to adopt healthy lifestyles, such as poverty and media pressure. Added to this is the suggestion that although the correlation between healthy lifestyles and good health outcomes is strong, it is not conclusive. Social factors, for instance, may have a large part to play in health. From this perspective the emphasis on individual responsibility is seen as scapegoating the sick and blaming them for their own misfortune. Such a debate has implications for the allocation of resources.

Associated with the dilemma relating to the allocation of resources is a suggestion that changes in social policy relating to resourcing of services and the prioritizing of need have a profound impact on those requiring rehabilitation programmes. Elliot (1995) talks of the stresses experienced by health carers in the conflict between the identification of those in greatest need when allocating resources and the belief in the right to equal assess to care and treatment and provision of resources to all in need.

- *Is it possible to deliver a rehabilitation programme when care is based on availability of resources rather than the needs of patients*
- *What should be the nurse's response in such circumstances?*

Within the general sphere of health care the individual's right to choose how his or her care is managed and the possible lack of clarity as to the right or wrong of a situation (for example, whether or not to provide care for someone with heart disease who continues to smoke) may leave the practitioner unsure about how to act and moral dilemmas arise. The same is true in the arena of rehabilitation, particularly in relation to goal setting. There may be times when the goals of the health professional and those of the client are diametrically opposed.

There is a need for health professionals to enter into open debate concerning an appropriate response to dilemmas such as those identified here, but ultimately the decision about the appropriate action must lie with individual practitioners.

DECISION MAKING

Gordon Hill is a 29-year-old sales representative. Recently, following a road traffic accident, he has become severely disabled. He sees life as worthless and a rehabilitation programme to maximize his abilities and independence as useless. The nurse, believing that disability does not devalue the individual, views the development of skills to promote independence as vital.
- *Explain why Gordon feels this way.*
- *Gordon and the nurse have differing views on rehabilitation. What are the consequences of accepting each view?*
- *How might the nurse acknowledge Gordon's feelings, but also encourage him to take a more positive outlook?*
- *Devise a plan to reinforce Gordon's self-esteem by using appropriate goals?*

REFLECTIVE KNOWLEDGE

Rehabilitation is a complex activity. It requires an understanding of the psychological and social impacts illness has on an individual and how these can influence a client's progress to optimum functioning. The nurse must also consider policy issues in relation to the provision of care and address ethical dilemmas. The role of the nurse within the rehabilitation process is therefore multifaceted and requires a dynamic approach. The nurse must draw on wide ranging knowledge to promote the wellbeing of clients, facilitate multidisciplinary teamwork and deliver individualized care. The main points covered in this chapter were as follows:

- rehabilitation is a process aimed at enabling an individual to gain his or her optimum level of functioning through a multidisciplinary approach;
- the nurse's role is multifaceted and requires a breadth and depth of knowledge relating to clients' physical, social and psychological needs and care management and delivery issues;
- communication is a central factor in the effectiveness of rehabilitation programmes;
- integral parts of the nurse's role are those of health educator (this includes the identification of risk factors associated with various disorders) and as a facilitator of change;
- rigorous assessment is essential in providing a baseline from which to work, identifying what is achievable and in monitoring progress;
- appropriate goal setting is a prerequisite to the identification of desired outcomes of care, ensuring effective communication, teamwork and the maintenance of client and carer motivation;
- social and psychological issues have a profound influence on the individual's experience of illness, provision of services and delivery of care.

▶ CASE STUDIES

Four case studies now follow, one from each branch of nursing. Use the knowledge you have gained from this chapter to answer the questions set in each.

▶ CASE STUDY: MENTAL HEALTH

Kevin is 20 years old and has been diagnosed as schizophrenic. He is an only child, has very few friends and normally lives with his elderly parents. Kevin was attending university, but had to leave because of his illness. He has had a number of admissions to his local acute psychiatric unit, usually when his parents feel they can no longer cope with his 'odd' behaviour. Following his most recent admission he has been referred to the rehabilitation team with a view to placing him in a rehabilitation hostel. It is hoped to enable Kevin to live independently in the community.

■ **What are the immediate problems that confront Kevin and the rehabilitation team?**

■ Consider the examples of motivation theories and suggest how these could be used to motivate Kevin to participate in his rehabilitation programme.

■ Select one of the problems you have identified and construct a rehabilitation programme encompassing short-term and long-term goals.

▶ CASE STUDY: ADULT

Edna is 64 years old and lives with her 72-year-old husband, Sidney. They have three daughters, June aged 44 years, Mary aged 42 years and Joan, aged 40 years, all of whom are married and live some distance away. Edna is the main carer for her husband who has dementia. She suffers a severe stroke and is admitted to hospital with a left-sided hemiplegia. Initially she is very reliant on the nursing staff for many of the basic requirements to sustain life. Gradually her condition improves.

■ Identify the changes in body image Edna may experience following her stroke.

■ What sort of labels may be applied to Edna and what impact could these have on her self-concept?

■ What impact may the recent developments in welfare provision have on the planning of a rehabilitation programme for Edna?

■ Identify and prioritize the services that Edna may require to enable her to live in her own home following her recovery.

▶ CASE STUDY: LEARNING DISABILITIES

John is 45 years old, has a moderate learning disability and lives in a staffed group home with three other residents. Before this he lived in the local large institution, which closed seven years ago. He is a popular member of the home, and takes part in many social activities. John is overweight, having a 'sweet tooth' and taking very little exercise. While attending the social education centre John has a heart attack and is admitted to hospital.

■ What personal characteristics may be attributed to John and how might these affect his care?

■ What changes might John need to make because of his myocardial infarction?

■ How could you use change theory to facilitate John's wellbeing?

■ John is to undertake a fitness regimen. Identify a possible long-term goal and the sequential short-terms goals to meet such a requirement.

▶ CASE STUDY: CHILD

Susan is eight years old and is the middle child of three. Her family live in a three-bedroom semi-detached house on the outskirts of the city. Both her parents work: her father Paul is a police officer, her mother Sarah works part time as a nurse. While on her way home from school Susan is knocked down by a car. As she has suffered severe head injuries she is transferred from the local hospital to the nearest neurosurgical ward some 40 miles away.

■ **What barriers to communication may be present for Susan and how could you overcome these?**

■ **Susan is referred to a rehabilitation team. What data would be needed to develop her rehabilitation programme and how could this be collected?**

■ **Identify a selection of assessment tools that will aid this process?**

▶ ANNOTATED FURTHER READING

BRENNAN, J. (1994) A vital component of care. The nurse's role in recognising altered body image. *Professional Nurse* **February**: 298.
  This paper offers the reader insight into the nurse's role in caring for clients with altered body image.
GIBBON, B., THOMPSON, A. (1992) The role of the rehabilitation nurse. *Nursing Standard* **6(36)**: 32–35.
HESLOP, A., KING, M. (1994) Let's treat body and mind. *Professional Nurse* **10(3)**: 188–190.
  These two articles identify the collaborative nature of rehabilitation and the role of nurses from differing specialities within this.
HAYNES, S. (1992) Let the change come from within, The process of change in nursing. *Professional Nurse* **July**: 635–638.
  This provides an insight into change theory and a comprehensive discourse on the management of change and nursing practice
SCUT, H.A., STAM, H.J. (1994) Goals in rehabilitation teamwork. *Disability and Rehabilitation* **16(4)**.
  Provides an in-depth discussion of goal setting in the rehabilitation setting
WORDEN, J.W. (1991) *Grief Counselling and Grief Therapy* (2nd edition). London. Routledge.
  Every change involves a loss and many people grieve or mourn, because of change. This is an area where people may be helped through the process of change. Worden identifies four tasks of mourning that must be completed for successful resolution. Although this was written with the bereaved in mind the principles may be applied to most loss. By identifying that a person may be grieving we may assist them through the grieving process and consequently facilitate their successful adaptation to change.

▶ REFERENCES

APPLETON, R. (1994) Head injury rehabilitation for children. *Nursing Times* **90(22)**: 29–31.

ARGYLE, M. (1969) *Social Interaction.* London. Methuen.

ATKINSON, R.L., ATKINSON, R.G., SMITH, E.E., BERN, D.J. (1993) *Introduction to Psychology* (11th edition). London. Harcourt Brace College Publishers.

BAKHEIT, A.M.O., McLELLAN, D.L. (1995) The impact of the Community Care Act on bed turnover in a rehabilitation unit. *Clinical Rehabilitation* **9(1)**: 70–73.

BERCHEID, E., WALSTER, E.M. (1974) Physical attractiveness. In BERKOWITZ, L. (ed.) *Advances in Experimental Social Psychology.* New York. Academic Press.

BINNIE, A., BOND, S., LAW, G., LOWE, K., PEARSON, A., ROBERTS, R., TIERNEY, A., VAUGHAN B. (1984) *A Systematic Approach To Nursing Care.* Milton Keynes. Open University.

BRENNAN, J. (1994) A vital component of care. The nurse's role in recognising altered body image. *Professional Nurse* **9(5)**: 298.

COSTELLO, J. (1995) Helping relatives cope with the grieving process. *Professional Nurse* **11(2)**: 89–92.

DAVIS, A., DAVIS, S., MOSS, N., MARKS, J., McGRATH, J., HOVARD, L., AXON, J., WADE, D. (1992) First steps towards an interdisciplinary approach to rehabilitation. *Clinical Rehabilitation* **6**: 237–244.

DEPARTMENT OF HEALTH (1990a) *NHS and Community Care Act.* London. Her Majesty's Stationery Office.

DEPARTMENT OF HEALTH (1990b) *Community Care in The Next Decade and Beyond*: Policy Document. London. Her Majesty's Stationery Office.

DEPARTMENT OF HEALTH (1991) *The Health of the Nation.* London. Her Majesty's Stationery Office.

DEPARTMENT OF HEALTH (1994) *Working in Partnership: A Collaborative Approach to Care. Report of the Mental Health Nursing Review Team.* London. Her Majesty's Stationery Office.

DOUGHTY, C. (1991) A multidisciplinary approach to cardiac rehabilitation. *Nursing Standard* **5(45)**: 13–15.

EASTON, K.L., RAWL, S.M., ZEMEN, D., KWIATOWSKI, S., BURCZYK, B. (1995) The effects of nursing follow-up on the coping strategies used by rehabilitation patients after discharge. *Rehabilitation Nursing Research* **4(4)**: 119–127.

EGAN, G. (1986) *The Skilled Helper – A Problem-Management Approach to Helping.* Pacific Grove, California. Brooks/Cole.

ELLIOT, M. (1995) Care management in the community: a case study. *Nursing Times* **91(48)**: 34–35.

FORM, A.F. (1994) Disability in dementia: assessment, prevention, and rehabilitation. *Disability and Rehabilitation* **16(3)**: 98–109.

GIBBON, B., THOMPSON, A. (1992) The role of the nurse in rehabilitation. *Nursing Standard* **6(36)**: 32–35.

GOEPPINGER, J. (1982) Changing health behaviours and outcomes through self-care. In LANCASTER, J., LANCASTER, W. (eds) *Concepts for Advanced Nursing – The Nurse as a Change Agent.* St Louis. C.V. Mosby.

GOFFMAN, E. (1963) *Stigma: Notes on the Management of a Spoiled Identity.* Englewood Cliffs, N.J. Prentice Hall.

HAFFER, A.. (1986) Facilitating change. *Journal of Nursing Administration* **16(4)**: 18–22.

HUCZYNSKI, A., BUCHANAN, D. (1985) *Organisational Behaviour; An Introductory Text* (2nd edition). London. Prentice Hall.

KELLEY, D., CONNOR, D.R. (1979) The emotional cycle of change. In JONES, J.E., PFEIFFER, J.W. (eds) *Annual Handbook for Group Facilitators.* California. University Associates.

KEYSER, D. (1986) Using nursing contracts to support change in nursing organisations. *Nurse Education Today* **6(3)**: 103–108.

KNAPP, M., LAWSON, R. (1995) Community care and the health service. In GLYNN, J.J., PERKINS, D.A. (eds) *Managing Health Care: Challenges for the 90s.* London. Saunders.

KUBLER-ROSS, E. (1970) *On Death and Dying.* New York. Macmillan.

LANCASTER, J., LANCASTER, W. (1982) *Concepts for Advanced Nursing – The Nurse as a Change Agent.* St. Louis. C.V. Mosby.

LEMERT, E. (1951) *Social Pathology.* New York. McGraw Hill.

LEWINTER, M., MIKKELSEN, S. (1995) Patients' experience of rehabilitation after stroke. *Disability and Rehabilitation* **17(1)**: 3–9.

MAINMAN, L.A., BECKER, M.H. (1974) The health belief model: Origin and correlation in psychological theory. *Health Education Monograph* **2**: 336–353.

MASLOW, A.H. (1970) *Motivation and Personality*, 2nd edition. New York. Harper.

McGRATH, J.R., DAVIS, A.M. (1992) Rehabilitation: where are we going and how do we get there?. *Clinical Rehabilitation* **6**: 225–235.

O'CONNOR, S. (1990) Removing barriers to communication. *Nursing Standard* **6**: 26–27.

PARSONS, T. (1951) *The Social System.* London. Routledge and Kegan Paul.

PRICE, B. (1990) *Body image: nursing concepts and care.* London. Prentice Hall.

PRIEST, V., SPELLER, V. (1991) *The Risk Factor Manual.* Oxford. Radcliffe Medical Press.

ROYAL COLLEGE OF NURSING (1991) *The Role of the Nurse in Rehabilitation of Elderly People.* London. Scutari Press.

SCUT, H.A., STAM, H.J. (1994) Goals in rehabilitation teamwork. *Disability and Rehabilitation* **16(4)**: 223–226.

SHEPPARD, B. (1994) Client's views of rehabilitation. *Nursing Standard* **9(10)**: 27–29.

SMITH, D.S., CLARK, M.S. (1995) Competence and performance in activities of daily living of clients following rehabilitation from stroke. *Disability and Rehabilitation* **17(1)**: 15–23.

SQUIRES, A., WARDLE, P. (1988) To rehabilitate or not? In SQUIRES, A.J. (ed.) *Rehabilitation of the Older Client.* London. Croom Helm.

STERNBERG, R.J. (1995) *In Search of the Human Mind.* London. Harcourt Brace College.

THURGOOD, A. (1990) Seven Steps to Rehabilitation. *Nursing Times* **86(25)**: 38–41.

TUCKMAN, B.W. (1965) Developmental sequences in small groups. *Psychological Bulletin* **63**: 384–399.

VAUGHAN, B., PILLMOOR, M. (1989) *Managing Nursing Work.* London. Scutari Press.

WATERS, K.R. (1994) Getting dressed in the early mornings: styles of staff/client interaction on rehabilitation hospital wards for elderly people. *Journal of Advanced Nursing* **19**: 239–248.

WILLIAMS, J. (1993) Rehabilitation challenge. *Nursing Times* **89(31)**.

WILLIAMS, S. (1987) Goffman, interactionism, and the management of stigma in everyday life. In SCAMBLER, G. (ed.) *Sociology Theory and Medical Sociology.* London. Tavistock.

WING, J. (1983) Schizophrenia. In WATTS, F.N., BENNET, D.H. (eds) *Theory and Practice of Psychiatric Rehabilitation.* Chichester. Wiley.

Index

Note: material in boxes, figures and tables is indicated [in this index] by *italic page numbers*